CLINICAL USE OF LABORATORY DATA

A PRACTICAL GUIDE

D. ROBERT DUFOUR, M.D.

Chief of Pathology and Laboratory Medicine Service

Veterans Affairs Medical Center

Professor of Pathology

George Washington University Medical Center

Washington, D.C.

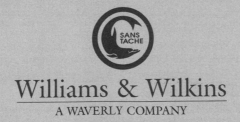

Williams & Wilkins

A WAVERLY COMPANY

BALTIMORE • PHILADELPHIA • LONDON • PARIS • BANGKOK
BUENOS AIRES • HONG KONG • MUNICH • SYDNEY • TOKYO • WROCLAW

Editor: Charles W. Mitchell
Associate Managing Editor: Grace E. Miller
Production Coordinator: Felecia R. Weber
Project Editor: Robert D. Magee
Designer: Mario Fernandez
Illustration Planner: Ray Lowman
Cover Designer: Mario Fernandez
Typesetter: Maryland Composition Co., Inc.
Printer/Binder: Walsworth Publishing Co.

Accurate indications, adverse reactions and dosage schedules for drugs are provided in this book, but it is possible that they may change. The reader is urged to review the package information data of the manufacturers of the medications mentioned.

Printed in the United States of America

Library of Congress Cataloging-in-Publication Data

Dufour, D. Robert.
    Clinical use of laboratory data : a practical guide / D. Robert Dufour.
       p.   cm.
    Includes index.
    ISBN 0-683-18017-7
    1. Reference values (Medicine)—Interpretation.   2. Diagnosis,
Laboratory—Evaluation.   I. Title.
    [DNLM: 1. Diagnosis, Laboratory. 2. Reference Values. QY 4
D861c 1998]
RB37.D84 1998
616.07′56—dc21
DNLM/DLC
for Library of Congress   97-12909
                                 CIP

The publishers have made every effort to trace the copyright holders for borrowed material. If they have inadvertently overlooked any, they will be pleased to make the necessary arrangements at the first opportunity.

To purchase additional copies of this book, call our customer service department at **(800) 638-0672** or fax orders to **(800) 447-8438.** For other book services, including chapter reprints and large quantity sales, ask for the Special Sales department.

Canadian customers should call **(800) 268-4178,** or fax **(905) 470-6780.** For all other calls originating outside of the United States, please call **(410) 528-4223** or fax us at **(410) 528-8550.**

Visit Williams & Wilkins on the Internet: http://www.wwilkins.com or contact our customer service department at **custserv@wwilkins.com.** Williams & Wilkins customer service representatives are available from 8:30 am to 6:00 pm, EST, Monday through Friday, for telephone access.

98 99 00 01
2 3 4 5 6 7 8 9 10

DEDICATION

To the two most important women in my life:
My mother, Claire, for her nurture and encouragement
My wife, Mary, for her love, understanding and support

Preface

Laboratory testing generates approximately 10% of all expenditures for health care in the United States. Physicians use tests to screen asymptomatic patients for disease; this growing segment of the testing market is used widely during a patient's pregnancy (α-fetoprotein and β-HCG to evaluate risk of neural tube defects and chromosomal abnormalities) and in her neonatal period to identify such congenital metabolic diseases as phenylketonuria and hypothyroidism. Screening is used increasingly in adults to identify individuals who are likely to have such serious disorders as carcinomas of the colon (fecal occult blood) and prostate (prostate specific antigen), or to evaluate the risk of coronary artery disease (cholesterol). Testing is also widely used in diagnosis of patients who present with symptoms that may be caused by a variety of disorders. A typical hospital laboratory may perform several hundred tests regularly, with several thousand tests being available from more specialized laboratories. Laboratory tests are playing an increasing role in the followup of patients with established diseases. In diabetics, regular monitoring of blood glucose at home has become a standard part of patient care in the past 15 years, and regular determination of glycated proteins and urinary microalbumin has been shown to help achieve better control, which lowers the rate of complications. The increasing use of laboratory tests has played a role in improving the quality of health care by providing more accurate diagnostic information to physicians.

With the expense and extent of laboratory testing, a casual observer would assume that there would be extensive instruction provided to physicians in the appropriate use of clinical laboratory. Unfortunately, few medical schools have extensive curricula in laboratory medicine. Most physicians learn to use laboratory tests by experience, which is usually practically oriented, aimed at knowing how to select the panels of tests that the laboratory offers and interpreting the most common laboratory tests. While this type of training is usually adequate for the majority of routine situations, it does prevent the physician from understanding the basic principles behind changes in laboratory test results and limits the utility of such testing in helping to establish a diagnosis in a patient with a difficult clinical problem.

In almost 25 years of working in the Clinical Pathology laboratory, I have had frequent opportunities to notice the unintended effects of such a fragmented approach to education on laboratory medicine. While still a medical student working in a hospital laboratory, I had gained a limited understanding of the clinical significance of laboratory tests. At the same time, there were two other medical students who were doing clinical electives at the hospital. I remember one patient who had undergone surgery for gallbladder disease. After surgery, he became progressively more jaundiced, and was thought to perhaps have developed halothane hepatitis. While his transaminases, SGOT and SGPT had risen, there was also a gradual and progressive rise in alkaline phosphatase. I remember discussing the possibility of obstructive jaundice with the other students, but was told that the cholangiogram did not disclose obstruction. When the patient died about 2 weeks after surgery and was found to have had a common duct gall stone at autopsy, my decision to enter pathology training was made. Since that time, in rounds with physicians of all specialties and in interactions with internal medicine residents undertaking electives in laboratory medicine, I have seen a familiarity with laboratory tests that is not always associated with an understanding of the physiologic factors that produce altered test results. In many cases, a clearer understanding of the science involved has led to a diagnosis that might have been delayed or missed had a less scientific study of the results been used.

Where is the physician to go for help in appropriately selecting and interpreting laboratory tests? At present, there are two basic options. Textbooks of laboratory medicine tend to have extensive discussions of the chemical principles underlying the laboratory tests, and usually contain extensive discussions of the physiologic principles, but are limited in their discussions of how the tests can be used by the practicing physician. Clinical medicine textbooks tend to contain detailed descriptions of illnesses, along with a listing of the labotory abnormalities found in each disorder. Missing is a discussion of the science involved, and a discussion of how tests could be used to differentiate similar disorders is often lacking. Subspecialty texts in such areas as gastroenterology, hematology, or endocrinology, among others, offer extensive coverage of laboratory testing in their areas of interest, and are a source of useful information for the practicing primary care physician in complicated cases, but they do not provide a consolidated, easy-to-use text for learning about use of laboratory tests in daily practice.

Laboratory medicine is a branch of medicine that evaluates laboratory tests for utility in patient diagnosis and performs laboratory tests in a way that minimizes the possibility of errors in test performance that may lead to erroneous treatment of patients. Laboratory medicine is based on the basic science disciplines of analytical chemistry, biochemistry, immunology, microbiology, and physiology. Laboratory tests are indicators of the physiologic status of a patient at a given point in time. A textbook of use to primary care physicians should explain those basic scientific principles that underlie the relationships between laboratory test results and disease. Other physiologic factors that affect laboratory test results would feature prominently in such a book. Such a textbook should also, where appropriate, summarize the methodologies used to measure given substances and the situations in which the method may produce misleading or erroneous results. Such useful information would provide the practicing physician with a scientific basis for interpretation and selection of laboratory tests. I have had the opportuntity to provide such information in a major textbook of endocrinology, and have received many favorable comments from practicing physicians in that specialty on the utility of the information provided. I have also prepared handouts for medical student that outline these general principles; these have been widely duplicated by students at several regional medical schools, and are commonly in use on the wards of our teaching hospitals. From the comments received from the students, this approach seems to meet their need for understanding the scientific basis for analysis of laboratory tests.

What is needed is a comprehensive textbook that combines the basic science that underlies laboratory tests, to allow the physician to recognize the advantages and limitations of laboratory tests and practical information on selection and interpretation of laboratory tests in common and uncommon clinical situations to serve as an introduction to the science of laboratory medicine for the practicing primary care provider by explaining in word, picture, and clinical example the appropriate uses of laboratory tests. A tabular collection of information on factors commonly affecting laboratory test results would provide a convenient way to use this book in the day to day practice of medicine. This book is organized in such a fashion. The introductory chapters describe general concepts that apply to all areas of laboratory testing, such as reference values, preanalytical variation, and statistical approaches to laboratory test interpretation. The middle section, the largest portion of the book, contains chapters that explain the biochemical and physiologic basis of laboratory tests for a given problem or organ system, describe patterns of abnormalities and use of tests in common diseases. The final section contains a large table that, for most common tests, lists reference values, the nature and extent of intra individual variation, diseases commonly affecting test results, and any other factors altering test results.

This book, an outgrowth of earlier teaching efforts focused on medical students, internal medicine and pathology residents, and graduate medical education courses for laboratory scientists, is an attempt to provide a resource to the practicing physician. It is intended primarily for the primary care physician and physician in training, who will encounter the widest range of clinical problems in their practices. Because of the attempt to provide breadth, it is necessarily briefer in its coverage than specialty texts in either Clinical Pathology or Internal Medicine subspecialties. It is not meant to replace such textbooks for those practitioners who specialize in Clinical Pathology or medical subspecialties. Rather, this textbook is intended to serve the needs of the primary care physician who must select, from the thousands of tests available, those most likely to help establish a diagnosis in their patients, and who must then interpret the results of those tests in a way that minimizes the likelihood of inaccurate diagnoses. I hope that this text will meet the needs of this audience.

Contributors

Linda G. Baum, M.D., Ph.D.
Associate Professor
Department of Pathology and Laboratory
  Medicine
Associate Division Chief of Hematopathology
UCLA School of Medicine
Los Angeles, California

Joseph M. Campos, Ph.D.
Director, Microbiology Laboratory and
  Laboratory Informatics
Department of Laboratory Medicine
Children's National Medical Center
Professor
Departments of Pedicatrics, Pathology,
  Microbiology/Immunology
George Washington University Medical
  Center
Washington, D.C.

D. Robert Dufour, M.D.
Chief of Pathology and Laboratory Medicine
  Service
Veterans Affairs Medical Center
Professor of Pathology
George Washington University Medical
  Center
Washington, D.C.

Scott J. Graham, M.D.
Head, Hematopathology
Naval Medical Center
Portsmouth, Virginia

John F. Keiser, M.D.
Chief of Microbiology/Serology Laboratories
George Washington University Medical
  Center
Washington, D.C.

Richard A. McPherson, M.D.
Professor, Department of Pathology
Chairman, Division of Clinical Pathology
Medical College of Virginia
Virginia Commonweath University
Richmond, Virginia

Salome Mendoza, M.T. (ASCP)
Technical Specialist
Clinical Microbiology/Serology Laboratories
George Washington University Medical
  Center
Washington, D.C.

James T. Rector, M.D.
Head, Division of Hematopathology
Department of Laboratory Medicine
National Naval Medical Center
Bethesda, Maryland

Contents

IV. DIAGNOSIS AND MONITORING OF INFECTIONS

V. IMMUNOLOGY

VI. FACTORS AFFECTING LABORATORY TESTS

SECTION I.
INTRODUCTION

CHAPTER 1

Reference (Normal) Values

D. ROBERT DUFOUR

WHY DO WE NEED REFERENCE VALUES?

Laboratory tests are monitors of physiologic processes, much as are pulse, respiration, and blood pressure. Practitioners have become accustomed to accepting a certain range of values for each of these as indicative of health; such results are commonly termed "normal." They serve as a basis of comparison in each patient encounter, to assess patient status; in this sense, they form a "reference" for comparison. If such values were not available, it would be impossible for the new practitioner to determine whether the values obtained in each patient were indicative of a healthy state or not. With time and experience, the practitioner would gain a general sense of what values to expect, recognizing that those far from these typical values are indicative of disease. It may not be possible, however, to empirically determine exact cutoff values to distinguish health and disease.

Definitions of Normal

While many differing definitions of normal can be found in dictionaries, two major ones apply to physiologic parameters. The definition most commonly considered in the medical sense is "free from disease; healthy." A second, perhaps easier to determine, definition is "average, typical, or usual." These two definitions do not always produce the same results. For example, while "typical" diets contain over 35% fat, few practitioners would consider this "healthy."

Determination of "Normal" Values

To determine "typical" results, a common approach is to take a random sample of "typical" members of a population, and to consider the central 95% of results as allowable limits for "normal"; in a gaussian distribution (see "The Gaussian ("Normal") Distribution"), this is calculated as the average result ± 1.96 standard deviations (SD). Blood pressure serves as an example of how these limits may not be identical to healthy examples. In the United States, 95% of the adult population has blood pressure values that are from 70 to 160 (systolic) over 60 to 105 (diastolic). Since such values are obtained from a statistical sample of "apparently" healthy individuals randomly selected from the population, they are statistically valid; because they were scientifically determined, they may seem appropriate for use. In the late 1960s, prospective, randomized studies showed that complications in patients with blood pressure between 140/90 and 160/110 were similar to those in persons with higher blood pressures. We now have blood pressure reference limits indicative of low risk of hypertensive complications, which exclude the 15 to 20% of the population that we now consider to have hypertension.

REFERENCE LIMITS FOR LABORATORY TESTS

The same two general methods could be used to establish reference values for laboratory tests: a randomized approach in which an arbitrary percentage of the population is considered to be "normal," or a clinically validated approach in which values correlated with health are identified. Unfortunately, for most laboratory tests, there is little clinical information on which to base clinically validated reference intervals. In most cases, therefore, reference values are established by laboratories using randomly (or, in some cases, non-randomly) selected individuals who appear healthy. The remainder of this chapter will discuss the approaches used by laboratories to establish reference values, the assumptions made in using such an approach, and the situations in which such reference values may cause apparently "abnormal" results that are of no clinical significance (or "normal" results which mask clinically important disease). The practitioner who understands the approaches used by laboratories to attempt to provide reference ranges will have a much better chance of recognizing those situations in which another reference interval should be sought.

BASIC STATISTICAL ASSUMPTIONS AND THE PROBLEMS THEY CREATE

The Gaussian ("Normal") Distribution

In taking repeated measurements of a fixed value, there is a degree of random error in the measurement. A curve of the number of observations of each result plotted against the value obtained will produce a symmetrical, bell shaped curve (Fig. 1.1); this is termed a gaussian or normal distribution. Among the statistical properties of such a distribution are: 1) the mean (average), mode (most frequent), and median (middle) results will be the same; 2) there is a predictable pattern of dispersion of results in which 3) the standard deviation (SD), a measure of the average absolute difference between each individual observation and the average observation, describes the dispersion such that 4) the mean ±1 SD includes 68% of results, mean ±1.96 SD includes 95% of results, mean ±2 SD includes 95.5% of results, and mean ±3 SD includes 99.7% of results. With a gaussian distribution, one can predict the proportion of results included within a given range by knowing the mean and SD of the distribu-

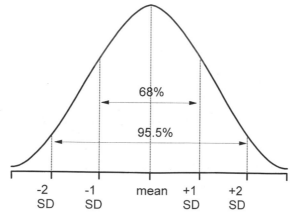

Figure 1.1. The "Normal" Distribution. In this symmetrical distribution, there is only random error in measurement. The standard deviation, which can be calculated easily with hand calculators or computers, describes the spread of results.

tion, using statistical tables. Many biological variables do not follow a gaussian distribution, but they commonly can be transformed mathematically (usually by taking the logarithm of the result) to values which do have that distribution. Many statistical tests for difference, such as the t-test, assume that data follow a gaussian distribution.

Effects of Assuming a Gaussian Distribution When One Does Not Exist

Figure 1.2 illustrates results obtained from measurement of bilirubin and creatine kinase in medical students. When distribution of results is highly skewed, mean ±2 SD will include significantly less than 95% of results. This would result in a higher percentage of healthy individuals being termed "abnormal" for that particular test. Most, but not all, laboratories manually inspect results of tests using graphs such as these, or use statistical tools to evaluate whether the data actually conform to a gaussian distribution. A simple approach that can be taken on data that do not follow a gaussian

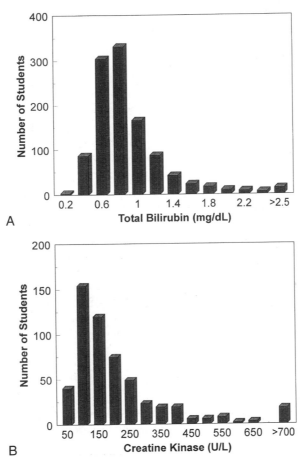

Figure 1.2. Skewed Distribution of Test Results. These two graphs show the results of total bilirubin (**A**) and creatine kinase (**B**) in 1404 medical students. The tendency for a greater number of high results is common for many laboratory tests. Had a gaussian distribution been assumed, reference ranges would have been −0.1 to 1.7 for bilirubin and −730 to 1175 for creatine kinase; the actual central 95% was 0.3 to 2.2 for bilirubin and 35 to 910 for creatine kinase. In addition to having inaccurate upper reference limits, the assumption of a gaussian distribution results in the lower reference limits below zero—an impossible situation.

Table 1.1.
Chance of All Results Being Normal in Test
Panels of Varying Size When Reference Range
Includes Only 95% of Results

Number of Tests	All "Normal"
1	95%
2	90%
6	74%
10	60%
12	54%
15	46%
20	36%
24	29%

distribution is to manually rank the data or use statistical tools to calculate percentiles which can then be used to identify the central 95% of results.

Effects of Classifying 95% of Results as "Normal"

By convention, laboratories typically use one of the above approaches to establish the reference limits for a laboratory test, including the central 95% of results in their reference range. This excludes 5% of the group originally tested, meaning that they have "abnormal" results for that test. Because many laboratories offer tests in panels, the same is true for each individual test as well. This can lead to results being outside reference values in a high percentage of healthy individuals. Table 1.1 lists the theoretical frequency of such an occurrence for several common panel sizes offered by laboratories, assuming that each of the tests varies independently of all other tests. (In reality, this does not commonly occur; many panels have test groupings of related parameters such as BUN and creatinine, total protein and albumin, AST (SGOT) and ALT (SGPT), and calcium, phosphate, and magnesium.)

Many medical schools incorporate teaching exercises for medical students which use their own laboratory results to illustrate the effects of using statistical reference ranges on the frequency of "abnormal" results in apparently healthy individuals. Table 1.2 illustrates the frequency of abnormalities in a panel of 12 tests (glucose, calcium, phosphate, BUN, uric acid, cholesterol, total protein, albumin, AST, alkaline phosphatase, LDH, and total bilirubin). Reference ranges were determined from the students' own results, including the central 95% of results as the reference range. "Abnormal"

Table 1.2.
Frequency of "Abnormal" Results in 694 Medical
Students with Reference Limits Including 95% of
Results for Each of 12 Tests

Number Abnormal	Percentage
0	66
1	26
2	6
3	2
4 or more	1

results occurred in a slightly lower percentage of students than would be expected from 12 independent tests, but over one-third of students had at least one "abnormal" result. This same phenomenon will occur in any population in which reference ranges are established in this fashion.

POPULATION SAMPLING AND PROBLEMS IT CREATES

To establish a reference range, a laboratory must take a sample of the population, obtain samples, and perform tests before applying the statistical procedures discussed earlier. The method the laboratory uses to obtain this sample will profoundly affect the utility of the reference ranges by various groups of practitioners. The statistical tools outlined in the previous section calculate what are termed *descriptive statistics*, implying that they describe the population tested. If the population is not representative of the persons subsequently tested, then reference values may not be an accurate reflection of expected results. An obvious example would be reference values for vital signs such as pulse, respiratory rate, and blood pressure obtained in adults; they would be totally inappropriate for use in infants and young children.

WHO COMPRISES THE SAMPLE?

The laboratory will typically establish their own reference values using a statistically valid sample size (usually over 100 persons), or validate reference values determined by the manufacturer of the reagents or equipment they use with a somewhat smaller sample size. There are several approaches often used by laboratories to obtain a sample; it is important for the practitioner to determine what sample the laboratory used to develop or validate their reference values, in order to determine how applicable they will be to the practitioner's patients.

Easily Recruitable Group

Most laboratories choose this simple approach, sampling persons who are readily accessible by the laboratory staff. Some of the groups which may be sampled in this way include medical students, laboratory or hospital employees, or blood donors. The problem with such an approach is that the sample may not be representative of the population of patients served by the laboratory. For example, the author's institution is a Veterans hospital, where the patients are over 90% male, predominantly African-American, and with an average age over 60. None of these easily recruitable groups are similar in composition to our patients. Use of a non-representative sample produces very misleading reference values (Fig. 1.3).

Random Sample of the Population

Some laboratories attempt to randomly sample a cross-section of the population that they serve. This is often accomplished by conducting health fairs or using random mailings to the community offering free blood screening for cholesterol in return for donating samples for reference value testing. If the persons recruited are truly representative of the healthy population, this approach may be the most valid method for obtaining reference values in a closed community, as may occur in smaller towns served by only one or two laboratories. Often, however, those responding to the campaign are more likely to have some signs or symptoms of illness, and thus are more interested in learning the results of their blood tests than asymptomatic individuals.

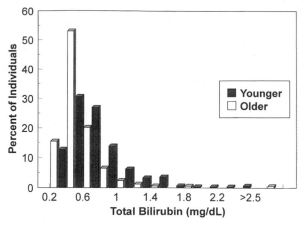

Figure 1.3. Effect of Age on Serum Bilirubin. Bilirubin concentration is significantly higher in younger vs. older women, with the upper reference limit approximately 0.3 mg/dL higher in the younger women. Similar differences occur for many other laboratory tests, including total protein, albumin, alkaline phosphatase, and liver related enzymes.

Elective Hospital Admissions

Another approach used by some laboratories, including our own, is the use of patients who are admitted to the hospital for elective surgical procedures, or are being seen for routine physical examinations. Such an approach is more likely to produce a representative group in urban areas; in addition, since all patients will have a history and physical performed, those with evidence of medical illnesses which may affect test results can be excluded.

Who Is Included and Excluded?

The criteria used for including and excluding individuals from the sample make an important contribution to the validity of reference values. Many laboratories rely on reported history of illnesses to exclude persons from the population sampled to determine reference values. Some exclude those receiving any prescription medications, while others exclude only certain categories of medications. Some take detailed histories and exclude individuals who drink alcohol above a certain level, smoke, etc. This approach has both advantages and disadvantages. Excluding anyone who is not "perfectly healthy" (as defined by the screening procedure) will usually result in tighter reference values. This may improve the ability of a test to pick up one of the conditions excluded, such as alcohol abuse; however, it will also increase the likelihood of persons with trivial clinical abnormalities having "abnormal" results. The practitioner needs to be aware of what approach was used by the laboratory where most tests are submitted to be able to accurately interpret results.

What Range of People Are Represented in the Reference Range?

The vast majority of laboratories publish a single reference range for most tests. This may be very appropriate if a large range of ages and ethnic groups are included in the sample; however, it may obscure trends in test result differences between groups. The most easily tested for are differences between adults and children, or between men and women. Many laboratories that test a wide range of patients publish different reference ranges for children and adults for most laboratory tests; however, laboratories which rarely see one or the other group may publish only a single reference range. This is an important consideration when seeing a child or adolescent in a hospital where adults are the usual patients. For a number of other tests, including alkaline phosphatase, total protein, uric acid, and others, values change significantly with advancing age in adults. Most laboratories publish different reference ranges for men and women for hemoglobin and hematocrit, for sex hormones, and for a few other tests such as PSA and uric acid. A number of other tests appear to correlate with lean body mass, which is significantly higher in men than women. Numerous studies have documented differences between different ethnic groups for some laboratory tests. Significant differences have been found in reference values for tests such as cholesterol, enzymes, and hormones between those of European, African, or Asian ancestry. Practitioners need to be aware of who was included in the reference sample to help evaluate whether their patient may fall outside the reference limits solely for this reason.

How Effectively Are Diseased Individuals Excluded?

For diseases that are symptomatic early, careful histories can exclude persons who are ill. Uncommon asymptomatic diseases can often be detected by using statistical techniques which detect "outliers," values that are unlikely to belong to the "normal" population by chance alone. A problem exists in detecting diseases which are common and asymptomatic for long periods of time. The classic illustration of this problem is the linkage between cholesterol and heart disease. While prospective studies have long recognized that cholesterol levels are linked to risk of atherosclerosis, laboratories established reference ranges for cholesterol based on values encountered in apparently healthy individuals. Because the incidence of atherosclerosis in our population is so high, reference values were often quite wide. Figure 1.4 illustrates cholesterol values obtained from medical students; the central 95% produces a reference range from 123–258 mg/dL (3.19–6.68 mmol/L). Such reference ranges were commonly reported

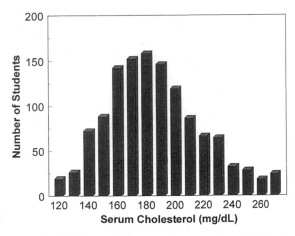

Figure 1.4. Serum Cholesterol in 1403 Medical Students. There is a broad distribution of cholesterol concentrations even within this relatively homogeneous group of students with an average age of 23 years; there were no differences between men and women. The 95% range includes values from 123 to 258 mg/dL. Almost 35% of the students had total cholesterol over "desirable" NCEP values, while 7.5% had values designated as "high" by the NCEP.

by laboratories until the late 1980s, when the National Cholesterol Education Program (NCEP), using data from the Framingham study, determined cholesterol values associated with increased risk of coronary artery disease. A similar situation exists in testing blood donors for risk of transmission of viral hepatitis. While reference values for ALT (SGPT) commonly reach 60 to 70 U/L, studies showed that risk of transmission of virus increased sharply when ALT was over 35 U/L. In both these instances, reference values obtained by any of the methods outlined above include a substantial number of patients with disease, and cause reference values to be insensitive to the presence of disease. A similar problem likely exists for other common diseases or conditions such as alcohol abuse, diabetes, and hypertension.

How Are Individuals Prepared for Collection?

As discussed in Chapter 2, many factors affect results of laboratory tests. In establishing reference intervals, laboratories may choose to control for none, some, or most of these variables. A common approach is to have individuals used for reference purposes report to the laboratory early in the morning in a fasting state, have them seated for a standard period and use tourniquets for only a specified length of time. This approach produces reference limits that are relatively tight, and which eliminate many variables known to affect test results. While this approach is recommended by standardization bodies, it creates many practical problems for the practicing practitioner who is required to evaluate an increased number of "abnormal" results. A problem with this approach is that most patients subsequently tested by the laboratory will not have had such careful control of these variables, and thus are more likely to have test results fall outside the reference limits. It is important for the practitioner to be aware of whether the laboratory reference values were determined using the recommended standard approach in evaluating "abnormal" results. If they were, repeat testing after the patient is prepared in a similar fashion to the reference population can help to determine whether the variation was due to differences in patient preparation. If, as in the author's laboratory, these variables were deliberately not controlled for, then an "abnormal" result carries much greater significance. For some tests, control of variables is vitally important to appropriate interpretation of results. For example, many endocrine tests show pronounced diurnal variation; reference values may be significantly different at different times of day. Renin and aldosterone levels change rapidly in response to changes in blood volume, as may be induced by changes in posture. In menstruating women, sex hormone concentrations change markedly throughout the menstrual period, as do concentrations of other substances such as cholesterol. During pregnancy, hormone levels vary significantly depending on duration of gestation. Alpha-fetoprotein concentration in maternal serum varies not only with duration of gestation, but also with maternal weight. For such tests, laboratories commonly publish more than one reference range. It is essential that the protocol used by the laboratory be known to the practitioner, so that the necessary patient preparation and clinical information can be provided to allow for accurate interpretation of test results in such circumstances.

LIMITATIONS OF POPULATION-BASED REFERENCE VALUES

While we need a frame of reference for comparing results in an individual, reference values often have limited usefulness. Most importantly, practitioners need to understand that results within reference values do not exclude disease, nor do results outside reference limits always indicate pathology. Standard reference values indicate typical or usual values for persons in the population tested; however, they fail to recognize that populations are composed of unique individuals whose results often vary less than those of the population as a whole. For example, a distance runner may have a resting pulse rate of 45, which is below the reference limits for the population; a pulse rate of 80 in this person may be highly abnormal, yet fall within the reference limits. Practitioners must be aware of which commonly measured tests may be subject to this problem.

RELATIVE DEGREE OF VARIATION IN TEST RESULTS

For many laboratory tests, as for other physiologic parameters, there is much less variation in an individual over time than there is from one person to another. Harris introduced the term "index of individuality" which is calculated as:

$$\frac{Average\ Variation\ Within\ One\ Person\ (Intraindividual\ Variation)}{Average\ Variation\ Between\ Persons\ (Interindividual\ Variation)} \qquad (1.1)$$

He proposed that, if the ratio is less than 1.4, standard reference ranges will not be sensitive to actual changes in the state of an individual. Examples of highly individual tests are cholesterol and alkaline phosphatase. For each of these tests, variation within a single person (*intraindividual variation*) over time averages about 5-7%; however, reference values have a variation of 15-25% around an average result for the population (*interindividual variation*). Changes that remain within the broad reference range for each of these tests would be missed, even though they may represent clinically important changes in the patient's condition. Table 1.3 lists the index of individuality for some common laboratory tests.

Individual Reference Ranges

An ideal approach to detecting changes in patient condition for tests with little intraindividual variation would be to use the patient's own previous results as a basis for comparison. In a practitioner's private practice, such an approach may be readily attainable, since earlier laboratory results become a part of the patient's medical record. In large HMO organizations, including systems such as the military and VA hospital systems, patients are commonly tested in only one laboratory over a long period of time. Computer storage of laboratory data allows practitioners ready access to earlier laboratory results on patients, even those who are being seen by a new practitioner for some medical problem. At the author's institution, use of a patient's previous results has become a common part of medical care, as many outpatient clinics print complete

Table 1.3.
Index of Individuality for Common Laboratory Tests

Test	Index
Calcium	1.3
Sodium	1.4
Magnesium	0.8
Phosphorus	0.9
Total protein	0.8
Cholesterol	0.6
Alkaline phosphatase	0.5

summaries of a patient's laboratory results over the previous three to four years at each clinic visit. With increasing use of computer networks and ability to transfer data across the country via the Internet, use of intraindividual reference values will likely expand for common tests. It is unlikely, however, that such an approach will ever become feasible for tests that are not part of general screening panels because of the tremendous cost of such an approach.

Disease-Specific Reference Values

For a few tests, large scale studies have helped to define test results which indicated risk or status of disease. Perhaps the most obvious example is cholesterol, where data on relative risk of coronary artery disease have been used to define cholesterol levels that are borderline high or high. The development of ranges of hemoglobin A_{1c} values that correlate with good, fair, and poor diabetic control, and the use of CD4 levels to monitor progression of HIV infection are other examples of using laboratory test results to monitor disease status. This approach will be useful for selected test/disease combinations, but is unlikely to be practical for the majority of laboratory tests.

Methodology Used by the Laboratory to Perform the Test

Most practitioners are aware that reference values differ from one laboratory to another. While some of the variation is due to the factors discussed earlier in the chapter, a major source of variation is the difference in methods used from one laboratory to another. There is no method, for measuring any substance, which is free from all interferences. In addition, for many substances, there is no "gold standard" which can be used by the laboratory to determine that its results match perfectly with those of all other laboratories. For some tests, particularly enzyme assays, the activity of the enzyme that is measured depends on the conditions used to measure it; variation in test conditions will change the results and therefore change the reference values. Practitioners must always check test results against the reference values for the laboratory where the test was performed; failure to do so may occasionally lead to serious errors in interpretation of test results. Figure 1.5 illustrates the difference in LDH

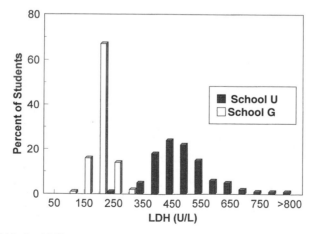

Figure 1.5. Effect of Method Differences on LDH Results. In two groups of medical students, testing was done in two laboratories that used different methodologies to measure LDH. In the laboratory for School U, results are approximately two–times higher than on the same specimens when tested in the laboratory for School G.

Approach to Unexpected Abnormal Laboratory Results

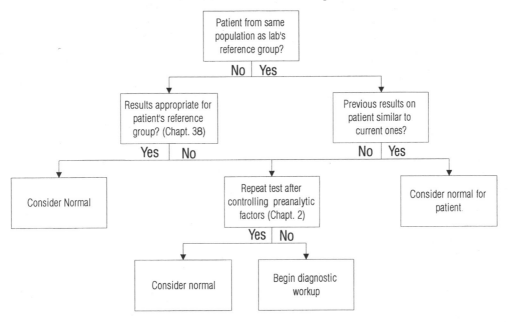

Figure 1.6. Approach to Unexpected Abnormal Laboratory Results. In a patient with unexpected abnormal results, first see if the appropriate reference range was used. If different from previous results, repeat under controlled conditions before further work-up.

results between medical students tested in two different laboratories, due to differences in methodology. This did not cause a problem for practitioners using either of the two laboratories, since few practitioners practiced at both institutions; however, consultants from one institution seeing patients in the other needed to be careful to avoid mistakes in interpretation.

APPROACH TO USE OF REFERENCE VALUES

This chapter highlighted some of the principles underlying the concept of reference values, the methods used by most laboratories to establish reference ranges, and some of the problems which may result from use of reference values as synonyms for "healthy." How, then, should practitioners use reference values in reviewing the results of laboratory tests performed on their patients? First, practitioners need to become familiar with the methods and population used by the laboratory to establish reference ranges. When unexpectedly abnormal results are encountered, the algorithm given here (Fig. 1.6) offers general guidelines for evaluation of the need to perform further diagnostic testing or accept the results as normal.

It is vital that practitioners develop a good working relationship with the laboratory where most of their patients' testing is performed. While most practitioners will develop familiarity with the limitations of reference values for tests which they commonly order, the same may not hold true for tests which they occasionally or seldom order. Most laboratories have consultants available, either from the professional staff or on an as needed basis, who can provide additional information which the practitioner can use to interpret unusual test results.

CHAPTER 2

Causes for Variation in Laboratory Testing

D. ROBERT DUFOUR

VARIABILITY—A CONSTANT IN NORMAL PHYSIOLOGY

From the time that practitioners began measuring vital signs, it was recognized that these were not constants, but that they changed in response to a variety of factors. For example, textbooks on physical diagnosis point out that temperature is highest in the evening and lowest in the early morning; ingestion of hot and cold beverages affect temperature readings; and that variation during the day is less in elderly patients. In women, the rise in temperature associated with ovulation is well known and is used as a test to detect its occurrence. Harrison's textbook of Internal Medicine discusses seasonal variation, postprandial changes, age, and pregnancy as factors which affect temperature. Pulse measurements are affected by respiration, markedly in children but to a lesser extent in adults, while stress and exercise increases pulse rate. A pulse rate below 50 is common in physically fit young adults, but is seldom representative of normal physiology in the elderly. The World Health Organization recommends that blood pressure be measured only after a patient is seated comfortably for several minutes to avoid false readings. Blood pressure is subject to significant variability between observers; many individuals have higher blood pressure when examined by a practitioner compared to other settings ("white coat hypertension").

It should not be surprising that such factors as diet, stress, patient preparation, exercise, diurnal variation, and physiologic states such as pregnancy could affect the results of laboratory tests as well as other physiologic variables. Laboratory tests are good markers of the patient's physiologic status under most circumstances, and this is the reason for their utility; this may, however, produce "abnormal" test results when the patient's physiologic state changes. In addition to physiologic factors, there are three other major causes of variation in laboratory tests. The specimen obtained from the patient may not be representative of the patient's actual state. Factors which can produce a non-representative specimen are usually related to the actual technique of collection, and include use of tourniquets, contamination with intravenous fluids, and contamination by anticoagulants or preservatives. Even if a representative specimen was obtained, the concentration of one or more substances in the specimen may change after collection. These changes are usually the result of metabolism in the specimen, occur with delay in delivery of specimens to the laboratory, and mainly affect substances used in metabolism, products of metabolism, or substances which leak from blood cells which can no longer maintain their integrity. Finally, actual errors in the process of measurement in the laboratory may produce results which are "abnormal" but obviously of no clinical importance. This chapter will detail all of the common factors and major tests which are affected, and offer suggestions on how to limit this type of variability.

PHYSIOLOGIC FACTORS AND THEIR EFFECTS ON LABORATORY TESTS

Diet and Laboratory Tests

Absorption of Dietary Components

Substances absorbed into blood from food are increased after a meal. For example, glucose and triglycerides increase shortly after food ingestion and remain elevated for as long as food continues to be absorbed; this may take several hours to be complete. While a glucose tolerance test produces marked increases in glucose, this does not occur after a meal because food glucose is primarily in starches, which must be digested before glucose is absorbed. In fact, average post-meal glucose is only slightly higher than fasting levels in young persons, although post-meal glucose concentration increases with age. Triglycerides start to rise within one-half hour of eating and peak at about two hours; synthesis of new lipoproteins by the liver results in another rise in triglyceride levels, which remain elevated for an average of 9–12 hours. For this reason, triglycerides should only be measured after a fast of at least 12 hours. Amino acid content of various foods is a major cause of fluctuation in plasma and urine amino acid concentrations; this must be controlled for in those instances where amino acids are measured. For example, hydroxyproline (an amino acid found only in collagen) is sometimes measured as a marker of collagen turnover in bone. In the diet, collagen is found principally in meat and in gelatin (used as an additive to many processed foods). Failure to control dietary intake of meat and gelatin can cause falsely high urinary hydroxyproline.

Hormonal and Metabolic Changes Following Food Ingestion

Meals directly stimulate a twofold to threefold increase in gastrin production; gastrin levels are thus best evaluated in fasting patients. Stimulation of gastric acid production leads to loss of HCl, increasing blood pH and lowering plasma chloride concentration. These changes secondarily alter renal acid handling, causing a marked rise in urine pH after meals, with pH often above 7.0. Glucose absorption stimulates insulin release, producing a several-fold rise in plasma levels. Insulin facilitates entry of potassium and phosphate into cells, causing a significant drop in plasma levels after eating. Many other hormones are also affected following a meal; glucose inhibits the production of both ACTH and growth hormone, while certain amino acids stimulate growth hormone production. The most reproducible laboratory results are therefore obtained when patients are fasting for 8–12 hours; all routine laboratory tests will show more correlation with the actual physiologic state when drawn in this fashion. This obviously is practical for hospitalized patients, but not for ambulatory care settings. Practitioners must recognize that persons whose blood is drawn when not fasting may have "abnormal" results. This represents a major concern for so few tests, however, that as a practical matter we require fasting specimens only for glucose (in diabetics only), triglyceride, and gastrin.

Effects of Prolonged Fasting

Failure to eat causes alteration in many laboratory tests, although changes often require several days to weeks to become apparent. A few tests are affected quickly. Bilirubin starts to increase after a fast of as little as 24 hours; this has been proposed as a diagnostic test to recognize Gilbert's syndrome, a congenital disorder with decreased bilirubin clearance. This increase in bilirubin may be of some concern in a patient following biliary tract surgery. Carotene, used as a test of gastrointestinal absorption, is cleared rapidly from blood with fasting; measurement of carotene to assess normal absorption should obviously not be carried out in a patient who is not eating. Stool fat measures the efficiency of the biliary tract, pancreas, and gastrointestinal tract in breaking down and absorbing dietary fat; in a defective system, over 7% of dietary fat is excreted in the stool. To perform and interpret this test, therefore, there must be a known amount of fat in the diet. With longer fasting, a number of endocrine adaptations occur. Most pituitary hormones are decreased, which decreases the levels of hormones regulated by pituitary hormones (such as thyroid hormone, testosterone, and estrogens). Levels of many plasma proteins decrease, as amino acids released from protein turnover are used for glucose production instead. Levels of lipids such as cholesterol also decrease as liver synthesis is impaired. While some of these tests may thus be useful as markers of nutritional state (Chapter 20), measurement of hormones or bilirubin may provide misleading information in malnourished patients.

Stress

Stress represents the response of the body to alteration in the normal physiologic state, leading to adaptations which may alter results of laboratory markers of normal physiology. In general, biologic changes of stress are due to a combination of hormonal adaptations. In most types of stress, there is increased production of a variety of neurotransmitters, including serotonin and catecholamines, which produce such physiologic changes as heightened awareness, increased pulse and blood pressure, and sweating. These hormones also have effects on other physiologic processes; increased glucose and cortisol are two well known effects of stress. Inflammation, another form of stress, is also associated with production of "hormones," also known as cytokines or interleukins. Accumulating evidence shows that these hormones have many effects on normal physiology. Interleukins increase the production of some plasma proteins, such as ceruloplasmin, fibrinogen, and haptoglobin, while inhibiting the production of transferrin and albumin; they also stimulate the production of granulocytes and platelets. Interleukins also have potent effects on the pituitary and hypothalamus, decreasing the production of most pituitary hormones but increasing ACTH production. The more intense and longer the inflammation is, the greater the degree of these changes. Interleukins markedly increase the rate of uptake of cholesterol by macrophages and blood vessel walls; it is not uncommon for plasma cholesterol to fall by 40% in patients with severe tissue damage as occurs after surgery, with severe infections, or following a myocardial infarction. Mental stress, as occurs with panic disorders and in psychiatric illness, may also produce significant changes in many laboratory tests, particularly those of the endocrine system. Before an examination, for example, catecholamine levels rise significantly. Changes in plasma volume often accompany acute stress of various sorts; the increase in blood volume dilutes plasma proteins, such that some (such as HDL cholesterol) decrease by as much as 15%. For these reasons, endocrine and lipid testing should never be performed electively when a patient is under stress, and must be interpreted with caution in a patient with signs or symptoms of endocrine disease and coexisting acute stress.

Patient Preparation

This is an important, but seldom considered, variable in laboratory testing. In the upright position, water and electrolytes are lost from the vascular space, causing proteins and protein bound substances to become relatively concentrated. Plasma proteins, enzymes, hematocrit, calcium, iron, hormones, and many drugs will be increased in concentration by an average of 5–8% in the upright position. When an individual takes a sitting position after being upright, it takes approximately 15 minutes for redistribution of water to the vascular space. When going from a sitting to a supine position, water and electrolytes move back into the vascular space, reducing the concentration of proteins and protein bound substances by 10–15%. If patients are seen in an ambulatory care setting, failing to require a period of sitting of at least 15 minutes will introduce significant variability into test results. Many other tests require more specific patient preparation. In glucose tolerance testing, for example, eating a high carbohydrate diet for three days prior to testing is necessary to "prime" the pancreas; failure to take in at least 150 g of carbohydrates during this time commonly produces a diabetic pattern of glucose tolerance. Patients taking thyroid hormone replacement commonly have measurements of TSH to evaluate the appropriateness of the dosage. Although thyroxine (T_4) has a half-life of approximately one week, it is absorbed relatively quickly from the intestinal tract after a dose. Consequently, patients taking T_4 in the morning prior to having blood drawn commonly have transiently increased T_4 and lowered TSH, which could lead to inappropriate adjustment of dosage. There are many other examples of the effects of patient preparation discussed in Chapter 38.

Exercise

Physical exercise produces both short term and long term changes in laboratory tests. In those who exercise on a regular basis, there are increased levels of plasma enzymes found in muscle, such as creatine kinase (CK), aspartate aminotransferase (AST or SGOT), and lactate dehydrogenase (LDH). Since many of these enzymes are also found in liver, this pattern is often confused with liver disease. Although CK is not commonly measured, increases in CK are often dramatic, reaching 10–20 times the normal upper reference limit in persons who engage in contact sports, body building, or distance events. Cessation of exercise for several days will normalize enzyme levels if due to this cause. Exercise also decreases estrogen concentration, probably due to lower gonadotropin production by the pituitary, while it increases uric acid (in men), most likely due to decreased excretion. There is also a transient increase in urine protein following a period of exercise. Those who engage in endurance exercise often develop profound endocrine changes, with decreased production of FSH, LH, and prolactin; sex hormone levels (testosterone, estradiol, progesterone) will also decrease. It is generally not necessary to have patients stop exercise before having blood drawn; however, if there is a suspicion of liver or endocrine disease, repeating the tests after a period without exercise should help to clarify whether disease is present.

Cyclic Variation

Reproducible patterns of alteration in physiologic state, including laboratory tests, occur at specific times of the day, month, or year. Many pituitary hormones (and, to a lesser extent, the endocrine hormones which they control) show *ultradian* variation, changes occurring over a period less than one day. These hormones are released in episodic bursts (Fig. 2.1), causing a pattern of peaks and valleys of concentration in plasma. All pituitary hormones also show *diurnal* variation, changes occurring during a day. Melatonin, a hormone produced by the pineal gland when there is no light reaching the brain, stimulates the production of pituitary hormones. Although the

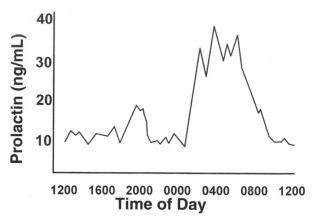

Figure 2.1. Diurnal Variation. Prolactin, as with most pituitary hormones, is released in episodic spikes during the day, with most hormone produced during sleep. A single pituitary hormone level provides little information unless markedly abnormal.

exact pattern varies for each hormone (see Chapters 13–15), in general levels begin to rise about 1–2 hours after sleep begins and peak around the middle of a sleep period before starting to fall shortly before waking. The pattern becomes "fixed," so that short term changes in when an individual sleeps do not alter this normal rhythm. When an individual changes this pattern for several days to weeks, as with shift work or when moving to another time zone several hours different from the original one, the body adjusts its internal clock to the new pattern. Other tests which show a pronounced diurnal variation are acid phosphatase and iron. When performing these tests, a reproducible time of collection is important; we recommend early morning collection. Any abnormalities should be checked against the patient's hours of work to assure that they are not due to comparison with an inappropriate reference range.

Changes may also occur over a longer period of time. In menstruating women, the hormonal changes of a normal menstrual cycle are associated with monthly variability in a number of laboratory tests. Standardization of time of collection within a menstrual cycle is not usually suggested for any tests other than estradiol or progesterone. Cholesterol is 25% higher during the second half of the menstrual cycle. If a woman is being treated for hypercholesterolemia, measurement of cholesterol during the period of menstruation will reduce variation and allow more accurate evaluation of the effects of treatment. Variation over a longer period of time, such as annual variation, occurs for a few laboratory tests. It should not be surprising that levels of vitamin D, which is produced by sunlight, are higher in the summer and lower in the winter; slight variation in parathyroid hormone and calcium occur in a similar fashion. Several pituitary hormones show lower production rates in winter than summer, perhaps a residual of hibernation responses.

Pregnancy

A number of physiologic changes are necessary to support a developing fetus. The earliest are hormonally mediated, due to markedly increased concentrations of estrogen and progesterone with rapidly rising HCG levels. Later, the placenta produces another hormone, *chorionic somatomammotropin*, with similarities in structure and action to growth hormone and prolactin. Together, these hormones cause progressive alteration in the physiologic state of the mother. Glucose tolerance decreases and postprandial glucose concentrations gradually rise during normal pregnancy to assure adequate glucose availability for the fetus. There is a decreased production of thyroid hormone, of unclear etiology, particularly in the first trimester of pregnancy, causing a gradual rise in TSH concentration. Increased estrogens increase the production of a number of plasma proteins, such as ceruloplasmin and thyroid binding globulin. Lipid levels rise gradually during pregnancy, with total and low-density lipoprotein cholesterol approximately doubling. Plasma volume rises progressively during pregnancy, diluting plasma proteins and lowering hematocrit in the first trimester; after about the 20th week, RBC mass also increases, although not to as great an extent as plasma until the last several weeks of pregnancy. In early pregnancy, glomerular filtration rate increases markedly, reaching values about 50% higher than baseline by the end of the first trimester, with a resulting fall in BUN and creatinine levels in blood. The placenta produces other substances, including alkaline phosphatase (which can increase by 100% near term), which appear in the mother's blood during the third trimester. A number of clotting factors increase significantly during pregnancy, including fibrinogen, which rises by an average of 50%. There are many additional laboratory results which change during pregnancy; these are detailed Chapter 38.

Drug Effects

Medications frequently cause altered laboratory test results. Most commonly, this is due to the direct or indirect pharmacologic actions of a drug on normal physiology. Many commonly ingested chemicals, including caffeine, nicotine, and ethanol may affect laboratory test results in a similar fashion. While it is impossible to document the effects of every drug on every laboratory test, Chapter 38 summarizes the effects of the most commonly used drugs on frequently ordered laboratory tests. Here, only the most commonly encountered drugs are summarized.

Caffeine

Like other methylxanthines such as theophylline, caffeine has effects mainly on the endocrine system. Marked increases in catecholamine production occur with caffeine ingestion (Fig. 2.2); this has indirect effects on glucose production, insulin levels, and glucose tolerance. Caffeine is a potent stimulus to gastrin production, with levels rising as much as 500% over baseline. Caffeine also increases the production of cortisol and 5-hydroxyindoleacetic acid, a metabolite of serotonin.

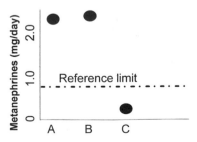

Figure 2.2. Effect of Caffeine on Catecholamine Metabolites. In this patient, initial urine levels of the catecholamine metabolite metanephrine were about twice normal on two occasions (**A, B**). On questioning, the patient admitted to drinking nine cups of coffee daily. Repeat measurement after he reduced his coffee intake to two cups daily was normal (**C**).

Nicotine

Whether from tobacco or patches, nicotine has many of the same effects as caffeine; it also stimulates catecholamine, gastrin, and cortisol production. Growth hormone markedly increases after nicotine exposure, and may reach levels ten times higher than baseline. Glucose tolerance is often improved by nicotine. Smokers often have higher levels of carboxyhemoglobin, which may produce an increase in hematocrit. Smoking decreases immunoglobulin and vitamin B_{12} levels.

Ethanol

The effects of ethanol depend on dose and duration of ingestion. Chronic alcohol ingestion is often associated with increased triglycerides and decreased glucose, due to the direct effects of ethanol on the liver. Ethanol stimulates the production of γ-glutamyl-transferase (GGT) by the liver. This has often been used as an indirect measure of alcohol intake; however, binge drinkers tend to have lower levels than do maintenance drinkers for the same amount of alcohol intake, and levels remain elevated for many weeks after abstinence begins. HDL cholesterol is increased by ethanol intake, roughly in proportion to the amount ingested.

Oral Contraceptives

This class of drugs is often considered as a single drug in medical publications; however, the relative amounts of estrogens and progestins cause significant variation in effect from one preparation to another. In general, oral contraceptives high in estrogen cause an increase in HDL cholesterol, thyroid binding globulin (causing increased total T_4 and low T_3 resin uptake (T_3RU)), ceruloplasmin, and certain coagulation factors. Progesterone causes decreased HDL cholesterol and increased LDL cholesterol, but does not alter most of the other tests mentioned for estrogen.

SPECIMEN COLLECTION FACTORS

The process involved in collecting specimens, particularly blood specimens, may cause the sample to not accurately represent the concentrations of substances that were present in the patient's blood. Since most educational programs do not discuss these factors, this section will outline the most important factors and their effects.

Tourniquet Use

When a tourniquet is placed on the arm, venous drainage is prevented, causing dilatation of the vein. As long as the volume of blood collected does not exceed the actual amount in the vein, this will not produce any changes; however, this is generally true only if a single tube of blood is obtained. Those tubes that are collected last in the process will be most affected. Blood that is still in the capillary bed will be affected by the increased pressure and decreased flow in two major ways.

Loss of Fluid

As venous pressure remains high, the return of water and electrolytes to venous blood from tissue is impaired. This produces an increase in the concentration of proteins and substances bound to proteins. The increase in concentration is directly related to duration of tourniquet use; it begins at about 1 min, causes a 5% concentration increase after about 3–5 min, and can produce a 15% higher concentration after 10–15 minutes, as may occur with a difficult blood draw.

Leakage of Cell Contents

As venous pressure remains high, circulation of fresh blood to the tissue diminishes. Cells continue their metabolic processes, resulting in a fall in the concentration of substances used in metabolism, and increasing the concentration of various metabolic products such as lactate. Potassium will leak from cells as acidosis occurs with lactate accumulation. Because muscle tissue is the most active metabolically, having the patient clench and unclench their fist while trying to draw blood will accelerate the rate at which these metabolic changes occur. Active fist clenching can increase apparent plasma potassium by 1.0–1.5 mmol/L within one minute (Fig. 2.3). There have been several reports in the literature of patients hospitalized for evaluation of hyperkalemia which was an artifact induced by this technique of specimen collection.

Contamination with Intravenous Fluids

Because of the extensive connections between veins in the forearm, blood drawn from one vein may show contamination from intravenous fluid entering another vein. Blood should never be drawn from an arm with intravenous fluid being infused unless a tourniquet can be placed between the line and the site of phlebotomy; even this technique can produce contamination in some cases. Blood may be drawn from an intravenous or intraarterial line, as long as a volume of blood equal to the volume of the catheter is removed prior to specimen collection. This produces a reliable sample of blood, except for measurement of any substance being given through the catheter at a concentration many times higher than that in blood (as often occurs with glucose, potassium, drugs, and heparin). For example, the concentration of glucose in 5% dextrose solutions is 5000 mg/dL, compared with a normal plasma glucose of approximately 100 mg/dL. In the case of heparin, many indwelling catheters have heparin in a coating on the catheter. Coagulation tests are notoriously unreliable in specimens

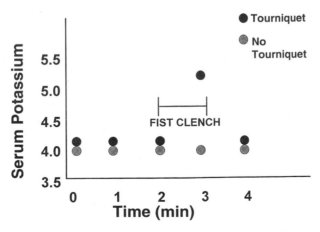

Figure 2.3. Fist Clenching Related "Hyperkalemia." Potassium was measured in specimens collected in patients with a tourniquet in place with and without fist clenching. Within one minute of fist contraction, potassium increased an average of 1.5 mmol/L. (Data from Don et al. N Engl J Med 1989;322:1291)

Table 2.1.
Anticoagulants and Preservatives Used for Blood Specimens

Color Stopper	Anticoagulant/ Preservative	Uses
Red	None	Most chemistry tests; produces serum
Green	Heparin	Most chemistry tests; produces plasma
Lavender	EDTA	Blood counts, some hormone tests, can also be used for lipids
Light Blue	Citrate	Coagulation tests
Black	Oxalate	Coagulation tests
Navy Blue	Acid washed	Trace metal analysis
Gray	Sodium fluoride	Glucose, lactate when specimen delays likely

taken from catheters for this reason. Many chronically ill patients have multilumen catheters to eliminate the need for venipunctures to obtain blood samples. If specimens are drawn while the fluid is being infused through another lumen, the specimen collected will be significantly diluted by the fluid administered; a more reasonable approach is to stop the flow of fluid for several minutes prior to specimen collection.

Contamination by Anticoagulants

Each of the different evacuated tubes used by laboratories has a different preservative or anticoagulant and purpose, as summarized in Table 2.1. In addition, some tubes contain gels that are used to separate serum (or plasma) from red cells and prevent metabolism from changing test results (discussed below).

The most obvious type of contamination results from collecting a specimen into an inappropriate tube. Most laboratories immediately recognize this problem, and reject such specimens. Occasionally, we have seen specimens which have apparently been poured from one type of tube into another to prevent the laboratory from rejecting the specimen; this can produce markedly abnormal and non-physiologic results, as illustrated in Table 2.2.

This problem can be prevented by following the laboratory's guidelines for proper tube selection. When multiple tubes of blood are collected at the same time, either using adapters which allow direct drawing into evacuated tubes or by filling multiple tubes with blood drawn by syringe, contamination from one specimen to another can occur. Even a small drop of blood from lavender top tubes, which contain high concen-

Table 2.2.
Effect of Anticoagulants on Routine Tests

Test	Red Top	Lavender Top (K EDTA)	Light Blue Top (Na Citrate)
Sodium (mmol/L)	142	137	194
Potassium (mmol/L)	4.2	24.8	3.7
Chloride (mmol/L)	106	102	67
Bicarbonate (mmol/L)	25	22	7
Calcium (mg/dL)	9.8	0	6.7
Magnesium (mg/dL)	1.9	0	1.7
Alkaline Phosphatase (U/L)	97	0	45
Creatine Kinase (U/L)	205	0	155

trations of potassium EDTA as an anticoagulant, will produce a marked increase in potassium along with markedly decreased calcium and magnesium (which replace K^+ on the EDTA) and low levels of enzymes such as CK and alkaline phosphatase (which need these metals for their measurement). Specimens for coagulation testing should never be the first drawn, since tissue fluid can initiate the clotting process and cause falsely low levels of coagulation factors. The preferred order of collection or filling of tubes is: tubes with no preservatives (red top tubes); tubes with mild anticoagulants (green, gray, blue, black); and lavender top tubes last. Finally, samples for trace metal analysis (aluminum, zinc, copper, and lead) require special collection tubes and, in some cases, needles to prevent contamination of specimens, which can increase metal concentrations many-fold.

Labeling Errors

Studies have shown that if specimens are drawn in one location and then carried to another site for labeling, the incidence of mislabeled specimens is many times higher than when specimens are labeled at the actual time and site they are obtained from a patient. In one hospital, initiating a policy requiring specimen labeling at the bedside in a unit where mislabeled specimens were common virtually eliminated this problem. At the least, receiving results for a patient that were drawn from someone else is an irritation, since they often indicate a change in condition of the patient when one did not occur. In some instances, especially where results are changed in a direction that could represent an expected change in patient condition, they could lead to inappropriate treatment of a patient. While careful attention to a policy of labeling specimens at the bedside minimizes these errors, it is wise to consider whether a change may be due to a specimen error and repeat any suspicious results before initiating therapy.

Technique of Collection

The most important artifact induced by collection is hemolysis, which causes leakage of hemoglobin (which can interfere with many laboratory tests) and red cell contents (such as potassium, phosphate, and enzymes, including lactate dehydrogenase (LDH), and to a lesser extent AST and ALT). Hemolysis is most commonly caused by turbulent blood flow. This often occurs with evacuated tubes when blood is trickling into the tube from a poorly flowing venipuncture. It occurs more commonly with large bore than with small bore needles, although there is a common misconception that the opposite is true. When skin is cleansed with an alcohol solution, failure to allow the alcohol to dry prior to venipuncture can produce hemolysis. If blood is collected with a syringe, forcibly pulling the barrel back to its full extent to speed the process of collection, or forcibly pushing down on the stopper to more rapidly fill evacuated tubes will frequently produce hemolyzed specimens.

Source of Specimen

Arterial blood differs from venous blood in having higher concentrations of energy substrates (glucose, oxygen) and lower concentrations of waste products (ammonia, K^+, H^+, lactate). In most circumstances, these differences are minimal and need not be considered in interpreting results; in our laboratory, reference values for venous and arterial lactate are identical. In states of hypoperfusion, the differences between arterial and venous blood are magnified; for example, patients in shock may have normal arterial glucose and undetectable venous glucose. Capillary blood, which is often used for glucose measurements, is closer to arterial than to venous blood.

CHANGES IN SPECIMENS AFTER COLLECTION

Post-collection artifacts are rarely a problem with blood tests, but represent a major problem for urine or stool specimens; variations in these fluids will be discussed in appropriate sections of the book.

Metabolism in Specimens

After collection, cells remain viable for many hours, and continue their metabolic processes. This leads to a fall in glucose and oxygen concentration in blood and an increase in acid production (leading to a decrease in pH) and CO_2. After glucose is depleted, cells can no longer generate energy, and so begin to leak their contents, such as K^+, Mg^{++}, and phosphate. Eventually, cells will begin to break down, releasing hemoglobin, enzymes, and iron, among many substances. To prevent these changes, specimens are brought to a laboratory as soon as possible after collection of blood, and the specimen is centrifuged to separate the liquid (serum if blood is allowed to clot first, plasma if an anticoagulant is used) from the cells. Once separated from cells, serum or plasma is relatively stable. The major factor producing abnormal results due to metabolism is a delay in specimens reaching the laboratory. This is most critical for blood gases and glucose; even a slight delay may cause marked changes in blood gas results, while glucose falls by 3% per hour at room temperature.

Enzymatic Processes

Plasma and serum contain a number of proteolytic enzymes which can cause degeneration of proteins, including peptide hormones and enzymes. For many hormones, specimens should be collected in lavender top tubes, because many proteases require ions which bind to EDTA. Samples for enzyme and hormone measurements must often be frozen to prevent change in concentration. Failure to follow these requirements may lead to grossly inaccurate results and inaccurate diagnoses.

Effects of Hematologic Disease

In normal blood, most metabolic activity is due to red blood cells, which are much less complex and less metabolically active that white blood cells. In patients with high white blood count, especially in leukemias, the rate of metabolism is markedly accelerated over normal, such that the metabolic changes discussed above occur in minutes, rather than hours. When platelets participate in clot formation, they release potassium into blood. Serum potassium is thus always higher than plasma potassium; this is not usually a problem, since the differences average only 0.2–0.3 mmol/L. In patients with increased platelet count, however, the difference between serum and plasma potassium increases by an average of 0.1–0.2 mmol/L for every 100,000/mm³ increase in platelet count; patients with markedly elevated platelet count may thus appear to have hyperkalemia when serum specimens are examined. In any patient with markedly abnormal white cell or platelet count, specimens should be collected in green top tubes, which will result in heparinized plasma rather than serum; specimens should be brought to the laboratory without delay so that separation of plasma from the abnormal cells can be accomplished rapidly.

CAUSES OF ERROR IN MEASUREMENT

While the factors discussed earlier are the most common causes for laboratory results to not reflect the actual status of the patient, occasionally errors in the actual measurement are the cause. Laboratories regularly perform "quality controls," in which specimens of known composition are tested by the same method to assure that the testing procedure is working properly. There are certain conditions, however, when results in an individual sample may produce inaccurate results. The most common of these are discussed for each test in the table at the end of the book; the general causes of such errors are discussed here.

Interference from Drugs or Chemicals

Drugs ingested by a patient are the most common cause of measurement errors. Many laboratory tests use chemical reactions which are not entirely specific for the substance to be measured; a good example is in creatinine measurements. Acetoacetate, one of the ketone bodies accumulating in diabetic ketoacidosis, cross-reacts in most creatinine assays, causing falsely elevated results which may lead to a suspicion of acute renal failure. Some cephalosporin antibiotics also cross-react in this assay, although to a much lesser extent. Iron commonly produces a false positive result for stool occult blood, as can substances found in meat and some vegetables. Drugs may also inhibit a chemical reaction; vitamin C causes falsely low results in urine dipstick tests for blood and glucose.

Problems in the Specimen

As already mentioned, hemolysis can occur during the collection process. Not only does hemolysis release red cell contents, but hemoglobin directly interferes in many different chemical reactions. Many tests in the laboratory use measurement of the amount of light passing through a specimen; specimens with increased hemoglobin, bilirubin, and lipids (which produce turbidity, preventing light's passage) often produce erroneous results. Abnormal proteins, as found in patients with multiple myeloma or cryoglobulinemia, may precipitate spontaneously, also producing turbidity. Increased lipids also reduce the amount of water in a sample; methods which take a fixed volume of plasma will have a lower concentration of all substances dissolved in water, which includes most laboratory tests of interest to practitioners. Usually, this will cause no more than a 5–10% underestimation of actual results, which is probably acceptable for most tests; however, for electrolytes such as sodium and chloride, this represents a serious error which has been termed "pseudohyponatremia." Some newer methods can measure sodium directly in plasma, and will not show this error. In fingerstick glucose testing, glucose is usually measured by an enzyme termed glucose oxidase; the amount of oxygen in the specimen is critical to the measurement of glucose. Patients with abnormal pO_2 or hematocrit, which changes oxygen in blood, frequently have errors in glucose measured by this method.

Mislabeled Specimens

Labeling problems rarely occur in the laboratory. Commonly, laboratories take small amounts of blood out of a tube for testing, and the sample obtained is then labeled with the same specimen number as the tube. Clerical errors at this step may result in results being reported for another patient.

CHAPTER 3

Evaluating Usefulness of Laboratory Tests

D. ROBERT DUFOUR

REASONS FOR DOING LABORATORY TESTS

While laboratory tests could be ordered for many reasons, most fall into three categories: screening, diagnostic, and monitoring. Each requires different assumptions about test usefulness.

Screening Tests

By definition, screening refers to testing for disease in asymptomatic individuals; common examples include neonatal testing for phenylketonuria, cholesterol to predict risk of coronary artery disease, and prostate specific antigen (PSA) to identify prostatic carcinoma. Closely related in principle is **case finding,** in which persons with symptoms of one disease are tested for another disorder; examples include thyroid testing in patients with atrial fibrillation, glucose testing in those with peripheral neuropathy, or vitamin B_{12} in persons with dementia.

Deciding Disorders Suitable for Screening

Several criteria are used in determining whether to screen for a particular disease. A screening test should be easy to perform, inexpensive, carry little risk to the patient, and detect disease in a high percentage of cases. The disease screened for must be treatable and have serious health consequences. Examples include blood pressure for hypertension and glucose during pregnancy for gestational diabetes. Many routine laboratory tests such as complete blood counts, urinalysis, and chemistry panels are done for screening or case finding.

Benefits of Screening Programs?

Additional factors determine the worth of screening programs, including benefits and the cost-benefit ratio. The most important is whether there is benefit to detecting asymptomatic disease, rather than waiting for signs and symptoms. While it might appear advantageous, this is not always the case. For example, sputum cytology and chest x-ray screening programs in asymptomatic smokers detect lung cancer and increase 5-year survival, but the same percentage of screened and unscreened patients died of lung cancer. This is due to biases introduced by screening (Fig. 3.1).

Justification for Screening?

For many diseases, there is little information on biases, making determination of screening's advantages difficult. In a comprehensive review of screening by the American College of Physicians, evidence supported screening for hypertension, hypercholesterolemia, breast cancer, and cervical cancer, but not for routine electrocardiograms,

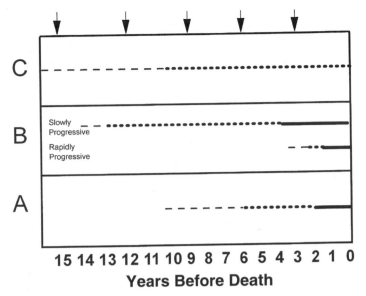

Figure 3.1. Biases introduced by screening programs. The natural history of disease is illustrated as representing undetectable disease (dashed line), asymptomatic stages detectable by screening (dotted line), and symptomatic stages (solid line). Screening is performed every three years (arrows). **Lead-time bias (A)** occurs in incurable diseases with a relatively long asymptomatic stage; detecting disease at this stage appears to improve survival over detecting symptomatic disease, but no patients are benefited. **Length bias (B)** occurs when some cases of disease are slowly progressive, while others progress rapidly through an asymptomatic stage and are quickly fatal. Screening programs are likely to detect only the slowly progressive cases, improving apparent survival. **Ascertainment (overdiagnosis) bias (C)** occurs with latent diseases (many cases of thyroid and prostate cancer) which are clinically silent, never causing clinical problems, but are detectable by screening. Patients with latent disease are diagnosed, treated, and "cured," although their disease would have remained undiagnosed (and had no effect on their survival) if screening were not done.

stress tests to detect coronary artery disease, or screening programs for osteoporosis, diabetes (except during pregnancy), thyroid disease, or lung cancer. The authors also found strong evidence against commonly performed screening tests such as hemoglobin, urinalysis, and chest x-rays. Even commonly performed case finding for thyroid disease was considered of questionable benefit, except in women over age 40 or in elderly inpatients.

Cost–benefit Analysis

If screening is to be beneficial, benefits should outweigh costs. Many studies question the cost–effectiveness of screening for many diseases, including prostate cancer and hypercholesterolemia. "Routine," relatively inexpensive laboratory tests are widely used during physical examinations. Multiphasic screening (a battery of clinical and laboratory tests combined with physical examination) has a minimal effect on improving outcomes after the initial examination. With the expansion of managed care, cost–benefit analysis will likely become a major consideration in deciding on the use of screening tests.

Diagnostic Tests

Another common type of testing aids in the diagnosis of patients with nondiagnostic signs and symptoms; for example, a patient presenting with jaundice, light stools, and dark urine could have hepatitis or a bile duct obstruction. Diagnostic testing helps narrow the differential and may establish the correct diagnosis. One limitation of diagnostic testing (discussed in detail later in this chapter) is that the likelihood of misleading information varies with likelihood of disease in the patient. Diagnostic testing provides the most benefit when uncertainty is highest, and provides little useful information (and an increasing likelihood of misleading results) as the likelihood of disease is either very high or very low.

Monitoring Tests

Tests performed to evaluate the course of disease or detect complications are referred to as monitoring tests; to be useful, several conditions must be met.

Relation of Test to Disease Status

The test selected must correlate with the natural course of a disease or its complications. Serum enzymes such as SGOT (AST) and SGPT (ALT) have relatively short half-lives in plasma, and correlate with rate of cell injury over the past 1–2 days (Chapter 11). With acetaminophen-induced liver disease, damage usually occurs over the first 1–3 days after ingestion; enzymes peak at 1–2 days, then fall at the same rate in all patients, even those who develop liver failure. In viral hepatitis with massive necrosis, AST and ALT levels gradually return to normal as most liver cells are destroyed. In both situations, plasma enzymes provide misleading information suggesting recovery, and do not correlate with disease activity.

Timing of Testing

For a test to be useful, the time course of change in results must parallel changes in disease activity. Many tests of liver function in hepatitis change at a different rate than does disease activity. Albumin, with a half-life of three weeks, falls slowly with liver injury and returns to normal slowly, lagging behind changes in other proteins with shorter half-lives (such as coagulation factors). The varied half-lives of the three major forms of bilirubin affect usefulness at different stages of liver injury. In early stages, bilirubin rises at a relatively constant rate as liver function declines, correlating well with disease activity. As the liver heals, conjugated and unconjugated bilirubin fall by about half each day for several days until only biliprotein (half-life of three weeks) remains; from this point, total bilirubin will fall very slowly and does not correlate with liver function.

Control for Other Factors Affecting Test Results

Blood sugar results are affected by a number of factors: anemia produces erroneous fingerstick glucose results; shock produces large discrepancies between venous and fingerstick glucose; collection of blood from an arm where intravenous dextrose is infusing causes markedly elevated glucose (Chapter 2). It is also important to consider differences representing a clinically significant change. For example, an average day to day variation in serum cholesterol is 13%. With a true average cholesterol of 200 mg/dL (5.18 mmol/L), cholesterol may go as high as 226 mg/dL (5.85 mmol/L) or as low as 174 mg/dL (4.51 mmol/L) without indicating real change in lipid status. It is important for practitioners to become familiar with the expected variation in commonly used tests (Chapter 38).

STATISTICAL CONCEPTS RELATED TO TEST INTERPRETATION

As discussed in Chapter 1, there is always overlap between results in healthy and diseased individuals. A practical approach to evaluating test results considers the sensitivity and specificity of a test along with likelihood that disease is present.

Sensitivity

The ability of a test to detect disease is termed sensitivity, which can be calculated from the results of a test in patients with a particular disease (Eq. 3.1).

$$Sensitivity = \frac{Abnormal\ Results\ in\ Patients\ With\ the\ Disease}{All\ Patients\ With\ the\ Disease} \tag{3.1}$$

Abnormal results are considered "positive" findings, while normal results are described as "negative." Results are considered true if they correctly identify that the patient does or does not have the disease, and false if they lead to the wrong interpretation. Patients with disease could, therefore, have either true positive or false negative results (Eq. 3.2).

$$Sensitivity = \frac{True\ Positive\ Results}{True\ Positive\ +\ False\ Negative\ Results} \tag{3.2}$$

In published papers, sensitivity is typically determined by testing patients with well established diagnoses recognized by a "gold standard" criterion. Patients with early or mild forms of disease may not have the same frequency of abnormal results, resulting in reduced sensitivity when the test is used in individuals with less advanced cases. Published sensitivity figures represent the highest possible figure, and are likely to be lower when all patients with the disease are included.

In some cases, a new diagnostic test is significantly more sensitive than the "gold standard." For example, current criteria for myocardial infarction require presence of two of these three findings: prolonged chest pain, new EKG changes, and elevated cardiac enzymes. In recent years, newer markers of myocardial damage (including troponin and myoglobin) detect patients with chest pain, normal EKGs, normal CK-MB, and elevation of the new marker. Such patients have a clinical outcome similar to those meeting accepted criteria for myocardial infarction, although technically these are "false positive" results.

Specificity

The ability of a test to give normal results in patients without a particular disease is termed specificity, calculated as (Eq. 3.3).

$$Specificity = \frac{Normal\ Results\ in\ Patients\ Without\ the\ Disease}{All\ Patients\ Without\ the\ Disease} \tag{3.3}$$

Patients without disease could have true negative results, or falsely positive results. Specificity thus can also be expressed as (Eq. 3.4).

$$Specificity = \frac{True\ Negative\ Results}{True\ Negative\ +\ False\ Positive\ Results} \tag{3.4}$$

In published papers, specificity is often determined by testing healthy persons; test performance is frequently worse in patients with disorders similar to the disease in question. For example, anti-nuclear antibody (ANA) testing was originally introduced as a diagnostic test for Systemic Lupus Erythematosus (SLE). While ANA specificity is reasonably high in the general population, the frequency of positive results in other autoimmune disease patients is also high, causing much lower specificity for SLE.

Evaluation of Positive Test Results—Predictive Value

Sensitivity and specificity are determined by using a test in patients known (by a "gold standard") to either have or lack disease. Typically, practitioners order tests because they do not know to which of these two groups their patient belongs. In this situation, information begins with knowledge of results rather than diagnoses. Once the result is obtained, the practitioner needs to know the likelihood that it indicates that this patient does (or does not) have a disease. The most commonly used statistical tool to answer this question is predictive value.

Mathematical Basis of Predictive Value

Predictive value expresses the mathematical likelihood that a particular result correctly classifies the patient as normal or abnormal. It is based on Bayes' theorem for determining the change in likelihood of making a correct conclusion when an additional piece of information is added; it was popularized for medical uses in the 1970s. Predictive value of a positive result (+PV) for disease is calculated as (Eq. 3.5).

$$+PV = \frac{Total\ true\ positive\ results\ (TP)}{Total\ positive\ results\ (TP\ +\ FP)} \tag{3.5}$$

The total number of positive results is dependent on the characteristics of the test (sensitivity and specificity) as well as the relative frequency (**prevalence**) of the disease. Although most texts use prevalence, this implies that testing is done for screening. In diagnostic testing, it is better to use an estimate of likelihood that disease is present given the signs and symptoms that are present. For example, in patients with chest pain and new EKG changes, likelihood of disease is about 50%. Likelihood can be substituted for prevalence in calculations. Total true positive results are equal to sensitivity times prevalence, while total false positive results equal $(1 - specificity) \times (1 - prevalence)$, with sensitivity, specificity, and prevalence expressed as fractions (Eq. 3.6).

$$+PV = \frac{Sensitivity \times Prevalence}{(1 - specificity) \times (1 - Prevalence)} \tag{3.6}$$

Table 3.1 illustrates the effects of changing prevalence (or likelihood) on +PV for a test with 95% sensitivity and 95% specificity. The differences occur because the relative number of true positive and false positive (*total* true positive, *total* false positive) results in changes along with disease prevalence.

While predictive value is widely used in medical publications, the practitioner should be aware of several limitations in its theory and the statistical approaches used in medical publications.

Table 3.1.
Predictive Value of a Positive Result (+ PV) for a
Test with 95% Sensitivity and 95% Specificity at
Varying Prevalence (Likelihood)

Prevalence (Likelihood)	Predictive Value of a Positive Result
95%	99.7%
70%	97.8%
50%	95.0%
30%	89.0%
10%	67.9%
5%	50.0%
1%	16.1%
0.1%	1.8%
0.01%	0.2%

Predictive Value Does Not Equal Utility

Predictive value indicates the relative likelihood that a test result indicates an individual has a given disease, based solely on that result. Some references state that low predictive value indicates screening should not be performed. In screening for rare congenital diseases such as phenylketonuria or hypothyroidism, the predictive value of screening tests is less than 5% even when test specificity is (as is usually the case) 99.8%. As discussed earlier, since both diseases are serious, treatable disorders with clear advantages to detecting the disease before it becomes symptomatic, screening is indicated. Low predictive value only indicates that diagnosis should not be based on this test alone; follow-up tests are used to establish the diagnosis. Attempting to find infants with these diseases without the screening test is akin to trying to find a needle in a haystack; recognizing affected infants in the group with an abnormal screening test is like finding a needle in a pin cushion, easily accomplished.

Predictive Value is a Poor Model of the Diagnostic Process

Predictive value theory requires that all test results be classified as "normal" or "abnormal"; this results in the loss of useful information. For example, serum calcium is considered equally abnormal at 10.6 mg/dL (2.65 mmol/L), 12.0 mg/dL (3.0 mmol/L), and 15.0 mg/dL (3.75 mmol/L); most practitioners would interpret each of these results in a different fashion. Additionally, predictive value establishes likelihood of a diagnosis based on a single test result; few findings are pathognomonic. Most experienced practitioners evaluate a variety of information in reaching a diagnosis, giving different weight to each variable.

Predictive Value Calculations are Often Made Erroneously

Calculation of predictive value requires knowledge of prevalence (or likelihood) of disease in a population. Many published articles instead test a small group of patients with disease and a sample of normal individuals (for example, 50 patients with disease and 100 normal individuals), then use the number of positive results in each group to calculate predictive value. This approach is valid only if actual disease prevalence is 0.333, typically significantly overestimating the actual predictive value of the test when used in the general population.

Other Mathematical Approaches to Interpretation of Test Results

In addition to the widely used predictive value model, there are several other mathematical approaches which can assist practitioners in interpreting laboratory test results.

Relative Operating Characteristic Curves

Predictive value considers a single point to be the dividing value between "normal" and "abnormal"; however, that point is often established arbitrarily. By graphing the relative ability of a test to separate healthy and diseased individuals at different cutoff points (Fig. 3.2), it is possible to select a value with maximum sensitivity, maximum specificity, or maximum efficiency (percentage of total patients correctly diagnosed). Relative operating characteristic (ROC) curves can also be used to compare performance of two or more diagnostic tests. While ROC curves are superior to simple predictive value, they suffer from most of the same limitations already discussed.

Likelihood Ratios

If data exist on a large number of patients, it is possible to calculate the relative likelihood of disease at any given test result (Fig. 3.3). Likelihood ratios eliminate the loss of information inherent in predictive value, and can be very helpful in interpreting results of numerical tests. The requirement for large numbers of individuals severely limits the ability to readily use likelihood ratios.

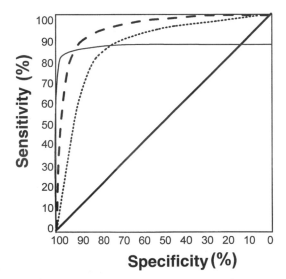

Figure 3.2. Relative Operating Characteristic (ROC) Curves. Sensitivity and specificity of different diagnostic tests can be compared to each other and to a random test (diagonal straight line) by plotting their ability to correctly classify patients at different values of the test. An ideal test will have a curve which stays on the top and left lines of the graph. In the example, Test A (dashed line) performs better than Test B (dotted line) at all values. Test C (solid line) performs better than Test A in terms of specificity, but never picks up more than 80% of the cases of disease. In this example, Test A might be used to screen for disease, and Test C could be used to confirm any abnormal result from Test A. Test B would not be useful.

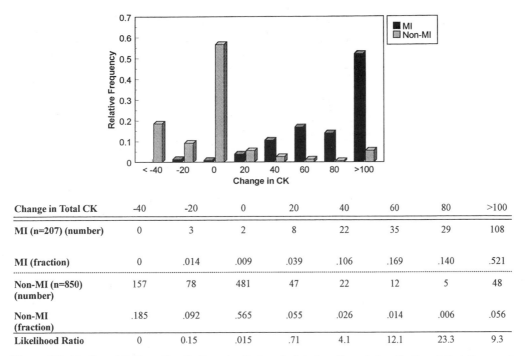

Change in Total CK	-40	-20	0	20	40	60	80	>100
MI (n=207) (number)	0	3	2	8	22	35	29	108
MI (fraction)	0	.014	.009	.039	.106	.169	.140	.521
Non-MI (n=850) (number)	157	78	481	47	22	12	5	48
Non-MI (fraction)	.185	.092	.565	.055	.026	.014	.006	.056
Likelihood Ratio	0	0.15	.015	.71	4.1	12.1	23.3	9.3

Figure 3.3. Likelihood Ratios. The likelihood ratio is calculated as the relative likelihood that the result indicates disease to likelihood that disease is not present. A likelihood ratio of 1 indicates equal likelihood of disease presence and absence; higher values mean disease is that many times more likely to be present than absent, while lower values indicate the opposite. Data from a large study of patients admitted to a coronary care unit with chest pain looked at the change in CK between the first and second specimen. The likelihood of myocardial infarction was low if the CK did not increase; became 35% if CK increased 20–39 U/L, and became strongly positive if CK increased more than 40 U/L. The study concluded that total CK could be used as a screening test to determine if other tests needed to be run. (Data from Dufour DR, et al. Am J Cardiol 1989;63:652)

Advanced Mathematical Models

A number of more advanced mathematical approaches to interpretation of laboratory data have been used to attempt to improve the diagnostic utility of laboratory tests; extensive discussion of these is beyond the scope of this textbook. Among these approaches are multiple regression analysis, expert systems, and neural networks. Numerous studies have shown that such expert approaches work better than predictive value and likelihood ratios, but are not adequate replacements for complete evaluation by an experienced practitioner. These limitations relate to the difficulty of putting a specific numerical weighting on individual laboratory or clinical observations.

SECTION II.
CHEMICAL PATHOLOGY

CHAPTER 4

Acid–Base and Blood Gas Disorders

D. ROBERT DUFOUR

Acid–base disorders are extremely common in hospitalized patients, and require laboratory tests for recognition, diagnosis, and management. Although plasma electrolytes and arterial blood gases are among the most commonly ordered tests, acid–base disorders are often difficult to diagnose correctly if they are assumed to occur singly; most patients with acid–base abnormalities have at least two, and in many cases, three or more different acid–base problems. This chapter will discuss general concepts of acid–base disorders, mechanisms for recognition of pathogenetic patterns of simple acid–base disorders, and approaches for recognition of multiple acid–base problems in a patient.

ACIDS, BASES, AND pH

Acid releases hydrogen ion (H^+), while base neutralizes H^+; the amount of H^+ depends on the relative amounts of acid and base present. The H^+ concentration in blood (normal value: 40 nmol/L) is commonly expressed as pH (normal value: 7.40), the negative logarithm of H^+ concentration. The use of pH instead of H^+ concentration hampers understanding of acid–base disorders; it obscures the actual changes in H^+ (pH changes in the opposite direction), and H^+ is logarithmically, not linearly, related to pH changes. For example, a change in pH of 0.3 is associated with a twofold change in H^+ concentration, since the log of 2 is 0.3. When pH changes from 7.4 to 7.7, H^+ concentration decreases from 40 nmol/L to 20 nmol/L. When pH changes from 7.1 to 7.0, a relatively small change in pH, H^+ concentration increases from 80 to 100 nmol/L, the same absolute change as in pH 7.4 to 7.7. This often causes problems in appreciation of the relative severity of acid–base disorders (Table 4.1).

Dissociation Constants

At equilibrium, there is a balance between the amount of an acid (HA) and its dissociation products, H^+ and A^-, described by a dissociation constant, K_a (Eq. 4.1), often described by its negative logarithm, pK_a. This equation can also be transformed by taking the negative logarithm of both sides, producing the general form of the Henderson–Hasselbalch equation (Eq. 4.2). These equations can also be used for any specific acid, such as carbonic. Under normal conditions, carbonic acid concentration is equal

Table 4.1.
Comparison between pH and H⁺ concentration

pH	7.75	7.7	7.65	7.6	7.55	7.5	7.45	7.4	7.35
H⁺ (nmol/L)	18	20	22	25	28	31	35	40	45
pH	7.3	7.25	7.2	7.15	7.1	7.05	7	6.95	6.9
H⁺ (nmol/L)	50	56	63	71	79	89	100	112	125

to the solubility of CO_2 in water, $(0.03 \times pCO_2)$. The two forms of the equation then become Equation 4.3.

$$H^+ = K_a \times \frac{HA}{A^-} \tag{4.1}$$

$$pH = pK_a - \log \frac{HA}{A^-} \; or \; pH = pK_a + \log \frac{A^-}{HA} \tag{4.2}$$

$$H^+ = 24 * \frac{pCO_2}{HCO_3^-} \; or \; pH = 7.6 + \log \frac{HCO_3^-}{pCO_2} \tag{4.3}$$

Buffers

Substances (or mixtures of substances) capable of resisting pH change when acid or alkali are added are known as buffers. Proteins have both acidic and basic side groups and can function as buffers. More typically, buffers are mixtures of a weak acid and its conjugate base, such as carbonic acid and bicarbonate. Buffers work best when approximately equal amounts of buffer acid and buffer base allow neutralization of both acid and base; this occurs when the H^+ concentration is near the K_a for the acid, (pH is near pK_a). **Buffering capacity** refers to the ability to resist pH changes, determined by both **relative** and **absolute** concentrations of buffer acid and buffer base. A buffer functions well when the concentration ratio of buffer components is between 10:1 and 1:10, (within 1.0 pH unit of the buffer's pK_a). At any given relative concentration, a mixture with 1 mole of each component would have greater capacity than one with 1 millimole of each.

Body Buffers

Hemoglobin, plasma proteins, carbonic acid–bicarbonate, and phosphate serve as the most important physiologic buffers. Hemoglobin (pK_a 6.8) represents 80% of the chemical buffering capacity of blood, while plasma proteins (pK_a (collectively) about 6.5) represent 14% of capacity. The carbonic acid–bicarbonate system (pK_a 6.1) represents 6% of buffering capacity; it is, however, the most important body buffer because of the capability to rapidly change (*compensation*) pCO_2 (altering respiratory rate) or the concentration of HCO_3^- (altering renal tubular reabsorption) to restore their ratio towards normal, which will normalize pH. In disorders such as lactic acidosis, concentrations of acid (and H^+) are often 5–10 mmol (mmol = 10^{-3} mole) per liter, compared to normal H^+ of 40 nmol (nmol = 10^{-9} mole) per liter. Total hemoglobin and proteins represent about 3–4 mmol of buffer, which would quickly be exhausted, leading to severe acidosis if compensatory changes in pCO_2 or HCO_3^- did not occur.

COMPENSATION

Acid–base disturbances are typically classified as either metabolic or respiratory. Compensation attempts to alter the other component (respiratory change in pCO_2 in a metabolic disorder which changes HCO_3^-).

Respiratory Compensation

Altered H^+ concentration in the brain's respiratory center changes respiratory rate; increases stimulate respiration, lowering pCO_2, while decreases will lower the respiratory rate, leading to increased pCO_2. Respiratory compensation begins quickly, and reaches a maximum after 12 hours.

Metabolic Compensation

When blood pCO_2 increases, renal tubular carbonic anhydrase increases production and reabsorption of HCO_3^-; the opposite changes occur with decreased pCO_2. Although this compensation begins quickly, it does not reach a maximum for 3–5 days.

Rules of Compensation

Compensation changes only respiratory excretion of CO_2 and renal handling of HCO_3^-

A patient with metabolic acidosis in which HCO_3^- is lost compensates by eliminating CO_2. Even though it would also "correct" an acidosis, compensation does **not** involve loss of HCl from the GI tract, for example. Thus, a decrease in plasma Cl^- in a patient with decreased HCO_3^- indicates a second acid–base disorder. (However, when renal HCO_3^- excretion is altered, there is an opposite change in Cl^- concentration to maintain the balance of electrical charges; this change is equal for both, so that if the HCO_3^- level decreases by 5 mmol/L, Cl^- concentration increases by the same amount).

Compensation is driven by how far H^+ is from normal

As H^+ concentration nears normal, compensation will begin to diminish. Marked changes in the compensating compound (HCO_3^- or pCO_2) at or near normal pH suggests the presence of another acid–base disorder.

Compensation does not overshoot, and will not take pH beyond normal

For example, in a patient with a high anion gap metabolic acidosis, a low H^+ and low pCO_2 indicate a coexistent respiratory alkalosis.

Rules for Evaluation of Adequacy of Compensation

Several "rules" exist for expected compensation in patients with primary acid–base disorders (Table 4.2). These rules describe the changes that occur with **simple** acid–base

---

Table 4.2.
Expected Compensation for Acid-Base Disorders

Metabolic Acidosis—CO_2 Excretion by Lungs
- pCO_2 decreases 1–1.3 mm Hg for every 1 mmol/L decrease in HCO_3^-
- pCO_2 within 2 of sum $(1.5 \times HCO_3^-) + 8$
- pCO_2 within 2 of last 2 digits of pH

Respiratory Acidosis—HCO_3^- Retention by Kidneys
- Acute: HCO_3^- increases 1 mmol/L for every 10 mm Hg increase in pCO_2
- Chronic: HCO_3^- increases 3.5 mmol/L for every 10 mm Hg increase in pCO_2

Metabolic Alkalosis—CO_2 Retention by Lungs
- pCO_2 increases 0.6 mm Hg for every 1 mmol/L increase in HCO_3^- (maximum of 60 mm Hg)

Respiratory Alkalosis—HCO_3^- Excretion by Kidneys
- Acute—No compensation, self limited
- Chronic—3–5 mmol/L decrease in HCO_3^- for every 10 mm Hg decrease in pCO_2 (minimum 14 mmol/L)

disorders, and can be used to help indicate the presence of mixed disorders when used with the points mentioned in the preceding paragraph. Because respiratory compensation reaches maximum quickly, only one pattern of expected compensation is listed; since metabolic compensation is more gradual, expected changes with acute and chronic respiratory disorders are listed separately.

THEORETICAL CONCEPTS IN APPROACHING ACID–BASE PROBLEMS

Acid*osis* and Alkal*osis* versus Acid*emia* and Alkal*emia*

Acid*osis* refers to a change in the amount of acid in the body, while acid*emia* refers to a change in the H^+ concentration. When a person has an acidosis, such as lactic acidosis, lactic acid is completely dissociated to lactate and H^+. We commonly use changes in the concentration of hydrogen ion as a measure of acidosis, but these are not equivalent. **Changes in H^+ are never as large as changes in amount of acid produced** because the body's buffering system neutralizes nearly all of the added acid or base to maintain pH close to physiologic levels. In a patient with acute lactic acidosis and blood lactate concentration of 7.5 $m$mol/L, 7.5 mmol/L of H^+ is also produced. This commonly changes pH from 7.4 to 7.1, which represents a change in H^+ concentration from 40 to 80 $n$mol/L; the remaining H^+ was neutralized by buffers. **Changes in H^+ reflect the ratio of acid and base.** In mixed acid–base disorders, which are commonly encountered clinically, H^+ concentration will change less than the change in either acid or base concentration, and may be normal if the changes produce a normal ratio of acid to base. The changes in the anions of acids directly reflect the amount of acid added.

Anion Gap

The difference between the major measured cation, sodium, and the major measured anions, chloride and bicarbonate $[Na^+ - (Cl^- + HCO_3^-)]$ is termed anion gap. A "gap" occurs because the concentrations of unmeasured anions (albumin, phosphate, organic acids, etc.) are much greater than those of unmeasured cations (immunoglobulins, calcium, magnesium, potassium). "Normal" values for anion gap vary significantly from one patient to another, and from one laboratory to another (primarily due to slight differences in measurement of sodium and chloride). Each practitioner must determine the normal limits of anion gap for the laboratory which they use, rather than using published figures. It is better to use previous patient results as individual "normal" values if available, since these correct for individual differences in unmeasured ions. Increased anion gap occurs with production of a metabolic acid, buffered by HCO_3^- (Eq. 4.4).

$$HA \rightarrow H^+ + A-$$
$$H^+ + HCO_3^- \rightarrow H_2CO_3 \rightarrow H_2O + CO_2 \qquad (4.4)$$
$$HA + HCO_3^- \rightarrow H_2O + CO_2 + A^-$$

For each mmol/L of acid added, there is a 1 mmol/L decrease in HCO_3^- mmol/L increase in A^- and anion gap. Anion gap directly indicates the presence of organic acids such as lactate and ketoacids, and directly quantifies the amount present. Unlike H^+ concentration, it is not affected by coexistent acid–base disorders. Anion gap should be the first result evaluated in investigation of a suspected acid–base disorder.

LABORATORY TESTS OF ACID BASE STATUS

The following tests are helpful to identify and characterize acid–base disorders.

Plasma Electrolytes

Initial evaluation of patients with suspected acid–base disorders can be done using plasma electrolytes and calculated anion gap. Bicarbonate is usually measured as total CO_2, which includes carbonic acid and other forms of soluble CO_2; this value is approximately 1–2 mmol/L higher than actual bicarbonate. Chloride normally changes in parallel with sodium; an independent change in Cl^- always indicates the presence of an acid–base disorder. Anion gap provides direct evidence of the presence and extent of some forms of acidosis. Normal values for bicarbonate, chloride, and anion gap rule out all acid–base abnormalities except acute respiratory disorders.

Blood Gases

Measurement of blood gases provides different information than electrolytes. Unfortunately, there are frequently problems with handling of blood gas specimens which lead to erroneous results (Table 4.3). Approximately 15% of specimens from locations with a low rate of performing blood gases have erroneous results; a difference of more than 2–3 mmol/L between calculated (from blood gases) and measured (from electrolytes) bicarbonate indicates a likely problem with the blood gas specimen, and suggests the need to repeat the test. Blood gases are usually performed on arterial blood, which is essential for evaluation of oxygen transport. Venous blood gases are adequate for evaluation of acid–base disorders; H^+ and pCO_2 are slightly higher than in arterial blood.

Second Line Tests

Almost all acid–base disorders can be recognized with electrolytes and blood gases. Second line tests are most useful in patients with metabolic acidosis and an increased anion gap; these include ketone bodies, lactate, and osmotic gap, which should identify virtually all of the causes of an increased anion gap as outlined in Table 4.4.

Ketone Bodies

When fatty acids are used for energy, the final products include β-hydroxybutyric acid, acetoacetic acid, and acetone, collectively termed ketone bodies. Anion gap measures

Table 4.3.
Effect of Specimen Handling Variables on Blood Gas Measurements

Factor	pH	pO_2	pCO_2
Not submersing specimen in ice slurry	Decrease up to 0.01 in 10 minutes	Decrease up to 5% in 10 minutes	Minimal change
Air bubbles not removed	Increase if sample agitated	Increase slightly, decrease in patients with high initial pO_2	Decrease
Excess liquid heparin added	Decrease with some forms; usually no effect	Increase slightly, decrease in patients with high initial pO_2	Decrease

Table 4.4.
Causes of Increased Anion Gap

"DUMP SALE"
Diabetic Ketoacidosis
Uremia (end stage renal failure)
Methanol
Paraldehyde
Salicylate
Alcoholic Ketoacidosis
Lactic Acidosis
Ethylene Glycol

all except acetone, while plasma or urine acetone does not measure β-hydroxybutyrate. At presentation with ketoacidosis, β-hydroxybutyric acid is the dominant form, representing about 95–98% of total ketone bodies. An empirical relationship exists at this point between total ketone bodies and ketones, as measured in most laboratories, such that the *ketone titer* (i.e., if positive in a 1:16 dilution, 16) will give an approximation of the total amount of ketoacids in mmol/L, which can be compared with anion gap. With treatment, β-hydroxybutyric acid is metabolized to acetoacetic acid, and ketone titer often rises even as total ketone bodies drop. In treating ketoacidosis, therefore, anion gap should be followed until it reaches normal, and then ketones should be measured on a regular basis (approximately every 4–8 hours) until undetectable, to prevent premature discontinuation of intensive therapy and relapse of ketoacidosis.

Lactate

Anaerobic metabolism of glucose produces lactic acid (lactate). To prevent false increases in lactate, blood should be collected without a tourniquet (to prevent lactate accumulation), put into tubes containing sodium fluoride, and placed in ice water (to prevent post-collection glucose metabolism). Arterial and venous lactate are usually almost equal; in shock, decreased oxygen delivery to tissues leads to increased lactate production. The difference between arterial and venous lactate is a measure of tissue perfusion. It can be measured in peripheral veins as an indicator of perfusion of a limb, or in central venous blood to evaluate adequacy of oxygen delivery to all tissues.

Osmotic Gap

Osmolality is discussed in more detail in Chapter 5. Osmotic gap is defined as the difference between the measured plasma osmolality and osmolality calculated from the molal concentrations of all major known solutes (Eq. 4.5).

$$\frac{1}{0.93} \times \left\{ (1.86 \times Na^+) + \frac{Glucose}{18} + \frac{BUN}{2.8} \right\} + \frac{EtOH}{3.8} \qquad (4.5)$$

Normal values for osmotic gap are between 0 and 10 mOsm/kg. An osmotic gap indicates the presence of millimolar amounts of an uncharged small molecular weight compound. For all practical purposes, the only substances which can produce an osmotic gap are alcohols (methanol, ethanol, isopropanol, and ethylene glycol), acetone, acetylsalicylic acid, and paraldehyde. Because ethanol is commonly ingested, ethanol should be included in calculated osmolality.

ACID–BASE DISORDERS—A PATHOPHYSIOLOGIC APPROACH

Acid–base disturbances are commonly divided into four categories (respiratory, metabolic, acidosis and alkalosis). While respiratory disorders have only one pathophysiologic cause for each, many different pathogenetic mechanisms underlie "metabolic" disturbances; an understanding of these simplifies the approach to and understanding of metabolic acid–base disturbances.

Mechanisms of Acid–Base Handling

Acid and base are produced and excreted each day, maintaining normal acid–base balance. Because of the nature of acid and base production shown (Fig. 4.1), net increase in acid (acidosis) can occur from four mechanisms: 1) increased production of acid; 2) addition of acid (exogenous acid); 3) decreased acid drainage; and 4) increased base drainage. Net increase in base (alkalosis) can result from three mechanisms: 1) addition of base (exogenous base); 2) decreased base drainage; and 3) increased acid drainage. Each mechanism produces a distinct laboratory picture which can be used to identify its presence.

Increased Acid Production

This is the most common form of acidosis, usually caused by increased generation of ketoacids or lactic acid. In children, congenital metabolic errors rarely produce this pattern. The acids generated fully dissociate at body pH, producing an increased anion gap. The vast majority of patients with an increased anion gap have lactic acidosis or ketoacidosis; evaluation should include measurement of lactate and ketone titer if the cause is not immediately apparent from clinical evaluation (e.g., lactic acidosis in cardiac arrest). If the change in anion gap is not equal to lactate or ketone concentration, further evaluation to rule out acid ingestion is indicated.

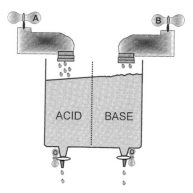

Figure 4.1. Pathogenesis of Acid–Base Disorders. Acid–base balance is altered by changes in production (faucets) or excretion (drains) of acid and base. The drains on both sides work normally, but the faucets are partially dysfunctional. The acid "faucet" (**A**) can open, releasing more acid, but cannot be completely shut (baseline state of acid production). The base "faucet" (**B**) is frozen, reflecting the limited ability to alter the normal low rate of base production. Acidosis occurs when the acid faucet is opened, the acid drain is closed, the base drain is opened, or exogenous acid is added to the system. Alkalosis occurs when the acid drain is opened, the base drain is closed, or exogenous base is added.

Lactic Acidosis

Anaerobic glycolysis leads to accumulation of lactic acid, usually due to decreased tissue oxygen delivery (**Type A**) from decreased blood flow (shock, septicemia) or decreased pO_2 (severe lung disease, respiratory arrest). Less commonly, local metabolic changes cause lactate production (**Type B**), such as increased muscle activity (severe exercise, status epilepticus), tumors (especially leukemias and lymphomas), or altered liver metabolic state (alcohol intoxication). Lactate is the metabolic product of propylene glycol, a solvent for many intravenous drugs (phenytoin, nitroglycerine); large amounts can accumulate with continuous infusions in patients with decreased renal function.

Ketoacidosis

Metabolism of fatty acids as an energy source produces ketoacidosis. Most commonly, this occurs when glucose can not be metabolized, usually with insulin deficiency (diabetic ketoacidosis), or impaired carbohydrate production (starvation, alcohol withdrawal). Ketoacidosis is often present with other acid–base disorders, especially metabolic alkalosis from vomiting.

Acid (or Acid Precursor) Ingestion

This uncommon acidosis is characterized by increased anion and osmolar gaps. In children, the most common form is accidental overdosage with salicylate; anion and osmotic gaps tend to be only mildly increased except in severe intoxication. Salicylate also stimulates the respiratory center, and respiratory alkalosis is often the more severe acid–base abnormality present. In adults, ingestion of methanol or ethylene glycol is more common than salicylate poisoning. In the early stages of intoxication, osmotic gap is elevated but anion gap is normal. As metabolism continues, acid products accumulate while osmotic gap falls. Plasma osmotic gap correlates well with the concentration of the parent compound; concentration can be estimated from the osmotic gap (concentrations in mg/dL: ethylene glycol, osmotic gap $\div$ 6.2; methanol, osmotic gap $\div$ 3.2). Paraldehyde, rarely used in North America, is recognized by a distinctive odor in sweat and breath.

Decreased Acid Excretion

Impaired ability of the lungs or kidneys to excrete acid is a common cause of acidosis.

Renal Failure

The kidneys clear organic (lactic acid, amino acids, etc.) and inorganic (phosphoric, sulfuric) acids from the blood; renal failure allows these to accumulate at a rate of 1–2 mmol/L daily, with a similar increase in anion gap. Ability to excrete these acids is impaired in oliguric acute renal failure; in chronic renal failure, anion excretion is preserved until plasma creatinine is 10–12 mg/dL (884–1060 μmol/L).

Respiratory Failure

Approximately 12,000 mmol of carbonic acid are produced daily (from carbohydrate metabolism) in a normal adult. Respiratory acidosis develops acutely with loss of gas exchange in pneumonia, adult and neonatal respiratory distress syndromes, airway obstruction, decreased respiratory rate, or decreased lung volume. With continuous air trapping (chronic obstructive pulmonary diseases such as emphysema), a well-compensated respiratory acidosis occurs. Respiratory acidosis differs from other forms of acidosis in that the plasma HCO_3^- and arterial pCO_2 are increased rather than decreased, and anion gap is normal.

Increased Base Excretion

Loss of HCO_3^- in either urine or stool is a less common cause of acidosis. To maintain a stable electrical charge, the kidneys reabsorb chloride to replace the lost HCO_3^-, producing a normal anion gap (**non-anion gap acidosis**) and increased plasma Cl^- (**hyperchloremic metabolic acidosis**). Chronic respiratory alkalosis is compensated for by renal bicarbonate loss, and will produce similar electrolyte changes; however, such patients will be alkalotic. It is important for the practitioner to rule out this disorder before diagnosing hyperchloremic metabolic acidosis. Clinical information is usually adequate to distinguish renal and non-renal causes of bicarbonate loss. When needed, urine electrolytes can be used to estimate relative amounts of ammonium ion (the form in which H^+ is excreted in urine) and bicarbonate. This can be done most simply by calculating the urine anion gap (Eq. 4.6).

$$Urine\ Anion\ Gap\ =\ (Na^+\ +\ K^+)\ -\ Cl^- \qquad (4.6)$$

A positive anion gap indicates the presence of another anion, typically bicarbonate; a negative gap detects large amounts of cations, typically ammonium.

Extrarenal Bicarbonate Loss

Biliary and pancreatic fluids contain large amounts of bicarbonate, normally reabsorbed in the distal small bowel and colon. Patients with diarrhea lose significant amounts of HCO_3^- in a short period of time. Rarely, patients with an ostomy will also have a similar picture.

Renal Bicarbonate Loss

Renal tubular acidosis (RTA) is due to abnormal acid–base handling (Fig. 4.2) at different portions of the nephron, with varying associated findings (Table 4.5); by definition, glomerular function is normal. Drugs blocking bicarbonate regeneration, such as carbonic anhydrase inhibitors used to treat glaucoma, cause reversible RTA. In patients with mild to moderate renal insufficiency, reduced glomerular filtration rate inhibits renal ability to maximally excrete K^+ and H^+, producing laboratory results that simulate Type IV RTA.

Base Ingestion

This is a rare cause of alkalosis; patient history is vital for correct diagnosis. In questionable cases, or if the patient denies ingestion, urinary electrolytes may be of value; the kidneys will attempt to excrete excess bicarbonate, resulting in a strongly positive urine anion gap. Common causes are administration of HCO_3^- (antacid abuse, excessive administration during resuscitation), other oral antacids, or citrate with massive blood transfusion (over 10 units per day) or impaired hepatic citrate metabolism (neonates, liver disease).

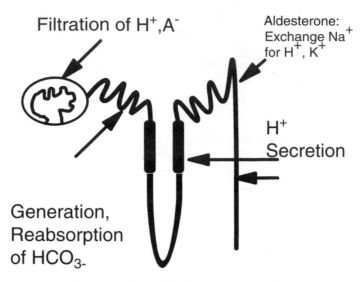

Filtration of H$^+$,A$^-$

Aldosterone:
Exchange Na$^+$
for H$^+$, K$^+$

H$^+$
Secretion

Generation,
Reabsorption
of HCO$_3$.

Figure 4.2. Renal Handling of Acid–Base Status. The kidneys have a variety of complicated mechanisms for maintenance of acid–base homeostasis. The glomeruli filter H$^+$ as well as any acid anions present. The proximal tubules reclaim bicarbonate with high effectiveness (80–90%), while the distal tubules and collecting ducts secrete H$^+$ as NH$_4$$^+$. Aldosterone acts on the proximal collecting duct to reabsorb Na$^+$ in exchange for H$^+$ or K$^+$.

Decreased Base Excretion

Underexcretion of HCO$_3^-$ commonly contributes to alkalosis, but is rarely the sole cause. In the distal tubule, Na$^+$ is passively reabsorbed along with an anion, usually Cl$^-$. When there is deficiency of Cl$^-$ (as in dehydration), another anion must be reabsorbed, typically HCO$_3^-$; this has been termed **contraction** (contraction of intravascular volume) or **chloride responsive** (corrected by Cl$^-$ administration) alkalosis. Common causes are dehydration and overtreatment with diuretics. This form can be identified in questionable cases by documenting an undetectable urine Cl$^-$, usually with orthostatic hypotension and low urine Na$^+$.

Acid Excretion

Increased acid excretion from lungs, kidneys, or stomach is the most common cause of alkalosis. Because the acids loss differ, each site of loss produces a distinct clinical and laboratory picture.

Table 4.5.
Types of Renal Tubular Acidosis

Type	Site of Defect	Associated Findings
I	Distal Tubule	Kidney stones, low K$^+$
II	Proximal Tubule	Defective reabsorption of many other substances
III	Both Proximal and Distal Tubule	Combines features of Types I and II
IV	Cortical Collecting Duct	Aldosterone deficiency or resistance, high K$^+$

Gastric Acid (HCl) Loss

Prolonged vomiting or nasogastric suction commonly produce alkalosis, usually readily recognized from the clinical history. Laboratory tests can suggest the diagnosis if the patient is unable to provide a history (as may occur with bulimia). Plasma Na^+ is normal, HCO_3^- is increased, Cl^- is decreased, and anion gap is normal. Urine Cl^- is usually undetectable, while urine Na^+ and K^+ will be high, resulting in a strongly positive urine anion gap.

Renal Acid Loss

Mineralocorticoids often contribute to alkalosis through renal H^+ excretion. In Cushing's syndrome and primary or secondary hyperaldosteronism, alkalosis is accompanied by high normal Na^+, decreased K^+, decreased Cl^-, and increased HCO_3^- in plasma, while urine shows detectable Cl^-, low Na^+ excretion (fractional excretion of sodium usually below 1%), and inappropriately increased K^+ excretion (fractional excretion of potassium usually greater than 40%, total urine K^+ more than 30 mmol/d). In dehydration, aldosterone causes alkalosis in a similar fashion. Diuretics also commonly cause alkalosis through this mechanism.

Pulmonary Acid Loss

Any factor stimulating the respiratory center produces respiratory alkalosis. Common causes include hypoxemia, chemicals (such as salicylates), pain, or psychogenic causes and alcohol withdrawal. Acute respiratory alkalosis is usually transient and self-limited. *Chronic* respiratory alkalosis occurs with prolonged hypoxemia, most frequently due to shunting of blood (cyanotic congenital heart disease, cirrhosis, recurrent pulmonary emboli) or with interstitial lung disease (early heart failure, pneumocystis or other interstitial pneumonias, interstitial fibrosis). If pH is not considered, chronic respiratory alkalosis can easily be misdiagnosed as renal tubular acidosis, as it causes decreased plasma HCO_3^-, increased plasma Cl^-, and strongly positive urine anion gap.

Approach to Suspected Acid–Base Disorders

Using the pathophysiologic principles defined above, the algorithm in Figure 4.3, the compensation rules in Table 4.2, and the expected changes listed in Table 4.6, the practitioner can identify most common simple and mixed acid–base disorders.

OXYGEN DELIVERY

Oxygen is poorly soluble in blood and is transported by hemoglobin. Hemoglobin with oxygen bound is called *oxyhemoglobin*, while hemoglobin without oxygen is termed *deoxyhemoglobin*; in normal blood, these make up about 98% of total hemoglobin. Molecules with ferric (Fe^{+++}) ion (rather than ferrous, Fe^{++} found in hemoglobin) are termed *methemoglobin*, which does not bind oxygen. Carbon monoxide combines with hemoglobin with an affinity 20-times that of oxygen, producing *carboxyhemoglobin*.

The relatively tight binding of oxygen to hemoglobin allows gradual release to tissues throughout the body. The sigmoidal shape of the **oxygen dissociation curve** (Fig. 4.4) causes oxygen delivery to be more dependent on the degree of saturation of hemoglobin than pO_2. Dissociation is also affected by type of hemoglobin present (hemoglobin F and some congenital hemoglobin variants have high oxygen affinity),

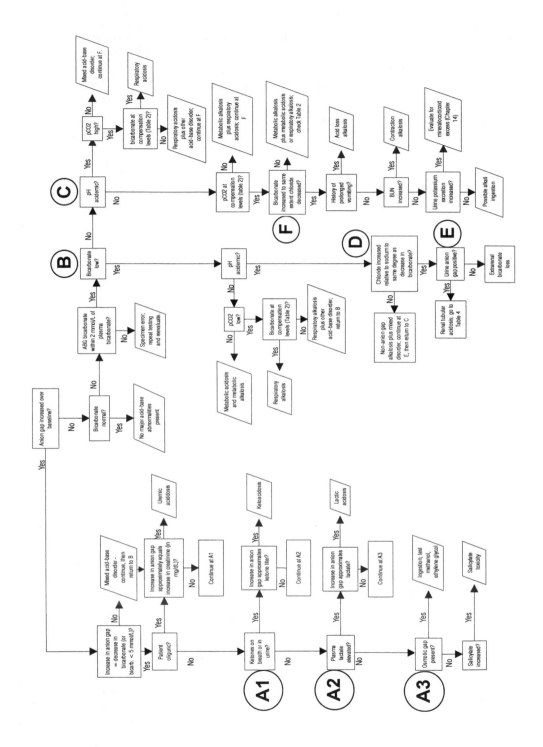

Table 4.6.
Expected Changes in Different Acid-Base Disorders

Pathogenetic Cause	Primary Abnormality	Associated Changes
ACIDOSIS		
Acid overproduction	↑ anion gap	↓ HCO_3^- in same amount as ↑ in anion gap; ↑ lactate or ketone titer = ↑ anion gap; normal osmolar gap in lactic acidosis, osmolar gap <25 in ketoacidosis
Acid ingestion	↑ anion and osmolar gaps	↓ HCO_3^- in same amount as ↑ in anion gap; normal lactate, ketones
Decreased pulmonary acid excretion	↑ pCO_2	Only compensation: ↑ HCO_3^-, ↓ Cl^-, change in each equal
Decreased renal acid excretion	↑ anion gap (1 mmol/L/d), oliguria	↓ HCO_3^- in same amount as ↑ in anion gap; normal lactate, ketones, osmolar gap
Stool bicarbonate loss	↓ HCO_3^-, normal anion gap; strongly negative urine anion gap	↑ Cl^- relative to Na^+; ↑ in Cl^- = ↓ in HCO_3^-; ↓ K^+
Renal bicarbonate loss	↓ HCO_3^-, normal anion gap; positive urine anion gap	↑ Cl^- relative to Na^+; ↑ in Cl^- = ↓ in HCO_3^-; K^+ may be ↑ or ↓
ALKALOSIS		
Base ingestion	↑ HCO_3^-, strongly positive urine anion gap, usually detectable urine Cl^-	↓ Cl^- relative to Na^+, plasma anion gap normal or slightly ↑
Decreased base excretion	↑ HCO_3^-, positive urine anion gap, undetectable urine Cl^-; volume depletion	↓ Cl^- relative to Na^+, plasma anion gap normal or slightly ↑; ↓ urine Na^+
Gastric acid Loss	↑ HCO_3^-, positive urine anion gap, undetectable urine Cl^-	↓ Cl^- relative to Na^+, plasma anion gap normal or slightly ↑; normal urine Na^+
Renal acid loss	↑ HCO_3^-, normal or ↓ urine anion gap, detectable urine Cl^-	↓ Cl^- relative to Na^+, plasma anion gap normal, ↓ plasma K^+; ↓ urine Na^+, ↑ urine K^+
Pulmonary acid loss	↓ pCO_2	Compensation only with chronic form: ↓ HCO_3^-, ↑ Cl^-, change in each equal; positive urine anion gap, normal plasma anion gap

2,3-diphosphoglyceric acid (2,3-DPG), pH, pCO_2, and temperature. Increases in H^+, CO_2, 2,3-DPG, and temperature increase oxygen delivery by decreasing oxygen binding to hemoglobin, shifting the oxygen dissociation curve to the *right*. Decreases in H^+, CO_2, 2,3-DPG, and temperature will all decrease oxygen delivery by increasing oxygen binding to hemoglobin, shifting the oxygen dissociation curve to the *left*.

pO_2

Arterial oxygen pressure is the most accurate measure of oxygen status, but requires arterial blood sampling; its measurement is used only when critical for patient care.

Figure 4.3. Approach to Acid–Base Disorders. In initial evaluation of a patient, anion gap and bicarbonate should be checked; if normal, no further investigation is needed. The algorithm indicates the need for continually comparing the observed compensation changes with those expected, as indicated in Table 4.2. Using this approach, up to three mixed acid–base abnormalities can be detected. Practically, although more may coexist, it is virtually impossible to determine their presence without sequential studies.

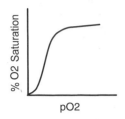

Figure 4.4. Oxygen Dissociation Curve. At high O_2 pressures, such as occur in the lung, hemoglobin saturation approaches 100%. As O_2 diffuses from blood vessels into tissue and pO_2 falls, O_2 is released from hemoglobin to replace it, slightly lowering saturation. The gradual slope at the right of the curve shows that this reservoir is not depleted easily at usual pO_2 values. When the curve is shifted to the right, O_2 is more easily delivered, but the "reservoir" is more rapidly depleted. The opposite occurs when the curve shifts to the left (see text for additional information).

Because of the shape of the oxygen dissociation curve, hemoglobin saturation will be virtually complete at a wide range of values for pO_2, making oxygen saturation (more commonly used) less sensitive than pO_2 for detecting problems with oxygen delivery, particularly with increased pO_2 (in patients on high amounts of inhaled oxygen).

Alveolar-arterial Gradient of pO_2

Calculation of differences in gas exchange are an approximation of the adequacy of pulmonary function, and can (along with pCO_2) provide a guide to the type of injury preventing adequate oxygenation. Normally, exchange of CO_2 is much more efficient than that of O_2; however, because of significant reserve, adequate pO_2 is maintained. There normally is a gradient between arterial and alveolar pO_2, calculated as (Eq. 4.7)

$$Alveolar\ pO_2 = [(P_{Atm} - P_{H_2O\ in\ alveoli}) \times \%O_2] - P_{Alveolar\ CO_2} \qquad (4.7)$$
$$A - a\ gradient = Alveolar\ pO_2 - arterial\ pO_2.$$

At sea level, atmospheric pressure is 760 mm Hg, water vapor pressure is about 45 mm Hg, and room air is 21% O_2. At normal respiratory rates, alveolar pCO_2 is approximately 20% lower than arterial; with hyperventilation they become approximately equal. The faster the respiratory rate, the lower the water pressure. In persons breathing room air, there is normally a 10–20 mm Hg A-a gradient; high gradients indicate decreased oxygen exchange caused by one of two major mechanisms.

Decreased Alveolar Ventilation

Decreased air exchange may be caused by decreased respiratory rate, decreased number of functioning alveoli (severe pneumonia), or with obstruction to ventilation (as in chronic obstructive lung diseases). In such states, there is decreased exchange of both O_2 and CO_2, leading to decreases in the former and increases in the latter in blood.

Decreased Oxygen Exchange

Impairment of gas diffusion may be due to interstitial thickening (interstitial fibrosis, interstitial pneumonias such as pneumocystis, or with pulmonary edema), or mismatching between ventilation and perfusion, as occurs with shunting of blood (pulmonary emboli, cirrhosis, and congenital heart disease). In both situations, hypoxemia stimulates a compensatory increase in ventilation. The more efficient excretion of CO_2 produces respiratory alkalosis.

Evaluation of Oxygen Saturation

Evaluation of oxygen saturation is widely employed in evaluation of oxygen transport. Not all methods produce equivalent results, and several may produce misleading results in certain clinical conditions. The most widely used methods for oxygen saturation include the following.

Pulse Oximetry

Use of bedside spectrophotometers to measure relative amounts of oxyhemoglobin and deoxyhemoglobin has become standard in monitoring patients in many hospitals. While pulse oximeters are generally reliable, they produce inaccurate results in some clinical settings, and the practitioner must recognize these situations. Accurate results cannot be obtained in hypotensive patients. Pulse oximetry cannot detect high pO_2, and cannot be used to prevent oxygen toxicity in infants. The method assumes that only oxyhemoglobin and deoxyhemoglobin are present; it overestimates oxyhemoglobin in the presence of carbon monoxide or methemoglobin, and cannot be used to detect carbon monoxide poisoning. With these limitations in mind, it is the quickest method to assure adequate oxygen availability to tissue.

Estimation from pO_2

Estimated hemoglobin saturation is done routinely with blood gas analyses by assuming the presence of a normal hemoglobin dissociation curve, and correcting for the effects of temperature, H^+, and pCO_2 on oxygen saturation. Decreased 2,3-DPG concentration (which occurs with transfused blood and with starvation), presence of methemoglobin or carboxyhemoglobin, and hemoglobin variants all alter hemoglobin saturation without changing pO_2 (and, therefore, *calculated* percent saturation). In these situations, oxygen saturation is overestimated by the formulas used on blood gas instruments.

Differential Spectrophotometry

Blood gas laboratories commonly utilize this technique, which directly calculates the concentrations of oxyhemoglobin, deoxyhemoglobin, methemoglobin, and carboxyhemoglobin. It provides accurate measurements in almost all situations, but is not as readily available as the first two techniques.

CHAPTER 5.

Water and Electrolyte Balance

D. ROBERT DUFOUR

NORMAL PHYSIOLOGY OF WATER AND ELECTROLYTES

Water Compartments

Approximately 50–60% of body weight is water, existing within three compartments. **Intracellular fluid** (ICF) represents about 1/2 to 2/3 of total body water, while **extracellular fluid** (ECF) comprises the remainder in two interchangeable locations. About 1/4 to 1/3 of ECF is in plasma, within the blood vessels; the volume of this compartment is closely regulated. Most ECF is in interstitial fluid, the volume of which is largely unregulated.

Interchange of Water between Compartments

Water enters the body from the intestine and passes into plasma. From there, it distributes to the other two compartments based on differences in pressure. **Osmotic pressure,** caused by a difference in the number of solute particles, regulates movement of water between plasma and ICF (Fig. 5.1). Cell membranes do not allow sodium, potassium, glucose (in most cells), or protein to cross the membrane, generating osmotic pressure. Some substances such as urea and ethanol readily cross cell membranes, and do not contribute to osmotic pressure. A difference of 1 mmol/L in the concentration of a solute creates a pressure of 17 mm Hg across the membrane. Hydrostatic and oncotic pressure are most important in regulating movement of fluid between plasma and interstitial fluid (Fig. 5.2). At the arterial side of the capillary bed, high pressure forces water and electrolytes from plasma into tissue. Vascular fluid loss increases tissue hydrostatic pressure and increases protein concentration, generating **colloid osmotic** or **oncotic** pressure (10–15 mm Hg at normal protein concentration). At the venous end of the capillary bed, tissue hydrostatic and oncotic pressure move water back to plasma. An increase in venous (or lymphatic) hydrostatic pressure, or a fall in plasma oncotic pressure, favor accumulation of interstitial fluid (edema).

Composition of Body Compartments

Differences in electrolyte and protein concentration regulate movement of fluid between body compartments (Table 5.1). Intracellular fluid contains potassium, magnesium, protein, and bicarbonate as major solutes; protein concentration in cells is much higher than in plasma. Interstitial fluid and plasma are similar in most ways, except that protein content is much higher in the latter. Extracellular fluid has sodium, chloride, and bicarbonate as major solutes. Changes in relative solute concentration alter osmolality and lead to fluid shifts from one compartment to another.

Regulation of Water and Electrolyte Status

Each day, 2–3 L of water is lost from the body, mostly in urine, with a minimum water excretion of about 500 mL per day. An average of 1 L of water is lost in sweat, stool,

52

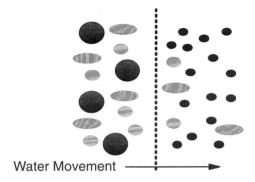

Water Movement ⟶

Figure 5.1. Osmotic Pressure. A difference in the concentration of *particles* on different sides of a membrane which allows passage of water (but not particles) generates pressure for the movement of water from the side with low concentration; particle size is irrelevant. In this example, water moves from left to right; movement will cease when the particle concentration is the same on both sides.

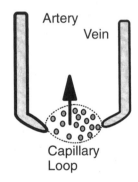

Figure 5.2. Factors Governing Movement of Fluid in the Capillaries. Differences in pressure govern the exchange of fluid between the intravascular and interstitial fluid compartments. At the arterial side, the higher hydrostatic pressure forces fluid through the permeable capillary walls. This increases the protein (circles) concentration, increasing oncotic pressure. When blood reaches the venous end, the low hydrostatic pressure and high oncotic pressure draw water back into the vessels. An increase in venous hydrostatic pressure, or a decrease in plasma proteins, increases fluid in the interstitial space; this is termed *edema*.

and breath (insensible fluid losses). Water must be taken in to replace these losses, or dehydration will result. The body has a complex regulatory system which detects changes in osmolality and volume to match water intake with losses (Table 5.2). Of these, the most important is thirst; inability to respond to water losses with water ingestion is the most common cause of dehydration and hypernatremia.

Table 5.1.
Composition of Body Fluid Compartments

Fluid Compartment	% Total Body Water	Major Cations	Major Anions	Protein Concentration
Intracellular	50–65	K, Mg	PO_4	Very High
Intravascular	10–12	Na, K, Ca	Cl, HCO_3	High
Interstitial	25–40	Na, K, Ca	Cl, HCO_3	Very Low

Table 5.2.
Regulators of Osmolality and Volume

Factor	Stimulus	Effect
Thirst	Increase in osmolality of 1%; decrease in volume >5%	Increase water intake; decrease osmolality
Antidiuretic hormone (ADH)	Increase in osmolality of 1%; decrease in volume >5%	Increase water reabsorption by kidney, sweat glands; decrease osmolality
Renin/angiotensin/ aldosterone	Decrease in volume; decreased electrolyte in urine	Increase blood pressure; increase plasma Na^+ (slightly), decrease plasma K^+, H^+, decrease urine Na^+, increase urine K^+, H^+
Atrial natriuretic hormone (ANH)	Increase in atrial blood volume	Increase urine Na^+, decrease blood volume; decrease aldosterone

Osmoregulators

These hypothalamic sensors respond to an increase in osmolality (usually sodium) of less than 1%, activating two types of protective responses. Thirst sensors stimulate water intake, returning osmolality to normal. Antidiuretic hormone (ADH; vasopressin) is synthesized in the hypothalamus and released from the pituitary in response to increased osmolality. ADH increases the permeability of renal collecting ducts to water, increasing urine osmolality and decreasing water losses; it can reduce total daily losses to a minimum of 1–1.5 liters. Osmoregulators are most important in day to day regulation of volume status.

Volume Regulators

These sensors require a greater percent change from baseline than osmoreceptors, but override the osmoreceptor signal if necessary to preserve plasma volume. ADH production increases as blood volume decreases by more than 5%, and becomes marked as volume decreases by more than 10%, even if plasma osmolality is decreased (Fig. 5.3). Thirst receptors also recognize a decrease in volume, although the effect is not

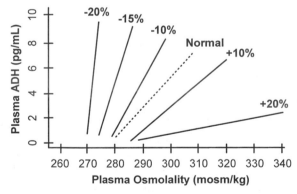

Figure 5.3. Effect of Osmolality and Intravascular Volume on ADH. In general, plasma osmolality is the most important factor controlling day to day production of ADH. At low plasma volume, however, ADH is produced even at relatively low plasma osmolality, while high volume inhibits ADH production even when plasma osmolality is moderately increased. Each line represents the ADH production curve for a different plasma volume, with curves from −20% (below normal) to +20% (above normal). (Adapted from Robertson, G. L. in Becker, K. L. (ed.): Principles and Practice of Endocrinology and Metabolism, 2nd ed. Philadelphia, Lippincott, 1995, p. 252.

as great as with ADH. With a decrease in renal blood flow or distal tubular sodium, renin is released, leading to production of angiotensin II (AG II), a potent vasoconstrictor. AG II stimulates aldosterone production, causing renal sodium retention in exchange for potassium or H^+. Atrial natriuretic hormone (ANH) is produced by the atrial myocardium in response to the stretching of fibers, indicating increased blood volume. ANH shunts renal blood flow to more cortical nephrons, decreasing maximum sodium reabsorption, and inhibits production of renin and aldosterone. These two effects decrease plasma volume and total body sodium. ANH is the only active factor preventing an increase in blood volume. Renal factors affecting water and electrolyte status are discussed more fully in Chapter 6. Final adjustment of urine electrolyte and water is accomplished through the actions of aldosterone and ADH. Urine reaching the sites of action of these hormones has an osmolality of approximately 100 mOsm/kg, but contains significant amounts of sodium. In the absence of aldosterone, approximately 3–5% of sodium reaching urine is lost, while ADH deficiency may allow as much as 10% of water to be excreted.

Plasma Electrolytes

Because plasma sodium concentration is the major factor affecting osmotic pressure, it is regulated closely, with average daily variation of less than 1.5%. Chloride concentration is passively regulated along with sodium, normally changing in parallel; discordant changes in sodium and chloride usually indicate the presence of an acid-base disorder (Chapter 4). Plasma potassium concentration is not closely regulated by hormones. Potassium is constantly lost as cells are shed from body surfaces. In the kidney, most potassium is reabsorbed in the proximal tubule, although about 5% escapes. Aldosterone causes additional potassium loss in the distal tubule.

LABORATORY TESTS USED TO EVALUATE FLUID AND ELECTROLYTE ABNORMALITIES

The most useful tests for evaluation of fluid and electrolyte status are measurement of plasma and urine electrolytes and osmolality, along with tests used to evaluate volume status. Many laboratories use serum (obtained when blood clots) and plasma (obtained when an anticoagulant such as heparin is used) interchangeably when measuring "plasma" electrolytes. For the most part, results are identical, so that comments made about "plasma" measurements also apply to serum. When there are important differences, serum and plasma will be discussed separately.

Plasma Sodium

Normally, only 93% of plasma is water; the remainder is comprised of solids, such as lipid and protein, which are suspended in and displace water. Sodium concentration in *plasma* is thus about 7% lower than sodium concentration in *water*, which is what affects osmoreceptors. In patients who have an increase in solids, either lipid (triglyceride) or protein (in patients with monoclonal or polyclonal gammopathies), the water content of a given volume of plasma decreases. For example, if protein is 7 g/dL and triglycerides are 7000 mg/dL (7 g/dL), then solids will make up 14 grams of every 100 grams of plasma, or 14%, while water will be only 86%. Plasma sodium will be falsely low in such a situation (**pseudohyponatremia**), although not markedly decreased. The highest triglyceride concentration encountered in our laboratory was 11 g/dL; this

reduce plasma water content to 82%, decreasing plasma sodium to 82/93 of
al concentration, or from an average of 140 to 123. Some laboratories perform
racentrifugation of lipemic specimens, which eliminates lipid related pseudohypo-
atremia. Increases in plasma protein rarely exceed 11 g/dL (110 g/L), which would
decrease apparent sodium concentration by only about 5–6 mmol/L. In some laboratories, particularly those that measure electrolytes and blood gases on whole blood specimens, sodium activity is measured, which is directly proportional to sodium concentration in water; using such methods, results are not affected by the amount of protein
or lipid.

Plasma Potassium

Of all laboratory tests, this is the one which is most subject to erroneously high results.
Potassium concentration in cells is approximately 35–40 times higher than in plasma,
so that release from cells under various circumstances can produce erroneous potassium results. Grossly hemolyzed specimens give erroneously high potassium. Platelets
release potassium when forming a clot; in patients with extreme thrombocytosis, serum
potassium is approximately 0.1–0.15 mmol/L higher than in plasma for each
100,000/mm^3 increase in platelet count. White cells metabolize glucose much more
rapidly than red cells; in patients with extreme leukocytosis, potassium may be released
in vitro within 30–60 minutes. Finally, allowing the blood to sit at room temperature
for a long time, or in a refrigerator for a short time before centrifugation of the blood
allows potassium to leak out of red cells and makes the plasma concentration appear
high. Potassium results may also be artifactually increased by problems occurring during specimen collection. Potassium EDTA is the anticoagulant in lavender top tubes;
it is common to see "plasma" specimens contaminated with EDTA when blood is drawn
with a syringe and injected into tubes, or if the lavender top tube is drawn before the
plasma specimen, frequently giving potassium concentrations over 10 mmol/L. Fist
clenching during blood drawing causes release of potassium from muscle, and can
increase potassium concentration by 1–1.5 mmol/L. Finally, contamination by intravenous fluids containing potassium may also falsely increase potassium.

Plasma Chloride

Measurement of chloride concentration is not of much benefit in evaluating patients
with fluid and electrolyte disorders, but it is important in recognizing and evaluating
patients with acid-base disorders (Chapter 4). Methods for chloride also are affected
by changes in water content, producing falsely low results in the same situations discussed for sodium.

Urine Electrolytes

Measurements of urine electrolytes are very helpful in patients with fluid or electrolyte
abnormalities. In normal individuals, urine electrolyte and water handling maintain
normal fluid and electrolyte status. Renal electrolyte handling is best understood in
terms of "appropriate," rather than "normal" values. For example, if a patient is dehydrated, an extremely dilute urine with an osmolality of 50 is inappropriate, even though
such a value could be found in a healthy person. Similarly, a urine sodium concentration
of 100 mmol/L in the same patient would also be inappropriate. In our own laboratory,
we do not publish reference values for urine osmolality or electrolyte concentrations.

It often is helpful to calculate the fractional excretion of electroly†
Chapter 6. These calculated parameters provide additional informa
lyte concentration, which are affected by differences in water excretic.
sodium excess, fractional excretion of sodium can reach greater than 5%, w
fall to less than 0.1% if maximal sodium retention is needed. With excess po.
intake or increased aldosterone production, fractional excretion of potassium .
exceed 50%; it is rare to see values less than 10%, even with severe hypokalemia.

Osmolality

Plasma osmolality can either be measured or calculated; in urine, only measured values
are reliable.

Plasma Osmolality

Since most adaptive mechanisms respond to changes in osmolality, it would seem
logical to measure plasma osmolality. In reality, plasma osmolality can be reliably
estimated from measurements of the major osmotically active substances (sodium, urea,
and glucose) (Eq. 5.1).

$$Calculated\ osmolality\ =\ \frac{1.86\ Na\ +\ \dfrac{GLUCOSE}{18}\ +\ \dfrac{BUN}{2.8}}{0.93} \tag{5.1}$$

This formula holds true unless measurements of sodium are erroneous, as may
occur with increasing amounts of protein or lipids, or if other osmotically active substances are present. Many textbooks suggest measuring plasma osmolality in every
patient with hyponatremia, to detect pseudohyponatremia. Because most laboratories
report specimens with markedly elevated triglycerides as "grossly lipemic," this cause
of pseudohyponatremia is easily detected. The presence of other osmotically active
substances causing hyponatremia can usually be suspected from the clinical history
and other laboratory results, such as glucose; these will be discussed in more detail later.
For these reasons, calculated osmolality is usually as reliable as measured osmolality in
plasma.

Urine Osmolality

Urine osmolality measurements are extremely valuable in the evaluation of fluid and
electrolyte disorders, as they directly indicate the degree of renal water conservation.
The osmolality of glomerular filtrate is approximately 270–290 mOsm/kg. In states of
water deprivation, ADH stimulates maximal water conservation, such that urine may
achieve an osmolality as high as 1200 mOsm/kg. With excessive water intake, maximal
dilution can produce an osmolality as low as 50 mOsm/kg. In childhood and with
increasing age, these values differ; those over the age of 65 often cannot achieve maximum concentrations over 700 mOsm/kg, while maximal diluting ability is often no
lower than 100–150 mOsm/kg. A less than maximally dilute urine means that ADH is
present; a very low osmolality (<100 mOsm/kg) indicates absence of or resistance to
ADH.

Hormone Measurements

Rarely, measurements of ADH, renin, or aldosterone are needed to evaluate patients
with electrolyte disorders; situations in which these measurements are important will

be covered below. Further discussions on renin and aldosterone are found in Chapter 14.

When Not to Do Tests of Electrolyte Status

Measurements of plasma electrolytes are among the most commonly performed laboratory tests. In general, there are few situations where plasma electrolyte tests should not be measured. In patients receiving intravenous fluids, care must be taken to avoid contamination of specimens with the fluid being administered. Contamination of specimens by anticoagulants or preservatives may produce grossly inaccurate results. In the case of potassium, the factors causing artifactual hyperkalemia should be controlled if electrolyte measurement is important in a patient. Urine electrolyte tests should not be ordered in patients receiving diuretics, since these will lead to erroneous results. Because of the rate of change in electrolytes, there is little reason to measure them more frequently than every six hours. In patients with hypernatremia, serum sodium often rises during therapy; this may be disconcerting. In hypernatremic patients, BUN serves as a better gauge of the adequacy of replacement of intravascular volume.

DISORDERS OF WATER AND SODIUM

Evaluation of a patient with suspected fluid or electrolyte disorders begins with an estimate of extracellular fluid volume. Patients are categorized as *hypervolemic* in the presence of edema, either generalized or ascites; *hypovolemic* based on presence of orthostatic hypotension, dry mucous membranes, and tenting of skin; or *euvolemic* if none of the above features are present. Orthostatic hypotension, the most sensitive indicator of hypovolemia, occurs with a decrease in plasma volume of 8–10%. Ascites or peripheral edema are usually detectable once extracellular fluid volume rises by 10–15%. Thus, the "euvolemic" category includes patients with decreased, increased, and normal volume status. As discussed earlier, hormonal changes begin with as little as a 5% decrease or 1–2% increase in plasma volume. Measurement of BUN and creatinine may be helpful in determining the direction of a change in volume status. With decreased plasma volume, BUN typically increases from baseline when ADH production is stimulated, at approximately 5% lower volume. Altered filtration occurs when ANH is produced in excess, such that BUN and creatinine often fall slightly from baseline in volume excess states. Comparison of values to previous results when electrolyte status was normal is particularly useful for detecting small changes from the patient's basal state.

Hyponatremia

Decreased serum sodium is a common electrolyte abnormality in hospitalized patients. Common classification systems for hyponatremia use the patient's volume status as the primary method of categorization. As discussed above, however, euvolemic patients may actually have mildly decreased or increased volume. There are four primary mechanisms for production of hyponatremia; in the vast majority of cases, one of the first two mechanisms is responsible. In almost all patients, compensation by the other mechanism may make it difficult to tell by laboratory tests which is the primary abnormality. For example, a patient may develop excessive perspiration, which causes loss of both water and sodium; the fluid lost is relatively hypotonic. Decreasing volume stimulates thirst and ADH production, which further dilutes the remaining sodium. Similarly, if

Table 5.3.
Summary of Clinical and Laboratory Features in Hyponatremia

Pathogenesis	ECF Volume	Plasma Osm	Urine Osm	FE_{Na}	Other
Extrarenal sodium loss	↓	↓	↑	1%	Typically due to sweat or diarrhea losses; ↑ BUN/Cr ratio
Renal sodium loss	↓	↓	↑	>1%	Tubular dysfunction; ↑ BUN/Cr ratio. Hyperkalemia with low aldosterone
Water overload	N to sl ↑	↓	<100	1%	Usually seen in psychiatric patients; ↓ BUN/Cr, uric acid
SIAD (Inappropriate Antidiuresis)	N to sl ↑	↓	>200	Varies	U_{Na} and FE_{Na} ↑ with sodium administration; ↓ BUN/Cr, uric acid
Osmotic dilution	N or ↑	N or ↑	Varies	Varies	Most common with glucose; mannitol, glycine rarely
Edema	↑	↓	↑	<1%	Edema may be systemic or localized, as in ascites

water excess is the initial pathologic event, an increase in plasma volume stimulates ANH production, leading to increased sodium loss. To accurately classify hyponatremic patients, it is usually necessary to use patient history, clinical evaluation of volume status, BUN and creatinine, urine electrolytes, and urine osmolality together to reach a correct interpretation of the pathogenetic cause, which will lead to appropriate treatment of the patient (Table 5.3, Fig. 5.4).

Decreased Sodium

Sodium losses occur from the kidneys or from extrarenal sources such as sweat and diarrhea. Rarely, a long term sodium deficient diet may cause hyponatremia; this is typically seen in alcoholic patients. Patients have decreased total body sodium, and are typically clinically hypovolemic or euvolemic, with increased BUN and high BUN/ creatinine ratio.

Extrarenal Sodium Losses

Diarrhea, fever, and exercise cause loss of sodium and water. While sodium losses from diarrhea are usually obvious from patient history, losses from sweat may not be clinically recognized by the patient. Such patients will typically have low urine sodium excretion (U_{Na} less than 10 mmol/L, FE_{Na} much less than 1%), and high urine osmolality (usually greater than 500 mOsm/kg).

Renal Sodium Loss

Most commonly, this is due to diuretic administration. Less commonly, sodium loss is due to renal tubular disease (salt wasting nephritis); common etiologies include the diuretic phase of acute tubular necrosis, tubular damage following prolonged urinary tract obstruction, and interstitial nephritis. Such patients tend to have high urinary sodium excretion (U_{Na} greater than 20 mmol/L, FE_{Na} greater than 1%) and high urinary osmolality (above 500 mOsm/kg). Rarely, renal sodium losses are due to a deficiency of renin and/or aldosterone (discussed more fully in Chapter 14). Patients with

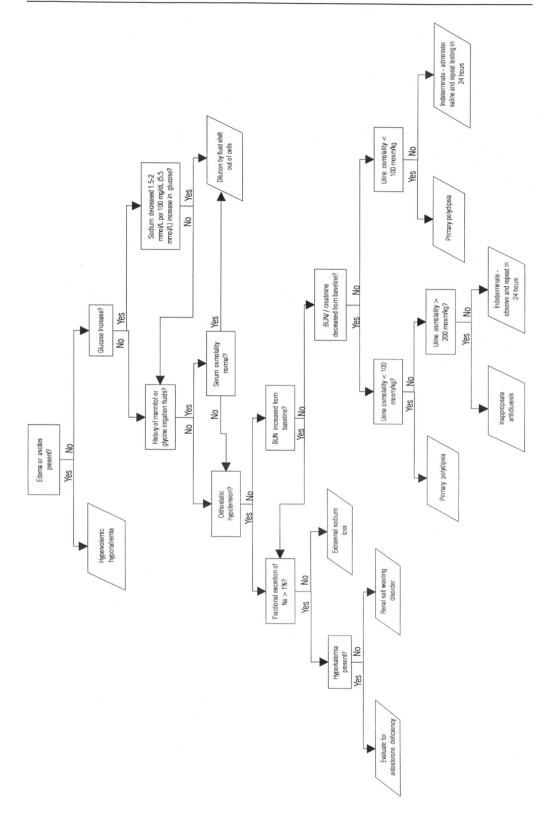

hypoaldosteronism resemble those with renal sodium losses in having high urine sodium and osmolality; however, they will also be hyperkalemic, and have inappropriately low urinary potassium excretion (FE_K below 20%).

Decreased Sodium Intake

Rarely, patients with extremely poor diets, especially alcoholics or anorectics, will present with hyponatremia. Occasionally, patients in hospitals may be maintained on hypotonic intravenous fluids for a prolonged period, eventually producing hyponatremia. Again, as in patients with extrarenal sodium losses, these patients will be hypovolemic, have low urine sodium excretion and high urine osmolality, and increased BUN; they may be recognized because of the lack of history of sodium loss and detailed dietary history

Increased Extracellular Fluid Water

A primary increase in ECF water is a common cause of hyponatremia. Such patients are typically euvolemic clinically, although BUN, creatinine, and uric acid are usually decreased from baseline.

Primary Polydipsia

Excessive water intake is an uncommon cause of hyponatremia. While most commonly seen in psychiatric patients, it also occurs in patients who drink excessive amounts of water to relieve a dry sensation in their mouth or to treat hiccups. Often, a history of increased water ingestion is not obtained from such patients, but can be diagnosed by extremely low urine osmolality (usually less than 100 mOsm/kg, and in most cases about 50 mOsm/kg) and very low concentrations of all urine electrolytes. Fluid restriction restores sodium concentration to normal quickly.

Syndrome of Inappropriate Antidiuretic Hormone

Syndrome of inappropriate antidiuretic hormone (SIADH), one of the most common causes of hyponatremia, is defined clinically by excretion of urine that is less than maximally dilute in a patient with decreased osmolality and normal or slightly increased intravascular volume (that is, there is no *appropriate* cause for ADH production). Urine osmolality greater than 200 mOsm/kg always indicates the presence of water conservation and ADH effect; urine osmolality between 100 and 200 mOsm/kg usually indicates ADH presence, but may represent maximal diluting ability in the very young or very old; urine osmolality below 100 mOsm/kg indicates absence of ADH and rules out this syndrome. SIADH is most commonly seen in lung disease, in many malignan-

Figure 5.4. Approach to Hyponatremia. Initial evaluation of hyponatremic individuals begins with evaluation of volume status. Patients clinically fluid overloaded (edema) require no further laboratory evaluation. History should be studied for risk factors for osmotic shifting of fluid (diabetes, use of mannitol or glycine irrigation fluids during surgery); normal to increased osmolality confirms this pathogenesis. Patients clinically hypovolemic have sodium losses; urine sodium excretion can clarify the source of losses. Clinically euvolemic patients are likely to be either slightly hypovolemic or hypervolemic. The BUN/creatinine ratio can help to clarify which change in volume is present. Patients slightly hypervolemic likely have either primary polydipsia or inappropriate antidiuresis. Slightly hypovolemic patients usually have salt losing disorders, and are studied in essentially the same fashion as clinically hypovolemic patients.

cies (most notably small cell lung carcinoma), and in many CNS abnormalities; other common causes are alcohol withdrawal, administration of drugs which can stimulate ADH production (such as carbamazepine), and deficiency of cortisol (which normally inhibits ADH secretion). U_{Na} is extremely variable, and depends on sodium intake; in most cases, U_{Na} is more than 20 mmol/L and FE_{Na} is above 1%. Patients with low sodium intake may have very low urine sodium excretion, which may suggest extrarenal salt loss as the etiology of hyponatremia. In questionable cases, administration of 2 L of normal saline over 24 hours and repeat measurement of U_{Na} and FE_{Na} can serve as a diagnostic test: both will typically reach the values given above in SIADH, but will remain low with sodium depletion. Measurement of ADH is seldom necessary. Many textbooks state that SIADH is a diagnosis of exclusion. While it is true that many other disorders produce hyponatremia with high urine osmolality, almost all differ from SIADH in that they are associated with either low plasma volume or edema. If clinical and laboratory features are consistent with a euvolemic or slightly hypervolemic state, the only other important clinical disorder producing this picture is hypothyroidism, in which maximal urine diluting ability is impaired. Only in extremely rare cases, however, is an SIADH-like picture the only clinical manifestation of hypothyroidism.

Shift of Water Out of Cells

This common cause of hyponatremia occurs in the presence of an osmotically active substance in plasma which cannot enter cells, causing water to shift from cells into plasma. In contrast to all other hyponatremic disorders, shifts of water are associated with normal or increased plasma osmolality. Patients with water shifts may have varying volume status, depending on the type of osmotically active substance present. The most common cause is diabetes mellitus, in which plasma sodium will fall by 1.5–2.0 mmol/L for each 100 mg/dL (5.6 mmol/L) increase in glucose; "correcting" sodium for the degree of elevation of glucose can predict, with relative accuracy, the sodium concentration which will be present after hyperglycemia has resolved. In the early stages of hyperglycemia, intravascular volume is slightly increased; as hyperglycemia persists, glucose acts as an osmotic diuretic, causing renal sodium and water losses, so that patients become hypovolemic. Less commonly, other solutes such as mannitol, hydroxyethyl starch, and glycine (used in irrigation during prostate and endometrial ablation) are responsible; with glycine, many liters of fluid may be absorbed (Fig. 5.5). Intravascular volume is typically slightly increased by these other osmotically active agents; with glycine, pulmonary and cerebral edema may develop. History is the most important means to identify this type of hyponatremia. Treatment with saline is not indicated, since this will cause fluid to leave cells and may worsen the patient's clinical picture.

Edema

Increased amount of interstitial fluid is a rare cause of hyponatremia, due to loss of sodium and water from plasma. Edema is caused by alteration in the normal balance of pressures between plasma and interstitial fluid; most commonly, it is due to high venous pressure in congestive heart failure, but less commonly may be caused by low oncotic pressure in nephrotic syndrome or high portal venous pressure. Loss of fluid from plasma leads to increased production of ADH and aldosterone, increasing total body sodium and lowering plasma osmolality. Diagnosis is based on clinical detection of edema; no laboratory tests are diagnostic. Patients with edema related hyponatremia

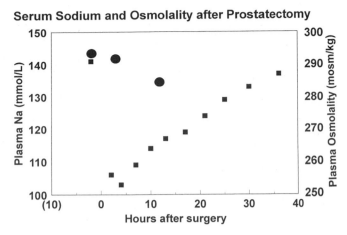

Figure 5.5. Effects of Glycine Absorption on Serum Sodium and Osmolality. During transurethral prostatectomy, this patient absorbed an estimated 26 L of glycine irrigation fluid (osmolality approximately 210 mOsm/kg). Although there was a marked decrease in serum sodium (squares), reaching a nadir of 103 mmol/L, serum osmolality (circles) decreased only slightly and did not leave the normal range.

have low urine sodium excretion and increased urine osmolality if untreated; with diuretic treatment, results cannot be interpreted.

Increased Plasma Sodium (Hypernatremia)

Hypernatremia is a relatively common condition in hospitalized patients. While there are three possible mechanisms for development of hypernatremia, only one is commonly encountered.

Loss of Fluid

Sodium losing disorders lead to loss of a fluid that is lower in osmolality than plasma; in patients without ability to respond to thirst signals, this will cause hypernatremia. Problems with thirst perception are common in neurologic disorders, especially dementia; lack of free access to water is common in infants and in institutionalized patients. The vast majority of cases of hypernatremia are due to this mechanism. Volume loss leads to increased BUN and creatinine, and patients are clinically hypovolemic. Urine osmolality is high, and FE_{Na} is low; however, the high amount of sodium filtered often causes urinary sodium concentration to be relatively high (often greater than 20 mmol/L). It is important for the practitioner to be aware of the effects of treatment on plasma sodium concentration. In response to loss of water, cells generate small molecular weight sugars within cells (sometimes termed *idiogenic osmols*), raising the osmolality of intracellular fluid. Intracellular fluid thus has an even greater increase in osmolality than extracellular fluid. To correct volume deficit and hypernatremia, it is necessary to administer both free water (to correct the intracellular fluid deficit) and sodium (to correct the extracellular fluid losses). Administration of normal or half normal saline causes all of the sodium to stay in the vascular space (since aldosterone production prevents any significant renal loss), while approximately 60% of the water enters cells. The result is that **plasma sodium concentration typically rises during treatment of hypernatremia.** This is often frustrating to the practitioner, who is expecting results to improve with treatment. It is better to monitor BUN and creatinine and clinical status of the patient; when volume status nears normal (as evidenced by return of BUN to near baseline and absence of orthostatic hypotension), plasma sodium will begin to fall.

Diabetes Insipidus

Absence of ADH or, less commonly, renal resistance to ADH effects produces diabetes insipidus (DI). Patients with DI excrete large volumes of extremely dilute urine (osmolality usually less than 100 mOsm/kg) with low urine sodium concentration. Because thirst is typically intact, patients are only mildly hypernatremic (plasma Na 143–146) even when fluid intake and urine output are over 10 L/d, and volume status is typically normal. If patients with DI cannot get water, they will rapidly become dehydrated. Even in the presence of dehydration, however, BUN does not increase relative to creatinine, since ADH is necessary for reabsorption of BUN to produce a high BUN/creatinine ratio. The diagnosis of DI can be confirmed by performing a water deprivation test. Patients are allowed to have no oral or intravenous fluids, and should collect all urine produced on an hourly basis. The test is continued until one of the following occurs: 1) body weight declines by more than 3%; 2) urine osmolality reaches a plateau, with three consecutive specimens within 30 mOsm/kg of each other; 3) plasma osmolality increases by more than 10 mOsm/kg. A normal response is for urine volume to fall and urine osmolality to increase to greater than 500 mOsm/kg. If a normal response is not obtained but one other end points occurs, ADH may be administered to determine whether the kidneys have a normal response. Failure to concentrate urine with an increase in concentration after ADH administration is typical of pituitary (central) DI, while lack of response even after ADH administration describes nephrogenic DI.

Administration of Hypertonic Fluids

This is an extremely rare cause of hypernatremia. Occasionally, patients are given hypertonic sodium intravenously, often as sodium chloride with sodium bicarbonate during resuscitation. Intake of sodium may occur in children with diarrhea given "chicken soup" as therapy, and with ingestion of salt water in those lost at sea or salt water drowning. Patients with excess sodium intake often have normal volume status clinically, and have extremely high urine sodium excretion. History is important in establishing the diagnosis.

DISORDERS OF POTASSIUM

Abnormal plasma potassium typically occurs without any change in body water or volume. Plasma potassium is controlled largely by the balance between intake and excretion, with shifts into and out of cells also contributing to variation in potassium. Because there is no hormonal regulation of plasma potassium, significant changes in intake, rate of loss, or both, cause abnormal potassium in a high percentage of patients. Potassium abnormalities are the most frequently encountered electrolyte disorders.

Decreased Plasma Potassium (Hypokalemia)

Hypokalemia can occur from three basic mechanisms: loss of potassium (the most common cause), decreased potassium intake, or shift of potassium into cells. Figure 5.6 illustrates an approach to hypokalemic patients.

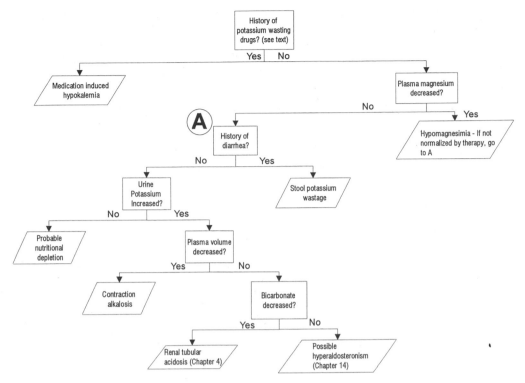

Figure 5.6. Approach to Hypokalemia. In hypokalemic patients, review of history for medications should be the initial step; patients on no medications should be checked for hypomagnesemia and history of diarrhea. If these are absent, low urine potassium indicates nutritional depletion. Low plasma volume (or high BUN/creatinine ratio) identifies contraction alkalosis as the likely cause. Plasma bicarbonate helps to classify renal potassium wasting states into renal tubular acidosis and probable aldosterone mediated hypokalemia; further details on evaluation for these states are included in Chapters 4 and 14, respectively.

Loss of Potassium

This is the most common cause of hypokalemia, usually due to urinary potassium loss. Drugs are a common cause of renal potassium wasting, either due to a direct effect on the tubules, as with diuretics, aminoglycoside antibiotics, amphotericin B, and cisplatinum, or complexing of potassium within the tubule with carbenicillin and ticarcillin. Magnesium deficiency impairs potassium absorption, as do some forms of renal tubular acidosis. Increased aldosterone causes sodium retention at the expense of potassium and also produces metabolic alkalosis in many patients. In all of these cases, FE_K will be inappropriately high, often over 40%. Diarrhea commonly causes loss of potassium which may be severe; patients with stool losses tend to have extremely low FE_K, often below 10%. Potassium may also be lost through vomiting.

Decreased Intake

Poor nutrition is an occasional cause of hypokalemia; in fact, hypokalemia is the most dangerous electrolyte abnormality in patients with marked malnutrition. Because there is an obligatory loss of potassium each day, hypokalemia usually develops after less than 30 days of deficient intake. Such patients have very low FE_K, typically below 5%.

Shift of Potassium into Cells

Alkalosis increases the activity of the sodium–potassium pump, causing potassium to enter cells and lowering plasma potassium; hypokalemia is corrected with resolution of the acid–base imbalance. Insulin causes potassium to enter cells along with glucose; hyperglycemic diabetic individuals often show a marked fall in plasma potassium when given insulin after a period of poor control. Similarly, patients who have been malnourished and who are started on parenteral nutrition commonly become hypokalemic.

Increased Plasma Potassium (Hyperkalemia)

Hyperkalemia usually results from one of three mechanisms. Before starting therapy or further diagnostic evaluation, it is always necessary to exclude an artifactual increase in potassium, as discussed earlier in the chapter. Patients with true hyperkalemia usually have a combination of increased intake and decreased renal excretion. In patients with normal renal function, leakage from cells should be investigated as an uncommon cause.

Increased Intake

This is rarely the sole cause of hyperkalemia; however, since the only mechanism for excreting excess potassium is in urine, ingestion of increased amounts of potassium is a common cause of hyperkalemia in patients with renal insufficiency. Common sources of potassium are salt substitutes, fruit, and potassium supplements. Potassium "supplements" may sometimes be occult, as in patients given Neutraphos (potassium phosphate) or Penicillin VK. Such patients tend to have a high FE_K, often over 50%, but relatively low total potassium excretion given their hyperkalemia.

Decreased Clearance

Renal failure is the most common cause of hyperkalemia, often in association with mild increases in potassium ingestion. Hyperkalemia due solely to renal failure does not reproducibly occur until late in the course of renal failure. In many patients with moderate renal insufficiency, particularly in diabetics and with alcohol abuse, ability to produce and/or respond to aldosterone is impaired, producing hyperkalemia and non-anion gap metabolic acidosis (Type IV renal tubular acidosis). In addition, certain drugs reduce renal potassium excretion; the most common are the potassium sparing diuretics such as triamterene and spironolactone. As mentioned above, patients with deficient aldosterone will have both hyponatremia and hyperkalemia; an increased FE_{Na} (above 1%) and decreased FE_K (under 20%) can be helpful in identifying these patients. Hypoaldosteronism may also be caused by drugs, most commonly nonsteroidal anti-inflammatory agents, angiotensin converting enzyme inhibitors, and heparin.

Shift Out of Cells

Acidosis reduces the activity of the cellular sodium–potassium pump, resulting in a shift of potassium out of cells and resultant hyperkalemia. Insulin deficiency prevents cellular potassium entry and can cause hyperkalemia even in the absence of ketoacidosis. Patients with rapid cell destruction, as with or tumor lysis syndrome (following chemotherapy of highly sensitive malignancies such as leukemia, lymphoma, and small cell cancers) or rhabdomyolysis, can rapidly leak large amounts of potassium into plasma and develop severe hyperkalemia. Affected patients will have increased plasma levels of other cellular contents, such as LDH, phosphate, and uric acid, and commonly develop acute renal failure due to uric acid precipitation in tubules.

Renal Function and Urinalysis

D. ROBERT DUFOUR

NORMAL STRUCTURAL PHYSIOLOGY

The kidney is composed of three functional areas: glomeruli, tubules/collecting system, and endocrine kidney. Each glomerulus drains into a single tubule, with associated endocrine cells, forming a **nephron.** Many disorders cause loss of entire nephrons, impairing all three functional components, while other diseases affect isolated components, producing distinct clinical and laboratory features.

Glomerulus

The glomeruli filter blood, allowing passage of water and dissolved solutes while retaining cells and suspended particles; substances with molecular weight below 35,000–40,000 pass through, while cells and most proteins are retained. In normal adults, approximately 180 L of plasma is filtered daily. Glomerular filtrate has the same osmolality as plasma and contains the same concentration of small compounds (electrolytes, glucose, urea, creatinine, etc.); it is virtually devoid of cells, most hormones, enzymes, and major plasma proteins.

Tubules

Renal tubules process glomerular filtrate, retaining needed compounds, excreting waste products, and ultimately producing an average of 1.5 L of urine daily. The segments of the tubule perform different functions, as illustrated in Figure 6.1. Tubular function is necessary for normal fluid, electrolyte, and acid-base balance.

Endocrine Function

The kidney produces several hormones and excretes or metabolizes other hormones. Among the major hormone products of the kidney are erythropoietin (Chapter 24), produced by interstitial cells; renin (Chapter 14), produced by the juxtaglomerular apparatus; and calcitriol (1,25-dihydroxyvitamin D) (Chapter 10), produced by the proximal tubular epithelial cells. The kidney is also important in metabolism of insulin.

THEORETICAL CONCEPTS USED IN DESCRIBING RENAL FUNCTION

Clearance

In renal clearance, a specific amount of substance is removed from plasma in a given period of time; this same amount is excreted in urine. The rate at which a volume of blood is "cleared" is termed **clearance rate.** The mathematical relationships involved are illustrated in Equation 6.1. A number of factors must be controlled to accurately use and interpret clearance (Table 6.1). In addition, there are relationships between

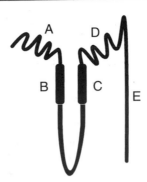

Figure 6.1. The renal tubule has several segments which control water and solute status. Initially, the proximal convoluted tubule (**A**) absorbs most solutes, about 2/3 of sodium and water, and little chloride. In the first half of the loop of Henle (**B**), water is absorbed in excess of sodium, increasing osmolality to as much as 1200 mOsm/kg. In the next segment (**C**), sodium and chloride absorption produces a fluid with a relatively low osmolality and virtually no potassium. The distal convoluted tubule and cortical collecting duct (**D**) can absorb sodium in exchange for potassium or hydrogen ion, mainly under the effects of aldosterone. The collecting duct (**E**) can, in the presence of ADH, absorb water and produce a very concentrated urine.

Table 6.1.
Considerations in Measuring Clearance

- Plasma concentration must be constant
- Accurate timing of urine collection
- Urine, plasma concentration in same units
- Urine flow rate in mL/min (24 h volume divided by 1440 min)
- 24 hour used to minimize diurnal variation
- Other times can be used if no variation

---

clearance and the individual variables measured (Table 6.2). Clearance is meaningful only if the mechanism for renal handling of a substance is known. If the substance is only filtered, clearance equals **glomerular filtration rate (GFR).** For substances filtered but reabsorbed, clearance relative to GFR can be used to evaluate tubular function. For substances filtered and secreted by tubules, clearance represents a sum of tubular and glomerular function.

$$Amount\ cleared\ =\ plasma\ concentration\ (P) \times clearance\ rate\ (C)$$

$$Amount\ excreted\ =\ urine\ concentration\ (U) \times urine\ flow\ rate\ (V) \qquad (6.1)$$

$$P \times C = U \times V \qquad C = \frac{U \times V}{P}$$

Table 6.2.
Mathematical Relationships in Clearance

- If amount excreted (U × V) is constant, clearance = constant × (1/P) (for creatinine, assumption valid in individual over time)
- If urine production constant, clearance = constant × (U/P) (for creatinine, more valid for comparing results between individuals)
- Many factors invalidate assumptions of constants; use of these estimates less reliable than measuring clearance

Fractional Excretion

The ratio of excretion to filtration is termed fractional excretion, calculated by comparing the clearance of compound x to glomerular filtration rate (Eq. 6.2). As discussed later, creatinine clearance is usually used to estimate GFR; the equation can be rewritten to substitute this for GFR (Eq. 6.2). By convention, results are multiplied by 100 and expressed as a percentage. For substances filtered and not altered by tubules, fractional excretion is 100. Substances not filtered, such as proteins, have no fractional excretion. Substances reabsorbed by tubules have fractional excretion between 0 and 100, depending on tubular function. Substances filtered and secreted have fractional excretion over 100.

$$Fractional\ excretion_x\ (FE_x) = \frac{Clearance_x}{glomerular\ filtration\ rate} \tag{6.2}$$

$$FE_x = \frac{U_x/P_x}{U_{Cr}/P_{Cr}} = \frac{U_x \times P_{Cr}}{P_x \times U_{Cr}}$$

Tubular Reabsorption

If a compound is reabsorbed, it is not excreted; tubular reabsorption represents the opposite of fractional excretion, and can be calculated with Equation 6.3.

$$Tubular\ reabsorption_x\ (TR_x) = 100 - FE_x \tag{6.3}$$

GLOMERULAR FUNCTION TESTS

Tests to evaluate glomerular function fall into two types: those which estimate the number of nephrons (GFR, plasma concentration of waste products), and tests of intact filtering function (urine protein, urinalysis).

Glomerular Filtration Rate

Many renal diseases cause loss of complete nephrons, manifested mainly by reduction in glomerular filtration rate (GFR). Clearance of substances filtered but neither reabsorbed nor secreted by tubules can be used to calculate GFR. No endogenous compounds fulfill this criterion, but inulin and iothalamate are used in research settings for precise measurement of GFR. Creatinine is filtered by glomeruli, but secreted by tubules; creatinine clearance overestimates GFR. At low plasma creatinine, 10% of urinary creatinine comes from tubular secretion, overestimating the numerator in Equation 6.1. Conversely, assays for plasma creatinine typically overestimate creatinine by 10%. Thus, at low plasma values, creatinine clearance is a reasonable estimate of GFR. As plasma creatinine increases, the fraction reaching urine by secretion also increases, while interferences in plasma creatinine are of less importance; these two factors cause creatinine clearance to overestimate GFR by 20–30% or more. Since absolute GFR is always low by this point, the error is of little clinical importance in determination of renal function.

Plasma Concentration of Filtered Substances

Plasma urea nitrogen (BUN) and creatinine are widely used to estimate renal function; the relationship between plasma values and GFR is shown in Figure 6.2.

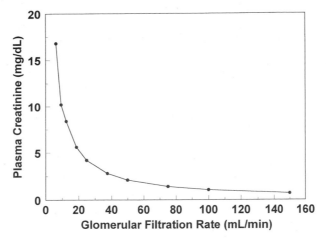

Figure 6.2. There is an inverse relationship between plasma creatinine and creatinine clearance, used as an estimate of glomerular filtration rate. As GFR initially declines, there is only a slight absolute increase in plasma creatinine. As renal damage progresses through its moderate stages (GFR between 60 and 20 mL/min), the curve is close to linear, making plasma creatinine a good measure of GFR. In the late stages of renal failure, small absolute changes in GFR cause large changes in plasma creatinine.

Creatinine

Irreversible degradation of muscle creatine produces the waste product creatinine. Major determinants of creatinine production are muscle mass and protein intake. With increasing age from 20 to 70 years, muscle mass declines steadily, plasma creatinine remains constant, but GFR declines significantly. The same plasma creatinine indicates significantly different renal function in young and old individuals. Several published formulas "correct" plasma creatinine for patient age; the easiest to use is shown in Equation 6.4. This formula applies to adult men; in adult women, values are multiplied by 0.85.

$$C_{Cr} = \frac{(140 - Age\ (yrs)) \times Wt\ (kg)}{72 \times Serum\ Creatinine\ (mg/dL)} \tag{6.4}$$

Most laboratories measure creatinine using the Jaffe reaction, which is subject to interference from ketone bodies and, less frequently, some cephalosporin antibiotics. The ketone interference may be substantial in some assays (with ketones positive at a 1:32 dilution, creatinine may be overestimated by 3–4 mg/dL) and less in other systems; practitioners should check with the laboratory they use most frequently. Some laboratories use a more specific enzymatic assay, which does not show these interferences.

Urea (blood urea nitrogen, BUN)

Amino acid metabolism in the liver produces urea as a waste product; rate of production is dependent on protein intake and liver function. In the kidney, urea is filtered and a variable percentage is passively reabsorbed along with water (mainly under the influence of ADH). Clearance of urea falls in states of volume depletion, leading to a more rapid increase in BUN than in creatinine, which may be helpful diagnostically. States with increased protein turnover (burns, infections, upper GI bleeding) lead to increased

Table 6.3.
BUN/Creatinine Ratio

- High Ratio
  Dehydration
  Upper GI Bleeding
  Acute obstruction
  Acute glomerulonephritis
- Normal Ratio
  Acute tubular necrosis
  Chronic obstruction
  Loss of nephrons
- Low Ratio
  Renal dialysis
  Severe skeletal muscle injury
  Liver disease
  Malnutrition

urea production and elevation in BUN without a change in renal function. Decreased amino acid turnover (malnutrition, liver disease) causes a fall in urea levels and underestimation of renal function. States with altered ADH activity cause unexpected changes in urea; in diabetes insipidus, urea is lower than expected for renal function, while falsely high values occur with inappropriate ADH production. Differences in the way BUN and creatinine are handled makes the BUN:Creatinine ratio useful in evaluating cause of abnormal results (Table 6.3).

Evaluation of Filtration Barrier

In many glomerular diseases, leakage of proteins is the first sign of glomerular injury, occurring months to years before a decrease in GFR.

Urine Protein

A small amount of plasma protein, primarily very low molecular weight proteins and traces of albumin, pass through the glomeruli; this is almost completely reabsorbed by tubules. Normal total urine protein is less than 150 mg/d and urine albumin is less than 40 mg/d. Increased loss of protein, particularly albumin, is the earliest indicator of glomerular damage. Transient increases in protein excretion occur in the upright state, with exercise, and in acute illness. In addition, bleeding and infection of the urinary tract cause protein leakage into urine.

Tests for total urine protein

Dipsticks use a method similar to that used to measure plasma albumin; results are falsely negative in Bence Jones proteinuria, and are insensitive to early renal damage. **Microalbumin** measures small amounts of albumin; microalbumin dipsticks are available, but the test is most commonly and more accurately performed in the laboratory. Total protein detects all urine proteins, and is preferred for diagnosis and follow-up of patients with multiple myeloma. Quantitation in a 24-hour urine specimen eliminates diurnal variation and is most widely used. Ratio of protein to creatinine in a random urine specimen correlates well with 24-hour total protein, and is easier to use in follow-

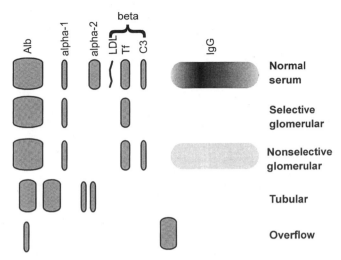

Figure 6.3. Patterns of proteinuria compared to a normal plasma reference pattern on top (Alb—albumin; LDL—low density lipoprotein; Tf—transferrin; C3—component of complement). With minimal damage to the glomerulus, only small M.W. proteins such as Alb, a_1-AT, and Tf will pass into the urine. With more severe glomerular injury, larger proteins such as immunoglobulins also appear. With tubular injury, Alb and other low M.W. proteins normally absent from plasma (retinol binding protein, β_2-microglobulin, and others) become apparent.

up after determining correlation in an individual; values greater than 0.5 suggest significant proteinuria.

Urine protein electrophoresis

Rarely, electrophoresis of urine proteins (Fig. 6.3) is useful in determining the nature of renal injury present. In children, selective glomerular proteinuria usually occurs in minimal change disease which has a good prognosis; non-selective proteinuria usually indicates a more significant disorder and may indicate need for a renal biopsy. In adults, the distinction is not helpful since many progressive renal diseases, including diabetes, produce selective proteinuria.

Hematuria

With severe glomerular damage, red cells can pass the glomerular filter and appear in the urine. Microscopic analysis provides additional information in patients with hematuria. RBC casts confirms presence of glomerular bleeding. Red cells become deformed (**dysmorphic** RBCs) while passing through the tubules; a high percentage of dysmorphic cells seen in Wright stained urine sediment can confirm glomerular bleeding in the absence of RBC casts.

EVALUATION OF TUBULAR FUNCTION

Evaluation of proximal tubular reabsorptive functions and concentrating ability of the loop of Henle are the most reliable methods to identify tubular damage.

Reabsorption of Solutes

Many important substances are filtered by glomeruli and reabsorbed in the proximal tubule, including glucose, phosphate, uric acid, bicarbonate, magnesium, and K^+. Low plasma levels of all of these except glucose, and high urine glucose with normal plasma glucose, may call attention to tubular damage. More sensitive tests of proximal tubular injury include measurement of small molecular weight proteins in urine, and measurement of the enzyme **N-acetylglucosaminidase (NAG),** present in high concentration in tubular epithelial cells. As noted above, small proteins filtered by glomeruli are normally reabsorbed by tubules; detection of these proteins in urine by electrophoresis indicates significant tubular damage. Other small proteins may be measured specifically, including amylase and β_2-microglobulin (Chapter 9).

Excretion of Water and Electrolytes

These tests measure function of the loop of Henle and distal nephron. In states of oliguria, with urine output less than 400 mL per day, urine osmolality and electrolyte concentrations can tell whether low urine production is an appropriate attempt to preserve plasma volume or represents renal tubular injury (acute tubular necrosis).

Free Water Clearance

Ability of the tubules to concentrate and dilute urine is a function of the loop of Henle and the collecting ducts; these are the sites of injury in many forms of tubular disease. Free water clearance (C_{H2O}) is the difference between total water "clearance" (urine volume) and required water clearance (osmolar clearance) (Eq. 6.5).

$$C_{H_2O} = V - C_{osm} = V - \frac{U_{osm} \times V}{P_{osm}} = V \times \left(1 - \frac{U_{osm}}{P_{osm}}\right) \qquad (6.5)$$

While exact calculation requires timed collection, since the volume term does not cancel out as in fractional excretion, practically this is not needed. If urine and plasma osmolality are virtually identical (as happens with acute tubular necrosis, ATN), the term in parentheses becomes zero and C_{H2O} is zero for any urine volume. In ATN, zero free water clearance develops within 1–2 hours of tubular injury. Decreased renal blood flow ("prerenal azotemia") causes water conservation by ADH and negative free water clearance.

Fractional Excretion of Sodium

Fractional excretion of sodium (FE_{Na}) measures the ability of tubules to conserve sodium. In dehydration, increased renin and aldosterone should lead to maximum conservation of sodium by the tubules; FE_{Na} is usually less than 1% (often less than 0.2%). In acute tubular necrosis, an inability to reabsorb sodium leads to high FE_{Na}, characteristically greater than 1% and often 3–5% or higher; however, it generally takes 18–24 h for FE_{Na} to exceed 1%, longer in those with high aldosterone (congestive heart failure, dehydration). FE_{Na} is falsely elevated following diuretic administration.

URINALYSIS

Substances reach urine by a combination of two possible mechanisms: concentration dependent excretion and abnormal renal function. Most essential filtered components (including glucose, bicarbonate, and K^+) are completely reabsorbed by tubules; high plasma concentration may exceed reabsorptive capacity and increase urinary excretion. Blood cells and plasma proteins do not pass glomeruli; their presence in urine indicates abnormal function. While glomerular disease is the most common cause, bleeding, tumors, and inflammation also cause leakage of protein and cells. Tubular disease may also cause loss of small compounds such as glucose. Casts and crystals may form directly in the tubular lumen as local concentration is increased by reabsorption of water. Such findings can point to the presence of intrinsic renal disease.

Routine Urinalysis

Physical, chemical, and microscopic analysis of urine are the oldest laboratory tests; traditional urinalysis includes all three components. Specimens should be tested soon after collection; casts and cells begin to deteriorate within 30 minutes, with faster breakdown in dilute urine specimens or those with very low or high pH. Longer delays also allow proliferation of bacterial contaminants from skin or urethra. Refrigeration preserves most urine elements, but may cause precipitation of crystals.

Gross Appearance

Normal urine is yellow due to urochrome pigment, with degree of coloration related to urine concentration. Abnormal colors indicate presence of colored chemicals (Table 6.4). Normal urine is transparent; cloudiness indicates the presence of particulate matter, such as crystals, red or white blood cells, mucus, or bacteria.

Concentration

Urine concentration differs markedly during the day; determination is of little value in routine urinalysis. Over 80% of urine solute consists of urea and creatinine. In patients with oliguria, polyuria, or fluid and electrolyte disorders, solute concentration provides an indication of tubular function and ADH levels. Several different methods are used to evaluate urine concentration; they do not always agree. Osmolality (Chapter 5) evaluates molar concentration of solutes; it is most the reliable, and should be used when highly accurate results are needed (water deprivation test for diabetes insipidus, suspected acute tubular necrosis). Specific gravity (SG) measures weight of urine solutes; in most instances SG and osmolality are closely related (osmolality of 300 mOsm/kg equals SG of 1.010). Results diverge when high molecular weight substances are present (glucose, protein, or radiologic contrast agents), causing higher specific gravity than osmolality. Ionic strength (electrolyte concentration) is used to measure "SG" with dipsticks; falsely elevated results occur with proteinuria or very abnormal pH. While in normal individuals there is a parallel relationship between electrolyte excretion and total urine solute, acute illness causes these to diverge, and results of "SG" from dipsticks and true SG or osmolality show poor correlation in hospitalized patients.

Table 6.4.
Causes of Abnormal Urine Color

Red—blood, hemoglobin, phenolphthalein, porphyrins, beets, rifampin, L-dopa, paraflex
Brown—hemoglobin, myoglobin, bilirubin, nitrofurantoin
Orange—urates, pyridium, urobilin (breakdown product of urobilinogen), sulfasalazine
Black—hemoglobin, myoglobin, alkaptonuria, L-dopa (all on standing)

Table 6.5.
Significance of Urine Chemical Tests

Test	Urinary Disease Affecting	Systemic Disease Affecting	Interferences
Specific gravity	Disorders of urine concentrating ability	Changes in fluid status	With salt retention, may differ markedly from true osmolality, since the test measures ionic strength; proteinuria, alkaline pH lead to incorrect results
pH	Rental tubular acidosis; urinary tract infections may produce alkaline pH	Acid–base disorders	None
Protein	Glomerular diseases; infection; tubular disorders	Infection, exercise, fever cause transient proteinuria	Alkaline pH may cause false positive; false negative with Bence Jones protein
Glucose	Tubular disorders (rarely)	Diabetes mellitus	Ascorbic acid produces falsely low results
Ketones	None	Ketoacidosis	Ascorbic acid rarely produces false negative
Blood	Any site of bleeding in urinary tract (glomerulonephritis, tumors, stones, infection)	Coagulopathy; hemoglobinuria in hemolysis; myoglobinuria with muscle damage	Ascorbic acid falsely lowers results; exposure to air may cause false negative. Highly concentrated urines may be falsely negative.
Bilirubin	None	Liver and billiary disease	False negative if exposed to light
Urobilinogen	None	Hemolysis; cirrhosis; resolution phase of liver/ biliary diseases	Many drugs produce false positive, especially sulfonamides
Nitrite	Infection with most Gram-negative organisms	None	Exposure to air, contamination cause false positive; ascorbic acid may produce false negative. Negative results expected with Gram-positive infections
Leukocyte esterase	Infection of GU system; interstitial nephritis	None	Ascorbic acid, aminoglycosides, heavy proteinuria produces false negative. Negative results expected with lymphocytic inflammation (as in tuberculosis)

Chemical Analysis

Dipsticks allow determination of many chemicals in urine quickly, efficiently, and inexpensively. The significance of various chemical findings is summarized in Table 6.5. A number of clinical studies have shown that 95–98% of clinically important urine abnormalities are detected by chemical examination; microscopic analysis adds little if urine is negative for the four tests usually indicating urinary tract disease: protein, blood, leukocyte esterase, and nitrite.

Microscopic Urinalysis

Many laboratories have abandoned urine microscopic examination as part of routine urinalysis, relying on gross examination and chemical analysis to detect specimens requiring microscopic analysis. Microscopic examination is most useful in patients with

Table 6.6.
Significance of Urine Microscopic Findings

Finding	Normal	Urinary Tract Disease	Systemic Disease
Crystals	Uric acid, calcium oxalate, triple phosphate	Cystine in some tubular disorders; uric acid, calcium oxalate rarely with nephrolithiasis	Tyrosine in liver disease; drug crystals
Epithelial cells	Squamous, transitional epithelial cells	Renal tubular cells with tubular injury (tubular necrosis, transplant rejection)	None
Red Blood Cells	3–5/high power field; higher in menstruating women	Glomerular injury; nephrolithiasis; inflammation (especially hemorrhagic cystitis), neoplasms	Rarely with sickle cell disease, coagulopathies
White Blood Cells	3–5/high power field	Infections of bladder, kidney; interstitial nephritis (eosinophils)	Infection of prostate, cervix, vagina
Hyaline casts	Expecially after exercise	Any cause of proteinuria, especially glomerular disease	Dehydration, fever; other causes of proteinuria (e.g., diabetes)
Granular casts	Rarely with exercise	Heavy proteinuria; pigmented granular casts with acute tubular necrosis	Rarely with nonglomerular causes of proteinuria
Cellular casts	Not found	RBC casts in glomerulonephritis; WBC casts in pyelonephritis	None
Organisms	Contamination or prolonged storage before examination	Cystitis, pyelonephritis	Prostatitis

abnormal chemical analysis and in patients with signs or symptoms of urinary tract disease. The significance of various microscopic findings is summarized in Table 6.6.

Method of Examination

A 10 mL urine sample is centrifuged, all but 0.5–1.0 mL is discarded, and sediment is resuspended and examined microscopically. This is adequate for identification of particulates, but not for precise quantitation; many laboratories have introduced reproducible techniques for performing sediment examination. Since relative concentration of particles varies with overall concentration of urine (which may vary by more than 20-fold), there is no obvious advantage to more reproducible techniques. Staining of sediment improves ability to distinguish cells from each other, and marginally increases identification of casts.

Crystals

Most crystals (Fig. 6.4) form when the sample temperature drops after specimen collection, and are rarely of clinical significance. Some laboratories do not report calcium oxalate, uric acid, triple phosphate, or amorphous crystals, comprising 99% of urine crystals. In cases where intratubular formation of crystals is suspected (uric acid or xanthine crystals in tumor lysis, calcium oxalate with ethylene glycol poisoning), urine should be kept at 37 C after collection and during centrifugation. Various drugs, notably sulfonamides, may form crystals in vivo, which sometimes cause acute renal failure. Increased amino acids form crystals: tyrosine (circular clusters of needles) with liver disease; cystine (flat, colorless hexagons) with renal tubular disorders and kidney stones. Bilirubin produces clusters of needle-shaped, yellow to brown crystals.

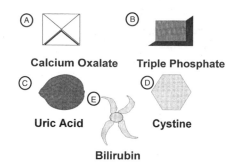

Figure 6.4. Common urine crystals (**A–C**) are seen in many normal urine samples, usually as a result of specimen cooling. While calcium oxalate and uric acid occur in acidic urine, triple phosphate is found in alkaline urine. Cystine crystals (**D**) are uncommon, but always indicate significant disease; in children, they suggest inherited renal tubular dysfunction; in adults, they occur with renal injury. Bilirubin crystals (**E**) are common with increased conjugated bilirubin; they are gold-brown and confused with drug crystals.

Cells

Epithelial cells (Fig. 6.5) from the vagina, urethra, and bladder are normally shed, and are of no significance. Renal tubular epithelial cells, if present in increased numbers, indicate tubular damage (tubular necrosis, interstitial nephritis, or transplant rejection). Tubular cells can be difficult to distinguish from transitional epithelial cells; they can be reliably identified by staining with labeled antibodies to Tamm–Horsfall protein produced exclusively by tubular cells. Red blood cells are a normal finding in menstruating woman, and up to 5–10 per high power field (HPF) may be found in young persons without indicating pathology. Increased numbers indicate bleeding in the urinary tract (or, in women, vaginal bleeding). Dysmorphic red cells (discussed earlier) usually occur with glomerular disease, but may form in highly concentrated urine. Prolonged contact with very dilute urine causes red cell lysis. White blood cells may be normal if less than 3–5 per HPF are seen. Prolonged contact with very dilute urine leads to white cell breakdown. Increased white cells indicate inflammation in the urinary tract (cystitis, pyelonephritis) or genital tract (cervicitis and vaginitis in women, prostatitis in men). Eosinophils are found in many drug reactions (drug-induced inter-

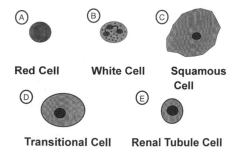

Figure 6.5. Common Urine Cells. Squamous and transitional epithelial cells (**C, D**) are commonly encountered and are normal. Only rare renal tubular cells (**E**) occur in normal urine; increased numbers indicate tubular damage. Normal red blood cells (**A**) are biconcave disks; they indicate bleeding after the kidney. Small numbers are often of no significance. Deformed (dysmorphic) red cells usually indicate glomerular bleeding. White cell (**B**) granules typically move, causing cells to "glitter" and making them readily recognizable. As with red cells, small numbers are often insignificant findings.

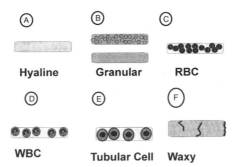

Figure 6.6. Urinary Casts. Hyaline casts (**A**), composed of Tamm–Horsfall protein, are seen in dehydration, after exercise, and with renal injury. Granular casts (**B**) contain plasma proteins or, less commonly, degenerated cells; they usually are seen in renal disease. Pigmented granular casts occur with ATN, and less commonly with hemoglobin and myoglobin casts. Cellular casts indicate the type of injury present. RBC casts (**C**) are found in glomerulonephritis, while WBC casts (**D**) occur in pyelonephritis. Tubular cell casts (**E**) are rarely seen, usually with transplant rejection and less commonly with ATN. Waxy casts (**F**) are typically broad, and form with very slow urine flow in renal failure; they often appear fractured with cracks extending across them.

stitial nephritis). They are extremely labile, so sediment should be examined within one hour of collection. Values greater than 10% of white blood cells in urine are considered abnormal.

Casts

Tamm–Horsfall protein, secreted by tubular cells, may form a gel when urine concentration is increased by water reabsorption or urine flow rate slows; the gel makes a cast of the inside of the tubule in which it forms, and traps any particles present in the urine. Casts allow a non-invasive "biopsy" of the renal tubules (Fig 6.6).

Microorganisms

Bacteria accumulate in urine unless examined rapidly; some bacteria and many yeast can even grow at refrigerator temperatures. If uncentrifuged, fresh urine is examined, a count of two or more bacteria per HPF correlates well with a culture result of greater than 100,000 colonies per mL. In various studies, this technique recognizes urinary infection in 95% of symptomatic patients, but only 75% of asymptomatic infections.

WHEN NOT TO DO RENAL FUNCTION TESTS

There are no situations when measurement of plasma BUN and creatinine should not be done; because they increase only slowly with changes in renal function, they should not be measured more than once a day. Creatinine results should be interpreted with caution in patients with ketoacidosis or on cephalosporins unless measured by enzymatic methods. GFR should not be measured when plasma creatinine is increasing or decreasing, as results will be inaccurate. Measurement of microalbumin should only be done on first morning or 24-hour urine specimens to eliminate posture and exercise effects; it should not be done in acutely ill patients or in the presence of urinary tract infection or bleeding. Testing for suspected nephrotic syndrome can be done at any time, since very high protein does not occur in other states. Urinalysis should not be

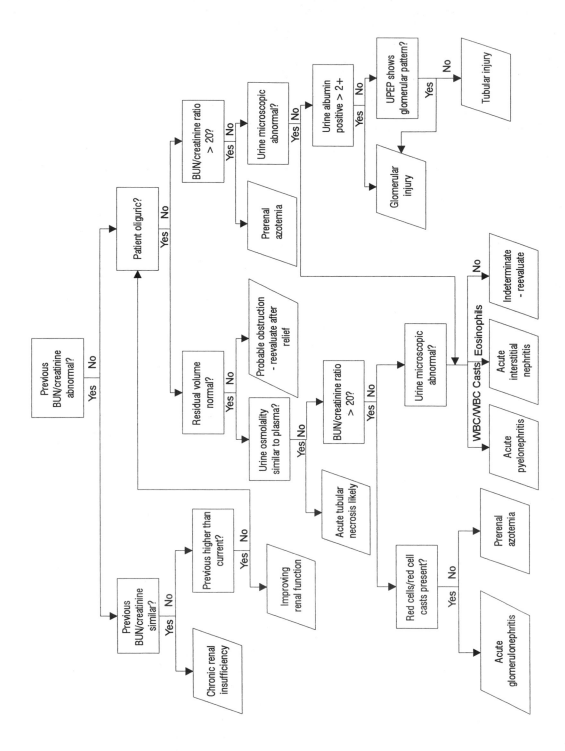

done unless signs and symptoms of urinary tract disease are present or there is a high risk of asymptomatic urinary tract disease (diabetes, hypertension, elderly patients, or pregnant women). Microscopic urinalysis need not be done unless dipstick is positive for protein, blood, nitrite, or leukocyte esterase. Urine electrolytes should not be used to test for tubular damage in patients receiving diuretics or in nonoliguric patients; results are often misleading.

PATTERNS OF RENAL DISEASE AND THEIR LABORATORY DIAGNOSIS

While there are a large number of diseases which may affect the kidney, they produce characteristic patterns of injury which cause recognizable clinical and laboratory patterns (Table 6.7). In patients detected with elevated BUN and/or creatinine, an approach to laboratory evaluation is outlined in Figure 6.7.

Decreased Renal Blood Flow = Prerenal Azotemia

With shock, renal blood flow diminishes causing a fall in GFR. To compensate for decreased blood volume, ADH and renin are produced, causing maximum retention of salt and water; FE_{Na} is typically less than 0.5%, and free water clearance is strongly negative. BUN and creatinine both rise, but water reabsorption causes greater increase in BUN, producing a high BUN:creatinine ratio.

Mild Glomerular Injury = Proteinuria

Increased urine albumin is the most common means of detection of mild glomerular injury. Transient glomerular dysfunction is common with febrile illness and after exercise; testing should not be done when these are present. In diabetes mellitus and hypertension, the first sign of glomerular injury is microalbuminuria in a first morning specimen or 24-h urine (greater than 30 μg/min (40 mg/d), greater than 32 mg/g creatinine). With more progressive injury, total protein exceeds 150 mg/day, and "protein" dipsticks are persistently positive. After months to years, nephrons are lost and plasma BUN and creatinine begin to rise.

Moderate, Chronic Glomerular Injury = Nephrotic Syndrome

With more severe glomerular injury, protein loss of more than 3 g/day exceeds liver synthetic capacity; this causes a progressive fall in the concentration of small plasma proteins, especially albumin. Liver synthesis of all proteins increases, and large proteins (a_2-globulins, lipoproteins) are increased in blood. Reduction in albumin often leads to edema.

Figure 6.7. Approach to Renal Disease. In patients with increased BUN or creatinine, comparison to previous results can prevent unnecessary testing. With apparent acute increases, presence or absence of oliguria helps focus the differential diagnosis. With oliguria, evaluation for obstruction should be done early, followed by evaluation of urine concentrating ability to recognize ATN. If osmolality is increased and BUN/creatinine ratio is high, urinalysis is often helpful in determining a likely cause. In non-oliguric patients, urinalysis is again the most useful test. With normal microscopic urinalysis and proteinuria, UPEP may help differentiate glomerular and tubular injury. Although not shown on the diagram, imaging studies for obstruction should be performed if an obvious cause for renal dysfunction cannot be identified.

Table 6.7.
Clinical–Laboratory Patterns of Renal Disease

Disorder	Major Laboratory Findings	Other Laboratory Abnormalities	Tests for Differential Diagnosis
Prerenal azotemia	Increased BUN, creatinine with high ratio; $FE_{Na} \ll$ 1%, negative free water clearance	High renin, aldosterone	None
Mild glomerular injury (diabetes, hypertension)	Microalbuminuria, normal BUN, creatinine early	None	None
Chronic glomerular injury (Nephrotic syndrome)	Marked proteinuria (>3 g/day)	Decreased serum albumin, elevated cholesterol; BUN, creatinine normal early	None usually in children; complement in adults to detect immune damage
Acute glomerulonephritis	Slight increase in BUN, creatinine, often with high ratio; hematuria, red cell casts, moderate proteinuria	Complement (C_3, C_4) low in most forms; normal with Goodpasture's syndrome; C_4 normal in type II membranoproliferative	ASO-post-infectious ANCA-Wegener's (c-ANCA), polyarteritis/vasculitis (p-ANCA) ANA-systemic lupus Anti-GBM-Goodpasture's
Interstitial nephritis	Slight increase in BUN, creatinine (ratio normal), urine eosinophils	Tubular pattern of proteinuria	None usually
Acute tubular necrosis	Increased BUN, creatinine (ratio normal), free water clearance zero; FE_{Na} >1%	Hyaline, granular casts often present	None
Obstruction	Increased BUN, creatinine: ratio high early, normal later; FE_{Na} <1% early, >1% later; free water clearance negative early, zero later	Dilated urinary system on imaging studies	None
Urinary tract infection	Leukocyte esterase positive, nitrite positive with most gram negative infections; white cells in urine. BUN, creatinine usually normal	WBC casts in pyelonephritis	None
Chronic renal failure	Increased BUN, creatinine (ratio normal), anemia, hypocalcemia, hyperphosphatemia, metabolic acidosis, hyperkalemia	Increased anion gap in late stages	None
Nephrolithiasis	Urine crystals may or may not be present; hematuria when stones break free	Urine calcium, oxalate, citrate, uric acid if stones cannot be recovered	Stone analysis

Glomerular Inflammation = Nephritic Syndrome

Inflammation impairs all glomerular functions, causing reduced GFR, often with decreased urine output; damaged glomeruli leak protein and red cells. Low GFR prevents the rate of loss from exceeding the synthetic rate, so plasma proteins are typically normal. Edema develops due to decreased salt and water excretion. Complement levels are usually low in nephritic syndrome. The most common cause is postinfectious glomerulonephritis, particularly due to streptococci; in the absence of a specific history of streptococcal infection, antistreptolysin O (ASO) can be diagnostic. A variety of immunologic diseases often cause nephritic syndrome, and can be recognized by specific autoantibodies: lupus nephritis (anti-double-stranded DNA), Wegener's granulomatosis (antineutrophil cytoplasmic antibodies, ANCA), and Goodpasture's syndrome (antiglomerular basement membrane antibodies) are the most common.

Mild Tubular Inflammation = Interstitial Nephritis

Most cases of interstitial nephritis are due to reactions to drugs, typically associated with prominent eosinophilic response and increased eosinophils in urine. Tubular function is typically impaired, and BUN and creatinine rise with a normal ratio; urine output is usually normal. The proximal tubule is the most common site of injury; impaired solute absorption causes tubular proteinuria, glucosuria, increased FE_{Na}, hypokalemia, and non-anion gap metabolic acidosis. In some cases, renin production is affected, causing hyperkalemia and, less commonly, hyponatremia.

Severe, Acute Tubular Injury = Acute Tubular Necrosis

The two main causes of acute tubular necrosis (ATN) are drugs, usually damaging proximal tubules, and shock, damaging the loop of Henle. Many cases of drug-induced ATN have normal urine output (nonoliguric), while most cases of shock-induced ATN have decreased urine output (oliguric). BUN and creatinine invariably rise, with a normal ratio; creatinine usually increases by about 1 mg/dL each day. Within hours of onset of ATN, free water clearance approaches zero. Urine sodium losses typically follow after about 24 hours, with FE_{Na} over 1%. In severe cases, urine composition begins to resemble plasma, with Na greater than 100 mmol/L, K less than 10 mmol/L, and creatinine less than 20 mg/dL. In most cases, renal function returns; however, during recovery the tubules are not able to concentrate or to dilute urine (diuretic phase of ATN) and large amounts of water and electrolytes are lost in the urine. During this time, measurement of urine electrolytes is useful to match replacement to losses.

Urinary Tract Obstruction

Obstruction of outflow to one kidney causes gradual loss of function of that kidney, but laboratory abnormalities are usually absent. With gradual obstruction of outflow to both kidneys, urine output may remain normal, but BUN and creatinine will slowly rise. In early stages, BUN rises faster than creatinine, causing a high BUN:creatinine ratio; as obstruction persists, tubular dysfunction prevents BUN absorption and the ratio becomes normal with elevations of both. FE_{Na} and free water clearance initially resemble those in prerenal azotemia, but chronically high pressure leads to tubular dysfunction and a picture resembling ATN. With relief of chronic obstruction, a picture similar to the recovery phase of ATN occurs (postobstructive diuresis); urine electrolytes can be used to guide therapy. Urethral obstruction leads to dilatation of and inability to empty the bladder, which can be detected by measuring residual volume at catheterization after the patient empties the bladder. Obstruction at higher levels leads to dilatation of the ureters and renal pelvis, and later to hydronephrosis (due to renal atrophy), which can be detected on imaging studies.

Suspected Urinary Tract Infection

In patients with symptoms suggestive of urinary tract infection (frequency, urgency, burning, fever) (Chapter 28), urine dipstick for leukocyte esterase and nitrite has a high sensitivity for detecting infection, and treatment can often be given based on these results. Culture and sensitivity is still often recommended before treatment is started in patients with positive dipstick, but is not needed if dipstick is negative. In asymptomatic patients at high risk for urinary tract infection (such as pregnant women), dipsticks have a sensitivity of about 70%, so that urine culture should be performed even if dipstick is negative. White blood cell casts indicate infection involving the kidney (pyelonephritis).

Chronic Renal Insufficiency or Failure

Gradual loss of functioning nephrons is typically asymptomatic; it can only be detected by measuring a reduction in GFR. Initially, BUN and creatinine may be within the reference range, but will gradually increase as more nephrons are lost. Once the amount of renal tissue declines to less than 25–30% of normal, other renal functions, such as calcitriol production and acid excretion are impaired, so that hypocalcemia, nonanion gap metabolic acidosis, and hyperkalemia are often present. As GFR declines to less than 20% of normal, deficient erythropoietin often results in mild anemia. Progressive loss of renal function is usually inevitable by this point, and worsening renal function is often manifested by hypertension, edema, severe anemia, or metabolic bone disease induced by the hypocalcemia. Decreased urine concentrating ability often results in nocturia. In late stages (GFR less than 5% of normal), increased anion gap metabolic acidosis often occurs. Oliguria is uncommon in chronic renal failure; GFR of 1% of normal is adequate to allow a normal urine output. In monitoring patients with chronic renal failure on dialysis, a number of laboratory tests can be useful in detecting important complications. Renal osteodystrophy is a combination of changes, largely related to abnormal parathyroid hormone (PTH) and vitamin D function (Chapter 10). Excess PTH production is common and a major contributor to bone disease; PTH levels, measured every 6–12 months, should be between 3 and 5 times the upper reference limit of normal. Aluminum contamination of dialysis water often contributes to toxicity in dialysis patients (Chapter 19); aluminum should also be measured every 6–12 months.

Nephrolithiasis

When the concentration of solutes in the loop of Henle exceeds their solubility, crystals form. With markedly increased concentrations (uric acid in tumor lysis, calcium oxalate with ethylene glycol poisoning), a picture resembling obstruction occurs as multiple tubules are obstructed. More commonly, a single tubule is obstructed; the crystals gradually enlarge as more solute is deposited on the edge, and may eventually break loose and enter urine (kidney stone). Stones can be analyzed if recovered to determine which components have precipitated. Most stones are calcium oxalate or calcium phosphate; less commonly, uric acid or cystine stones form. If stones cannot be recovered, urine quantitation of excretion of solutes can suggest the etiology. With calcium oxalate stones, the fundamental problem may be excess urine calcium or oxalate or decreased urine citrate (which complexes calcium and prevents precipitation); measurement of each of these solutes often suggests appropriate therapy. A small fraction (5%) are caused by chronic hypercalcemia, usually due to hyperparathyroidism (Chapter 10); serum calcium should be measured in all patients with calcium containing stones.

CHAPTER 7.

Carbohydrate Metabolism

D. ROBERT DUFOUR

Carbohydrates are the major source of energy for most cells. The major carbohydrate of medical importance is glucose; other carbohydrates are discussed briefly at the end of the chapter.

NORMAL GLUCOSE METABOLISM

Glucose is obtained from three major sources. Dietary polysaccharides are digested by amylase (in the mouth and intestine) to release glucose. This is the major source during waking hours. **Glycogen,** polymerized glucose found primarily in liver and muscle, maintains glucose levels during short-term fasting. **Gluconeogenesis,** synthesis of glucose from amino acids mainly in liver, maintains glucose levels during more prolonged fasting.

Hormonal Regulation

Several hormones help maintain glucose concentration within relatively narrow limits by altering rates of clearance and release of glucose (Fig. 7.1).

Insulin

The major glucose lowering hormone is produced by pancreatic islet β-cells when cellular glucose concentration increases above a threshold level; a transporter protein allows glucose entry into β-cells. Insulin is produced and stored as **proinsulin;** when glucose concentration rises, proinsulin is cleaved to insulin and inactive **C-peptide,** and further proinsulin is synthesized. While insulin is cleared rapidly from plasma (half-life about 4 min), C-peptide is removed slowly (half-life 20–30 min) and the half-life of both insulin and C-peptide is prolonged in patients with renal failure. Insulin promotes glucose uptake by most cells, promotes glucose metabolism, and inhibits gluconeogenesis, all lowering plasma glucose. Insulin promotes triglyceride accumulation and inhibits its breakdown, favoring storage of energy as fat. Only 10% of the amount of insulin needed to maintain normal plasma glucose inhibits fat breakdown and prevents ketoacidosis.

Glucagon

Produced by pancreatic islet α-cells in response to low plasma glucose or low insulin, glucagon stimulates glycogenolysis and gluconeogenesis, increasing plasma glucose. It also stimulates triglyceride breakdown and metabolism of fatty acids to form ketone bodies. Several intestinal hormones with a similar structure, termed **glicentins,** have unclear functions.

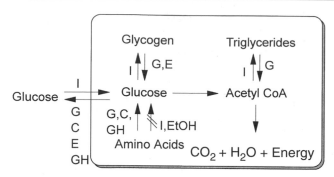

Figure 7.1. Factors Affecting Glucose Metabolism. The liver cell shown illustrates the effects of alcohol (EtOH) and the hormones insulin (I), glucagon (G), epinephrine (E), cortisol (C), and growth hormone (GH) on glucose use and production. Insulin allows glucose entry into cells, and favors production of glycogen and triglycerides to store energy; it also inhibits gluconeogenesis from amino acids. Glucagon has essentially the opposite effects. Cortisol and growth hormone stimulate gluconeogenesis, while epinephrine stimulates glycogen breakdown. These last four hormones make glucose available to cells in the absence of insulin. Alcohol inhibits gluconeogenesis and glycogen breakdown, and may cause hypoglycemia when alcohol ingestion stops.

Insulin-like Growth Factors

The insulin-like growth factors (IGFs) have structural and physiologic similarities to insulin; there are separate receptors for insulin and each of the IGFs. Their importance in regulating serum glucose under normal circumstances is not clear, however, tumors producing IGF-2 have been associated with hypoglycemia. IGF-1 is discussed more fully in Chapter 15.

Other Hormones

Cortisol (and synthetic glucocorticoid hormones) increases gluconeogenesis, catecholamines stimulate glycogen breakdown, and growth hormone antagonizes insulin receptor binding and inhibits tissue glucose utilization. Plasma glucose modifies production of both ACTH and growth hormone: high levels inhibit production, low levels have the opposite effect. Catecholamines stimulate glycogenolysis, raising glucose concentration. Disease states with increased production of any of these hormones may cause hyperglycemia, while deficiency of growth hormone or cortisol is commonly associated with hypoglycemia.

MEASUREMENT OF GLUCOSE

Tests for glucose can be performed using whole blood or plasma. The results are usually set to agree with each other. It is important for the practitioner to understand the relatively common causes of erroneous results for glucose.

Interferences in Measurement of Glucose in Blood, Plasma, and Urine

Glucose is most commonly measured by glucose oxidase in the laboratory, in test strips for home and bedside glucose monitoring, and in urinalysis. In bedside and home testing when using whole blood, the intensity of the color (or, in some strips, an electri-

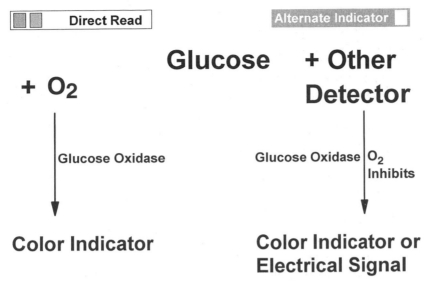

Figure 7.2. Effects of Oxygen on Blood Glucose Test Strips. The oxygen content of blood alters the apparent glucose concentration in whole blood glucose oxidase test systems. With direct read methods, low oxygen or hematocrit causes falsely low glucose, while high values cause erroneous increases. Many newer methods use an alternate indicator; in these methods, low oxygen or hematocrit falsely increases glucose, while high values have the opposite effect. The exact magnitude of the change and the range of acceptable pO_2 and hematocrit values varies from method to method. Newer glucose dehydrogenase methods are not affected by oxygen content.

cal signal) is affected both by glucose and oxygen content (Fig. 7.2), and altered by changes in hematocrit and pO_2. In serum tests and urine dipsticks, very low and constant atmospheric oxygen allows consistent results not affected by blood oxygen content. Deterioration of urine and whole blood glucose strips by exposure to air and inhibition of urine glucose measurement by ascorbic acid are common problems which cause falsely low glucose results. More recent bedside glucose assays use different enzymes and are not subject to these interferences. Whole blood glucose assays are only accurate within a relatively narrow limit [usually 40–50 mg/dL (2.2–2.8 mmol/L] on the low end, 350–400 mg/dL [(19.4–22.0 mmol/L) on the high end]. Patients with values beyond these limits must have serum glucose performed.

Other Causes of Erroneous Glucose Results

Glucose metabolism after collection

Glucose is metabolized by blood cells until plasma is separated from cells. Glucose falls by 3–5% per hour at room temperature in normal blood, faster with elevated white blood cell count and slowed with refrigerator storage. Glucose metabolism can be prevented by sodium fluoride, but these specimens cannot be used for other laboratory tests. Sodium fluoride tubes may be needed if blood will not reach the laboratory for several hours, if storage temperatures are high, or if white blood count is above $100,000/mm^3$.

Arterial–Venous Glucose Differences

Under most circumstances, venous blood glucose is similar to arterial blood glucose (capillary glucose, used in fingerstick measurements, is similar to arterial blood). After meals, venous blood glucose may be 15% lower than capillary glucose because insulin increases tissue glucose uptake. In patients in shock, tissue glucose use causes markedly decreased venous blood glucose, especially when collected from arms or legs; values may be less than 10 mg/dL (0.6 mmol/L). In such situations, patients have no symptoms of hypoglycemia because arterial and capillary glucose are normal. Low venous blood glucose with normal fingerstick glucose strongly suggests critically low perfusion.

OTHER LABORATORY TESTS OF CARBOHYDRATE METABOLISM

Glucose Tolerance

Administration of a large amount of glucose tests β-cells' ability to increase insulin production. In contrast to meals, when glucose is released slowly from starch and other complex sugars, pure glucose (usually 75 g, but 100 g in pregnant women) is given orally over five minutes, allowing rapid absorption. In addition to a fasting glucose specimen, samples are drawn at regular intervals after glucose administration (usually at 0.5, 1, 1.5, and 2 h; extending testing beyond two hours is not useful except during pregnancy). The test is used to diagnose diabetes in patients without classic signs and symptoms of diabetes with normal fasting glucose. Except during pregnancy, glucose tolerance tests are seldom required to establish a diagnosis of diabetes.

Insulin and C-peptide

Measurements of these compounds are most commonly needed to evaluate hypoglycemia. Many patients using nonhuman insulin have insulin antibodies, causing falsely high or falsely low insulin levels. C-peptide is more stable than insulin and has a longer half-life, making it a more useful indicator of endogenous production; insulin antibodies do not interfere. C-peptide half-life (and plasma concentration) is increased by renal failure. C-peptide is not increased when insulin is injected, making it a useful test for recognition of insulin-producing tumors.

Glycation of Proteins

Amine groups react with glucose and other chemicals after protein synthesis, producing irreversibly modified proteins. Among the reactive chemicals are urea, salicylates, bilirubin, acetaldehyde from ethanol metabolism, and glucose (Fig. 7.3). The major blood proteins modified are albumin and hemoglobin. The modified protein can be distinguished from native protein in a variety of ways. Modified protein concentration is directly related to protein life span and average chemical concentration during this time. It essentially integrates the area under the curve of chemical concentration versus time of protein life. In normal circumstances, modified hemoglobin measures average chemical concentration over the past 6–8 weeks, while modified albumin measures average chemical concentration over the past 10–14 days. Glucose–modified proteins are termed **glycated,** although many publications use the term **glycosylated** instead. Glycated protein concentrations must be interpreted in light of factors which affect their levels.

Effects of Acute Changes in Glucose Concentration

An acute, marked increase in glucose persisting for several days produces the same increase in glycated protein concentration as moderate increases over 1–2 weeks or mild increases for many weeks (Fig. 7.4).

Hemoglobin A β-chain Modifications

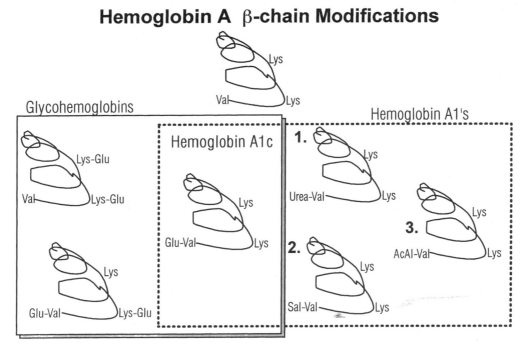

Figure 7.3. Nomenclature of Modified Hemoglobins. Hemoglobin can be modified by attachment of chemicals to reactive sites: the N-terminal valine and lysine residues on the β-globin chain. Glucose attached to N-terminal valine produces hemoglobin A_1c, while other compounds attaching produce other hemoglobin A_1s. Any hemoglobin with glucose attached, whether to valine or lysine or a combination, is termed a glycohemoglobin.

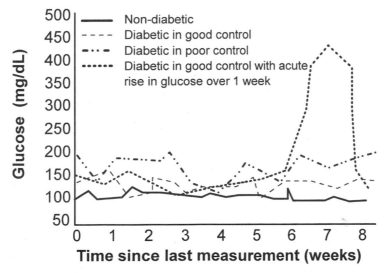

Figure 7.4. Effect of Changes in Glucose Concentration on Hemoglobin A_1c. Hemoglobin A_1c level integrates the area under the curve of glucose versus hemoglobin life; this practically approaches eight weeks. Normal patients and patients with good diabetic control will usually have normal areas under the curve and normal hemoglobin A_1c. Patients with poor control have increased area under the curve and high hemoglobin A_1c. If there is a marked rise in glucose in a patient with previously good control, area under the curve and hemoglobin A_1c are markedly increased.

Table 7.1.
Factors Altering Half-life of Glycated Proteins

Decreased hemoglobin half-life
   Hemolysis (hemoglobinopathies, immune hemolytic anemia, renal failure, thalassemia)
   Bleeding
Increased hemoglobin half-life
   Splenectomy
   Iron Deficiency Anemia
Decreased serum protein half-life
   Protein losing states (nephrotic syndrome, diabetic renal damage, protein losing enteropathy, burns)
   Catabolic states (hyperthyroidism)
Increased protein half-life
   Hypothyroidism

Altered Protein Life Span Changes Relationship of Glucose to Glycated Protein

If protein half-life is decreased, glycated protein is lower for the same average glucose concentration. If protein clearance is retarded, glycated protein concentrations increase. Situations which alter the half-life of hemoglobin and albumin are listed in Table 7.1.

Assays for Glycated Hemoglobin

Several methods for measuring glycated hemoglobins vary in the forms of modified hemoglobin actually measured; most are reported as "hemoglobin A_1c." *It is important for the practitioner to know which glycated hemoglobin assay is used in order to properly interpret results.* The tests used, their nomenclature, and difficulties in use are listed in Table 7.2. Assays which measure total hemoglobin A_1 have been most commonly used, although total glycohemoglobin assays are becoming most common. Methods actually measuring hemoglobin A_1c are still infrequent. The American Diabetes Association recommends use of true hemoglobin A_1c results, with 7.25% the upper limit of acceptable glucose control. All assays provide misleading information on average glucose levels when red cell life span is significantly altered (Table 7.1).

Table 7.2.
Glycated Hemoglobin Assays in Routine Use

Type of Assay	Compound(s) Measured	Advantages	Disadvantages
Total Hemoglobin A_1	All hemoglobin A_1's	Inexpensive, widely available, easy to perform	Falsely low with hemoglobin S, C; falsely high with hemoglobin F, other hemoglobin A_1's (alcohol abuse, renal failure, salicylates)
Total Glycohemoglobin	Any glucose modified hemoglobin	Not affected by hemoglobin variants, can be automated, can be converted to true hemoglobin A_1c	Does not have same correlation with glucose control in very poorly controlled patients
True Hemoglobin A_1c	Hemoglobin A_1c	Not affected by hemoglobin variants, recommended by Am Diabetes Assn	Tends to be most expensive, usually difficult to perform compared to other assays

Fructosamine

Glucose attached to lysine residues on serum proteins, mainly albumin, is measured by the fructosamine assay, which measures glucose control over a shorter period of time (10–14 days) than hemoglobin A_1c. This may be useful in following recent compliance after a period of poor control, or when patients are being seen at frequent intervals after changing therapy. It is of less use than hemoglobin A_1c when patients are seen infrequently. An abnormal ratio of other proteins to albumin, especially IgA, falsely increases fructosamine.

DIABETES MELLITUS

Approximately 4% of the United States population is affected by diabetes, a major cause of morbidity and mortality. Diabetes is caused by deficiency of insulin, either absolute or relative, which causes hyperglycemia.

Classification

There are two major types of diabetes mellitus, with two minor ones classified separately.

Type I (Insulin Dependent, IDDM)

An absolute deficiency of insulin caused by autoimmune destruction of β-cells produces IDDM (10% of diabetics). Cell-mediated immunity to islets and plasma antibodies to islet cell antigens such as insulin and glutamic acid decarboxylase (GAD) can be found for up to 10 years before clinical diagnosis of IDDM, causing a gradual decrease in insulin production with normal glucose. Eventually, the insulin reserve is exhausted; over a few months, the affected individual develops abnormal glucose tolerance, fasting hyperglycemia, and finally ketoacidosis (often triggered by an acute illness). About 25% of IDDM patients have a brief period of not requiring insulin after an initial episode of ketoacidosis (sometimes termed the "honeymoon" period). They will have low–normal insulin and C-peptide during this time.

Type II (Non-insulin Dependent, NIDDM)

Inadequate insulin production caused by a relative decrease in insulin production and by peripheral insulin resistance (exacerbated by increased body fat) produces NIDDM. Relative absence of insulin causes increased glucagon production, increased gluconeogenesis, and increased glycogenolysis. Ketoacidosis usually does not develop since some insulin is available; 10–20% of patients do require insulin to control blood sugar.

Gestational Diabetes

Hyperglycemia developing during pregnancy and resolving after delivery is termed gestational diabetes. The incidence of pregnancy-related complications of diabetes in gestational diabetes is intermediate between that of normal and previously diabetic women.

Secondary Diabetes

Hyperglycemia due to another condition, such as Cushing's syndrome, acromegaly, hyperthyroidism, medications toxic to islet cells (pentamidine), or pancreatic destruc-

Table 7.3.
Criteria for Diagnosis of Diabetes

Adults:
 Random glucose >200 mg/dL (11.1 mmol/L) AND signs or symptoms of diabetes OR
 Fasting glucose >140 mg/dL (7.8 mmol/L) on two or more occasions OR
 Glucose tolerance test: 2 hr PLUS 0.5, 1, or 1.5 hr value >200 mg/dL (11.1 mmol/L) on two or more
   occasions
Children:
 Fasting glucose >140 mg/dL (7.8 mmol/L) on two or more occasions PLUS
 Glucose tolerance test: 2 hr PLUS 0.5, 1, or 1.5 hr value >200 mg/dL (11.1 mmol/L) on two or more
   occasions
Pregnancy:
 Screen: 50 g glucose: 1 hr value >140 mg/dL (7.8 mmol/L) PLUS
 Glucose tolerance test: Two or more of the following values: Fasting >105 mg/dL (5.8 mmol/L); 1 hr
   >190 mg/dL (10.6 mmol/L); 2 hr >165 mg/dL (9.2 mmol/L); 3 hr >145 mg/dL (8.1 mmol/L)
Amount of glucose administered for glucose tolerance test: Adults, 75 g; Children, 1.75 g/kg (maximum 75
 g); Pregnancy, 100 g. Proper preparation, as discussed in text, is essential for correct interpretation.

tion (surgery, chronic pancreatitis) is referred to as secondary diabetes. In some cases, hyperglycemia resolves with treatment of the underlying disorder, but many patients develop permanent diabetes.

Diagnosis

Currently accepted diagnostic criteria are given in Table 7.3. Diagnosis is based on blood glucose levels and signs and symptoms of diabetes (polyuria, polydipsia). Some have suggested use of glycated protein measurements instead. Elevated true hemoglobin A_1c is diagnostic of diabetes but less sensitive than a glucose tolerance test. Glycated protein measurements *should not* be used to diagnose gestational diabetes.

Recognizing, Monitoring, and Preventing Metabolic Complications of Diabetes

Ketoacidosis

With IDDM, ketoacidosis (Chapter 4) occurs when insulin is discontinued or when insulin requirements increase (stress–related increases in cortisol and catecholamines). Hyperglycemia is accompanied by fatty acid metabolism, producing ketone bodies. Tests for recognizing and monitoring ketoacidosis are shown in Table 7.4. Serum

Table 7.4.
Recognition and Monitoring of Ketoacidosis

Recognition:
 Moderate–marked hyperglycemia
 Increased anion gap acidosis
 Positive ketones (titer approximates anion gap)
 Often increased K^+, PO_4, BUN/creatinine indicating dehydration
 Dilutional hyponatremia (Na^+ ↓ 1.5–2.0 mmol/L for every 100 mg/dL (5.5 mmol/L) ↑ in glucose
Monitoring
 Glucose every 2 hours until normal, every 4 hours until ketones negative
 Anion gap every 4 hours till normal
 K^+, PO_4 every 2–4 hours for first 12 hours; treat low values
 Ketones every 4–6 hours after anion gap normalized until negative

Table 7.5.
American Diabetes Association Target Values for
Treatment of Diabetic Patients

Fasting glucose: 80–120 mg/dL (4.4–6.7 mmol/L)
Bedtime glucose: 100–140 mg/dL (5.6–7.8 mmol/L)
True hemoglobin A_1c: <7.25%

glucose measurements are preferable until glucose is less than 400 mg/dL (22.2 mmol/L); below this level, bedside glucose measurements are reliable and results are available more readily, helping to prevent hypoglycemia.

Hyperosmotic Nonketotic Coma (hyperosmolar coma)

When insulin is present but is inadequate for demand, glucose increases without development of ketoacidosis, typically reaching a plateau at 300–400 mg/dL (16.7–22.2 mmol/L), where renal excretion equals rate of production. From this point, high urinary glucose causes polyuria, water loss from brain cells impairs thirst perception, loss of water from other cells produces dehydration, and glucose gradually increases to markedly elevated levels which may reach 1000–1500 mg/dL (55–83.3 mmol/L).

Preventing Complications Related to Chronic Hyperglycemia

Many of the complications of diabetes, including renal injury, peripheral neuropathy, retinal disease, and cataracts, are believed to be caused by poor control of glucose. The Diabetes Control and Complications Trial (DCCT) documented that improved control of glucose prevented retinopathy and glomerular disease. The goals of treatment are based upon maintaining near normal glucose without producing hypoglycemia. Target values for treatment of diabetic patients recommended by the American Diabetes Association are listed in Table 7.5. This group has also recommended annual measurement of urine microalbumin (Chapter 6) in patients with NIDDM, or with IDDM for longer than five years, to detect early renal injury. Patients with microalbuminuria may benefit from more specific measures to prevent renal injury. A discussion of such measures is beyond the scope of this book.

WHEN NOT TO DO TESTS OF GLUCOSE METABOLISM

Blood Glucose

Ideally, glucose should be measured only in the fasting state to screen for diabetes. Screening should only be done on healthy, ambulatory patients, because stress hormones increase glucose during acute illness. In patients with diabetes, controversy exists as to how many daily glucose measurements should be done; the American Diabetes Association suggests fasting and bedtime glucose. There is little evidence that more frequent measurements of glucose in hospitalized patients is more important than in home monitoring, except in patients with ketoacidosis or hyperosmolar states. In hospitalized patients, whole blood glucose measurements should not be used when a patient has anemia or polycythemia until it can be determined that the method is not affected by the change in oxygen content.

Table 7.6.
Preparation for GTT

High carbohydrate intake (>150 g/d) for 3 days
Cancel if vagal reaction occurs when glucose given
Fasting overnight; no caffeine in same period
Testing done only in early morning
Discontinue drugs affecting glucose tolerance (diuretics, oral contraceptives, β-blockers, salicylates, INH, nicotine) if possible
Defer testing during hospitalization, acute illness

Glucose Tolerance Test

Fasting blood glucose is more reliable than the glucose tolerance test (GTT) for diagnosis of diabetes. If fasting glucose is normal and GTT is needed to screen for diabetes, particularly in pregnant women, careful patient preparation is critical to assure accurate results (Table 7.6). GTT should never be performed in hospitalized patients, and should be deferred for at least one month after recovery from acute illness.

Glycated Protein Measurements

As discussed earlier, marked elevations in plasma glucose significantly increase both glycohemoglobin and fructosamine; results will be affected when glucose is greater than 300 mg/dL (16.7 mmol/L). Fructosamine will return to baseline within about two weeks. Hemoglobin A_1c will show a rapid fall over about two weeks, and then will return gradually to baseline by about two months. If interim diabetic control needs to be tested at a follow-up appointment within two months of the episode, fructosamine should be used. Hemoglobin A_1c results will be falsely decreased following an episode of bleeding or hemolysis, and are unreliable after blood transfusion. Results are falsely increased in iron deficiency anemia. In those situations, fructosamine can be used instead. Fructosamine is falsely low with protein losing states; it should not be used in patients with 1+ or greater protein on urine dipsticks.

Microalbumin Measurements

Testing for microalbumin should not be done during acute illness. In patients with signs or symptoms of urinary tract infection or bleeding, testing should be deferred until the condition is resolved.

HYPOGLYCEMIA

In normal humans, decreasing glucose concentration inhibits insulin production and stimulates glucagon production, which usually prevents glucose from falling below 60

⟶

Figure 7.5. Approach to Hypoglycemia. Initial evaluation should be based on whether the patient is diabetic, as antidiabetic therapy is the most common cause. In non-diabetics, patients should be classified as acutely ill or otherwise well. In acute illness, hypoglycemia is often due to organ dysfunction or endocrine diseases such as adrenal and pituitary insufficiency. In well patients, hypoglycemia should be confirmed during a 72–hour fast, with insulin measured during hypoglycemia. If insulin is elevated, C-peptide separates endogenous from exogenous insulin administration. Elevated insulin with low C-peptide indicates surreptitious insulin use.

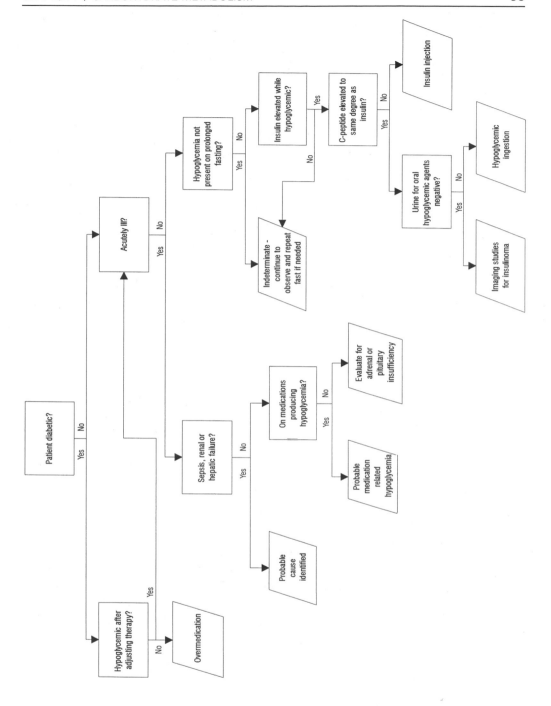

mg/dL (3.3 mmol/L), even with prolonged fasting. Hypoglycemia is defined by plasma glucose concentration below 40 mg/dL (2.2 mmol/L). Symptoms of hypoglycemia (autonomic symptoms such as diaphoresis and neurologic symptoms such as confusion and headache) may occur in patients with relatively rapid fall in glucose, and may be absent in patients with frequent hypoglycemic episodes. The etiology of hypoglycemia varies between patients with other major medical problems and otherwise healthy individuals (Fig. 7.5). In ill patients, hypoglycemia is often due to medications (especially pentamidine), sepsis, shock, renal failure, or endocrine diseases such as hypopituitarism or adrenal insufficiency. Diabetic patients on insulin often become hypoglycemic with change in food intake or in shock (due to decreased insulin clearance and delayed insulin absorption). In otherwise healthy patients, insulin-induced hypoglycemia is the most common cause, and such patients should be evaluated for a possible insulin producing tumor. Rare causes are beyond the scope of this presentation.

72–Hour Fast

The recognized standard approach for suspected insulinoma is to evaluate for hypoglycemia during a prolonged fast. The test is continued until the patient develops plasma (not whole blood) glucose below 40 mg/dL (2.2 mmol/L) or until the fast has continued for 72 hours. Well over half of patients with insulinoma actually become hypoglycemic within 24 hours, and over 95% develop hypoglycemia during the 72 hours. Samples should be obtained for glucose and insulin every 6 hours until the glucose falls below 50 mg/dL (2.7 mmol/L), and then hourly. Specimens are sent for insulin and C-peptide only on the lowest glucose result or the first glucose below 40 mg/dL (2.2 mmol/L). The test is usually interpreted on the basis of the insulin/glucose ratio, which should be greater than 0.3 (when insulin is reported in μU/mL and glucose in mg/dL) in insulin-mediated hypoglycemia. Some have suggested taking the ratio as insulin/(glucose − 30) to correct for the "baseline" glucose level; then levels over 1.0 suggest insulinoma. Insulin should be evaluated along with C-peptide to rule out hypoglycemia due to self-administration of insulin, which is at least as common as insulinoma. Elevated insulin with low C-peptide establishes the diagnosis of insulin injection.

OTHER CARBOHYDRATES

While glucose is the only carbohydrate of interest in adults, metabolic disorders involving other carbohydrates may be present in children. Since most carbohydrates are "reducing substances," these sugars may be detected in urine by older tests for glucose which measured the amount of reduction of copper salts (Benedict's test, Clinitest).

Galactose

Lactose (the major carbohydrate in milk) contains both glucose and galactose. Galactosemia describes several congenital abnormalities of galactose metabolism, usually due to deficiency of galactose-1-phosphate uridyl transferase, causing accumulation of galactose-1-phosphate and damaging several organs. All states screen for this disorder by measuring blood galactose after infants have been fed milk; abnormal screening tests are followed by measurement of enzymes involved in galactose metabolism.

Fructose

Sucrose ("sugar") contains both glucose and fructose, which may accumulate with congenital enzyme deficiency. **Essential fructosuria** (deficiency of liver fructokinase) is associated with high fructose but no clinical symptoms. **Fructose intolerance** (deficiency of fructose-1-phosphate aldolase) prevents the use of fructose-1-phosphate, inhibiting glucose metabolism. Affected individuals develop vomiting and hypoglycemia after ingestion of fructose, often associated with renal tubular dysfunction causing aminoac-iduria and high serum uric acid.

Lactose

Milk must be digested by intestinal lactase into galactose and glucose prior to absorption. Deficiency of lactase is relatively common, but most patients avoid milk and other products containing lactose and have no problems. Rarely, malabsorption may be the initial manifestation of lactase deficiency. Lactase deficiency can be documented, if required, by administration of 25 g of lactose orally ("lactose tolerance test"), with measurement of glucose at 0, 1, and 2 hours. Normally, glucose increases with absorption of liberated glucose. Patients with lactase deficiency often develop significant abdominal discomfort after administration of lactose, and this formal test is not commonly required to establish a diagnosis.

CHAPTER 8

Lipids

D. ROBERT DUFOUR

BLOOD LIPIDS

Lipids are required for many purposes: cholesterol is needed for steroid synthesis and is a critical component of cell membranes; phospholipids are a key element in cell membranes, myelin, and surfactants; triglycerides provide long-term energy storage. Because lipids usually enter the blood stream from the intestine or the liver, these water insoluble compounds must be transported to sites of storage or use within transport packets termed **lipoproteins.** The major lipoproteins and their composition are shown in Table 8.1.

The protein portion of these molecules, termed **apolipoproteins,** perform a variety of functions necessary for normal lipid metabolism (Table 8.2). Blood lipid levels represent the balance between absorption and synthesis on the one hand, and use and clearance on the other. It is easier to understand the various lipoproteins and apolipoproteins in terms of their normal metabolic pathways, as illustrated in Figure 8.1.

Transportation of Dietary Lipid

Absorption of dietary lipid takes place within the small intestine, where free fatty acids and other lipid compounds are taken up into the cytoplasm of epithelial cells, triglycerides are resynthesized, and lipid is incorporated into **chylomicron** particles. On the chylomicron surface is *apo C-II*, an activator of lipoprotein lipase (LPL) (present in muscle and fat), which hydrolyzes the triglyceride. The released free fatty acids enter fat cells for resynthesis into triglycerides, or muscle cells for energy production. Also present is *apo E*, a surface protein which is recognized by liver receptors (apo-B/E receptors) after removal of a large portion of the triglyceride, allowing removal of chylomicron remnants from the blood. Apo E is discussed in more detail later.

Transportation of Liver Synthesized Lipid

The liver is the major organ involved in intermediate metabolism and synthesis of cholesterol and triglycerides. Excess free fatty acids are removed by the liver, and excess dietary calories are converted by the liver into triglyceride molecules. Cholesterol is synthesized in the liver from acetate; while some of the cholesterol is used locally for production of bile acids, the remainder is available for transport. The rate of synthesis of cholesterol in the liver is inversely proportional to dietary cholesterol and directly related to dietary saturated fat. The liver packages both cholesterol and triglyceride into **very low density lipoprotein** (VLDL). As with chylomicrons, apo C-II is present on the surface and activates LPL to release free fatty acids to the tissues. As both triglyceride and apo C-II are gradually lost, the VLDL is converted to smaller **intermediate density lipoprotein** (IDL).

Table 8.1.
Composition and Function of Lipoproteins

Lipoprotein	Lipids	Apoproteins	Function
Chylomicrons	90% triglyceride (TG) 10% cholesterol (C)	1% of weight; apo B48, C-II, E	Delivers dietary triglyceride from intestine to fat cells, muscle; delivers dietary cholesterol to liver
Very Low Density Lipoprotein (VLDL)	60% TG, 20% C	10% of weight; apo B100, C-II, E	Delivers triglyceride from liver synthesis to fat cells, muscle
Intermediate Density Lipoprotein (IDL)	35% TG, 35% C	15% of weight; apo B100, E	Remnant of VLDL metabolism; normally transiently present in circulation
Low Density Lipoprotein (LDL)	10% TG, 50% C	20% of weight; apo B100	Delivers cholesterol from liver synthesis to cells; inhibits further synthesis when binding to receptors
Lipoprotein (a)	10% TG, 50% C	20% of weight; apo B100, apo(a)	No known normal function
High Density Lipoprotein (HDL)	<5% TG, 20% C	50% of weight; apo AI, AII	Converts cholesterol to cholesterol esters; returns cholesterol to liver

Fate of IDL

After removal of most of the triglyceride and apo C-II, some IDL molecules are converted to **low density lipoprotein** (LDL), while others bind to apo-B/E receptors in the liver and inhibit cholesterol synthesis. There are three major inherited variants of apo E. Individuals may be homozygous for one variant (for example, E3/E3), or have one of each of two different types (for example, E3/E4). The most common variant, apo E3, has average affinity for B/E receptor binding. Apo E2 has a substitution which greatly limits receptor binding. Persons homozygous for this form have low levels of LDL, but usually have markedly increased levels of IDL. Apo E4 has a substitution which enhances receptor binding, and inhibits clearance of LDL. Persons homozygous for this variant have increased levels of LDL. Familial forms of Alzheimer's disease

Table 8.2.
Location and Function of Apolipoproteins

Lipoprotein	Found In	Function
AI	HDL, Chylomicrons	Activates LCAT:HDL receptor binding to allow cholesterol extraction from cells
AII	HDL	Not known
B48	Chylomicrons	Structural support
B100	LDL, VLDL	Structural support; receptor binding to deliver cholesterol to target cells; feedback inhibition of liver cholesterol synthesis
CII	Chylomicrons, VLDL; early HDL molecules	Activation of lipoprotein lipase
E	Chylomicrons, VLDL, IDL; some HDL molecules	Receptor binding to clear lipoprotein remnants from circulation
(a)	Lp(a)	Binds to LDL; homology with plasminogen; may inhibit clot lysis, facilitate cholesterol uptake by scavenger receptors

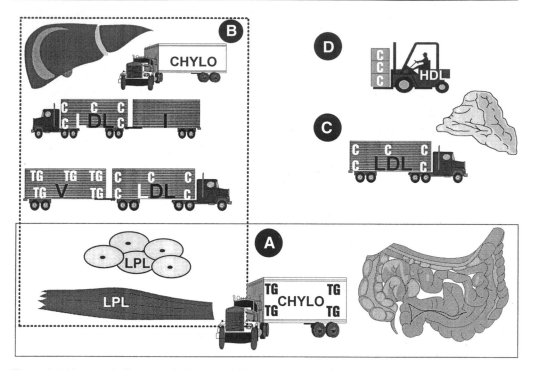

Figure 8.1. Lipoprotein Transport Pathways. Lipids are transported from sites of entry into blood by lipoproteins. Exogenous lipid from food, mainly triglyceride (**A**) is transported to fat and muscle tissues by chylomicrons, where lipoprotein lipase (LPL) breaks down triglyceride for transport into cells. Endogenous lipid, both triglyceride and cholesterol, is synthesized in the liver and released (**B**) as very low density lipoproteins (VLDL). After removal of triglyceride, chylomicron remnants and VLDL remnants (intermediate density lipoproteins, IDL) are recognized by liver receptors and cleared from the blood, inhibiting further cholesterol synthesis. Some IDL are converted to low density lipoproteins (LDL), which deliver cholesterol to tissues (**C**) by both receptor mediated mechanisms in most tissues and scavenger pathway in macrophages, which may lead to atherosclerosis. Cholesterol is returned to the liver (**D**) by high density lipoproteins (HDL).

have been linked to inheritance of the apo E4 variant, and in non-familial forms, those having the gene have an increased risk of developing Alzheimer's disease (higher in E4/E4 persons than in those with one E4 gene).

Transport of Cholesterol to Tissue

After conversion of IDL to LDL, virtually all of the cholesterol remains present, while apo E and apo C-II are lost. Apo B-100, the only structural protein of LDL, is now exposed on the surface and recognized by specific receptor proteins on cells. LDL is taken into cells, the protein degraded, and cholesterol released. In most tissues, cholesterol is used for synthesis of essential components. In the liver, cholesterol additionally inhibits synthesis of cholesterol as well as synthesis of LDL receptor proteins. Thus, LDL normally serves as a feedback mechanism to regulate cholesterol production (however, excess dietary saturated fat or cholesterol overcomes this inhibition). LDL cholesterol can also be removed by **scavenger receptors** on the surface of macrophages and other cells. These receptors react primarily with LDL which has been modified (by oxidation of lipids or attachment of glucose to the apoprotein), and lead to cellular accumulation of lipid. Unlike LDL receptors, these scavenger receptors do not decrease synthesis of cholesterol. An additional factor in the transport of cholesterol is the trace lipoprotein **Lp(a),** which contains both LDL and a specific apoprotein, *apo (a)*. The amount of apo (a) in an individual is determined by genetics, and the apo (a) concentration varies over a range of 1000-times between individuals. Apo (a) has structural homology to plasmin, and can apparently attach to fibria. This produces problems in two ways: by competing with plasmin, it appears to retard breakdown of fibrin; in addition, Lp(a) facilitates LDL accumulation in blood vessels. LP(a) increases risk of both atherosclerosis and arterial thrombosis.

"Reverse" Transport of Cholesterol

High density lipoprotein (HDL), as produced by the liver, contains relatively little lipid; these particles have been termed "nascent" HDL. The two major proteins found in HDL are *apo AI* and *apo AII*. Apo AI is an activator of the enzyme lecithin–cholesterol acyltransferase (LCAT), which produces cholesterol esters (less likely to enter cells). Apo AI also appears to be important in binding to cellular receptors and facilitating the release of cholesterol from cells for uptake by HDL. Apo AII, which is increased by alcohol, has no known function as of yet; however, particles which contain both apo AI and apo AII have decreased ability to remove cholesterol from cells, and may thus be less beneficial to the body. HDL transports cholesterol from peripheral tissues to the liver, where it can be removed from the circulation and excreted.

LIPOPROTEINS AND ATHEROSCLEROSIS

Atherosclerosis is an extremely common disorder, found in virtually 100% of Americans. It causes most cases of heart disease, the most common cause of death in Europe and North America. Numerous studies have shown a strong, direct correlation between total cholesterol and LDL-cholesterol levels and incidence of atherosclerosis, but a strong inverse relationship with HDL-cholesterol. IDL are also considered atherogenic, as they are taken up by the scavenger pathway. Triglyceride levels generally are not considered to be an independent risk factor for atherosclerosis, although high triglycerides correlate with lower HDL-cholesterol concentrations; high triglycerides do increase the risk of pancreatitis. Lipid levels are one of several risk factors for atherosclerosis, making direct prediction of atherosclerosis based on lipid levels alone impossible. The proposed pathogenetic sequence of atherosclerosis (Fig. 8.2) illustrates how other factors affect the rate of progression of atherosclerosis. Lipid levels must be considered along with other risk factors (Table 8.3) in determining risk of atherosclerosis, and on deciding whether and how to treat a patient.

Reference Ranges for Plasma Lipids

Because of the prevalence of atherosclerosis in the United States population, population-based reference ranges for lipids are of little benefit in identifying persons likely to develop atherosclerosis, as discussed in Chapter 1. Until adolescence, lipid values in boys and girls are roughly equal. At puberty, total and HDL cholesterol decrease in males relative to females. With increasing age, cholesterol increases an average of 5–10 mg/dL (0.13–0.26 mmol/L) each decade. Currently, classification of total, LDL-cholesterol, and HDL-cholesterol levels in the United States are based on the recommendations of the National Cholesterol Education Program (NCEP), which determined the relative risk associated with various cholesterol levels.

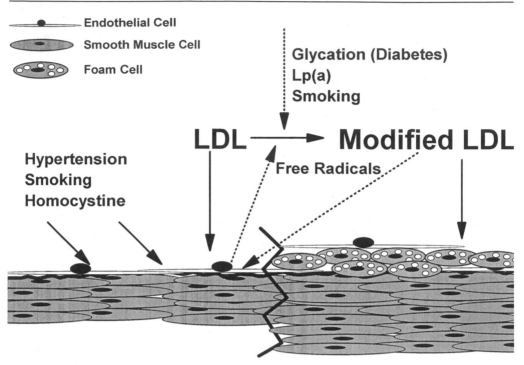

Figure 8.2. Pathogenesis of Atherosclerosis. The current hypothesis on pathogenesis of atherosclerosis highlights the importance of endothelial injury in the initiation of pathologic changes. Among other factors causing damage to endothelial cells are hypertension, various chemicals found in cigarette smoke, and homocystine; increased amounts of LDL may also be directly toxic. Damaged endothelial cells incite an inflammatory response, releasing free radicals which can oxidize the lipid component of LDL. Various cytokines released in response to injury cause accumulation of macrophages, and also stimulate proliferation of smooth muscle cells. Oxidized LDL may also be generated by chemicals found in cigarette smoke. Attachment of carbohydrate in diabetes, and attachment of apoprotein (a) producing lipoprotein (a), are additional modifications which may occur within the LDL molecule. All forms of modified LDL are preferentially taken up by the scavenger pathway found in macrophages, converting them to foam cells.

Lipid Measurements

Tests for lipids have become extremely reliable in most laboratories. It is important for the practitioner to be aware of some of the inherent variation in lipid levels which may affect interpretation about compliance with or response to treatment.

Table 8.3.
Risk Factors for Atherosclerosis

Age (>45 in men, >55 in women)
Family history of premature CAD (MI or sudden death <55 in men or <65 in women)
Current smoking
Hypertension
Diabetes mellitus
HDL cholesterol <35 mg/dL (0.9 mmol/L)
Negative Risk Factor
HDL cholesterol >60 mg/dL (1.6 mmol/L)

Cholesterol

In contrast to the comments made in Chapter 1 regarding the need to evaluate each laboratory's results differently, total cholesterol results are usually very similar when determined in different laboratories. Concentration is relatively unaffected by diurnal variation, and shows no significant change after meals; therefore, specimens for cholesterol can be drawn at any time of day, even after meals. In an average person, cholesterol values vary by an average of 6.5% from one day to the next. Reference values for cholesterol are based on atherosclerosis risk, and are illustrated in Figure 8.3.

Triglyceride

Average daily variation in fasting triglyceride concentration is approximately 25%. Following a meal, triglycerides rise markedly in as little as 15–30 min, due to chylomicrons entering the bloodstream. Triglyceride concentration does not return to baseline until at least 9–12 h following the last food ingestion in an average person; thus, an overnight fast is essential. Classification of triglyceride levels has also been based on clinical significance: levels lower than 200 mg/dL (2.3 mmol/L) are considered normal,

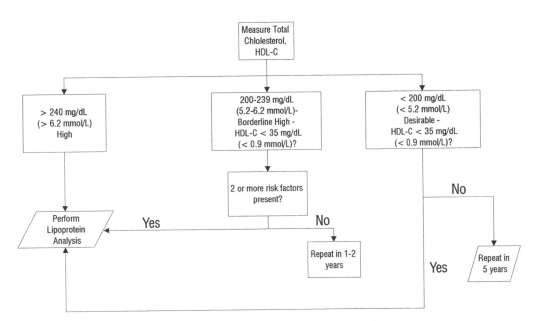

Figure 8.3. National Cholesterol Education Program (NCEP) Guidelines for Screening for Hyperlipidemia in Adults. The NCEP recommends screening of all adults for potentially dangerous levels of lipids to prevent development of critical arterial occlusion by atherosclerosis. Patients with previously diagnosed atherosclerosis based on clinical findings such as coronary artery disease, cerebrovascular disease, or peripheral vascular disease require lipoprotein analysis (Fig. 8.4). Initial screening is done by means of total cholesterol (TC) and high density lipoprotein cholesterol (HDL-C). The major test used in initial classification is TC, with risk classified as desirable (below 200 mg/dL, 5.2 mmol/L), borderline high (200–239 mg/dL, 5.2–6.2 mmol/L), or high (above 240 mg/dL, 6.2 mmol/L). HDL-C results are used for secondary classification, with values below 35 mg/dL (0.9 mmol/L) classified as low. Patients with desirable TC and normal HDL-C are given advice about a healthy life style, with repeat testing recommended after five years. If HDL-C is low, lipoprotein analysis is performed. Patients with borderline high TC, normal HDL-C, and fewer than two other risk factors are also given advice, but are advised to be tested again within two years. All other patients with borderline high or high TC are referred for lipoprotein analysis.

those 200–399 mg/dL (2.3–4.5 mmol/L) are borderline high, values 400–1000 mg/dL (4.5–11.3 mmol/L) are classified as high, and those greater than 1000 mg/dL (11.3 mmol/L) are termed very high.

Lipoprotein

Measurements of lipoproteins show considerable day-to-day variation. Estimates of LDL-cholesterol and HDL-cholesterol variation average over 10% for each.

LDL-cholesterol

In most laboratories, LDL-cholesterol (LDL-C) is not actually measured, but is calculated based on total cholesterol (TC), triglycerides (TG), and HDL-cholesterol (HDL-C) (all concentrations in mg/dL) using the Friedewald Equation (Eq. 8.1).

$$LDL-C = TC - HDL-C - \left(\frac{TG}{5}\right) \tag{8.1}$$

This estimate of LDL-C is reasonably accurate as long as there are no chylomicrons or IDL present, and triglyceride concentration is less than 400 mg/dL (4.5 mmol/L). LDL-C can also be measured directly, but the assay tends to overestimate LDL-C when increased chylomicrons or VLDL are present. Day to day variation is approximately 10%; for this reason, NCEP recommends that decisions on treatment be based on an average of two results performed within 1–8 weeks of each other. If there is a difference of more than 30 mg/dL (0.76 mmol/L) between the two values, then a third determination should be made and the three values averaged. Reference values are based on the risk of atherosclerosis, and are described in Figure 8.4.

HDL-cholesterol

Measurements of HDL-C are less well standardized than total cholesterol tests. In most laboratories, an attempt is made to precipitate all other lipoproteins, and the remaining cholesterol is considered to represent HDL-cholesterol. Although this technique over-estimates HDL-cholesterol when chylomicrons or VLDL are present in increased amounts, it is considered the most reliable measurement for routine use. The effect of chylomicrons means that the test should be performed on fasting specimens. The NCEP has suggested routine measurement of HDL-cholesterol regardless of whether the patient has been fasting. Because falsely high HDL-cholesterol leads to underestimation of LDL-cholesterol and, therefore, of risk of atherosclerosis, our recommendation is to only perform lipid testing in patients who are fasting. HDL-cholesterol values below 35 mg/dL (0.9 mmol/L) are associated with increased risk of atherosclerosis, while values greater than 60 mg/dL (1.6 mmol/L) are associated with reduced risk.

Apolipoprotein

Measurements of apo AI and apo B can be made more accurately than lipoprotein cholesterol concentrations, and may actually correlate better with risk of atherosclerosis. Because there has been no prospective validation of appropriate "risk values" for apolipoproteins, they are not commonly used at present. Lipoprotein (a) has been associated with hypercoagulable states, and has been used for evaluation of patients with arterial thrombosis.

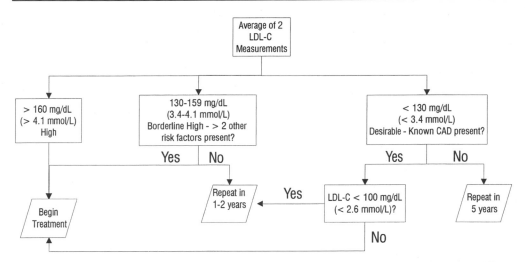

Figure 8.4. National Cholesterol Education Program (NCEP) Guidelines for Lipoprotein Analysis and Treatment Decisions in Adults. Lipoprotein analysis involves measurement of total cholesterol (TC), triglycerides, high density lipoprotein cholesterol (HDL-C), and either measurement or calculation of low density lipoprotein analysis (LDL-C) on two occasions 1–8 weeks apart. The results of the two tests are averaged. If the two LDL-C values differ by more than 30 mg/dL (0.76 mmol/L), a third measurement is performed and the three values averaged. As with screening TC values, LDL-C results are classified into three risk groups: desirable (below 130 mg/dL, 3.4 mmol/L), borderline high (130–159 mg/dL, 3.4–4.1 mmol/L), and high (above 160 mg/dL, 4.1 mmol/L). Patients with known atherosclerosis are considered separately, with target LDL-C values less than 100 mg/dL (2.6 mmol/L). Patients with desirable LDL-C are educated on a healthy life style and asked to return within five years for repeat testing. Those with borderline high LDL-C are evaluated on the presence of other risk factors. If fewer than two others are present, education is given and the patient is asked to return within one year for repeat testing. A similar approach is used for patients with known atherosclerosis and LDL-C below 100 mg/dL (2.6 mmol/L). All other patients are begun on treatment, with dietary therapy and exercise usually recommended initially.

When Not to Do Lipid Testing

Acute tissue injury causes a marked fall in total and LDL-cholesterol values. This decrease begins within one day of myocardial infarction, surgery, or septicemia, and can cause as much as a 40% decline in total and LDL-cholesterol values. VLDL increases by as much as 25%. Lipid values do not return to baseline for at least three months. HDL-cholesterol may fall by as much as 15% with even elective hospital admission. For these reasons, lipid values should not be done at the time of acute illness or for at least three months later for assessing the risk of atherosclerosis. Pregnancy causes a marked rise in lipid concentration, with values approximately doubling for total and LDL-cholesterol. Lipid values in prepubertal children are not well correlated with lipid concentrations seen in adulthood; many children with high cholesterol will not have high risk cholesterol as adults, and many adults with high cholesterol did not have high cholesterol as children. These observations have caused many to question the benefits of screening for cholesterol abnormalities in prepubescent children. The NCEP does not support routine lipid screening in children, but recommends testing children whose parents have clearly elevated cholesterol or in whom there is a strong family history of premature atherosclerosis. In high risk children, decision levels for desirable, borderline high, and high total cholesterol and LDL-cholesterol are 30 mg/dL (0.76 mmol/L) lower than the comparable values in adults given in Figures 8.3 and 8.4. A number of medications, listed in Chapter 38, are known to alter cholesterol

Table 8.4.
NCEP Target Levels for Treatment of High LDL Cholesterol

Risk Factors	Total Cholesterol Target	LDL Cholesterol Target
Less than two other risk factors	<240 mg/dL (6.2 mmol/L)	<160 mg/dL (4.1 mmol/L)
Two or more risk factors	<200 mg/dL (5.2 mmol/L)	<130 mg/dL (3.4 mmol/L)
Known coronary artery disease or other form of atherosclerosis	Not recommended	<100 mg/dL (2.6 mmol/L)

concentration. Patients who will be on these medications for only a brief period should not have lipid testing performed during the time they are taking these medications. Patients who will be receiving therapy with these agents for a prolonged period should not be tested until approximately three months after achieving a stable dosage regimen.

What Lipid Tests Should be Used for Atherosclerosis Risk Assessment?

The NCEP recommends measurement of total and HDL-cholesterol for initial evaluation of risk of atherosclerosis. These results are interpreted based on the lipid levels and presence of other risk factors listed in Table 8.3, using the algorithm given in Figure 8.3. For patients with increased risk, lipoprotein analysis is performed by measuring fasting cholesterol, triglycerides, HDL-cholesterol, and either a measured or calculated LDL-cholesterol. Decisions on treatment are based on LDL-cholesterol values and the presence of other risk factors (Fig. 8.4).

What Lipid Tests Should be Used for Follow-up of Treatment?

If treatment for high lipid levels is needed, the NCEP has established target values for LDL-cholesterol to determine adequacy of therapy. Patients should be on a specific form of therapy (diet, exercise, or medications) for at least 3–6 months before repeating lipid levels. Details on treatment are beyond the scope of this book. While decisions on whether to change treatment are based on LDL-cholesterol, the NCEP recommends the use of total cholesterol as a screen, with measurement of LDL-cholesterol only when the cholesterol is below the target values. Practically, however, this requires the patient to return for a second visit, which may outweigh the savings of doing only cholesterol as the initial test; we perform both tests simultaneously. The recommended target goals for therapy vary depending on the presence of other risk factors, and are listed in Table 8.4.

LIPID AND LIPOPROTEIN ABNORMALITIES

The importance of various lipid disorders has become widely recognized in the past 30 years. The work of Fredrickson and Levy in the late 1960s called attention to the *patterns* of lipoprotein abnormalities which can be seen with inherited lipid disorders; their classification system is still used by some practitioners (Table 8.5). Because many (if not most) lipoprotein abnormalities are either multifactorial or acquired, this system is no longer in widespread use as a classification scheme, although some still use it as a descriptive system. The NCEP does not currently classify lipid disorders beyond determining which lipoprotein is the cause of elevated cholesterol. It does, however,

Table 8.5.
Fredrickson-Levy Classification of Lipid Disorders

Type	Lipoprotein Increased	Lipids Increased
I	Chylomicrons	Triglyceride (T:C ratio >10:1)
II	LDL (Also VLDL in IIb)	Cholesterol (T:C ratio <1); Triglyceride also increased in IIb (T:C ratio about 1)
III	IDL	Triglyceride, cholesterol (T:C ratio 1)
IV	VLDL	Triglyceride, sometimes cholesterol (T:C ratio 2:1–5:1)
V	VLDL, Chylomicrons	Triglyceride, cholesterol slightly increased (T:C ratio 5:1–10:1)

recommend evaluation for possible familial or secondary hyperlipidemia when clinically indicated. The major causes of familial and secondary hyperlipidemia are discussed below.

Hypercholesterolemia

Increased cholesterol is due, in most cases, to a combination of high dietary intake of fat and mild genetic differences in lipid metabolism, with perhaps 5% of cases having secondary or familial disorders as the primary cause. The most important of these are discussed below.

Familial Hypercholesterolemia

This inherited defect in LDL receptors leads to defective feedback inhibition, increased cholesterol uptake by the scavenger pathway, and premature atherosclerosis. Heterozygous individuals (prevalence about 1 in 500 in Europe and North America) have half the normal LDL receptors, and have cholesterol concentrations in the 300–500 mg/dL (7.6–13 mmol/L) range. They typically develop myocardial infarction by their 30s or early 40s. Homozygous individuals, about 1 in 1,000,000, completely lack LDL receptors, have cholesterol concentrations in the 800–1000 mg/dL (20.8–26 mmol/L) range, often have eruptive tendon xanthomas, and suffer myocardial infarction before age 20.

Familial Hyperbetalipoproteinemia

This entity probably represents a variety of disorders, at least some of which are associated with a change in LDL or LDL receptor structure. Cholesterol concentrations are usually between 250–400 mg/dL (6.5–10.4 mmol/L) and premature atherosclerosis often presents in the 40–50 year range.

Familial Hyperalphalipoproteinemia

An autosomal dominant trait is associated with marked increase in HDL-cholesterol. Affected persons have a slight to moderate increase in total cholesterol, but normal LDL-cholesterol. These individuals have mild or no atherosclerosis and often live to be over 90.

Secondary Hypercholesterolemia

A variety of acquired disorders increase lipoprotein synthesis (e.g., nephrotic syndrome, obstructive jaundice) or decrease their catabolism (e.g., hypothyroidism), in-

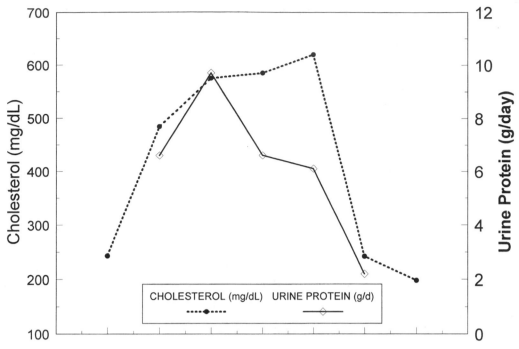

Figure 8.5. Effects of Nephrotic Syndrome on Plasma Cholesterol. In this patient with nephrotic syndrome, serum cholesterol increased markedly with development of proteinuria, and returned to baseline when proteinuria diminished. At its peak, when urine protein was approximately 10 g daily, serum cholesterol reached values over 600 mg/dL (15.6 mmol/L).

creasing plasma cholesterol. Many patients with secondary hypercholesterolemia have cholesterol concentrations of 600–800 mg/dL (15.2–20.8 mmol/L) or higher. Successful treatment of the underlying disorder typically causes a marked fall in cholesterol, often to normal or baseline values (Fig. 8.5).

Increased Triglyceride

High triglyceride concentration is generally of less significance than increased cholesterol and is often not treated. There is an inverse correlation between triglyceride concentration and HDL-cholesterol concentration, and marked increases in triglyceride concentration (over 1000 mg/dL, 11.3 mmol/L) can precipitate intermittent abdominal pain, lipid deposits in skin, and pancreatitis. As with cholesterol, most cases of high triglycerides are due to diet, although secondary increases due to alcohol abuse, diabetes mellitus, and renal failure are also common. Only rarely is increased triglyceride due to inherited disorders of lipid metabolism, as discussed below.

Increased IDL

Familial dysbetalipoproteinemia is a relatively rare cause of increased triglyceride, virtually always associated with homozygosity for apo E2, preventing hepatic IDL clearance. The increased IDL is cleared by the scavenger receptors and leads to premature atherosclerosis. Triglyceride concentrations are moderately elevated, and cholesterol concentration tends to be similar to that of triglyceride (both usually in the 300–400 mg/dL range).

Increased Chylomicrons

Chylomicron elevations rarely are responsible for increased triglycerides, but produce the most dramatic elevations. Although rare inherited deficiencies in apo CII and LPL occur, virtually all cases of increased chylomicrons are secondary. Disorders in metabolism of lipids which cause increased VLDL, such as diabetes and alcohol abuse, tend to overload LPL. A decrease in activity can lead to enzyme saturation; further dietary intake causes a rapid increase in triglyceride concentration. It is not uncommon for such individuals to have triglyceride concentrations over 5,000 mg/dL (56.5 mmol/L), and for increases of 2,000–4,000 mg/dL (22.6–45.2 mmol/L) to occur over the course of a few days. Such persons often develop abdominal pain and/or pancreatitis. They respond promptly to cessation of oral food intake; concentrations can fall from over 10,000 mg/dL (113 mmol/L) to less than 1,000 mg/dL (11.3 mmol/L) in 24–48 hours.

CHAPTER 9

Plasma Proteins

D. ROBERT DUFOUR

NOMENCLATURE OF PROTEINS

The term "plasma protein" refers to those polypeptides present at concentrations greater than 10 mg/dL (0.1 g/L). Furthermore, these proteins have a function in plasma, rather than a transient presence following release due to cell injury (as enzymes and "tumor markers," for example). There are approximately 20 peptides which meet this definition and form the basis for this chapter. Although all of these proteins except fibrinogen are present in both serum and plasma, serum is usually tested.

Protein Nomenclature

Proteins are classified in two different ways. The older nomenclature, which still persists, describes the physicochemical characteristics of proteins, grouping them on the basis of migration in electrophoresis (prealbumin, albumin, α_1-globulin, α_2-globulin, β-globulin, and γ-globulin). Most bands actually consist of several proteins, so that a newer classification system was created, based on the chemical name and function of each protein. The older system is still employed when protein electrophoresis is ordered. The major proteins comprising each of the electrophoretic bands are given in Table 9.1.

Source and Function of Plasma Proteins

Almost all plasma proteins are produced in the liver, the exceptions being peptide hormones, von Willebrand factor, and immunoglobulins. Major protein functions are outlined in Table 9.1. Proteins serve three major functions. Most are transport proteins, carrying a substance from cell to cell; examples include transferrin, lipoproteins, and albumin. Some are involved in protection of the body, serving to limit inflammatory damage or to attack foreign antigens; immunoglobulins, α_1-antitrypsin, haptoglobin, and complement are examples of this class. The final function is to provide oncotic pressure, necessary to prevent loss of fluid from the vascular space to interstitial fluid; albumin is the major protein of this type.

Factors Affecting Protein Levels

The regulation of plasma protein synthesis is not totally understood. Because most proteins are produced in the liver from dietary amino acids, liver disease and protein malnutrition lead to decreased levels of most proteins (although immunoglobulins are not low in liver disease). Cytokines such as *interleukin-1* and *interleukin-6* (IL-1, IL-6) stimulate hepatic synthesis of proteins which modify inflammatory response. These are often termed **acute phase reactants.** Synthesis of some transport proteins, including albumin, transthyretin, and transferrin, is inhibited in acute inflammatory states. Hepatic protein synthesis is stimulated by a fall in oncotic pressure, but only if adequate

Table 9.1.
Proteins Responsible for Electrophoretic Bands

Band	Protein(s)	Function	Factors Affecting Levels
Prealbumin	1. Retinol binding protein 2. Transthyretin	1. Transport for vitamin A 2. Reserve binder for thyroxine	1. 2: INC: GC DEC: LD, MN, AI, CI, NS
Albumin	Albumin	Transport for drugs, endogenous chemicals; oncotic pressure; amino acid source	DEC: LD, MN, AI, CI, NS, GC
α_1-globulin	1. α_1-Antitrypsin	1. Protease inhibitor; inactivates trypsin, other proteolytic enzymes from inflammatory cells	1. INC: AI, CI DEC: LD, MN, NS
	2. Orosomucoid	2. Immune response modifier, drug binder for acidic drugs such as lidocaine	2. INC: AI, CI, GC DEC: LD, MN, NS
	3. High density lipoprotein (HDL)	3. Reverse transport of cholesterol	3. INC: ES DEC: AI, LD, MN
α_2-globulin	1. α_2-Macroglobulin	1. Protease inhibitor	1. INC: AI, CI, NS DEC: LD, MN
	2. Haptoglobin	2. Hemoglobin binding protein	2. INC: AI, CI, NS, GC DEC: LD, MN, ES
	3. Ceruloplasmin	3. Ferroxidase, needed for iron transport; copper binding protein	3. INC: AI, CI, ES DEC: LD, MN
β-globulin	1. Transferrin	1. Iron transport and delivery to cells	1. INC: Fe deficiency, ES DEC: AI, CI, LD, MN, NS
	2. Low density lipoprotein	2. Cholesterol delivery to tissue	2. INC: NS, Androgen DEC: ES, LD, MN, CI
	3. C3	3. Complement component; inflammatory mediator	3. INC: AI, CI DEC: MN, LD
	4. IgA	4. Immunoglobulin involved in secretions	4. INC: LD, CI DEC: MN
	5. Fibrinogen	5. Coagulation factor (found only in plasma, not serum)	5. INC: AI, CI DEC: LD, MN
γ-globulin	1. IgG	1. Major immunoglobulin; long term immunity	1,2. INC: CI DEC: MN
	2. IgM	2. Initial response immunoglobulin	
	3. C-reactive protein	3. Inflammatory response mediator	3. INC: AI DEC: LD, MN

INC: Increased; DEC: Decreased; LD: Liver disease; MN: Malnutrition; AI: Acute inflammation (acute phase response); CI: Chronic inflammation; ES: Estrogen; GC: Glucocorticoids; NS: Nephrotic syndrome

amino acids are present. When oncotic pressure decreases due to renal protein loss in nephrotic syndrome, plasma levels of large molecular weight proteins [including low density lipoprotein (LDL), α_2-macroglobulin, and haptoglobin] will increase since they are too large to pass into the urine. States of increased protein breakdown, as may occur following burns or with high levels of glucocorticosteroids, will lead to reduced concentration of most proteins (although transthyretin, orosomucoid, and LDL are increased by glucocorticosteroids). Sex hormones alter synthesis of several transport proteins; in general, these effects are more apparent with estrogen, and affect primarily high density lipoprotein (HDL) and ceruloplasmin. Table 9.1 summarizes the effects of these various factors on plasma protein levels.

TESTS FOR DETERMINATION OF PLASMA PROTEINS

Total Protein and Albumin

Total protein and albumin measurements are widely used, and commonly available in chemistry panels. By subtracting albumin from total protein, **globulins** (a summation of all proteins other than albumin, mainly immunoglobulins) can be calculated. These tests are capable of detecting gross abnormalities in plasma proteins, as may occur with common conditions such as cirrhosis, severe protein malnutrition, multiple myeloma, autoimmune disease, and AIDS. Subtle changes in individual proteins or early diseases of these types are not usually recognizable. Hemolysis and very high triglycerides interfere with both tests.

Plasma Protein Electrophoresis

The main indications for performing plasma protein electrophoresis are follow-up of abnormal globulins identified from total protein and albumin for possible monoclonal

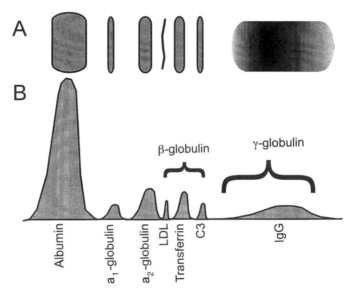

Figure 9.1. Normal Protein Electrophoresis. Proteins are separated in an electrical current, allowing identification of protein **bands (A)** after staining. Examination of the gel in a densitometer allows determination of the relative amounts of protein present, converting each of the bands to **peaks (B)**. These two terms occasionally lead to confusion; laboratory textbooks refer to monoclonal bands, while clinical textbooks describe monoclonal peaks or "spikes." The tallest peak in the scan is arbitrarily set to extend the full height of the scan. Laboratories usually send out copies of the tracing produced, although visual inspection of the gel provides more information; scans can be misleading, since the *relative* amount of individual proteins (compared to albumin) is actually expressed. The major proteins identifiable on protein electrophoresis are indicated. While most proteins are single chemical compounds and form discrete bands, immunoglobulins vary in makeup and form a broad ("polyclonal") staining pattern. With monoclonal proliferation of plasma cells, a single protein type is produced, and there is a discrete ("monoclonal") band similar to that seen with other proteins.

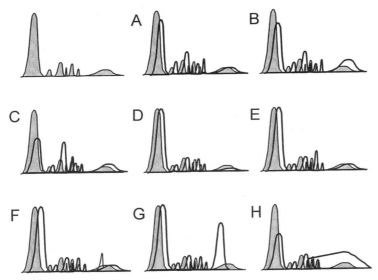

Figure 9.2. Abnormal Protein Electrophoresis Patterns. A normal protein electrophoretic pattern is shown in the upper left hand corner; abnormal patterns are shown relative to this as white tracings on the normal grey background. (**A**) Acute inflammation causes increase in α_1-globulin, α_2-globulin, and C3, while albumin (Alb) and transferrin (Tf) decrease. (**B**) In chronic inflammation, these changes are accompanied by a polyclonal increase in γ-globulins. (**C**) With protein losing states such as nephrotic syndrome, large proteins (α_2-globulin, LDL) increase while small proteins (Alb, Tf, α_1-globulin) decrease; γ-globulins may also be decreased. (**D**) In hypogammaglobulinemia, all other proteins are normal. (**E**) In iron deficiency, Tf is increased while other proteins are normal. (**F**) In monoclonal gammopathy of undetermined significance, a small, narrow band (spike) is present in addition to normal immunoglobulins in the γ-globulin region. (**G**) In multiple myeloma and Waldenstrom's macroglobulinemia, a monoclonal band (spike) replaces the normal γ-globulins. (**H**) In cirrhosis, liver produced proteins (all except the γ-globulins) are decreased; a polyclonal increase in IgG and IgA causes increased γ-globulins and β-γ bridging (IgA fills in the usual space between the β-band and γ-bands).

gammopathy, and follow-up of patients with known monoclonal gammopathy. Separating proteins in a gel (using electrical current) allows evaluation of several different proteins (Fig. 9.1). In general, an experienced interpreter can comment (in a semiquantitative fashion) about albumin, α_1-antitrypsin (α_1-AT), α_2-globulins, transferrin, C3, and IgG, as well as recognize the presence of monoclonal immunoglobulins. Several patterns of changes in proteins can be recognized, as illustrated in Figure 9.2. Electrophoresis is very useful for detecting the presence of abnormal proteins, such as monoclonal immunoglobulins, but of limited utility for other purposes.

Quantitation of Individual Proteins

Quantitation of individual proteins is preferred for all proteins except immunoglobulins, where protein electrophoresis separates monoclonal from polyclonal increases and can detect smaller amounts of monoclonal proteins than can quantitative immunoglobulins. Quantitative methods for IgM and IgA frequently produce erroneous results in patients with monoclonal proteins (Fig. 9.3). Patients with monoclonal IgM have monomeric forms which cause overestimation, while monoclonal IgA exists as polymers, producing falsely low results. The proteins commonly analyzed by quantitative assays are listed in Table 9.2.

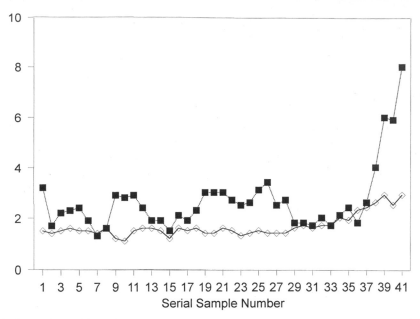

Figure 9.3. Comparison of Results of Monoclonal IgM. Serial results from this patient with Waldenstrom's macroglobulinemia compare results from the electrophoretic scan (open diamonds) with results from "quantitative" IgM assays (solid squares). Variation in the amount of monomers, normally absent from serum, causes significant overestimation of IgM using quantitative assays. Polymers of IgA cause false underestimation with quantitative IgA assays in patients with IgA myeloma.

Immunofixation Electrophoresis and Immunoelectrophoresis

These techniques are used to confirm the presence and identity of monoclonal immunoglobulins. Most laboratories use immunofixation (Fig. 9.4) because it is more sensitive and much easier to interpret. In many institutions, these tests are only done for initial evaluation if protein electrophoresis identifies a monoclonal band; they are not useful for follow-up.

Table 9.2.
Proteins Commonly Measured by Quantitative Assays

Albumin
α_1-Antitrypsin
β_2-Microglobulin
Ceruloplasmin
Complement components (C3, C4)
C-reactive protein
Haptoglobin
High Density Lipoprotein (as HDL cholesterol or apolipoprotein A)
Immunoglobulin E
Immunoglobulnis A, G, M (studied by electrophoresis if monoclonal protein suspected or previously confirmed)
Low Density Lipoprotein (as LDL cholesterol or apolipoprotein A)
Prealbumin (transthyretin)
Retinol-binding protein
Transferrin (or as Total Iron Binding Capacity)

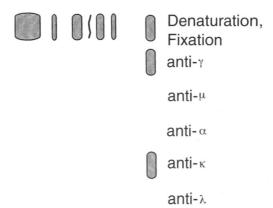

Figure 9.4. Immunofixation Electrophoresis. This is the most widely used technique for determining the type of monoclonal immunoglobulin present. Several repeated samples of the same serum are put on a single gel, after which the top-most is subjected to denaturation, "fixing" proteins onto the gel. In the remaining samples, an antiserum to one immunoglobulin chain is incubated with the serum, and then the plate is washed. When stained, only the proteins in the top sample and any antigen–antibody complexes will be "fixed" to the gel. In the example illustrated, the patient's serum is "fixed" by anti-γ and anti-κ sera, indicating a monoclonal IgG kappa protein.

PHYSIOLOGY AND PATHOPHYSIOLOGY OF INDIVIDUAL PLASMA PROTEINS

This section discusses the clinical significance of most major proteins. Complement levels are discussed in the section on immunology, while lipoproteins are discussed in the chapter on lipids (Chapter 8). Immunoglobulins are discussed separately later in this chapter.

Albumin

Albumin, the most abundant plasma protein, is synthesized by the liver, with a rate inversely related to oncotic pressure. It is a relatively small protein (M.W. 66,000) with a strong negative charge, which allows it to bind a wide variety of positively charged molecules (Ca^{++}, Mg^{++}), as well as having non-polar binding sites for drugs, lipids, bilirubin, and hormones. There are no disease states that cause albumin overproduction, elevated levels occur with hemoconcentration only. Hypoalbuminemia is common in hospitalized patients (Table 9.3).

α_1-Antitrypsin

α_1-Antitrypsin, a protease inhibitor (P_i) of both plasma and tissue enzymes, is important in limiting damage from white blood cell products such as elastase. α_1-AT synthesis is

Table 9.3.
Approach to Decreased Albumin

If Albumin is:	and Globulins are:	Consider:
Low	Low	Malnutrition; protein losing states (albumin reduced more)
Low	Normal	Protein losing states; acute inflammatory disorders
Low	High	Cirrhosis, AIDS, chronic inflammation, monoclonal gammopathy

increased by IL-1. The major cause for decreased α_1-AT is congenital. Inherited variants differing in a single amino acid can be separated by isoelectric focusing. Some variants prevent release from the liver, causing decreased protease inhibition and hepatocyte inclusions of α_1-AT. Unopposed proteases cause tissue injury, most notably in: the lungs, producing emphysema; the liver, producing hepatitis in both children and adults which may progress to cirrhosis; and less commonly affecting other organs. Quantitative α_1-AT or plasma protein electrophoresis (α_1-AT is the major α_1-globulin) can be used to screen for this disorder. Measurement should not be done during any inflammatory disease, since increased production may cause levels to fall within the reference range. If levels are low, the P_i type is determined by isoelectric focusing (phenotyping) to determine which variant or variants the patient possesses. These have been named based on their relative migration, with M (medium) being the most common, S (slow) being rare but usually not significant, and Z (for very slow) being the most dangerous. Patients who have only the Z phenotype (ZZ) constitute the vast majority of cases clinically associated with emphysema and liver damage, although patients with SZ, MZ, or SS types may rarely develop disease. Low levels also occur in malnutrition, cirrhosis, and protein losing states, but phenotype is normal.

β_2-Microglobulin

β_2-Microglobulin is a very small protein (M.W. 11,800), and is found on the surface of nucleated cells as the light chain of the Class I HLA antigen. Although present on all cells, levels mainly reflect proliferation or turnover of lymphocytes. As a small protein, it is freely filtered by the glomerulus, and in normal circumstances almost totally reabsorbed by the proximal tubules. High levels are usually due to decreased renal clearance (renal insufficiency or failure) or increased immune activity (acute or chronic inflammation, especially autoimmune diseases and AIDS; response to "foreign" antigens, as in tumors or transplant rejection; and B-cell neoplasms such as multiple myeloma and B-cell lymphomas). It is most commonly used as a prognostic marker in hematologic malignancies and for evaluating transplant rejection. In renal transplants especially, levels must be interpreted in light of the patient's renal function, with a baseline value serving as a good means for comparison as long as renal function remains stable. Urine β_2-microglobulin has been used to detect renal tubular injury. It is unstable if urine pH is kept above 6.0.

Ceruloplasmin

Ceruloplasmin (ferroxidase) is an enzyme that converts Fe^{++} to Fe^{+++}, allowing transferrin to bind iron. It contains approximately six copper ions per molecule of protein, mainly serving as enzyme activators. Ceruloplasmin is increased in all inflammatory diseases; its synthesis is also stimulated by estrogens. Levels are also increased in patients with Hodgkin's disease and with biliary tract obstruction. Low levels occur with liver disease, malnutrition, and in nephrotic syndrome, but the most important cause is Wilson's disease, an autosomal recessive disorder associated with copper accumulation in tissues. Only about 80% of patients with Wilson's disease have clearly decreased ceruloplasmin concentration; it is important to not measure ceruloplasmin when inflammation or estrogens cause falsely high concentrations. Other tests which are abnormal in Wilson's disease include a reduced plasma copper (also affected by estrogens or inflammation) and increased urine copper excretion. Plasma and urine copper are also increased by active liver disease, since the liver contains most copper stores in the body. Urine copper excretion is also increased when there is proteinuria, because almost all copper in plasma is protein bound.

C-Reactive Protein

C-Reactive protein (CRP) is a large protein involved in defense against foreign antigens; it has the ability to bind to a large number of compounds and can activate complement. Synthesis of CRP increases within 4–6 h of onset of inflammation, reaching peak values within 1–2 days at concentrations that may be many hundreds of times normal. This is many times the increase in other "acute phase response" proteins, which seldom increase by more than 3–5 times normal. CRP levels also fall quickly after resolution of inflammation, since its half-life is 6 h. The main use for CRP is as a marker of inflammation which rises before an increase in granulocyte count. Its main limitation is in its non-specific response.

Haptoglobin

Haptoglobin, a large protein structurally similar to immunoglobulin, binds hemoglobin entering the circulation. The hemoglobin–haptoglobin complex is cleared with a half-life of minutes. Haptoglobin is increased in acute inflammation, in protein losing states, and with glucocorticosteroid treatment, while levels are decreased by hemolysis, liver disease, malnutrition, and high estrogen states. Several genetic variants cause a wide range of "normal" results, and about 4% of African–Americans congenitally lack haptoglobin. Practically, a single haptoglobin level is of little use in evaluating a patient with suspected hemolysis. A baseline measurement should be obtained using specimens from before suspected hemolysis; if this is not possible, serial measurements of haptoglobin while hematocrit is falling and once it has stabilized can help to clarify the picture. Patients with hemolysis should show an acute decrease in haptoglobin which remains low while red cell destruction is continuing, then returns to normal in about one week after resolution. Stable values during and after a suspected hemolytic episode rule out that diagnostic possibility. If serial measurement is not possible, plasma protein electrophoresis or measurement of CRP could help to identify the presence of other states which might affect haptoglobin levels.

Immunoglobulin E

Immediate hypersensitivity reactions such as allergies often involve immunoglobulin E (IgE). Normally, only trace amounts are found in the circulation; almost all is bound to tissue mast cells. Increased IgE is found in many patients with allergic diseases, including bronchopulmonary aspergillosis and in many parasitic infections. IgE levels between one and five times normal are found in about one-third of non-allergic individuals and about one-third of patients with allergies, making this a gray zone for interpretation. Levels more than five times normal are found almost exclusively in persons with allergy. RadioAllergoSorbent Testing (RAST tests) for IgE antibodies against specific antigens are highly specific, and correlate with the importance of individual antigens better than do skin tests in patients with asthma. Patients who have undergone desensitization often have falsely negative RAST tests (IgG antibodies induced by immunization prevent detection of IgE). The tests can be expensive if a large panel is ordered; the use of patient history to select antigens to test can reduce costs.

Prealbumin

Prealbumin (transthyretin) is a trace protein (M.W. 55,000) that binds both thyroxine and retinol binding protein. It has a half-life of about 1–2 days, and its production is directly related to the availability of amino acids. For this reason, prealbumin is advocated as a marker of short-term nutritional status, and as a means to monitor the adequacy of amino acid administration in patients receiving nutritional support. Two other major factors affect prealbumin levels, however, which may make interpretation difficult. In acute inflammation, there is a marked fall in prealbumin, which may reduce levels to 20% or less of normal. Glucocorticosteroids cause increased prealbumin production.

Retinol-Binding Protein

Retinol-Binding Protein (RBP) is a very small protein (M.W. 21,000) which transports vitamin A. In normal circumstances, almost all RBP is bound to prealbumin with a half-life of the complex of about 12 h. When circulating free, it is rapidly cleared by glomerular filtration (half-life less than 4 h), and then degraded in tubular epithelial cells. The rate of production of RBP is less dependent on amino acid levels than on adequate vitamin A.

Transferrin

The iron transport protein transferrin (M.W. 77,000) is produced by the liver and, in small amounts, by several other organs. It has a half-life of about one week. Its production is mainly influenced, in an inverse fashion, by iron stores within the body; high levels occur with decreased iron stores and low levels are seen in iron excess. Inflammatory states cause lowered concentrations. While transferrin can be measured directly, as with other proteins, many laboratories perform Total Iron Binding Capacity (TIBC), since most iron is bound to transferrin. Several formulas for conversion of TIBC to transferrin have been published; the most widely used is:

$$\text{Transferrin (in mg/dL)} = [0.8 \times \text{TIBC (in mg/dL)}] - 44.$$

WHEN NOT TO DO PROTEIN TESTS

Total protein and albumin do not provide much useful information in ambulatory individuals, and screening in ambulatory patients is not recommended. Normal globulins (from total protein and albumin) eliminate the need for serum protein electrophoresis in patients suspected of having multiple myeloma, since such patients typically have moderate to marked elevation of total globulins. In high risk patients, normal urine protein eliminates the need for urine protein electrophoresis to rule out the 15% of cases of myeloma with only a monoclonal urine band. Serum protein electrophoresis is often misleading in patients with acute illness; testing should be deferred until after acute illness unless total protein is markedly elevated (more than 9 g/dL, 90 g/L).

IMMUNOGLOBULINS AND THEIR DISORDERS

The major plasma immunoglobulins (IgG, IgA, and IgM) are produced by plasma cells in response to stimulation by specific antigens in the presence of T-helper cells. A plasma cell typically produces IgG or IgA for secretion, but also has IgM on its surface; only one light chain type, either kappa (κ) or lambda (λ), is produced. Both the secreted immunoglobulin and the surface IgM are directed against the same antigen. Each molecule has identical light chains, and one of two heavy chains (mu (μ) in IgM and either gamma (γ) in IgG or alpha (α) in IgA).

Normal Immunoglobulins and Their Structure

Immunoglobulin synthesis and structure are discussed in more detail in Chapter 36. Each individual plasma cell (or clone of plasma cells) produces an antibody against only one antigen. In the course of B lymphocyte differentiation, a necessary precursor to plasma cell formation, the genes producing both heavy and light chains undergo rearrangement, such that each antigen recognizing cell produces an immunoglobulin of a distinct chemical nature which recognizes a unique antigenic site. It would be possible to *prove* that immunoglobulin molecules came from the same clone of plasma cells (**monoclonal immunoglobulin**) if they had identical antibody combining sites (*idiotypes*). This is not usually possible in clinical laboratories; instead, several features, if present, are considered diagnostic of a monoclonal immunoglobulin. If protein molecules show a highly compact band on the electrophoretic gel, this suggests a single chemical type of protein molecule as occurs with a monoclonal band. In addition, since each plasma cell produces only one type of light chain, demonstration that the band has only one heavy and one light chain type is considered diagnostic of a monoclonal immunoglobulin. Most commonly, the presence of protein of a single chemical type ("monoclonal" band or spike) is used to recognize proliferation of one clone.

IgG

The most abundant immunoglobulin, IgG is the major "memory" immunoglobulin. It is composed of two γ heavy chains and two light chains in each molecule. There are four subtypes of IgG, termed IgG_1, IgG_2, IgG_3, and IgG_4. In normal plasma, they are present in decreasing concentrations, but all four forms are normally found. Half-life of most subtypes of IgG is about 21 days. IgG represents the bulk of protein in the γ-globulin region on electrophoresis.

IgM

The rapid response immunoglobulin IgM is produced first in immune responses, and also the first immunoglobulin produced after birth. In normal plasma, it exists exclusively as pentamers, composed of five units of two μ heavy chains and two light chains, joined together by small peptides termed J-chains. IgM is present in only one major form.

IgA

IgA is a secretory immunoglobulin produced mainly near mucosal surfaces as protection against organisms in body cavities. Most IgA is produced by plasma cells in the lymphoid tissue of oral and intestinal mucosa. In secretions, IgA exists as dimers with two units of two α heavy chains and two light chains, joined by J-chains and containing another protein termed the secretory piece. In normal plasma, however, IgA exists in monomeric form, lacking J-chains and the secretory piece. There are two major subtypes of IgA in plasma, IgA_1 and IgA_2, in approximately a $9:1$ ratio. IgA has a half-life of six days.

γ-Globulin

On electrophoresis, the γ-globulin region is almost exclusively immunoglobulins. While other serum proteins are distinct chemical compounds which produce discrete protein bands (spikes), the varying chemical types of immunoglobulin molecules produces a diffuse pattern of staining. This pattern, reflecting production by many clones of plasma cells, has been termed **polyclonal.** A large amount of antibody directed against a single antigen (produced by a single clone of plasma cells) would produce a distinct band or peak on electrophoresis (**monoclonal band** or "spike").

Polyclonal Gammopathy

The polyclonal gammopathy pattern is caused by states in which there is general stimulation of the immune system. Common causes include chronic inflammatory disorders, such as autoimmune diseases and sarcoidosis; chronic infections, particularly tuberculosis and AIDS; and chronic antigenemia, as occurs in patients with portal hypertension, especially that due to cirrhosis. In some cases, there is a predominance of antibodies directed against a few specific antigens; this will produce small, distinct bands (*oligoclonal banding*). This pattern is seen most commonly in cerebrospinal fluid (CSF) with immunologic disorders involving the brain, and will be discussed in more detail in Chapter 19. In plasma, this pattern occurs with autoimmune and infectious diseases, notably HIV and Lyme disease.

Monoclonal Gammopathy

The term "monoclonal gammopathy" is technically inaccurate, since monoclonal immunoglobulins often migrate in electrophoretic regions other than the γ-globulin region; it is used here to comply with convention. IgA usually migrates in the β-globulin region; a monoclonal IgA may be missed by an inexperienced interpreter, since it may resemble an increased transferrin or an increased complement (Fig. 9.2E). Monoclonal IgM and IgG sometimes migrate closer to the β-globulin region than the γ-globulin region. Light chains, being much more variable in their charge, can migrate almost anywhere on electrophoresis, but seldom migrate as γ-globulins. A monoclonal plasma band in the γ-globulin region can usually be identified by visual inspection of gels at concentrations above 0.1 g/dL (1.0 g/L), but requires much higher levels to be detectable if it migrates in a fashion identical to that of other, normal plasma proteins such as complement or transferrin. Monoclonal gammopathies are relatively common; small monoclonal bands are found in 25–50% of patients with acute inflammation. In otherwise healthy individuals, the prevalence of monoclonal gammopathy increases with increasing age (3% over age 70, 10% over 80 years). Monoclonal gammopathy is more frequent in African-Americans than in those of European ancestry. Once a monoclonal gammopathy is identified, it is usually typed by immunofixation. Alternate approaches are to use immunoelectrophoresis or to quantitatively measure γ, α, μ, κ, and λ chains individually.

Monoclonal Gammopathy of Undetermined Significance

Monoclonal gammopathy of undetermined significance (Fig. 9.2F) (MGUS), also sometimes termed benign monoclonal gammopathy or essential gammopathy, refers to a monoclonal gammopathy in a person with no other evidence of a malignant proliferation of plasma cells or B lymphocytes. It represents the vast majority of monoclonal

Table 9.4.

Features Separating Malignancy of Plasma Cells (Multiple Myeloma [MM], Waldenstrom's Macroglobulinemia [WM]) from Monoclonal Gammopathy of Undetermined Significance (MGUS)

Feature	MM/WM	MGUS
Concentration of monoclonal protein	>2 g/dL	<2 g/dL
Concentration of other immunoglobulins	Decreased	Normal
Presence of free light chains (Bence Jones protein) in urine	50–70%	<20%
Anemia	Present	Absent
Bone lesions, Hypercalcemia	Present (MM) Absent (WM)	Absent
Change in monoclonal protein concentration over time	Increase	None

gammopathies. Features which distinguish MGUS from malignant disorders (discussed below) are listed in Table 9.4; however, except for bone marrow biopsy, none are 100% accurate. Approximately one-third of patients will develop a malignant proliferation, usually multiple myeloma, an average of ten years after initial recognition. No features at the time of recognition allow prediction of progression; regular follow-up is required. We suggest protein electrophoresis every six months for the first one to two years; if monoclonal protein concentration increases, a repeat bone marrow biopsy is indicated. After this period, yearly monitoring is performed as long as the patient remains asymptomatic. Some patients show gradual increase in concentration without other evidence of multiple myeloma.

Multiple Myeloma

Multiple myeloma (Fig. 9.2G) is a malignant proliferation of plasma cells which causes destructive bone lesions with resultant hypercalcemia. Typically, there is replacement of normal plasma cells, producing marked deficiency of all other immunoglobulins. Usually the monoclonal immunoglobulin is IgG, although about 15% of cases have monoclonal IgA and 15–20% produce only light chains (sometimes termed **light chain disease**). In perhaps 2–3% of cases, there is more than one clone of plasma cells present, producing **diclonal gammopathy.** In less than 1% of cases, the tumor does not secrete any monoclonal protein, and is termed non-secretory myeloma. Extremely rarely, tumors produce monoclonal heavy chains (termed **heavy chain disease**), or monoclonal IgD or IgE. There is no significant difference in the clinical features or course in any of these variants with the possible exception of non-secretory myeloma, which may have a worse prognosis. A monoclonal urine protein occurs in over 50% of cases of myeloma. It is important to determine whether or not this band represents free light chain (Bence Jones protein), since positively charged IgG may pass through the glomerular basement membrane. Free light chains are small enough to pass freely into urine. Quantitation of Bence Jones protein excretion, when present, is important in follow-up (the amount excreted is proportional to tumor mass).

Waldenstrom's Macroglobulinemia

The chronic lymphoproliferative disorder Waldenstrom's macroglobulinemia is characterized by the combination of a lymphoma-like clinical picture, IgM monoclonal gammopathy, bleeding problems, and increased blood viscosity producing headache and visual symptoms. Certain features of myeloma are absent, including hypercalcemia and lytic bone lesions. Bence Jones protein is present in at least half of cases, but is not as useful in following the disease as with multiple myeloma. As mentioned above, monomeric forms of IgM cause quantitative IgM assays to overestimate IgM concentration.

Hypogammaglobulinemia

Hypogammaglobulinemia denotes reduction of all immunoglobulins. Affected patients experience recurrent infections with bacteria. In children, many cases are inherited, such as **Bruton's agammaglobulinemia** (an X chromosome linked recessive trait with failure of B cell development), but in the majority of cases immunodeficiency develops later in life, termed **common variable immunodeficiency,** in which B cells are present but cannot mature to plasma cells. In this disorder, many patients develop intestinal malabsorption and evidence of autoimmune disease, which also occurs with increased frequency in family members. All immunoglobulins are decreased in both disorders, more severely in the congenital form. In adults, hypogammaglobulinemia is occasionally due to increased loss of immunoglobulins in nephrotic syndrome, or decreased production in malnutrition. Most commonly, however, the cause is a malignant proliferation of abnormal lymphocytes, usually chronic lymphocytic leukemia or multiple myeloma which does not produce intact immunoglobulins. **If hypogammaglobulinemia is present in an adult with normal plasma albumin,** urine protein electrophoresis should be ordered to exclude the possibility of light chain disease.

Selective IgA Deficiency

Selective IgA deficiency is the most common immunodeficiency, present in about 1 in 700 individuals. The majority of patients are asymptomatic, but some have evidence of abnormal immune function such as autoimmune diseases, allergy, and intestinal disease. Plasma protein electrophoresis is normal; this can be detected only with quantitative IgA measurement.

OTHER PROTEIN PATTERNS OCCASIONALLY OF USE

Plasma protein electrophoresis is seldom useful for diagnosis of other clinical disorders. Rarely, a pattern detected on protein electrophoresis may provide a clue to the presence of a disorder which had not been clinically suspected.

Chronic Portal Hypertension

The portal vein delivers amino acids from the intestine to the liver for protein synthesis, as well as immune complexes and bacterial antigens which should be removed from the circulation. Because of lack of raw materials, patients with hypertension in the portal vein, usually due to cirrhosis, will have decreased concentrations of albumin, α_1-globulin, α_2-globulin, and normal β-globulin (Fig. 9.2H). Portal hypertension prevents this normal function from occurring and results in polyclonal increases in IgA and IgG. The increased IgA causes increased staining in the region between the β-globulin and γ-globulin regions, termed β-γ **bridging.**

Protein Losing States, Especially Nephrotic Syndrome

This group of disorders known collectively as protein losing states is associated with greater decreases in the concentration of small sized proteins, such as albumin, transferrin, and positively charged proteins such as IgG (Fig. 9.2C). Levels of these proteins fall, which stimulates the liver to synthesize all proteins. Large proteins, including haptoglobin and LDL, will be present in plasma in increased amounts.

Inflammation

Cytokines produced by inflammation stimulate the production of a variety of proteins, as discussed earlier. With acute inflammation (Fig. 9.2A), the increases are apparent most commonly in the α_1-globulin and α_2-globulin; albumin and transferrin bands frequently decrease due to impaired synthesis. In chronic inflammation (Fig. 9.2B), stimulation of B-lymphocytes causes increased production of immunoglobulins and a polyclonal increase in γ-globulins; while albumin and transferrin remain low, the relative increases in the two α-globulin bands is not as great as with acute inflammation.

CHAPTER 10

Laboratory Evaluation of Mineral and Bone Metabolism

D. ROBERT DUFOUR

NORMAL BIOCHEMISTRY OF MINERALS AND BONE

Calcium

Most calcium (about 99%) is in bone; about 1–2% of skeletal calcium can be released rapidly without removing bone tissue. The remaining 1% of body calcium is almost exclusively extracellular, existing in three forms. **Free** (ionized) calcium (40–50% of total calcium) is physiologically active and maintained within a narrow concentration range (4.7–5.2 mg/dL, 1.17–1.29 mmol/L) by calcium regulating hormones. Protein-bound calcium (40–45% of total calcium) is biologically inactive. Acidosis displaces calcium from protein, while alkalosis increases protein-bound calcium. Albumin is responsible for 80% of protein binding, with most of the remaining 20% attached to IgG. Some patients with multiple myeloma may have high total calcium due to increased IgG binding. Inactive complexes of calcium (with bicarbonate, phosphate, citrate, or free fatty acids) comprise the remaining 5–10% of total calcium.

Phosphate

Approximately 80% of phosphate is found in bone. Most extraskeletal phosphate is within organic compounds such as nucleotides, phospholipids, and high energy compounds. Only 1% of total phosphate exists as free inorganic phosphate, with concentration approximately equal in intracellular and extracellular fluid. Inorganic phosphate is needed for bone mineralization and glycolysis.

Magnesium

Approximately half of body magnesium is located in the skeleton. Over 98% of extraskeletal magnesium is intracellular, with only 1% of total magnesium in extracellular fluid. Within cells, magnesium is a necessary catalyst for energy transfer and metabolic enzymes. The gradient between extracellular and intracellular magnesium is essential for normal cell membrane potential, and equilibrium between intracellular and extracellular magnesium occurs very slowly. Plasma magnesium exists in three forms: protein bound (approximately 33% of total), complexed to anions (about 5–10%), and free, which is physiologically active (about 60%).

Bone

Bone is formed by osteoblasts which synthesize structural proteins, collectively called **osteoid matrix,** that combine with minerals (predominantly calcium and phosphate). Approximately 20% of skeletal mineral is exchanged yearly in adults. Osteoid matrix is primarily type I collagen (95%); other proteins include **osteocalcin,** a vitamin K dependent calcium-binding protein. Osteoblasts also elaborate a bone-specific isoenzyme of alkaline phosphatase. Osteoblasts are converted to less active osteocytes, which control day-to-day bone maintenance and exchange calcium with extracellular fluid. Bone is removed by osteoclasts, multinucleated cells derived from blood monocytes, which release acid and degradative enzymes, including acid phosphatase, to dissolve mineral and degrade osteoid matrix.

PHYSIOLOGY OF MINERAL AND BONE STATUS

Calcium and Phosphate

Plasma free (ionized) calcium concentration is maintained within a relatively narrow range by several hormones, which facilitate interchange of calcium between extracellular fluid and bone, urine, and intestinal contents (Fig.10.1, Table 10.1).

Hormonal Regulation of Plasma Calcium

Parathyroid hormone (PTH), produced by the parathyroid glands, works along with calcitriol (1,25-dihydroxyvitamin D), the active renal product of metabolism of "Vitamin D" obtained from diet or sunlight (Fig. 10.2). In normal circumstances, these two hormones maintain normal free calcium concentration and bone mass. With increasing

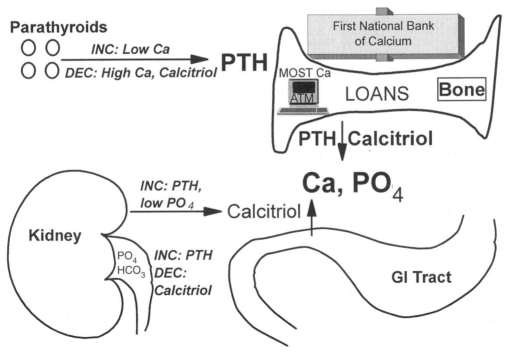

Figure 10.1. Maintenance of Plasma Calcium. With short-term needs for calcium, PTH mediates removal from the rapid exchange pool in bone, and also causes renal excretion of anions, displacing free calcium. With a longer term need, calcitriol increases intestinal calcium absorption; in the short term, it also assists PTH in mobilization of calcium from bone. With return of calcium to normal, and an increase in calcitriol, feedback inhibits further PTH production.

Table 10.1.
Effects of Calcium Regulating Hormones on Organs and Mineral Levels

Hormone	Intestine	Kidney	Bone	Serum
PTH, PTH-RP	No direct effect	↑ Ca reabsorption; ↓ PO_4, HCO_3^- absorption; ↑ 1-hydroxylase	[a]↑ reabsorption, mobilize Ca and PO_4	↑ Ca, Cl^-; ↓ PO_4, HCO_3^-
Calcitriol (1,25-$(OH)_2^-$ vitamin D)	[a]↑ Ca, PO_4 absorption	Slight ↑ Ca, PO_4 reabsorption	↑ effect of PTH on bone reabsorption	↑ Ca, PO_4
Calcitonin	Probably no direct effect	↓ Ca, PO_4 reabsorption	↓ bone reabsorption	↓ Ca, PO_4

[a] Most important action of hormone with respect to mineral metabolism.

age, decreased renal function, decreased calcium intake, decreased efficiency of calcium absorption, and decreased exercise lead to net loss of calcium from bone and lower bone mass.

Other Hormones Potentially Affecting Plasma Calcium

Calcitonin, produced by thyroid C-cells in response to high plasma calcium, seems to have no major role in calcium metabolism in humans, although its inhibition of bone reabsorption seems important. **PTH–related Peptide (PTHrP)** is produced by the fetal parathyroid, squamous epithelial cells, and breast epithelial cells, and is similar to PTH in its activity. In addition, PTHrP seems to facilitate calcium transfer across the placenta and into breast milk; its functions in adulthood are currently unknown.

Magnesium

Plasma magnesium primarily reflects balance between intake and loss. Several hormones affect plasma magnesium: PTH and aldosterone increase renal magnesium excretion and decrease plasma magnesium, while vitamin D increases intestinal magnesium absorption and plasma magnesium.

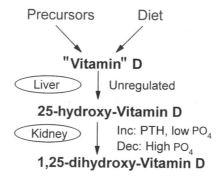

Figure 10.2. Formation of calcitriol (1,25-dihydroxyvitamin D). Dietary intake and sunshine provide "Vitamin D," converted in the liver to relatively inactive 25-hydroxyvitamin D (unregulated) and by the kidney to active calcitriol when stimulated by PTH or low phosphate. Synthesis is inhibited by high calcitriol and increased plasma phosphate.

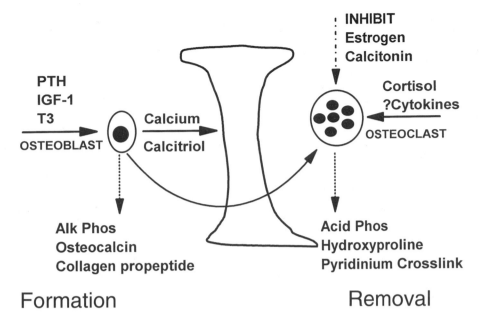

Figure 10.3. Normal Bone Physiology. In adults, bone physiology is governed by the balance between mechanical support needs (determined by bone use), and hormones controlling osteoblasts or osteoclasts. Because of the production of "coupling factors," osteoblasts typically activate bone formation and removal simultaneously. The relative balance between these determines an increase or decrease in bone mass.

Bone Physiology

Bone status is determined by a balance between formation and turnover (Fig. 10.3). Bone formation by osteoblasts requires raw materials (amino acids, calcium, and phosphate) and mechanical or hormonal stimulation. Insulin–like growth factor I and thyroid hormone are both required for normal bone growth in children. After puberty, PTH and mechanical stress are more important stimuli to osteoblasts. Low levels of PTH increase the rate of bone formation, but higher PTH levels increase production of "coupling factor" by osteoblasts, activating osteoclasts and causing bone removal. Bone removal by osteoclasts is dependent on both mechanical and hormonal stimuli, most importantly coupling factor and cytokines. Osteoclast activity is inhibited by estrogen and calcitonin.

LABORATORY TESTS OF MINERAL AND BONE METABOLISM

Plasma Calcium

Total calcium (measuring all forms of calcium) is the most common calcium test. Total calcium is affected by changes in physiologically active forms, so it does not provide direct information about active calcium if pH, protein levels, or calcium complexes are abnormal. If pH and complexing anion levels are normal, and the patient is not ill, it is possible to normalize the total calcium for low serum albumin (Eq. 10.1).

$$\text{Adjusted Ca (mg/dL)} = \text{Total Ca (mg/dL)} + 0.8 \times (4 - \text{Albumin (g/dL)})$$

$$(10.1)$$

Free calcium should be measured directly whenever critical information is needed. Specimens must be handled the same as blood gas specimens to prevent changes in pH which alter free calcium; free calcium measurements are often included with blood gases.

Phosphate

There is marked diurnal variation in phosphate concentration, with levels falling throughout the day and after meals; a single phosphate assay therefore provides little useful information. Since phosphate is largely cleared by the kidney, phosphate levels must be interpreted in light of renal function; "normal" phosphate is inappropriately low in a patient with renal failure. Phosphate measurements are often inaccurate in patients with monoclonal gammopathies, usually producing falsely high or, rarely, falsely low results.

Magnesium

Plasma total magnesium (few laboratories measure free magnesium) equilibrates slowly with cell magnesium, making it a poor indicator of total body magnesium. Plasma magnesium is falsely increased in hemolyzed specimens.

Parathyroid Hormone

The normal production and clearance of parathyroid hormone (PTH) is shown in Figure 10.4. **Mid-molecule or C-terminal** assays measure the long-lived, inactive metabolite of PTH. Results are falsely increased in renal failure and in hypercalcemia. **Intact** PTH assays measure active hormone released and do not cross react with PTHrP.

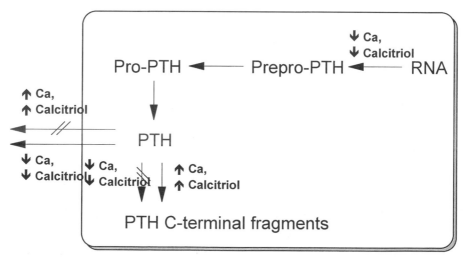

Figure 10.4. Production of Parathyroid Hormone. Low calcium stimulates production of both PTH and its precursors. PTH is cleaved in liver and kidney (half-life 5 min) to an active N-terminal fragment (half-life 5 min) and a larger inactive C-terminal fragment. This latter molecule is excreted by glomerular filtration; normally, its half-life is about 2 h, but is markedly prolonged in renal insufficiency. High calcium or calcitriol decreases the rate of release of intact PTH more than synthesis of pre-pro-PTH, causing an increased release of C-terminal fragments.

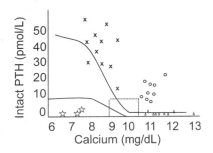

Figure 10.5. Relationship of PTH to Plasma Calcium. The dotted box illustrates the usually reported reference range for plasma PTH. The solid lines indicate the actual relationship between serum calcium and PTH as determined by Lepage et al. (Clin Chem 1992;38:2129). The reference range is appropriate only over a very narrow range of calcium values. PTH results in patients with hypoparathyroidism (star), chronic renal failure and secondary hyperparathyroidism (×), primary hyperparathyroidism (circle), and hypercalcemia of malignancy (triangle) are illustrated. Correct diagnosis is possible using the "dynamic" reference range; inappropriately high or low PTH for serum calcium indicates disease.

Intact PTH is not affected by renal failure and is appropriately low in all cases of hypercalcemia except hyperparathyroidism. Intact PTH assays should be chosen whenever PTH determination is needed, but must be interpreted in light of plasma calcium (Fig. 10.5).

Vitamin D

Assays for vitamin D metabolites are poorly reproducible, technically extremely difficult, and of less than ideal specificity. In evaluating vitamin D levels, it is better to interpret the general direction of changes than the absolute level. **25-Hydroxyvitamin D** is produced in direct proportion to available "Vitamin D"; testing is useful in suspected dietary vitamin D toxicity or deficiency. **1,25-Dihydroxyvitamin D** (calcitriol) measurements are useful in suspected ectopic vitamin D production (granulomatous disease, lymphoma) or end organ unresponsiveness to vitamin D.

Parathyroid Hormone-related Peptide

Levels of PTHrP are extremely low in normal persons, making interpretation of results difficult. PTHrP measurement may occasionally be helpful in patients with hypercalcemia, low PTH, and no clinical evidence of malignancy; elevated levels suggest an occult tumor. PTHrP levels are not markedly elevated in many cases of malignancy-related hypercalcemia.

Urinary Mineral Excretion

Urine mineral excretion can be measured as a total amount in a timed urine, but is better expressed as the fractional excretion (Chapter 6). Urinary excretion reflects net flux of each of these elements. Virtually all patients with hypercalcemia have normal to increased urinary calcium excretion, while patients with hypocalcemia have low urine calcium. Urinary phosphate has greater utility; most patients with increased PTH or PTH-like activity have high fractional excretion of phosphate (greater than 20%) despite low plasma phosphate, while most other causes of low phosphate have low urine phosphate excretion. Fractional excretion of magnesium above 30% in a patient with low plasma magnesium implies renal wasting.

Laboratory Tests of Bone Metabolism

While radiographs can estimate bone density and photon absorptimetry determines bone calcium content, they cannot evaluate relative activity of bone formation and turnover. Laboratory tests provide a measure of activity of bone at a specific time and are of particular value in recognition and treatment of patients with metabolic bone diseases. Reference values vary tremendously in children, due to periods of bone growth and the continuous bone turnover that accompanies growth.

Alkaline Phosphatase

Bone alkaline phosphatase is elevated whenever osteoblastic activity is increased. Alkaline phosphatase also comes from other tissues, and plasma levels vary widely from person to person; total alkaline phosphatase is an insensitive marker of bone formation. The bone and liver isoenzymes can be separated by a number of relatively inaccurate methods (heat fractionation, γ-glutamyl transferase (produced by liver), electrophoresis). Immunoassay of bone alkaline phosphatase is the best test, but still shows some cross-reactivity with the liver isoenzyme.

Osteocalcin

The vitamin K-dependent calcium binding protein osteocalcin (bone Gla protein) is produced by osteoblasts. Values are 50–100% higher at night, and day to day variation is 50%; mild abnormalities may not be clinically significant. Results from different labs vary because they measure active and inactive forms differently. To improve interpretation, osteocalcin levels should always be drawn in the morning.

Hydroxyproline

Since hydroxyproline is only found in collagen, it has been used as a marker of bone turnover. Urinary excretion shows marked diurnal variation, and is greatly affected by dietary intake of collagen (meat, gelatin, many prepared foods). Specimens of 24 hour urine should be collected only after the patient has been on a low collagen diet for several days. This test has limited sensitivity and specificity for metabolic bone disease.

Collagen Fragments

Pyridinium crosslinks (pyridinoline, deoxypyridinoline, and type I collagen telopeptides) are found exclusively in extracellular type I collagen. Although present in other tissues such as cartilage, the major site of type I collagen turnover is bone; deoxypyridinoline crosslinks and telopeptides are found almost exclusively in bone. Because of distinct diurnal variation, 24-hour urine collections are usually needed to accurately interpret results. High levels are usually seen in high turnover metabolic bone diseases.

Table 10.2.
Laboratory Tests in Mineral Disorders

State	T Ca	F Ca	PO$_4$	Mg	PTH	Alk Phos	Other
Hemoconcentration	sl–mod ↑	Nl	Nl	Nl	Nl	Nl	
Primry Hyperparathyroidism	sl–mod ↑	sl–mod ↑	Nl–sl ↓	Nl–sl ↓	1–2x Nl	Nl	Nl–sl ↑ 1,25 D
Humoral hypercalcemia of malignancy	mod–mk ↑	mod–mk ↑	sl–mod ↓	Nl	↓	Nl–mod ↑	
Metastases to bone	sl–mk ↑	sl–mk ↑	Nl	Nl–sl ↑	↓	sl–mk ↑	
Hypoalbuminemia	sl–mod ↓	Nl	Nl	Nl–sl ↓	Nl	Nl	
Chronic renal failure	Nl–mod ↓	Nl–mod ↓	Mod–mk ↑	Sl–mod ↑	Mod–mk ↑	Mod–mk ↑	Mkd ↓ 1,25 D
Hypoparathyroidism	sl–mod ↓	sl–mod ↓	sl–mod ↑	Nl–sl ↑	Nl–sl ↓	Nl–sl ↓	↓ 1,25 D
Mg Deficiency	sl–mod ↓	sl–mod ↓	Nl–sl ↓	sl–mod ↓	Nl–sl ↓	Nl	
Acute Illness	mod–mk ↓	mod–mk ↓	sl–mod ↑	Nl	Nl–sl ↓	Nl	
Ketoacidosis	Nl	Nl	↑ early, ↓ later	↑ early, Nl later	Nl	Nl	

T Ca = total calcium; F Ca = free calcium; PO$_4$ = inorganic phosphate; Mg = magnesium; PTH = intact parathyroid hormone; Alk Phos = alkaline phosphatase; 1,25 D = 1,25 dihydroxyvitamin D; sl = slight; mod = moderate; mk = marked; Nl = normal.

WHEN NOT TO DO TESTS OF MINERAL AND BONE METABOLISM

A summary of common laboratory patterns of mineral abnormalities is given in Table 10.2. Tests of mineral metabolism are not indicated as screening tests in asymptomatic patients. Case finding in hospitalized patients may be of benefit because of the higher prevalence of abnormalities. Free calcium levels are not indicated if total calcium and albumin are normal, except following administration of large amounts of anions (blood transfusions, bicarbonate) or in critically ill patients. Total calcium changes slowly in most disease states; in general, tests should not be performed more than twice in a day, and once daily is usually adequate. Plasma magnesium will normalize rapidly when magnesium is administered, but cannot be used to determine adequacy of replacement of total body magnesium. A repeat measurement two days after discontinuation of magnesium supplementation will be more useful. Tests of bone turnover should not be done in acutely ill patients or those at prolonged bed rest, since they will be transiently elevated during this time. Osteocalcin should not be used in patients receiving coumadin, since results will be falsely low.

HYPERCALCEMIA

A common metabolic problem, hypercalcemia is found in 0.1% of outpatients and 1% of hospital patients. Clinical symptoms are nonspecific, including irritability, mental status changes, hypertension, polydipsia, and polyuria. The degree of symptoms is dependent on the degree of elevation of free calcium. An approach to the patient with hypercalcemia is shown in Figure 10.6.

Artifactual (Protein Bound) Hypercalcemia

The most common cause of elevated protein bound calcium is hemoconcentration due to dehydration, posture, or tourniquet effects. In general, hypercalcemia is mild, with

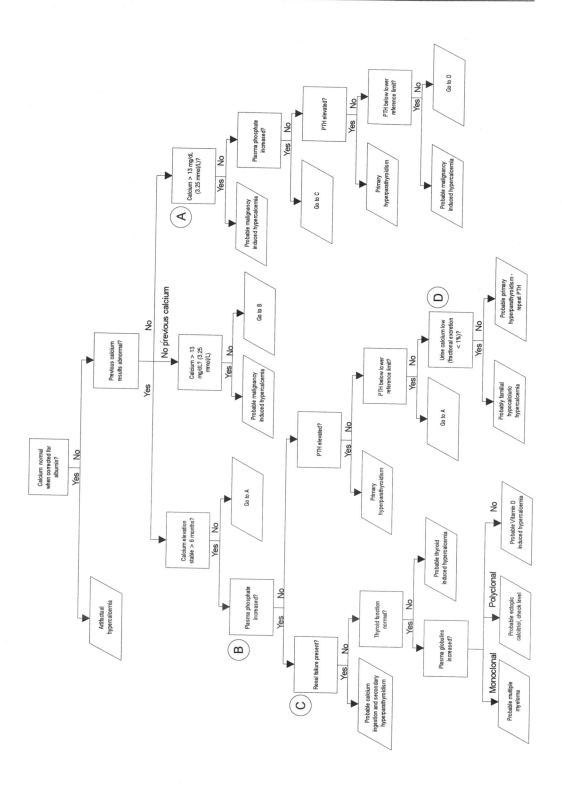

calcium usually <11.2 mg/dL (2.8 mmol/L). It should be suspected if plasma albumin is >4.5 g/dL (45 g/L), and assumed to be present if albumin >5.0 g/dL (50 g/L). In one series, 15% of all patients referred to endocrinologists for "hypercalcemia" had artifactual hypercalcemia. Less commonly, myeloma proteins bind calcium and cause increased total calcium with normal free calcium. This should be suspected if the patient is asymptomatic, or if a symptomatic patient initially responds to therapy but plasma calcium reaches a plateau; free calcium is normal. Such patients must be followed with free calcium measurements.

Primary Hyperparathyroidism

Inappropriate production of PTH is a fairly common (prevalence 1 in 1000) cause of chronic hypercalcemia, and the most common in outpatients. Most cases are asymptomatic and due to benign tumors. Calcium feedback on PTH production occurs, but requires higher plasma calcium than normal to suppress PTH, shifting the curve in Figure 10.5 to the right. Hyperparathyroidism is characterized by stable elevations of calcium lasting years. The hypercalcemia is usually mild (10.6–12.0 mg/dL, 2.65–3.0 mmol/L); severe hypercalcemia (greater than 13.0 mg/dL, 3.25 mmol/L) occurs in less than 5% of cases. Hypercalcemia is associated with relatively low plasma phosphate (average below 3.0 mg/dL, 0.94 mmol/L) in 80% of cases; because of marked diurnal and day to day variation, individual values are less useful than average values (Fig. 10.7). Plasma chloride is usually relatively high (greater than 103 mmol/L) in most cases, and the ratio of chloride to phosphate is typically greater than 33. Primary hyperparathyroidism can often be suspected from routine laboratory tests; diagnosis is based on inappropriate elevation of PTH. In most cases, PTH is 1–3 times normal, while in 5–10% of cases, PTH is "normal" but inappropriately high for hypercalcemia. Urine calcium and phosphate are usually elevated, and fractional excretion of phosphate is typically greater than 20%. Calcitriol is elevated in most cases, but is not needed to establish the diagnosis.

Hypercalcemia of Malignancy

Hypercalcemia in patients with malignancy is most commonly caused by production of PTHrP, activating bone reabsorption (**humoral hypercalcemia of malignancy, HHM**); it may also be due to bone metastases. Malignancy is the most common cause of hypercalcemia in hospitalized patients. In over 95% of cases, a tumor has either been diagnosed previously or is obvious at the time of presentation. HHM occurs in 1/4 to 1/3 of patients with squamous cell carcinomas, breast carcinomas, and renal cell carcinomas, and less commonly in other tumors. Hypercalcemia due to bone metastases is most frequent with multiple myeloma, breast carcinomas, and lung carcinomas (although rare in prostate cancer as bone metastases are usually osteoblastic). Release of skeletal calcium is not affected by feedback regulation; plasma calcium rises rapidly in many cases, often over a few days, and is greater than 13 mg/dL (3.25 mmol/L) in 50% of cases (Fig. 10.8). In HHM, laboratory abnormalities resemble those in primary

Figure 10.6. Approach to Hypercalcemia. Initial evaluation of hypercalcemic patients excludes an artifactual increase in calcium. Review of previous laboratory results can result in a high likelihood of correctly separating primary hyperparathyroidism (chronic, stable hypercalcemia) from other states. With recent increases in calcium or hospitalized patients, malignancy is far and away the most common cause. Elevated serum phosphate indicates less common causes which should be pursued before further patient work-up.

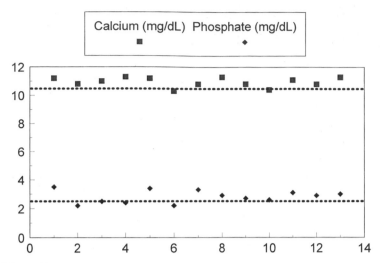

Figure 10.7. Primary Hyperparathyroidism. Results for plasma calcium (squares) and phosphate (diamonds) over a 30-month period in a patient with hyperparathyroidism are illustrated in relation to the upper (calcium) and lower (phosphate) reference limits (dotted lines). Over half of the phosphate values are actually "normal" although average phosphate is near the low end of normal, whereas calcium is almost always elevated. Typically, calcium varies little over time, reflecting feedback inhibition in this benign disease. Intact PTH was 1.5 times the upper reference limit. Hypercalcemia was cured by removal of a benign parathyroid adenoma.

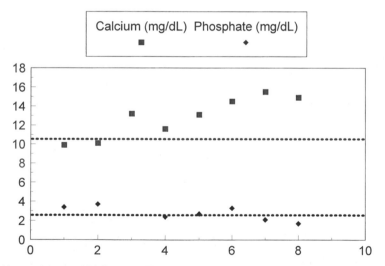

Figure 10.8. Hypercalcemia of Malignancy. Results for plasma calcium (squares) and phosphate (diamonds) over a two-month period in a patient with squamous cell carcinoma of the esophagus are illustrated in relation to the upper (calcium) and lower (phosphate) reference limits (dotted lines). Calcium often rises dramatically in as little as one week because of lack of feedback inhibition, as illustrated in this case. Phosphate is often much lower than typical for primary hyperparathyroidism. Intact PTH was below the lower limit of detection, while PTHrP was slightly elevated.

hyperparathyroidism, with increased calcium accompanied by decreased phosphate. Hypercalcemia from bone metastases is usually accompanied by low chloride (volume depletion from hypercalcemia), normal or high phosphate, and increased bone alkaline phosphatase, often with elevated total alkaline phosphatase. PTH is typically below normal in both forms of malignancy related hypercalcemia, but is not diagnostic. PTHrP is elevated in most patients with HHM.

Uncommon Causes of Hypercalcemia

Hemoconcentration, primary hyperparathyroidism, and malignancy cause over 95% of hypercalcemia. Other causes should be considered only if the three other disorders have been ruled out, except for drug-induced hypercalcemia, which is usually self-limiting if the offending medication can be discontinued. In most of these disorders, PTH is below normal.

Drug-induced Hypercalcemia

About 25–50% of patients with renal failure treated with high dose calcium carbonate and calcitriol will become hypercalcemic. This typically occurs early in treatment, and is more common in advanced renal failure. Lithium alters the level of calcium at which PTH is suppressed, commonly causing hypercalcemia; patients taking lithium may develop primary hyperparathyroidism after many years. Excessive intake of calcium carbonate, or moderate intake coupled with a drug inhibiting renal calcium excretion (such as thiazide diuretics) rarely produces severe hypercalcemia.

Familial Hypocalciuric Hypercalcemia

This autosomal dominant disorder, about 1/100 as common as primary hyperparathyroidism, causes chronic hypercalcemia with decreased urine calcium excretion (fractional excretion of calcium less than 1%). Joint problems and pancreatitis may occur in affected individuals. PTH is inappropriately elevated for hypercalcemia, typically in the middle of the reference interval, with slight overlap with values seen in primary hyperparathyroidism. In patients with a family history of hypercalcemia, or if PTH is not clearly elevated, fractional excretion of calcium (based on 24 hour urine) should be measured to exclude this disease before referring patients for surgery.

Systemic Disease

Hyperthyroidism and hypothyroidism are associated with hypercalcemia in fewer than 5% of cases. In hyperthyroidism, hypercalcemia is due to increased bone turnover, although the cause is not as clear in hypothyroidism. Sarcoidosis is often associated with ectopic production of calcitriol; about 25% of patients have increased urine calcium, but fewer than 5% become hypercalcemic. Other granulomatous diseases and some lymphomas also produce calcitriol inappropriately. A clue to the presence of sarcoidosis or hyperthyroidism is the presence of increased plasma phosphate, which is rare in other causes of hypercalcemia. Prolonged immobilization causes marked loss of skeletal calcium and may produce moderate to severe hypercalcemia, most commonly in younger individuals. In all systemic diseases, PTH is below normal.

HYPOCALCEMIA

Approximately 2–3% of hospitalized individuals and 0.1% of outpatients are hypocalcemic, although most have artifactual (protein bound) hypocalcemia. Symptoms of true

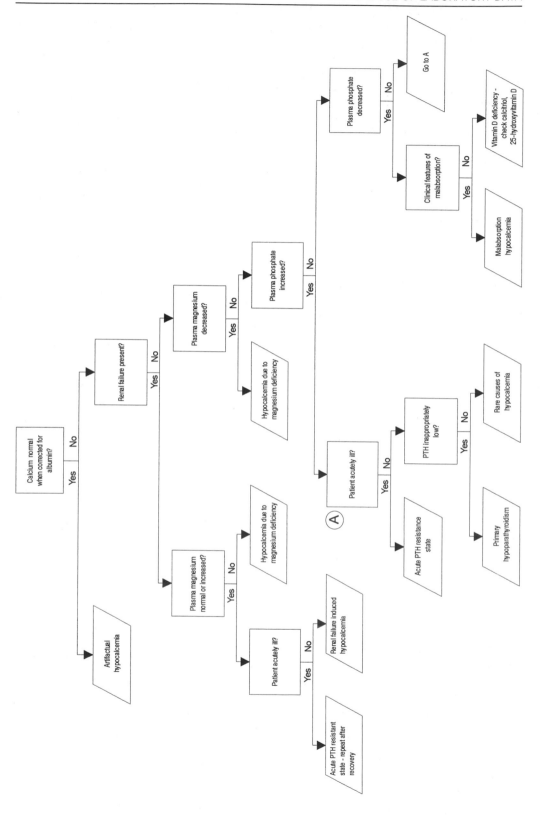

hypocalcemia depend on the rapidity of development. Chronic hypocalcemia, even if severe, is often asymptomatic, while patients with acute hypocalcemia often develop paresthesias, muscle spasms, and cardiac arrhythmias. Acute decreases in free calcium concentration with alkalosis, or with increased anions such as citrate, may also produce symptoms of hypocalcemia with normal total calcium concentration. Free calcium measurements are more important for evaluation of hypocalcemia than for hypercalcemia. A suggested approach to hypocalcemia is outlined in Figure 10.9.

Artifactual Hypocalcemia

Approximately 80% of cases of hypocalcemia are related to decreased albumin concentration (malnutrition, protein losing states, chronic liver disease). Affected individuals are asymptomatic, and no workup for calcium disorders is indicated.

Chronic Renal Failure

Patients with renal failure develop hypocalcemia due to decreased calcitriol production and decreased phosphate excretion. Calcium metabolism is usually normal until the glomerular filtration rate falls below 25–30 mL/min. Beyond this point, low free calcium and calcitriol lead to compensatory overproduction of PTH, termed **secondary hyperparathyroidism.** Inhibition of PTH production requires a higher calcium concentration in the absence of calcitriol, shifting the curve of PTH versus calcium (Fig. 10.5) to the right. In untreated patients, hypocalcemia, increased phosphate, and metabolic bone disease (**renal osteodystrophy**) develop as renal failure progresses.

Uncommon Causes of Hypocalcemia

Decreased albumin and chronic renal failure cause approximately 90% of hypocalcemia. If free calcium is low and the patient has normal renal function, one of the less common causes should be considered.

Hypoparathyroidism

A number of illnesses, including sepsis, shock, and pancreatitis, are associated with transiently low PTH, leading to low calcium and high phosphate. Less commonly, surgical removal of the parathyroid glands following neck surgery and autoimmune destruction may cause hypoparathyroidism. Rarely, hypoparathyroidism is due to congenital absence of the parathyroid glands, often accompanied by absence of the thymus and immune deficiency (Di George syndrome). Hypocalcemia is accompanied by high phosphate, decreased urine calcium excretion, and inappropriately low PTH.

Hypomagnesemia

Magnesium deficiency impairs PTH production and action, and also blocks release of calcium and phosphate from bone. Hypocalcemia is often accompanied by hypoka-

Figure 10.9. Approach to Hypocalcemia. Initial evaluation of hypocalcemic patients should exclude artifactual decreases due to low albumin, responsible for over 80% of cases. True hypocalcemia is caused by renal failure in over 50% of cases. If neither of these conditions is present, the clinical history often provides evidence for the mechanism. Acutely ill patients often develop PTH resistance, having rapidly falling calcium and increasing phosphate. In patients who are not ill, high phosphate suggests hypoparathyroidism. Normal or low phosphate should be followed by determining serum magnesium, a common cause of hypocalcemia. Malabsorption is a rare cause in adults but is more frequent in children.

lemia and low phosphate. Until magnesium is administered, hypocalcemia does not respond to calcium supplementation.

Malabsorption

In children, this is a relatively common cause of hypocalcemia (requirement for absorbed calcium to support rapid bone growth). In adults, malabsorption is a rare cause of hypocalcemia. Low calcium is usually accompanied by low phosphate. While generalized malabsorption may cause hypocalcemia, vitamin D deficiency is more commonly at fault. Low 25-hydroxyvitamin D is considered diagnostic; calcitriol is usually normal until late in deficiency.

HYPERPHOSPHATEMIA

Increased phosphate is often asymptomatic, in many cases is transient, and in most cases does not require any treatment. Chronic hyperphosphatemia or severe acutely increased phosphate may lead to precipitation of calcium phosphate salts in tissues termed metastatic calcification, which can also produce hypocalcemia.

Renal Failure

Most cases of hyperphosphatemia are due to renal failure; plasma phosphate rises in parallel with plasma creatinine in renal insufficiency.

Impaired Aerobic Glycolysis

Failure to use phosphate in glucose metabolism causes most cases of acute hyperphosphatemia; the transient rise may be extreme, reaching 4–5 times the upper reference limit. Both ketoacidosis and lactic acidosis are associated with hyperphosphatemia in the majority of cases. Treatment of the underlying disorder leads to rapid fall in phosphate, often producing hypophosphatemia (Fig. 10.10).

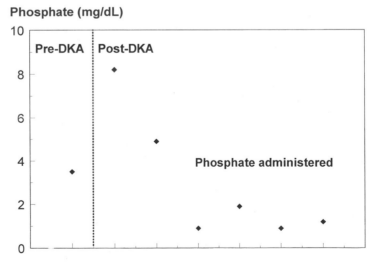

Figure 10.10. Phosphate in Ketoacidosis. This patient developed diabetic ketoacidosis while in the hospital. Although phosphate was markedly elevated on admission, it quickly fell after institution of insulin therapy, reaching normal values in 4 h and falling to 0.9 mg/dL after 12 h. Values remained low for almost 24 h despite prompt institution of phosphate supplementation.

Uncommon Causes of Hyperphosphatemia

In children, phosphate levels are significantly higher than in adults; values should be compared with an appropriate reference range before pursuing an extensive evaluation. In adults, artifactual hyperphosphatemia should be considered; delay in analysis of specimens often causes leakage of phosphate from cells after collection. Plasma protein and albumin should be measured to exclude interference from myeloma proteins.

Hypoparathyroidism

As mentioned above, PTH deficiency causes increased phosphate; values are usually only slightly elevated.

Vitamin D Toxicity

Excess vitamin D ingestion or ectopic production can cause hypercalcemia with increased plasma phosphate.

Hyperthyroidism

Increased phosphate is more common than hypercalcemia in hyperthyroidism. Results return to normal with control of thyroid hormone levels.

Cell Lysis Syndromes

Lysis of tumor cells or, less commonly, rhabdomyolysis, rarely causes hyperphosphatemia. Usually, the rate of phosphate release does not exceed renal ability to excrete phosphate; increased phosphate does not typically occur unless renal failure develops. Cell lysis can be recognized by association of hyperphosphatemia with hyperkalemia, increased uric acid, and increased LDH, as all are released in large amounts with cell lysis.

HYPOPHOSPHATEMIA

While mild hypophosphatemia is asymptomatic, severely decreased phosphate (less than 1 mg/dL, 0.3 mmol/L) may cause hemolysis, muscle weakness, and occasionally respiratory arrest and other neurologic problems. Restoration of aerobic glycolysis often is accompanied by hypophosphatemia, and may be severe in patients who have been malnourished for some time. Plasma phosphate should be monitored every 6 h for at least 24 h in malnourished patients being refed. Acute respiratory disorders are commonly associated with hypophosphatemia, although the mechanism has not been established. Rarely, renal tubular defects may cause urine phosphate losses and hypophosphatemia. Low phosphate is often associated with calcium and magnesium abnormalities (hyperparathyroidism, HHM, magnesium deficiency, vitamin D deficiency, and malabsorption).

HYPERMAGNESEMIA

Increased magnesium is the least common mineral abnormality and is rarely symptomatic; muscle weakness and cardiac arrhythmia occur with severely elevated magnesium. It is usually due to ingestion of magnesium in renal failure patients or treatment of toxemia of pregnancy. Rare causes of increased magnesium include adrenal insufficiency and absorption of magnesium from the GI tract in patients with intestinal injury. Artifactual hypermagnesemia occurs with hemolyzed specimens and with prolonged storage of whole blood.

HYPOMAGNESEMIA

Low magnesium is the most common mineral abnormality in hospitalized patients, found in up to 10%; it is often undiagnosed unless routine magnesium measurements are performed. Symptoms of hypomagnesemia are similar to those of hypocalcemia, and are often absent with chronic hypomagnesemia. Unexplained hypocalcemia or hypokalemia should lead to a plasma magnesium determination. Alcohol abuse is a common cause due to impaired renal magnesium reabsorption complicated by poor magnesium intake. Drug-induced renal magnesium wasting occurs in a high percentage of patients taking diuretics (thiazides, furosemide), cis-platinum, aminoglycosides, and amphotericin. Diarrhea commonly causes hypomagnesemia; stool magnesium is approximately 5 mmol/L, or five times higher than plasma. Symptoms of magnesium deficiency commonly occur with diarrhea because of the rapidity of magnesium loss. These three disorders cause 99% of hypomagnesemia; rarely, malabsorption, renal tubular defects, or hyperaldosteronism are responsible. Massive blood transfusions may cause decreased free magnesium with normal total magnesium.

METABOLIC BONE DISEASES

Disorders associated with abnormal bone formation, turnover, or mineralization are termed metabolic bone diseases. Radiographic findings can identify metabolic bone disease and quantify skeletal mass, but cannot determine rate of bone loss, disease activity, or pathogenesis. For example, osteopenia and decreased bone calcium are seen in osteogenesis imperfecta (decreased bone collagen formation), vitamin D deficiency (decreased bone calcium), osteoporosis (decreased bone formation), and hyperparathyroidism (increased bone turnover). Laboratory tests are helpful in identifying pathogenesis and rate of change in bone mass, useful both for diagnosis and in follow-up (Table 10.3).

Osteoporosis

Decreased bone formation in the face of normal bone turnover is the most common cause of osteoporosis, the most common metabolic bone disease. In some women, a

Table 10.3.
Laboratory Tests in Metabolic Bone Disorders

State	T Ca	PO$_4$	Bone AP	OC	HProl	X-links
Primary hyperparathyroidism	sl–mod ↑	Nl–sl ↓	Nl–sl ↑	↑	Nl–sl ↑	↑
Metastases to bone	mod–mk ↑	sl–mod ↓	mod–mk ↑	↑	↑	↑
Rickets	sl–mod ↓	sl–mod ↓	↑	↑	↑	↑
Renal osteodystrophy	sl–mod ↓	mod–mk ↑	mod–mk ↑	↑	N/A	N/A
Paget's disease	Nl	Nl	mod–mk ↑	↑	↑	↑
Osteoporosis	Nl	Nl	Nl	Nl	Nl	sl ↑
Hyperthyroidism	Nl–sl ↑	sl–mod ↑	sl–mod ↑	↑	↑	↑

T Ca = total calcium; F Ca:PO$_4$ = inorganic phosphate; Bone AP = bone isoenzyme of alkaline phosphatase; OC = osteocalcin (bone Gla protein); HProl = urine hydroxyproline; X-links = collagen crosslinks (including deoxypyridinoline); sl = slight; mod = moderte; mk = marked; Nl = normal.

rapid increase in bone turnover occurs immediately after menopause. Markers of bone turnover, such as pyridinium crosslinks, are slightly elevated in most patients and markedly increased in "high turnover" individuals. They are useful for initial evaluation of patients with reduced bone mass and for monitoring therapy of osteoporosis. Clinical manifestations occur only when bone mass has been critically reduced, many years after the process begins, with compression fracture of the vertebrae and fractures of long bones with minimal trauma. Typically, routine laboratory tests such as calcium, phosphate, and alkaline phosphatase are normal, as are markers of bone formation.

Vitamin D Deficiency

In addition to hypocalcemia and hypophosphatemia, vitamin D deficiency causes deficient mineralization of osteoid, accompanied by high rates of both bone formation and turnover. In the early stages, calcium and phosphate are normal, while markers of bone formation such as bone alkaline phosphatase and osteocalcin are increased; coupling usually causes an increase in bone turnover markers as well. In later stages, calcium and phosphate are usually low (except in renal failure). Measurement of bone turnover markers is useful in most patients; because urine excretion is used, this may be misleading with impaired renal function. Levels of bone alkaline phosphatase are thus the most useful test for following the adequacy of therapy.

Paget's Disease of Bone

Paget's disease of bone (also called osteitis deformans), a relatively common disease seen in 3–5% of the population, is asymptomatic in the majority of cases. It is characterized by abnormal bone formation and turnover, which leads to bone thickening. Laboratory tests of bone formation, notably osteocalcin and alkaline phosphatase (often 10–20 times normal) correlate well with disease activity; alkaline phosphatase is more commonly used to monitor therapy. Markers of bone turnover correlate poorly with disease activity; the average increase in pyridinium crosslinks is only about twice normal.

Renal Osteodystrophy

Various forms of bone injury occur in patients with chronic renal failure, collectively termed renal osteodystrophy; they include secondary hyperparathyroidism, vitamin D deficiency (osteomalacia), and aluminum-mediated toxicity of bone (Chapter 19). The most important is secondary hyperparathyroidism, detected by intact PTH. Levels of PTH less than four times the upper limit of normal are considered acceptable in renal failure patients. Many markers of bone metabolism are unreliable in patients with renal failure, with bone alkaline phosphatase the best test in this setting.

CHAPTER 11

Laboratory Diagnosis of Liver Disease

D. ROBERT DUFOUR

NORMAL LIVER FUNCTION

The liver, the largest internal organ, requires both normal numbers of hepatocytes and normal blood flow to perform its functions. The portal vein brings blood from the intestinal tract, delivering the raw materials needed for synthetic functions. The most important cells are hepatocytes, which perform most of the synthetic and metabolic functions. Excretory products (bile acids, waste metabolites including bilirubin) are secreted into canaliculi and then enter bile ducts to pass into the intestine. Diseases impairing portal blood flow (such as cirrhosis) impair protein synthesis more than metabolic functions (such as bilirubin metabolism). Diseases obstructing canaliculi, including hepatitis and bile duct obstruction, are associated with impaired excretory function and increased bilirubin, while protein synthesis is typically preserved. The liver has tremendous reserve capacity; most liver diseases are not associated with impaired hepatic function. Other functional liver cells include phagocytic Kupffer cells, responsible for removing antigen–antibody complexes and bacteria from the blood stream, and Ito cells, fat storing cells which can transform to collagen producing cells and cause scarring in chronic hepatitis and cirrhosis.

Summary of Liver Functions

Removal of metabolic substrates and toxic products occurs as blood passes through the liver. This is usually the last function lost with liver disease. Inability to extract waste products, such as unconjugated bilirubin, is a sign of severe liver dysfunction. Detoxification and excretion of toxic and waste products occurs by conversion of lipid soluble drugs and metabolic products (steroid hormones, bilirubin) to water soluble forms which can be more easily excreted. Plasma protein synthesis (Chapter 9) occurs mainly in liver; with impaired portal blood flow or hepatocyte injury, the rate of fall in plasma proteins depends on protein half-life. Metabolism of nutrients occurs as portal blood reaches the liver. The liver uses amino acids for protein synthesis, and detoxifies ammonia from amino acid metabolism by producing urea. The liver provides glucose (Chapter 7) during fasting by metabolism of glycogen, and later by gluconeogenesis. It manufactures most cholesterol and a significant proportion of triglycerides (Chapter 8), responding to changes in concentration of cholesterol and hormones to maintain adequate concentrations of both. Endocrine functions of the liver include synthesis of hormones (Insulin-like Growth Factors, angiotensinogen, T_3, and a small fraction of erythropoietin) and hormone inactivation (PTH, steroids, insulin). Binding proteins for many hormones are synthesized in the liver. Bile acids are produced in the liver and excreted into bile to facilitate micelle formation for intestinal fat absorption. The bile acids are then reabsorbed and extracted by the liver for reuse.

Laboratory Tests of Liver Function

Tests which evaluate liver functions are often used to identify significant liver disease, even though, as mentioned earlier, most liver diseases do not alter liver function. Along

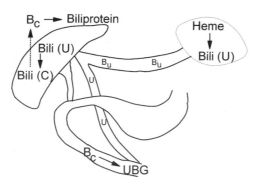

Figure 11.1. Bilirubin Metabolism. Bilirubin, the waste product of heme metabolism, is transported from the spleen to the liver as unconjugated bilirubin (B_u), loosely bound to albumin. Specific hepatocyte receptors transport B_u into the cell, where it is converted to water soluble conjugated bilirubin (B_c) by attachment of two molecules of glucuronic acid. The soluble B_c is secreted into bile ducts; this is the rate limiting step in handling bilirubin. A relatively constant percentage of intestinal B_c is converted by bacteria to colorless urobilinogen (U). A constant fraction of U is reabsorbed and subsequently excreted back into bile, with any excess U excreted in urine. If B_c excretion into bile is blocked, it diffuses into the plasma where a portion becomes covalently bound to albumin (termed biliprotein or δ-bilirubin).

with tests detecting liver cell injury (discussed later), they are widely used for this purpose.

Bilirubin

Normal production and metabolism of bilirubin is summarized in Figure 11.1. In normal plasma, only B_u is present. With liver disease, B_c may enter the plasma, where about 20% becomes bound to albumin, forming biliprotein. Presence of either B_c or biliprotein indicates liver disease. With recovery of liver function, B_u and B_c are cleared rapidly (half-life of 24 hours), while biliprotein remains elevated (half-life of 3 weeks). Most laboratories do not report the concentration of each bilirubin fraction, instead reporting bilirubin concentration as total, direct, and indirect. **Total bilirubin** measures all bilirubin fractions. **Direct bilirubin** measures bilirubin after directly mixing plasma and the reagent; this measures 5% of B_u, 70–90% of B_c, and 100% of biliprotein. **Indirect bilirubin** is indirectly calculated by subtracting direct bilirubin from total bilirubin; it measures primarily B_u and a small fraction of B_c. The following patterns of bilirubin abnormality suggest specific metabolic problems.

Mainly B_u (Indirect)

Increased bilirubin production is usually due to hemolysis, while hematomas and rhabdomyolysis are rare causes. Heme breakdown produces increased urine urobilinogen; LDH is usually increased. Decreased bilirubin conjugation is most commonly due to Gilbert's syndrome, a common insignificant congenital disorder (present in up to 5% of the population), recognized by its familial nature, normal LDH and urobilinogen, and significant increase in bilirubin after a 24 hour fast. Severe liver failure or far advanced portal hypertension prevent bilirubin conjugation and cause increased B_u.

Mainly B_c (Direct)

Normal individuals have essentially no B_c (and thus no biliprotein) in plasma, making direct bilirubin a sensitive marker of liver dysfunction. Increased B_c is usually due to liver disease or bile duct obstruction, typically associated with increased urine bilirubin and often with an absence of bile-derived pigments in stool (which becomes pale gray). Patients with hepatitis and obstruction have a similar ratio of direct to total bilirubin. Rarely, increased conjugated bilirubin is due to a congenital disorder of bilirubin excretion, which may be suspected from the family history.

Mainly Biliprotein (Direct)

This pattern can be recognized by elevated total and direct bilirubin, with direct almost equal to total, and absent or very low urine bilirubin. This pattern always indicates recovery from liver disease. Because of the long half-life of biliprotein, jaundice persists for several weeks after return of liver function.

Evaluation of Protein Synthesis

Plasma protein concentration depends on a constant rate of production. With decreased production, the relative decrease in plasma levels suggests the duration of liver dysfunction (e.g., albumin's half-life is three weeks, coagulation factor VII has a half-life of six hours). Factor VII is usually measured by the prothrombin time (Chapter 27); an abnormal prothrombin time is the most sensitive test of abnormal liver protein synthesis. Protein levels are also dependent on the patient's nutritional state, rate of loss, and cytokine levels, making them less specific for liver disease. Prothrombin time may also be abnormal with vitamin K deficiency, coumadin, or fat malabsorption (which also occurs with bile duct obstruction). Protein synthesis is usually normal in acute or chronic hepatitis or bile duct obstruction; abnormal protein levels in acute hepatitis indicate severe liver damage and high risk of liver failure. Low protein levels are the earliest abnormality in portal hypertension.

Other Metabolic Functions

With far advanced liver disease, other functions may be impaired. Any abnormalities in these functions indicate severe liver injury. Low urea (BUN) indicates markedly impaired synthetic ability. **Ammonia** accumulates in such cases; elevated ammonia is a late finding in liver failure. **Cholesterol** levels reflect mainly liver synthesis. A marked fall in cholesterol occurs with liver failure, and very low cholesterol indicates far advanced liver disease or severe malnutrition.

Tests of Liver Injury

In most cases, liver disease is recognized only by laboratory evidence of damage to liver cells, most commonly plasma enzyme levels. Enzymes are commonly called "liver function tests," but are more sensitive than tests of liver function. Most enzymes are also present in cells outside of the liver.

Normal Liver Enzymes

Hepatocytes contains many enzymes, only a few of which are routinely measured, and these are also found in other cells (Table 11.1). Within hepatocytes, enzymes are found in specific sites (Fig. 11.2), and the pattern of change indicates type of liver injury. With cell wall damage (most cases of hepatitis), AST, ALT, and LDH leak from cells. With damage to mitochondria (alcoholic liver damage), only AST is significantly ele-

Table 11.1.
Organ Locations of "Liver" Enzymes

Enzyme	Organs with High Concentrations	Relative Cell:Plasma Gradient (in liver)
AST (SGOT)	Liver, heart, muscle, kidney	7,000
ALT (SGPT)	Liver, kidney	3,000
LDH	Liver, RBC, heart, muscle, kidney, WBC, tumors	150
Alkaline-Phosphatase	Liver, bone, intestine, placenta	n/a
γ-Glutamyl transferase	Liver, pancreas, kidney, prostate	n/a

vated. Bile duct obstruction causes fragments of cell membrane to dissolve, leaking alkaline phosphatase and GGT into blood. Ingestion of microsomal enzyme inducing agents (alcohol, phenytoin, carbamazepine, barbiturates), will increase GGT.

The Transaminases

Liver, skeletal, and cardiac muscle contain large amounts of AST. The liver also contains large amounts of ALT, but other cells contain considerably less. With injury to the liver, the ratio of plasma AST to ALT is usually less than 2:1, while it is typically greater than 3:1 with damage to other organs, such as muscle. The differing half-lives of the two AST isoenzymes (cytoplasmic 6–8 hours, mitochondrial 10 days) and ALT (24–36 hours) explain many observed patterns in patients with liver disease. With hepatocyte injury, AST is transiently higher than ALT (because of higher cell concentration); within 24–48 hours, ALT becomes higher (because of its slower clearance). With mitochondrial damage (alcoholic hepatitis), AST will be higher than ALT and is stable over several days. ALT levels may be artifactually low in patients with renal failure due to a plasma protein which binds pyridoxal phosphate, a necessary activator.

Alkaline Phosphatase

Bone and liver are the major organs containing alkaline phosphatase on their cell surfaces; lesser amounts are found in intestine and placenta. These isoenzymes can be separated by a variety of methods (Chapter 10). In contrast to all other enzymes, alkaline phosphatase varies little from day to day. Damage to canaliculi by obstruction

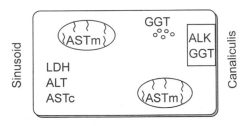

Figure 11.2. Location of Enzymes Within Hepatocytes. Enzymes have different locations within the cell, causing different patterns of abnormalities in various forms of liver disease. AST (SGOT) is found within both cytoplasm and mitochondria, while ALT (SGPT) and LDH are only within cytoplasm. GGT and alkaline phosphatase (ALK) are attached to canalicular membranes of the cell, apparently needed for energy generation to transfer substances into bile. GGT is also present in microsomes, with production enhanced by microsomal enzyme inducing drugs.

or directly in drug reactions causes a gradual increase in alkaline phosphatase for several days before reaching a plateau. The duration of the obstruction is roughly related to degree of elevation. Alkaline phosphatase requires cations (zinc, magnesium) for its actions, usually making results falsely low in patients with zinc deficiency, after blood transfusions (due to binding of cations by citrate in the preservatives), and with specimen contamination by EDTA from lavender top tubes.

Lactate Dehydrogenase

While most cells contain LDH in their cytoplasm, the gradient is much lower than for AST or ALT. The liver isoenzymes of LDH (LDH-4 and LDH-5) have a half-life of approximately 4–6 hours. These characteristics make LDH an insensitive test of liver injury.

γ-Glutamyl Transferase

In the liver, GGT is present on the canalicular surface and in microsomes. Increases in GGT are found with canalicular damage and exposure to agents inducing microsomal enzymes (ethanol, cimetidine, barbiturates, phenytoin, and carbamazepine). GGT shows considerable variation during the day, with levels increasing after meals. Specimens should ideally be drawn before breakfast.

α-Fetoprotein

During pregnancy, α-fetoprotein (AFP) levels are about 1,000,000 times adult levels (Chapter 22), gradually falling to adult levels by the sixth month. Regeneration or proliferation of liver cells causes increased AFP production. With recovery from liver injury and in chronic hepatitis, AFP levels are usually less than 50 times normal, and in most cases under 10 times normal. With neoplasms of hepatocytes (hepatocellular carcinoma, hepatoblastoma), AFP levels are also elevated in about 90% of cases, with levels greater than 500 times normal in about 70% of patients.

WHEN TO DO AND NOT DO TESTS OF LIVER STATUS

Screening for liver disease in most asymptomatic persons is not indicated. Screening is indicated in patient populations with a high prevalence of chronic viral hepatitis (homosexuals, intravenous drug abusers, alcohol abusers), or in geographic areas with a high prevalence of chronic hepatitis virus infection. Case finding in patients with nonspecific symptoms is reasonable, since most patients with liver injury have no liver-specific symptoms such as jaundice.

Testing Used for Case Finding

The most sensitive and specific screening tests are ALT, alkaline phosphatase, and direct bilirubin. When portal hypertension is suspected, prothrombin time is the most sensitive test. In patients at high risk for chronic viral hepatitis, ALT is the only screening test recommended; in alcoholics, AST should be added. AST, GGT, total bilirubin, and albumin are not recommended for initial testing because of low specificity and sensitivity.

Tests in Patients with Acute Jaundice

Initial Evaluation of Patients with Jaundice

AST, ALT, alkaline phosphatase, prothrombin time, and total and direct bilirubin are the most useful tests. Near normal alkaline phosphatase rules out obstruction unless symptoms have been present for less than 1–2 days. The relative elevation of AST and ALT can be useful for differential diagnosis of the cause of hepatitis. Total and direct bilirubin and prothrombin time indicate the degree of liver injury. If hepatitis appears likely and the pattern suggests immunologic injury (see below), serologic testing (IgM anti-HAV in children and young adults, anti-HB$_C$Ag in adolescents or adults, anti-HCV) should be performed. GGT in adults suggests alcoholic hepatitis. If obstruction is a possibility (particularly over age 40), imaging studies are better than laboratory tests for diagnosis.

Follow-up of Jaundiced Patients

AST and ALT do not correlate with clinical outcome or prognosis; they should not be used for follow-up after the initial diagnosis because they may be misinterpreted as indicating recovery. In patients with obstruction, a fall in alkaline phosphatase correlates with relief of the obstruction; alkaline phosphatase should not be checked more often than daily. Total and direct bilirubin usually do not increase more than 1 mg/dL (17 mmol/L) daily, and should not be checked more frequently than each day. The ratio of total to direct bilirubin may be useful in predicting prognosis, with a decreasing ratio indicating a poor prognosis. Once total bilirubin has begun to fall, plasma bilirubin is not useful as the slow rate of biliprotein clearance causes levels to remain elevated for weeks. Urine bilirubin is the best test for recovery of liver function. If prothrombin time is initially normal, repeat measurements should not be done unless the direct to total bilirubin ratio is decreasing.

Tests in Patients with Chronic Hepatitis

Chronic hepatitis is usually recognized by finding elevation of ALT, by case finding in patients with non-specific symptoms, and may even be detected by screening tests in asymptomatic high-risk individuals.

Initial Evaluation

Chronic hepatitis is usually discovered by increased ALT, which should be documented as elevated for six months before further workup is pursued. Initial evaluation should include HB$_S$AG and HCV measurement. If negative, measurement of anti–smooth muscle antibodies and iron and iron binding capacity should be performed to check for autoimmune chronic hepatitis and hemochromatosis, respectively. Serum iron should not be measured in HCV patients, as iron is typically high and may be misleading. Screening for Wilson's disease and α_1-antitrypsin deficiency should only be performed if other tests are negative in a patient younger than 40 years.

Follow-up of Chronic Hepatitis

ALT is the most useful test for monitoring disease activity, although values fluctuate from one measurement to the next. In untreated patients, no other liver tests are

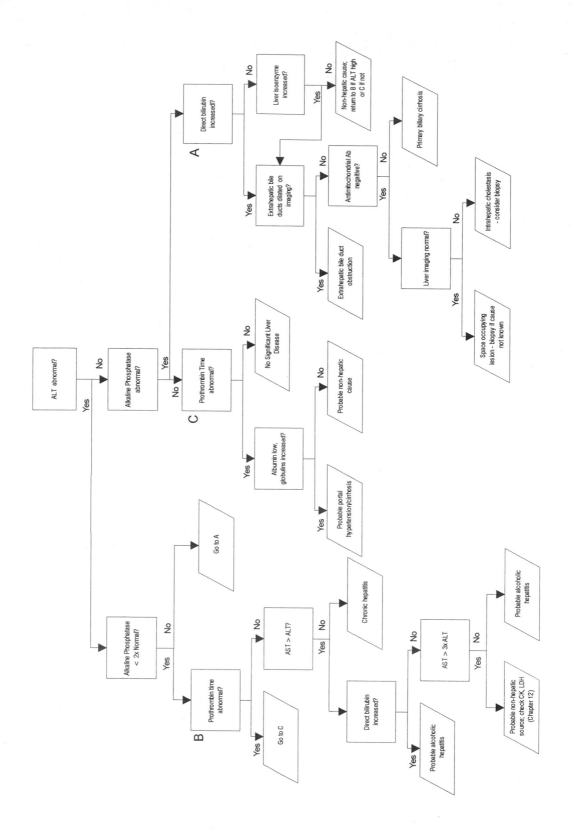

ALT abnormal?

Yes →

No →

Alkaline Phosphatase abnormal?

Yes →

No →

A

Direct bilirubin increased?

No → Liver isoenzyme increased?
- No → Non-hepatic cause; return to B if ALT high or C if not
- Yes → Primary biliary cirrhosis

Yes → Extrahepatic bile ducts dilated on imaging?
- Yes → Extrahepatic bile duct obstruction
- No → Antimitochondrial Ab negative?
  - No → Primary biliary cirrhosis
  - Yes → Liver imaging normal?
    - No → Intrahepatic cholestasis - consider biopsy
    - Yes → Space occupying lesion - biopsy if cause not known

C

Prothrombin Time abnormal?

Yes → Albumin low, globulins increased?
- Yes → Probable portal hypertension/cirrhosis
- No → Probable non-hepatic cause

No → No Significant Liver Disease

B

Alkaline Phosphatase < 2x Normal?

Yes → Prothrombin time abnormal?
- Yes → Go to C
- No → AST > ALT?
  - No → Chronic hepatitis
  - Yes → Direct bilirubin increased?
    - Yes → Probable alcoholic hepatitis
    - No → AST > 3x ALT
      - No → Probable alcoholic hepatitis
      - Yes → Probable non-hepatic source; check CK, LDH (Chapter 12)

No → Go to A

indicated unless jaundice develops. In chronic hepatitis B, HB$_e$Ag will remain present as long as infective virus is present; anti-HB$_e$Ag usually indicates recovery. Measurement of anti-HB$_e$Ag should not be performed more frequently than every 6 months. With treatment of hepatitis C infection, quantitative viral RNA by amplification techniques seems to correlate with treatment effectiveness better than does ALT. In patients with hemochromatosis, ferritin is used to follow the success of phlebotomies. In patients with chronic hepatitis of more than ten years duration, complications may be detected by laboratory tests. Prothrombin time can be checked annually, although it is less sensitive than biopsy to identify progression to cirrhosis. AFP is often used to identify progression to hepatocellular carcinoma; testing should be done every 6 or 12 months. If elevated, AFP levels should be repeated in 2–3 months if mildly (1–10 times) elevated, and followed by liver imaging if moderately (10–50 times) elevated or increasing. If the patient is experiencing an acute flare of chronic hepatitis, testing should be deferred until test results have returned to baseline.

APPROACH TO LIVER DISEASES

Many patients with liver disease are asymptomatic, with liver-related tests indicating liver injury. Figure 11.3 provides an algorithm for evaluation of liver related tests. Figure 11.4 outlines the approach to patients with jaundice.

Acute Hepatitis

The most common cause of jaundice is acute damage to hepatocytes, termed acute hepatitis. Approximately 80–90% of cases are due to viruses, alcohol causes 10%, and the remaining cases are due to drug reactions, toxic agents (acetaminophen, *amanita phalloides* mushrooms), or decreased liver blood flow in shock. The laboratory pattern falls into two major types: **immunologic** (viral, drug-induced, and alcoholic), with gradual prolonged damage and laboratory results changing little from day to day, and **direct injury** (toxic, ischemic), with damage occurring over a short period of time and laboratory results reaching maximal abnormality within one to two days, and returning to normal quickly (Fig. 11.5). In most cases, patients do not develop jaundice and have only laboratory abnormalities (**anicteric hepatitis**); only 10–15% become jaundiced (**icteric hepatitis**), and fewer than 1% develop liver failure (**massive necrosis**). Laboratory features of these three forms are illustrated in Figure 11.6. It is important to note that AST and ALT are not good indicators of recovery, as levels fall rapidly in patients with massive necrosis despite deteriorating liver function.

Laboratory Features

Features helpful in differentiating causes of acute hepatitis are summarized in Figure 11.4 and Table 11.2. Tests for follow-up of patients with hepatitis are summarized in Table 11.3.

◄——

Figure 11.3. Evaluation for Suspected Liver Disease. Initial evaluation of nonicteric patients with suspected liver damage can usually be performed with three tests: ALT, alkaline phosphatase, and prothrombin time. Normal values for all three rule out significant liver damage. Elevated ALT with normal results for the two other tests should be followed by measurement of AST and direct bilirubin. Elevated alkaline phosphatase with normal ALT and direct bilirubin should be investigated with alkaline phosphatase isoenzymes to determine the cause of elevation before proceeding further. Abnormal prothrombin time with normal albumin is usually due to nonhepatic problems.

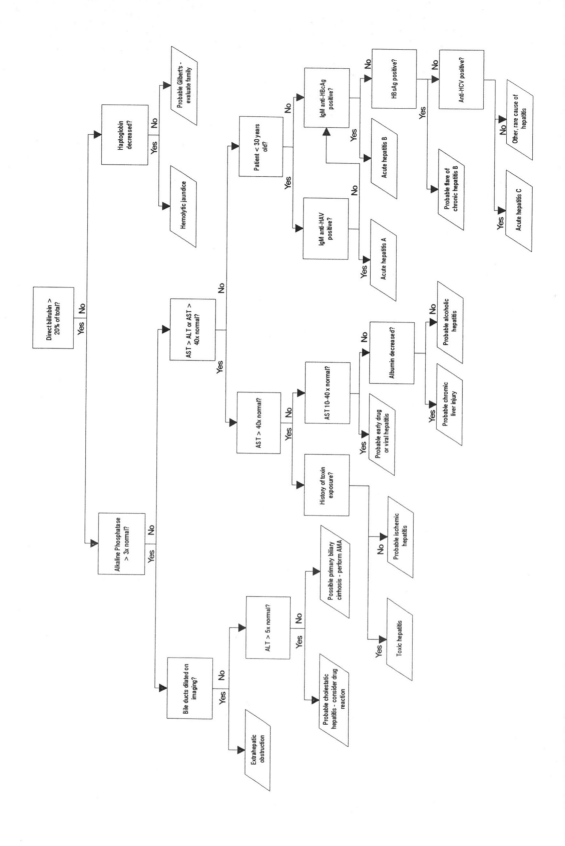

Figure 11.4. Evaluation of Icteric Patients. Jaundiced patients should initially be evaluated by determination of the relative amount of direct bilirubin; results below 20% of total typically indicate either hemolysis or Gilbert's syndrome. With increased direct bilirubin, alkaline phosphatase should be investigated initially; if over 3× normal, imaging of the bile ducts is indicated. With normal or mildly elevated alkaline phosphatase, AST and ALT should be measured. The relative and absolute values of these two enzymes usually provide a clue to the etiology of hepatic damage, while chronicity of injury can be evaluated with albumin. Viral serologies are useful for the determination of the cause of acute hepatic injury in patients with this pattern.

Increased Bilirubin

Usually, conjugated bilirubin is most elevated, with direct bilirubin 50–80% of total bilirubin. With massive necrosis, conjugation is impaired and indirect bilirubin increases to greater than 50% of total bilirubin. During recovery, biliprotein becomes the major form, and direct bilirubin approaches 100% of total bilirubin; recovery is indicated by disappearance of urine bilirubin.

Cytoplasmic Enzymes

In most cases, values of both AST and ALT are more than 10 times normal, and (except for the first 1–2 days) ALT is greater than AST. In alcoholic hepatitis, values are usually less than 10 times normal, and AST is typically more than twice ALT. In toxic and

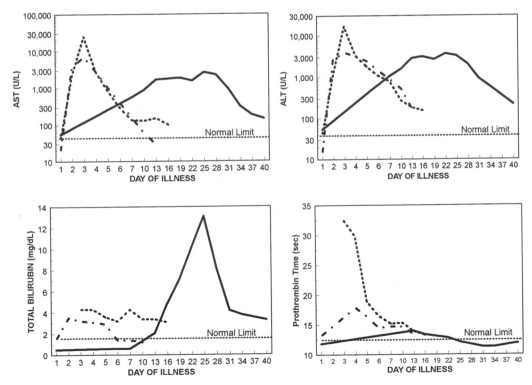

Figure 11.5. Results of Blood Tests in Differing Etiologies of Hepatitis. When damage to the liver is self-limiting, as occurs in toxic (dashed line) or ischemic (dot-dash line) hepatitis, there is a rapid increase in liver related tests, followed by a rapid return to normal. With immunologic injury, as typified by viral hepatitis (solid line), laboratory results show gradual worsening, reach a plateau, and slowly return to normal.

Table 11.2.
Key Features of Different Forms of Hepatitis

Features	Viral	Alcoholic	Toxic/Ischemic
AST/ALT ratio (at diagnosis)	<1	usually > 2	>1 (transient)
Peak AST (× normal)	10–100	1–10	>100
LDH (× normal)	1–2	1–2	10–40
Peak Bilirubin, mg/dL (mmol/L)	5–20 (85–340)	3–20 (51–340)	usually <5 (85)
Prothrombin time	NI	NI or sl. increased	usually >15 sec

ischemic hepatitis, values are typically greater than 100 times normal briefly and fall rapidly. LDH is usually normal, but may be elevated transiently in toxic and ischemic hepatitis.

Canalicular Enzymes

Alkaline phosphatase and GGT are usually only minimally elevated (less than twice normal). In alcoholic hepatitis, GGT is elevated in 70–80% of cases and alkaline phosphatase in increased in 5–10% of cases. In a small percentage of patients, most commonly with drug-induced liver injury, alkaline phosphatase and GGT are elevated along with AST and ALT (**cholestatic hepatitis**).

Proteins

Plasma albumin is normal in most cases. Prothrombin time is typically prolonged in toxic and ischemic hepatitis, and in about 25% of patients with alcoholic hepatitis. In patients with viral hepatitis, an abnormal prothrombin time occurs in only about 5% of cases and is considered a worrisome finding.

Viral Hepatitis

Most cases of hepatitis are due to infection with hepatitis A, B, and C viruses. Hepatitis A (HAV) is most common in children and adolescents; by age 30, 30–40% of the

Table 11.3.
Tests for Follow-up of Patients with Acute Hepatitis

Initial evaluation
   Prothrombin time (for severity evaluation)
   AST, ALT, alkaline phosphatase (for differential diagnosis)
   Total and direct bilirubin
Initial follow-up
   Total and direct bilirubin every two days until peak reached
   Prothrombin time daily (if initially elevated only)
Late follow-up (after peak bilirubin reached)
   Urine bilirubin daily until negative
High risk evaluation
   High risk state:
     Abnormal prothrombin time
     Direct bilirubin <50% of total
   High risk follow-up:
     Prothrombin time daily (until peak reached)

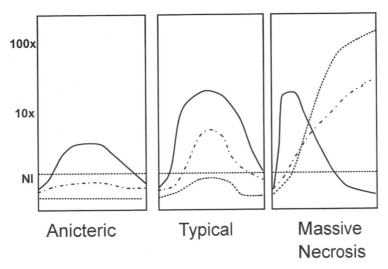

Figure 11.6. Results of Blood Tests in Hepatitis of Various Severities. The pattern of changes in bilirubin (dashed line), serum transaminases, AST and ALT (solid line), and prothrombin time (dotted line) are shown for the three major types of hepatitis. In patients with anicteric disease, serum AST and ALT rise slightly, but liver function remains normal. With typical icteric hepatitis, patients have more marked enzyme increases and become jaundiced with increased serum bilirubin; prothrombin time usually remains normal. With massive hepatic necrosis, the loss of all functioning cells causes AST and ALT to return to normal; however, liver function continues to worsen until the patient dies. Transplantation is the only effective treatment.

population has IgG anti-HAV indicating past infection. Acute hepatitis A is recognized by IgM anti-HAV. Hepatitis B (HBV) (most common in adults) has a complex structure, with several antigens which can be measured by laboratory tests (Table 11.4). Hepatitis C (HCV) causes most post-transfusion hepatitis and 15–20% of acute hepatitis. Current tests detect HCV antibodies 2–4 months after infection. Anti-HCV positive patients are usually infected, but false positive results can be excluded if the confirmatory RIBA (recombinant immunoblot assay) is positive.

Biliary Tract Obstruction

Jaundice occurs only with complete bile duct obstruction. In early obstruction, laboratory features resemble hepatitis, with AST and ALT transiently elevated (often 10–20

Table 11.4.
Serologic Markers of Hepatitis B Infection

Marker	Clinical Importance
Core antigen (HbcAg)	Not detected in serum; related to infectious viral particles.
Core antibody (HBcAb)	First host response to virus; IgM antibodies persist for 6 months, up to 18 months with chronic infection. IgG antibodies persist for life.
Surface antigen (HBsAg)	First marker, last antigen to disappear. Indicates presence of HBV DNA in body.
Surface antibody (HBsAb)	Last antibody to appear, usually indicates recovery. Also present after HBV vaccine. May become undetectable after many years.
e Antigen (HBeAg)	Related to core antigen, denotes infectious viral particles, correlates well with infectivity.
e Antibody (HBeAb)	Generally indicates viral clearance, predicts recovery from chronic hepatitis.
HBV DNA	Most sensitive test for infectious virus, usually available in research laboratories.

times normal), bilirubin predominantly conjugated (direct typically 50–80% of total), and alkaline phosphatase rising slowly. As complete obstruction persists, alkaline phosphatase rises, typically reaching 5–10 times normal, while AST and ALT fall toward normal. With space occupying lesions in the liver that do not completely obstruct drainage, total bilirubin is usually normal, direct bilirubin is slightly increased, alkaline phosphatase is usually increased, and AST and ALT are usually normal.

Chronic Hepatitis

Persistent evidence of hepatitis (defined by elevation of enzymes) for over six months defines chronic hepatitis. About 75% of cases have a definable etiology, most commonly HCV (50%), HBV (20%), and autoimmune disease (5%). Rarely, chronic hepatitis is due to congenital disease (hemochromatosis, Wilson's disease, or α_1-antitrypsin deficiency) or drug reaction. In some cases, no etiology can be determined. While historically chronic hepatitis was classified as chronic active or chronic persistent hepatitis, these terms have largely been abandoned. AST and ALT are usually mildly elevated (1–3 times normal) with ALT higher than AST. Alkaline phosphatase, GGT, total and direct bilirubin, and protein levels are usually normal, although globulins are elevated in the autoimmune form. Occasionally, particularly with hepatitis C, acute increases in AST, ALT, and total and direct bilirubin mimic acute hepatitis.

Cirrhosis

Chronic liver scarring in chronic hepatitis eventually leads to cirrhosis and its complication, portal hypertension. In early stages, diagnosis can only be made by biopsy. As portal hypertension worsens, the ability to synthesize proteins declines, first manifested by prolonged prothrombin time and later by decreased albumin and other liver produced proteins. Intestinal bacterial antigens stimulate increased IgG and IgA, producing polyclonal gammopathy with β-γ bridging on protein electrophoresis. By the time ascites develops, total bilirubin may be mildly elevated, and direct bilirubin is usually increased. In late stages, total bilirubin increases, with more than 50% being indirect bilirubin. Cholesterol and BUN fall, and ammonia rises.

Primary Biliary Cirrhosis

Primary biliary cirrhosis (PBC) is an autoimmune disease which destroys intrahepatic bile ducts, typically affecting middle aged women. It is often recognized by finding elevated alkaline phosphatase, accompanied by **antimitochondrial antibodies.** AST and ALT are usually mildly elevated, in the range seen in chronic hepatitis. Other autoimmune disorders are present in about 2/3 of patients, especially Sjogren's syndrome and rheumatoid arthritis, accompanied by positive rheumatoid factor. An increase in immunoglobulins (particularly IgM) is commonly present.

Liver Tumors

Metastases from tumors in other organs and benign vascular tumors (hemangiomas) are the most common liver tumors. They are frequently associated with mild to moderate elevation of canalicular enzymes (alkaline phosphatase, GGT); cytoplasmic enzymes such as AST and ALT and liver function tests are usually normal. Hepatocellular carcinoma (hepatoma) is the most common primary malignant tumor of the liver. It almost always arises in cirrhotic livers (60–70% of cases), especially following chronic hepatitis B or C infections or hemochromatosis, and is five times more common in males. α-Fetoprotein is elevated in 80–90% of patients, and is over 50 times normal in 60–70% of cases (nearly pathognomonic levels). Following surgical resection or chemotherapy, AFP levels can be used to monitor therapy. The normal half-life of AFP is approximately one week, so that levels should not be checked more often than monthly.

CHAPTER 12

Cardiac and Skeletal Muscle

D. ROBERT DUFOUR

NORMAL MUSCLE CONTENTS

Cardiac and skeletal muscle are similar in terms of biochemical composition, with both containing contractile proteins (actin, myosin, and troponins), enzymes (creatine kinase (CK), aspartate aminotransferase (AST or SGOT), and lactate dehydrogenase (LDH), and an oxygen binding protein (myoglobin). Muscle cells normally turn over at a very low rate, so their cell contents reach plasma in only small amounts. Upon irreversible damage, these proteins are released into the circulation. Smaller substances appear earlier than larger ones, and proteins that make up the contractile structures (such as troponin) are released slowly over many days (Fig 12.1).

Creatine Kinase

The major muscle enzyme, CK (sometimes called CPK), is present in high concentrations only in muscle (cardiac and skeletal) and the brain. Skeletal muscle contains 10,000 times as much CK as plasma, and 5–8 times as much as cardiac muscle, making CK much higher with skeletal muscle injury than with cardiac injury. Brain CK does not reach the circulation except following massive head trauma. In normal persons, plasma CK is derived from skeletal muscle. Levels are related to muscle mass and muscle activity, and are higher in younger persons, in men, and in those of African ancestry. Creatinine kinase is increased tenfold or more after strenuous exercise, particularly weight lifting, endurance exercise, and contact sports. Comparing CK to "reference" values is difficult, since there is a wide range of CK values in healthy individuals. Individual results are best interpreted based on changes from a baseline or by evaluation of level of exercise.

Isoenzymes

Creatinine kinase is a dimer, with muscle (M) and brain (B) subunits, producing three isoenzymes (MM, MB, and BB). The CK BB isoenzyme is found in brain, prostate, placenta, and fetal tissues. Creatinine kinase MB is a minor isoenzyme in skeletal muscle; it is typically less than 2% of total CK, but may be 5–10% in respiratory muscles and during muscle regeneration (with chronic muscle injury). In cardiac muscle (myocardium), MB averages 10–15% of total CK in most hearts. The major difference between skeletal and cardiac muscle is relative percentage of MB. In normal individuals, CK MB is usually under 1% of total CK. With skeletal muscle injury, MB is usually less than 3% of total CK, although in a small fraction of cases it is higher (but virtually never greater than 10% of total). With myocardial injury, MB is greater than 3% of total CK in 99% of cases, over 5% of total in 95%, and over 10% in 60%. Values between 3% and 10% of CK MB are indeterminate, although usually of cardiac origin; they should be confirmed as indicating myocardial damage by some other test or tests. In about 1–2% of those older than age 60 and in HIV infected individuals, CK BB is

156

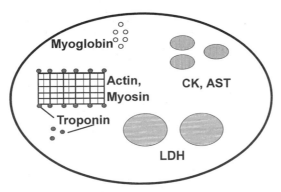

Figure 12.1. Relative Size of Myocardial Contents. Of the soluble cytoplasmic proteins, myoglobin is the smallest and released most rapidly with cell injury, while release of the relatively large LDH is delayed. Substances making up parts of the myofibrils, such as troponin and myosin, are released gradually and are detectable for many days.

bound to immunoglobulin (macro-CK 1). This form of CK BB may be measured as CK MB in some assays.

Several different methods are used to measure CK MB, with immunoassays specific for MB the most widely used. Results are reported in different units than total CK, so the percentage of total CK cannot be directly calculated (as units would not cancel out). However, a "relative index" is calculated by dividing CK MB by total CK and multiplying by 100 (the upper reference limit is usually less than 2.5%, which roughly corresponds to an actual percentage of 5%; most normal individuals lack CK MB). Levels of CK MB can also be measured by electrophoresis (upper reference limit 5%, with none detected in most normal individuals); a less sensitive and less accurate test than immunoassay. A few laboratories estimate CK MB by immunoinhibition: antibodies to CK M subunits inactivate all CK MM and half of CK MB, so the remaining CK is multiplied by two to give CK MB, which is then divided by total CK to calculate the percentage. This methodology assumes that no CK BB (or macro-CK) is present, and false positive results are relatively common. Hemolysis and liver injury also cause false positive results. This cross-reactivity leads to high "normal" values (up to 14–16 U/L). This in turn requires higher results to call a specimen abnormal, so false negative results are also common. Practitioners should be aware of these limitations if the laboratory they are using employs this technique for CK MB determination.

Creatine Kinase Isoforms

After tissue CK M subunits reach the circulation, they are rapidly modified (half-life of 3 hours) by plasma enzymes, altering their chemical structure and charge. The native and modified forms are termed "isoforms." There are three possible isoforms of CK MM, and two of CK MB. The relative ratio of the tissue and modified isoforms of CK MM and CK MB indicates how recently muscle injury has occurred, with a high fraction of tissue isoenzyme occurring for only a few hours after the onset of damage.

Lactate Dehydrogenase and Aldolase

These enzymes involved in glucose metabolism are present in most cells, with highest concentrations in liver, red blood cells, and cardiac and skeletal muscle. Lactate dehydrogenase and aldolase have the lowest cell gradient relative to plasma (150 times plasma), making them insensitive markers of muscle injury. With cell damage, LDH rises more slowly than CK or AST because it is a larger enzyme. Lactate dehydrogenase is a tetramer composed of heart (H) and muscle (M) subunits, producing five isoenzymes: LDH 1 is HHHH, while LDH 5 is MMMM. In normal plasma, LDH 2 is the dominant isoenzyme, followed by LDH 1, LDH 3, LDH 4, and LDH 5. Heart and red blood cells contain mainly LDH 1 and 2, which have half-lives of about 48 hours. Liver and skeletal muscle contain predominantly LDH 4 and 5, which have half-lives of about 4–6 hours. Aldolase isoenzymes differ from cell to cell, with skeletal muscle, cardiac muscle, and tumor cells containing the same isoenzyme. Older aldolase assays preferentially measured this isoenzyme, and many textbooks advocated aldolase as a useful marker of muscle injury. Current assays measure all isoenzymes equally. The low concentration and short half-life of aldolase make it inferior to CK for detecting muscle injury. Its measurement has been abandoned by many laboratories.

Aspartate Aminotransferase

Cardiac muscle contains twice as much AST (also called SGOT; see Chapter 11) as skeletal muscle. After muscle injury, AST reaches peak values 4–6 hours later than CK, but has a similar half-life. The CK/AST ratio takes advantage of the relative differences in CK and AST in skeletal and cardiac muscle to determine the source of increased CK. A ratio greater than 20 is typical of skeletal muscle injury.

Myoglobin

The muscle oxygen binding protein myoglobin appears rapidly in plasma after muscle injury, being detectable within 2–4 hours, peaking in 8–12 hours, and levels typically returning to normal by 24–30 hours. Myoglobin is cleared by the kidney and can be detected in urine shortly after muscle injury; however, most tests used to detect urine myoglobin (such as the "blood" dipstick) are much less sensitive than CK for detecting muscle damage. Plasma myoglobin levels are higher and remain elevated longer with renal insufficiency.

Troponin

Several small proteins (found in both cardiac and skeletal muscle) involved in activating muscle contraction are termed troponins. Two of these (troponin-T and troponin-I) are structurally different in skeletal and cardiac muscle, so that the cardiac-specific form can be separately measured by immunoassay. The cell to plasma ratio for troponin is much higher than for enzymes or myoglobin, making cardiac troponin a highly sensitive marker of myocardial injury. Most troponin is bound to muscle filaments, and is released slowly and remains elevated for one to two weeks after myocardial injury. Approximately 5% is free within the cytoplasm. This, and its small size, allows appearance in plasma within 3–4 hours of myocardial injury. The cardiac form of troponin-T is also produced by regenerating skeletal muscle, and levels are slightly increased in patients with renal failure; such changes have not been documented for troponin-I.

WHEN NOT TO DO TESTS OF MUSCLE INJURY

Laboratory tests are the major means to diagnose both myocardial infarction and skeletal muscle injury. There are few instances when these tests should not be done in patients suspected of having these disorders. Single specimens should never be used at initial presentation to decide whether patients with chest pain should be admitted or receive thrombolytic agents. The sensitivity of these tests when patients are first seen is usually less than 40%. In patients admitted for possible myocardial infarction, intramuscular injections should be prohibited to prevent difficulty in interpretation of the results. If total CK is used as a screening test, further testing need not be done if CK is stable or decreasing (Fig. 3.3). Tests for LDH isoenzymes should not be performed on hemolyzed specimens or in patients with hemolytic anemia, as red blood cells contain the same isoenzymes as does myocardium. Myoglobin and troponin-T should not be used in patients with renal failure, as both may be falsely elevated. Creatinine kinase is increased with even minor trauma to muscle; strenuous exercise can increase CK to 5,000–10,000 U/L, cardiopulmonary resuscitation commonly causes similar increases, and a single intramuscular injection may increase CK by over 1,000 U/L. Effects of these factors should always be considered before attributing an increased CK to intrinsic muscle disease.

MYOCARDIAL CELL DEATH

There is a spectrum of symptoms related to reduction in myocardial blood flow (ischemia) (Fig. 12.2). Myocardial cells are relatively resistant to ischemia: normal cells survive about 30 minutes of complete lack of oxygen, while chronically ischemic cells may survive up to one hour. After this time, myocardial cells begin to die (myocardial infarction). The number of cells dying increases rapidly over the next two hours, reaching maximum after six hours (Fig. 12.3). If the clot is dissolved, a **non-Q–wave myocardial infarction** typically results. Continued occlusion destroys essentially the complete thickness of myocardium (**Q–wave myocardial infarction**).

Diagnosis of Myocardial Infarction

WHO criteria for myocardial infarction require presence of two of three criteria: prolonged chest pain (more than 30 minutes), new ischemic EKG changes, and elevated plasma enzymes. In practice, however, enzymes are considered the gold standard for diagnosing myocardial infarction. Many cardiologists have adopted the use of the term "minimal myocardial damage" to recognize patients with chest pain, non-diagnostic EKG, and rises in plasma markers. Such patients are at increased risk for a major

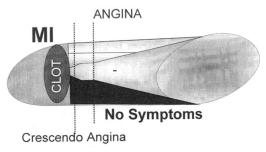

Figure 12.2. Spectrum of Symptoms Caused by Reduced Coronary Blood Flow. Gradual narrowing by atherosclerosis is typically asymptomatic until blood flow is less than 10% of normal when chest pain occurs with increased oxygen demand (exertional angina). Acute reduction in blood flow (usually from a clot) causes chest pain at rest. Often, a clot is not completely obstructing or is dissolved by the fibrinolytic system, producing unstable angina. If a clot persists, cells begin to die after about one hour (myocardial infarction).

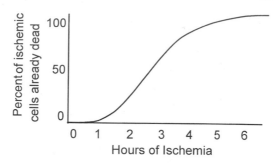

Figure 12.3. Fractional Survival of Myocardial Cells During Ischemia. With coronary artery occlusion, myocardial cells can survive for approximately 30 minutes, or up to an hour if previously deprived of oxygen by atherosclerosis. After this period, cells begin to die rapidly, with about 80% of cells at risk having already perished by three hours of occlusion. Approximately 100% of cells destined to die will have done so by six hours after onset of occlusion.

cardiac event, similar to patients with non-Q–wave myocardial infarction. The relative performance of criteria to detect myocardial infarction is illustrated in Figure 12.4 and in Table 12.1. The average peak CK level after myocardial infarction is approximately 1200 U/L, with an average MB of 11% (relative index 6%).

Laboratory Testing Strategies for Myocardial Infarction

Initial Evaluation of Patients in the Emergency Room

Laboratory tests have limited usefulness at the time of initial presentation. Only $\frac{1}{4}$ to $\frac{2}{5}$ of patients having myocardial infarction have abnormal laboratory tests when first seen in the emergency room. Normal results for initial tests should *never* be used to decide to discharge a patient from the emergency room, or to withhold thrombolytic agents.

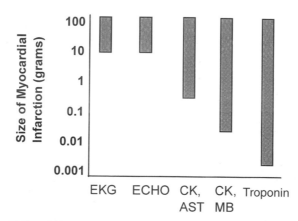

Figure 12.4. Relative Ability of Tests to Detect Myocardial Infarction. Theoretical minimum amounts of myocardial damage detectable are shown for each marker. Imaging techniques and EKG can detect injury to about 5–10 grams of myocardium. CK and AST will show a measurable increase with approximately 0.2 grams of myocardium damaged, while CK MB can detect injury to 1/10 that amount. With troponin, the extremely high cell content and low plasma levels lead to a theoretical sensitivity of about 0.003 grams of myocardial infarction. While pain is sensitive for all amounts of myocardial infarction, it is also present with reversible damage and is absent in as many as 20–30% of cases of myocardial infarction.

Table 12.1.
Relative Performance of Laboratory Markers of Myocardial Damage

Marker	M.W. (kd)	First Detected (hrs) (median)	Relative Increase (× NI)	Duration (hrs)	Sensitivity for MI (Q/non-Q)	Sensitivity for Unstable Angina
Myoglobin	18	2–3	12	18–24	100/100	?
Troponin I	23.5	4–6	50	>144	100/100	20
Troponin T	33	3–4	50	>240	100/100	40
CK	86	6–8	8	36–48	100/80	0
CK-MB mass	86	3–4	12	24–36	100/100	25
CK-MB immunoinhibition	86	6–8	6	24–36	100/85	0
CK-MB isoforms	86	3–4	n/a	8–12	100/100	25
AST	111	8–10	5	36–60	100/90	0
LDH	133	12–14	2.5	96–160	80–30	0

Use of Tests to Detect Myocardial Infarction

Serial measurements are needed to diagnose myocardial infarction; the sensitivity of markers reaches 98–99% by 6–10 hours after onset of symptoms. Troponin, CK isoforms, and CK MB immunoassay have similar sensitivity for detecting myocardial infarction; additionally, troponin-I is not affected by coexistent skeletal muscle injury. Any increase in these markers between two serial specimens which exceeds the reference limits indicates myocardial infarction. There is a rough relationship between the peak value of any of the markers and the amount of myocardium damaged.

Noninvasive Detection of Reperfusion

When myocardial infarction is diagnosed clinically within six hours of onset of pain, thrombolytic agents are used to remove the clot, restore myocardial blood flow, and limit infarct size. This therapy is successful in about $\frac{2}{3}$ of patients. Identification of patients without reperfusion could allow for use of other procedures (such as angioplasty or bypass surgery) to restore blood flow. Resolution of chest pain and elimination of EKG changes have traditionally been used to detect reperfusion. If blood flow is restored, rapid clearance causes a rapid rise in blood markers, an early peak, and more rapid return to normal (Fig. 12.5). Unfortunately, the accuracy of this technique does

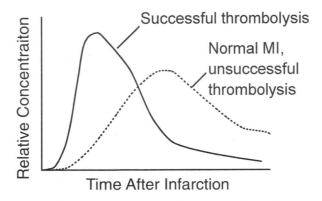

Figure 12.5. Time Course of Enzyme Changes with Normal Infarction and Reperfusion. If arterial circulation is reestablished, all soluble markers are released to the circulation more rapidly. This leads to earlier detection, a higher peak, and more rapid return to normal when compared to the pattern seen following typical myocardial infarction. A similar pattern occurs after cardiac surgery.

not approach 100% until 90 minutes after thrombolysis, which is not early enough to benefit patients who need other therapy (angioplasty or surgery to restore myocardial blood flow) to limit infarct size.

Detection of Myocardial Infarction with Coexistent Skeletal Muscle Damage

After surgery, cardiopulmonary resuscitation, or trauma, markers present in both cardiac and skeletal muscle (CK, CK MB, CK MB isoforms, myoglobin, and AST) are all increased, making detection of myocardial infarction difficult. In addition, dilution of the CK MB index by CK release from skeletal muscle causes frequent false negative results. Troponin is the test of choice for recognition of myocardial damage in such patients, with troponin-I slightly better than troponin-T.

Identification of Myocardial Infarction Following Cardiac Surgery

Release of myocardial proteins occurs in all cardiac surgery patients. After surgery, markers reach the circulation quickly (as with thrombolysis) through patent blood vessels. In perioperative myocardial infarction, markers are released more slowly, as with a typical myocardial infarction. The time course of markers is the best criterion for detecting myocardial infarction in this setting; in an autopsy controlled study, a CK MB of greater than 133 U/L at 15 hours after surgery had a sensitivity of 60% and a specificity of 100% for perioperative myocardial infarction.

Late Presentation

Patients presenting more than 24 hours after onset of symptoms often have nondiagnostic AST, myoglobin, CK, CK MB, and CK MB isoforms. In such situations, measurement of LDH isoenzymes has been used; an LDH 1 to LDH 2 ratio of at least 1 occurs in 30% of patients with non-Q–wave and in 80% with Q–wave myocardial infarction, and persists for 4–7 days. Troponin remains elevated for 7–10 days, and is more reliable than LDH isoenzymes.

DETECTING SKELETAL MUSCLE INJURY

Skeletal muscle disease usually presents with muscle pain or weakness. While laboratory tests are useful in detecting damage to skeletal muscle, they cannot differentiate varying causes of injury. The most reliable test is CK, capable of detecting damage to approximately 0.01 grams of muscle by producing a rise in total CK of 20 U/L. As discussed earlier, there is a wide range of normal values for CK: values over 1,000 U/L almost always indicate muscle injury, but may be due to benign forms of damage such as exercise, intramuscular injection, or mild trauma. With self-limited damage (including these benign forms), CK will typically fall after admission. A persistent elevation in CK indicates chronic, ongoing muscle damage.

Acute, Self-Limited Injury

The most classic form is rhabdomyolysis, in which muscle is damaged by physical agents (severe exercise, crush injuries, ischemia, ethanol, cocaine) or inflammation. Myoglobin and CK increase rapidly in plasma, reaching a peak in a relatively short period of time, and then falling gradually towards normal with a half-life of CK of approximately 18–24 hours. Urine myoglobin will often be present, and can be routinely detected by dipsticks when total CK is greater than 20,000 U/L. In patients who are dehydrated or who are exposed to other factors which decrease blood flow to the kidneys, myoglobin and other muscle contents may cause acute renal tubular necrosis and renal failure. If renal damage occurs, plasma levels of cell products such as potassium, phosphate, and uric acid may increase markedly and reach dangerous levels; in patients without renal damage, plasma levels usually remain normal. Patients with rhabdomyolysis should have a daily CK measurement until two consecutive days show a fall of 50% or more in results. Creatinine kinase isoenzymes are not needed when total CK is over 2,000 U/L, as clinical diagnosis of myocardial infarction is obvious in patients with this degree of elevation from cardiac sources. Patients with rising or elevated CK should have daily measurement of K^+, BUN, and creatinine to detect complications which require treatment. If BUN is increased or the patient is dehydrated, urine alkalinization can lessen likelihood of acute renal failure. This can be monitored by urine pH, which should be greater than 7.0.

Chronic, Ongoing Muscle Injury

Persistent muscle damage occurs with autoimmune disorders such as polymyositis, drug and ethanol exposure, or congenital degenerative diseases such as muscular dystrophy. Total CK is typically elevated, with the degree of elevation related to the extent of muscle damage; levels are stable or increase slowly over time. Patients with chronic muscle injury are less likely to have myoglobin in urine, and rarely develop acute renal failure. Levels of CK isoenzymes are not needed to establish the diagnosis in a patient with chronic CK elevation; if performed, CK MB is often 3% or higher, results rare with acute muscle damage.

CHAPTER 13

Laboratory Evaluation of Thyroid Function

D. ROBERT DUFOUR

NORMAL THYROID HORMONE PRODUCTION

Hypothalamic–Pituitary–Thyroid Axis

Thyrotropin-releasing hormone (TRH) is produced at many locations in the brain as a neurotransmitter at several sites (Figure 13.1). Production of TRH is largely independent of thyroid hormone levels. The production of thyrotropin (TSH) in response to TRH is inversely related to plasma thyroid hormone concentration because pituitary T_3 receptors control TSH production. The pituitary can convert thyroxine (T_4) to T_3 directly. Normally, 60% of pituitary T_3 is derived from pituitary conversion of plasma T_4. Thyrotropin production is exquisitely sensitive to small changes in T_4 level, showing a logarithmic response to altered thyroid hormone availability.

Thyroid Hormone Synthesis

Thyrotropin stimulates every step in the synthetic process, leading to storage of thyroid hormones as part of thyroglobulin and release of hormones from its breakdown (Figure 13.2). As long as TSH is relatively low, most thyroid hormone is fully iodinated, producing predominantly T_4. When TSH activity is high (as in hypothyroidism or in Graves' disease), iodine becomes slightly deficient, producing a much higher proportion of T_3.

Peripheral Fate of Thyroid Hormones

Transport

Thyroid hormones are transported by several plasma proteins, with 99.97% of T_4 and 99.7% of T_3 and reverse T_3 protein bound. The three major binding proteins are thyroid-binding globulin (TBG), albumin, and transthyretin (prealbumin). About 65% of T_4 and 75% of T_3 are bound to TBG, 10–15% of T_4 and 10% of T_3 are bound to albumin. Only T_4 is significantly bound to transthyretin. The high degree of protein binding causes an extremely long half-life for thyroid hormones (one week for T_4, one day for T_3). While only a small fraction of thyroid hormone exists in the free state, free hormone is considered metabolically active and is the only form which alters TSH production. The equilibrium for protein binding is illustrated in Equation 13.1.

$$T_4 \text{ (free)} + TBG \overset{k}{\vee} T_4 \text{ - } TBG$$

$$T_4 \text{ (free)} = k \times \frac{T_4 \text{ - } TBG}{TBG} \tag{1}$$

$$T_4 \text{ (free)} = k \times TBG \text{ Saturation}$$

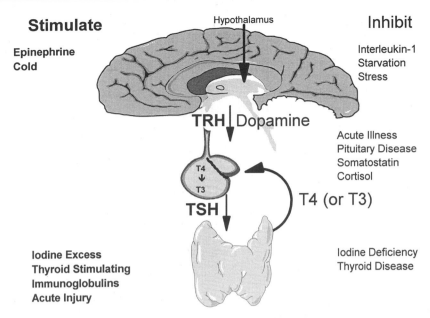

Stimulate

Epinephrine
Cold

Hypothalamus

Inhibit

Interleukin-1
Starvation
Stress

TRH Dopamine

Acute Illness
Pituitary Disease
Somatostatin
Cortisol

T4
↓
T3

TSH

T4 (or T3)

Iodine Excess
Thyroid Stimulating
Immunoglobulins
Acute Injury

Iodine Deficiency
Thyroid Disease

Figure 13.1. The Hypothalamic–Pituitary–Thyroid Axis. Hypothalamic production of TRH occurs at a relatively constant rate, inhibited by cytokines, starvation, and stress. TRH acts to stimulate TSH production by the pituitary; its response is inhibited by T_3 produced within pituitary cells from T_4. TSH production is also inhibited by dopamine, somatostatin, and cortisol. TSH stimulates production of thyroid hormone, which produces feedback inhibition of TSH production.

Changes in plasma total thyroid hormone concentration may be due either to changes in thyroid hormone production or changes in binding proteins. In physiologic states, free T_4 (and free T_3) and TBG saturation remain constant, even if the amount of binding proteins changes. With abnormal binding protein levels, slow change in concentration allows adaptation, resulting in a change in altered thyroid hormone production and total thyroid hormone levels but the same level of free T_4. If the equilibrium constant does not change, total thyroid hormone and binding protein concentrations can be used to estimate the concentration of free thyroid hormone; alterations in protein affinity invalidate this estimate.

Thyroid Hormone Metabolism

All thyroid hormones are metabolized by enzymatic removal of a single iodine by degradative enzymes known as monodeiodinases (Fig. 13.3). Cellular receptors respond primarily to T_3, with T_4 considered a prohormone. About 70% of circulating T_3 is produced in the liver. Tissue $3',5'$-monodeiodinase activity is extremely labile: activity is low in neonates and the elderly, and also falls with acute illness or malnutrition. These states are associated with low T_3 and increased reverse T_3 (rT_3) (due to decreased rT_3 clearance). This enzyme also shows increases in activity in hyperthyroidism and decreases in hypothyroidism.

Regulation of Thyrotropin Synthesis

Pituitary monodeiodinase is not as labile as that in other tissues. The pituitary responds primarily to changes in T_4 (and, to a lesser extent, T_3) production by the thyroid.

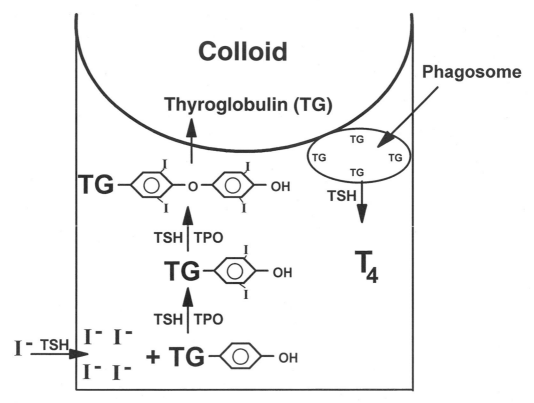

Figure 13.2. Thyroid Hormone Production. TSH stimulates all steps needed for the production of thyroid hormone. Initially, iodine is concentrated in the gland, where thyroid peroxidase (TPO) catalyzes its attachment to tyrosine residues on the already synthesized thyroglobulin (TG). TPO also catalyzes rearrangement of tyrosine side chains to produce iodothyronines, T_4 and T_3. Thyroglobulin is stored in follicles as a colloid. TSH stimulates formation of phagosomes which ingest and breakdown portions of the colloid, releasing active thyroid hormones T_4 and T_3 which enter the circulation. Under normal circumstances, the thyroid produces primarily T_4; when stimulated by TSH, T_3 production becomes more important.

LABORATORY TESTS EVALUATING THYROID FUNCTION

Assays for Total Thyroid Hormones

For many years, all assays measured total thyroid hormone, affected by levels of binding proteins. These total hormone assays are still the most widely used. Assays for total thyroid hormones are highly accurate, and show few interferences. Only rare patients with autoimmune thyroid diseases have antibodies which cause falsely low results in most assays.

Estimation of Thyroid-binding Globulin Concentration

When total thyroid hormone is measured, abnormal levels may be due to changes in the binding proteins. While binding protein levels could be measured directly, they are most commonly evaluated by the confusing T_3 resin uptake (T_3RU). Many laboratories now perform a newer version termed the T-uptake. Because the principles, results, and interpretation are exactly opposite, they are discussed separately. It is thus important for practitioners to know which of these tests their laboratory is using.

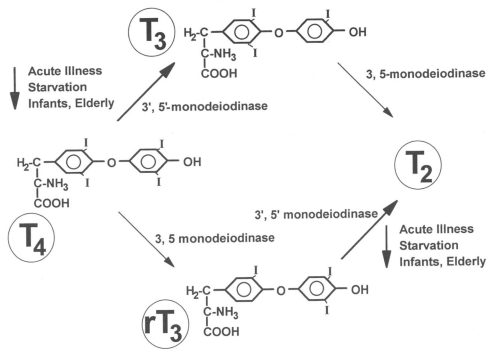

Figure 13.3. Thyroid Hormone Metabolism. T_4 is the major product of the thyroid gland, but T_3 is the active hormone. T_4 is metabolized by two different monodeiodinases, primarily in the liver and kidney, to produce two different isomers of T_3. If iodine is removed from the outer ring, T_3 is produced, while cleavage of an iodine from the inner ring generates inactive rT_3. Normally, activity of the former enzyme is several times that of the latter, and is responsible for further metabolism of rT_3. The enzyme removing iodine from the outer ring has reduced activity in infants and the elderly, and is decreased by acute illness and starvation; in these states, T_3 will fall but rT_3 will increase.

T_3 Resin Uptake (Fig. 13.4)

In most cases, T_3RU results are expressed as a percentage of T_3 added; however, some laboratories divide the result by a normal average, with a normal result being 1.0. Values of T_3RU are inversely related to unsaturated thyroid hormone-binding sites (Fig. 13.5). In primary thyroid diseases, T_4 and T_3RU levels change in the same direction, while with a primary change in TBG level, T_4 and T_3RU change in opposite directions. This simple rule is the easiest way to evaluate the commonly performed tests of thyroid function.

T-Uptake

In a T-uptake test (Fig. 13.6), results are divided by the average for the normal population, so that a normal result is 1.0. Values of T-uptake are directly related to the number of free binding sites. Therefore T_4 and T-uptake change in opposite directions with altered T_4 production, and change in the same direction with altered TBG (Fig. 13.7). T-uptake is less affected by changes in thyroid hormone concentration than by changes in TBG concentration, and tends to be normal in many patients with hypothyroidism or hyperthyroidism.

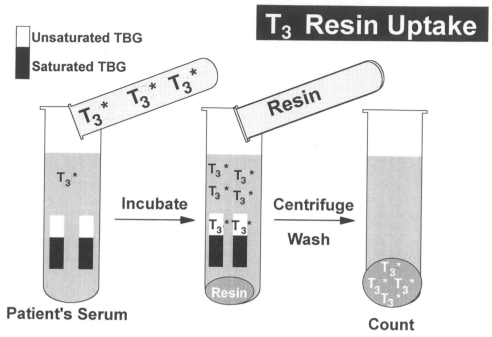

Figure 13.4. Principle of T_3 Resin Uptake (T_3RU). A known amount of labeled T_3 is added to patient plasma and allowed to come to equilibrium with available, unsaturated binding sites on TBG. To evaluate the amount absorbed by TBG, a resin is added to remove any remaining unbound labeled T_3. After centrifugation, the label in the resin is measured; this is inversely related to the available free binding sites on TBG.

Free Thyroid Hormone

For many years, the only test available to determine the free thyroid hormone level was equilibrium dialysis, a difficult and time consuming assay offered by few laboratories. More recently, a number of direct tests of free T_4 (and free T_3) have come on the market. An important assumption is that there is a normal thyroid binding equilibrium constant. In acute illness, there is a reduction in affinity constant, causing displacement of free thyroid hormone and an increase in its concentration. Some methods show this change, while others do not, causing different results in acutely ill patients. With equilibrium dialysis, about 10% of acutely ill patients have high free thyroid hormone levels, while about 25% have low levels with one step (analogue) assays. Results are usually normal with two step methods. Which of these methods is the most reliable is a matter of argument among experts. Practitioners must know which method is used by the laboratory to accurately interpret results.

One Step (Analogue) Assays

A labeled analogue of free T_4 competes with unlabeled T_4 in plasma for limited antibody binding sites; the amount of label bound is inversely proportional to plasma free T_4. Analogues also bind to albumin; if plasma albumin levels are abnormal, measured free T_4 is directly proportional to albumin concentration. If the affinity constant for the analogue is increased (antithyroxine antibodies or familial dysalbuminemic hyperthyroxinemia, discussed later), free T_4 is typically overestimated.

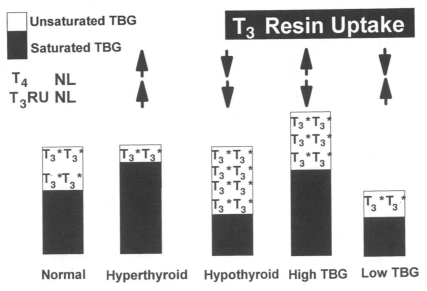

Figure 13.5. Effect of Changes in Thyroid Hormone and Binding Proteins on T_3RU. The bars represent TBG, with the solid portion depicting the proportion of binding sites occupied with T_4 produced by the thyroid. When thyroid hormone production is altered, saturation changes in the same direction, free binding sites will change in the opposite direction, and T_3RU changes in the same direction as total thyroid hormone. When the amount of binding protein changes, production of thyroid hormone will change as well, maintaining free T_4 at baseline levels but increasing total thyroid hormone. Saturation will remain constant, free binding sites will change in the same direction as total thyroid hormone, and resin uptake will change in the opposite direction. With primary thyroid disease, therefore, total T_4 and T_3RU change in the same direction; with alteration in amount of binding protein, total T_4 and T_3RU change in opposite directions.

Two Step Immunoassays

In this procedure, an antibody to T_4 is bound to a solid support and mixed with plasma, the solid support is washed, and a known amount of labeled T_4 is added. The amount of label bound is inversely proportional to plasma free T_4. Two site assays are less affected by changes in plasma albumin or altered affinity constants, and generally agree well with equilibrium dialysis.

Free Thyroxine Index

Free T_4 can be estimated indirectly from total T_4 and either T_3RU or T-uptake. If T_3RU is measured, T_4 is multiplied by T_3RU to get the free thyroxine index (FTI). Many laboratories divide this by the average T_3RU to get the same reference range as total thyroxine. Results diverge from measured free T_4 at the ends of the reference range. If T-uptake is measured, T_4 is divided by the T-uptake, with the reference range the same as for total T_4. Results using T-uptake agree better with free thyroxine than do those using T_3RU. Both methods give normal results in early thyroid disease, and produce misleading results in persons with both abnormal binding proteins and thyroid disease.

Radioactive Iodine Uptake

Thyroid iodine trapping is an active process, requiring TSH and an intact gland for normal uptake. Radioactive iodine uptake (RAIU) measures the fraction of radioactive

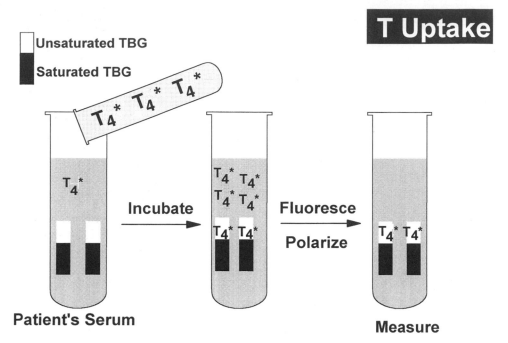

Figure 13.6. Principle of T-Uptake. A known amount of fluorescently labeled T_4 is added to patient plasma and allowed to come to equilibrium with available, unsaturated binding sites on TBG. Any T_4 bound to protein will not be able to rotate in solution. Thus when excited by polarized light, the bound T_4 will fluoresce in the same plane as the exciting light. The amount of polarized fluorescence is directly related to the number of unsaturated binding sites on TBG.

iodine taken up at specific times after ingestion, usually 6 or 24 hours (or both). Iodide, either dietary or from medications (amiodarone, radiographic contrast agents), saturates the gland and causes low uptake, while iodide deficiency produces increased radioiodine uptake. This test is a direct measure of thyroid activity in patients on normal iodide intake.

EVALUATION OF HYPOTHALAMIC–PITUITARY CONTROL

Thyrotropin

The pituitary responds to slight changes in thyroid hormone production. Thyrotropin becomes abnormal early in thyroid disease, and is the most sensitive test of thyroid function. Thyrotropin assays are referred to in "generations," with each resulting in a tenfold reduction of TSH detectable. First generation assays measured to 1 mU/L; 30% of normal patients had "low" TSH. Second generation assays detect 0.1 mU/L; "suppressed" TSH is found in almost all patients with hyperthyroidism, rarely in ambulatory patients, and in around 3% of euthyroid hospitalized patients. Third generation assays, with detection limits below 0.01 mU/L, have few falsely low results and identify hyperthyroid patients accurately, but few laboratories currently offer such tests. A number of assays detect 0.03 to 0.05 mU/L, and give few falsely suppressed results. We have found such assays to provide clinically usable information in almost all patients. Thyrotropin requires α and β subunits and carbohydrate for normal bioactivity; in secondary hypothyroidism, TSH with a reduced amount of carbohydrate is produced.

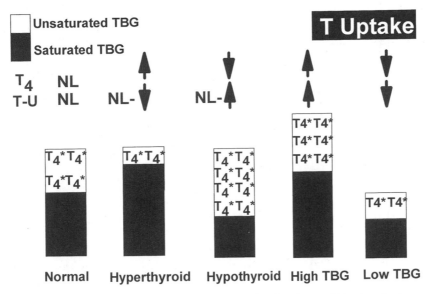

Figure 13.7. Effect of Changes in Thyroid Hormone and Binding Proteins on T-Uptake. The bars represent TBG, with the solid portion depicting the proportion of binding sites occupied with T_4 produced by the thyroid. When thyroid hormone production is altered, saturation changes in the same direction, but free binding sites and T-uptake will change in the opposite direction. When the amount of binding protein changes, production of thyroid hormone will change as well, maintaining free T_4 at baseline levels but increasing total thyroid hormone. Saturation will remain constant, and free binding sites and T-uptake will change in the same direction as total thyroid hormone. With primary thyroid disease, therefore, total T_4 and T-uptake change in opposite directions. With an alteration in the amount of binding protein, total T_4 and T-uptake will change in the same direction.

The resulting peptide has reduced TSH activity, but is measured in TSH assays, causing slightly increased TSH levels.

Thyrotropin Response to Thyrotropin-releasing Hormone

Before sensitive TSH assays became available, the increase in TSH after administration of 200 μg of TRH was used (normally, TSH increases 3–5 fold at 30 min). The pituitary response to TRH is inversely proportional to free T_4 concentration. Persons with hyperthyroidism have blunted responses, while hypothyroid patients show an exaggerated response. Patients with pituitary failure should theoretically show a blunted response. In fact, the test frequently produces inappropriately normal responses, and in one series, 70% had a normal or an increased response to TRH. Responses are also blunted with acute illness, and many older men have no response. Thyrotropin-releasing hormone infusion is seldom needed if TSH assays have a detection limit of less than 0.05 mU/L.

MISCELLANEOUS THYROID TESTS

Thyrotropin Receptor Antibodies

Antibodies against TSH receptors on thyroid cells are frequently present in autoimmune thyroid disease. Some are blocking antibodies, inhibiting TSH action; some stimulate thyroid growth without affecting function; and some activate receptors, causing hyperthyroidism. The TSH receptor antibody test detects all three types of antibodies. A more specific assay, thyroid stimulating immunoglobulin (TSI), detects only receptor-activating antibodies involved in the pathogenesis of Graves' disease. In equivocal cases, TSI may be of benefit, being most helpful in patients with a nodular goiter but high RAIU, in those having euthyroid ophthalmic manifestations suggesting Graves' disease, and in pregnant women with Graves' disease. In the last group, the TSI titer correlates with the degree of fetal thyroid enlargement.

Antithyroid Antibodies

The most useful of the thyroid antibodies are the antimicrosomal antibodies (being replaced in many laboratories with antithyroid peroxidase (anti-TPO) antibodies, detecting the major antigen found in microsomes). Such antibodies are characteristic of many types of thyroiditis, and the anti-TPO titer has been found useful in predicting the likelihood of progression in subclinical hypothyroidism. Anti-TPO is elevated transiently and in moderate titers in painless, subacute, and postpartum thyroiditis, but persists at high titers in Hashimoto's thyroiditis and, rarely, Graves' disease. Antithyroglobulin antibodies are also found in Hashimoto's and other forms of thyroiditis, although less frequently and less specifically than anti-TPO. Measuring antithyroglobulin is rarely of benefit.

Thyroglobulin

This storage form of thyroid hormone is produced solely in thyroid, with only trace amounts normally reaching plasma. Plasma thyroglobulin is related to thyroid mass; patients with goiter commonly have elevated results. Increased release of thyroglobulin occurs with thyroid damage from thyroiditis and in papillary and follicular thyroid carcinomas. Thyroglobulin is used to follow patients who are at high risk for recurrence following resection of differentiated thyroid carcinoma. If a subtotal thyroidectomy was performed, thyroglobulin should be measured when TSH is suppressed by replacement therapy in order to avoid confusion from production by residual normal thyroid tissue. After total thyroidectomy, thyroglobulin levels are most sensitive when TSH is elevated. About one-third of patients with increased plasma thyroglobulin develop antithyroglobulin antibodies, which interfere with measurement. Many laboratories routinely screen for the presence of antithyroglobulin when measuring thyroglobulin, and will not report results if antibodies are present.

Calcitonin

Calcitonin, the major product of thyroid parafollicular cells (C cells), is also produced in other organs, notably the lung. The major indication for calcitonin measurements is suspicion of malignancy or hyperplasia of C cells, including postoperative monitoring of patients with medullary thyroid carcinoma. Basal calcitonin measurements are adequate for follow-up of patients with known malignancy, but are relatively insensitive for early tumor detection. In families of patients with multiple endocrine neoplasia type II, screening identifies tumors in the early stages. An increase in calcitonin after known stimuli (pentagastrin, calcium, or both) has been used to detect increased parafollicular cells. Using both stimuli is the most sensitive provocative test (normal peak calcitonin is less than 300 pg/mL). Mutations in the *ret* oncogene are a more sensitive marker than the stimulated calcitonin test in detecting affected family members in familial forms of medullary thyroid carcinoma.

Table 13.1.
Thyroid Function Tests in Various States

State	T_4	FT_4	T_3	FT_3	T_3RU	T-U	TSH	RAIU	Other
Graves' disease	↑	↑	↑	↑	↑	NL-↓	S	↑	Anti-TPO, TSI ↑
Nodular goiter	↑	↑	Nl-↑	Nl-↑	↑	Nl-↓	S	Nl	
Hyperthyroid stage of thyroiditis	sl ↑	sl ↑	sl ↑	sl ↑	↑	Nl	S	↓	Anti-TPO ↑
Subclinical hyperthyroidism	Nl	Nl	Nl	Nl	Nl	Nl	S	Nl-↑	
Hashimoto's thyroiditis	↓	↓	Nl-↓	Nl-↓	↓	Nl-↑	↑↑	↓	Anti-TPO ↑↑
Hypopituitarism	↓	↓	Nl-↓	Nl-↓	↓	Nl-↑	Nl-↓	↓	
Subclinical hypothyroidism	Nl	Nl	Nl	Nl	Nl	Nl	↑	Nl-↓	
Nonthyroidal illness	Nl	Nl	↓	↓	Nl-↑	Nl	Nl-↓	Nl	
Severe nonthyroid illness	sl ↓	sl ↓	↓	↓	↑	Nl	Nl-↓	Nl-↓	
Increased TBG	↑	Nl	↑	Nl	↓	↑	* Nl	Nl	

T_4—total T_4; FT_4—free T_4; T_3—total T_3; FT_3—free T_3; T_3RU—T_3 resin uptake; T-U—T_4 uptake; RAIU—radioactive iodine uptake; TPO—thyroid peroxidase; TSI—thyroid stimulating immunoglobulins; Nl—normal; Sl—slightly; S—suppressed (undetectable); ↑—increased; ↑↑—markedly increased; ↓—decreased

LABORATORY APPROACHES TO EVALUATION OF THYROID DISEASE

General Screening Tests

For apparently healthy individuals, there is little need for measurement of thyroid function, with two exceptions. Congenital hypothyroidism is a common, preventable cause of mental retardation, and can be detected easily by umbilical cord blood tests. Thyroid disorders are common in the elderly, and in many cases do not produce classic metabolic changes. In both neonates and the elderly, routine screening appears justified. Published data do not support testing of asymptomatic persons in any other setting. There is good evidence to support case findings (testing patients with nonspecific symptoms) in certain settings. There is a relatively high incidence of unsuspected hyperthyroidism in patients with atrial arrhythmias. Dementia may be a presenting symptom of hyperthyroidism or hypothyroidism in the elderly. About 5% of patients with hypercholesterolemia have mild hypothyroidism, and treatment often improves cholesterol levels. While there is a relatively high incidence of unsuspected thyroid disease in patients with psychiatric symptoms, there is also a high incidence of transient thyroid dysfunction, particularly in depression; for this reason, some have questioned the wisdom of testing patients with acute psychiatric symptoms.

What Constitutes an Adequate Evaluation of Thyroid Function?

Thyrotropin is the best test for evaluation of thyroid function, changing earlier and more dramatically than thyroid hormone levels in thyroid disease. Most authorities suggest use of TSH alone for suspected thyroid disease; thyroid hormone (ideally free T_4) is measured only if TSH is abnormal. T_3 measurements are seldom of use in thyroid disease. We perform free T_3 measurements only with known or suspected hyperthyroidism. Patterns of change in thyroid function tests are illustrated in Table 13.1.

When Not to Perform Thyroid Function Tests

Routine testing for thyroid disease is not indicated in patients admitted with medical or surgical problems because of marked changes in thyroid function (see section on

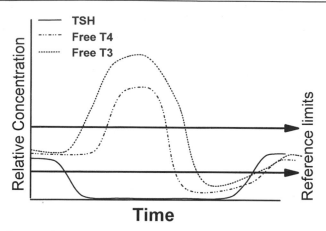

Figure 13.8. Time Course of Changes in Thyroid Function in Hyperthyroidism. Before development of symptoms, free T_3 and T_4 are within the reference limits while TSH is suppressed (subclinical hyperthyroidism). In early clinical hyperthyroidism, free T_3 is elevated but free T_4 is normal (increased T_3 production by stimulated thyroid gland, T_3 toxicosis). With recovery after treatment, T_4 and then T_3 will return to normal and often reach hypothyroid levels, while TSH production remains suppressed for some time before eventually returning to normal and restoring thyroid hormone production.

nonthyroidal illness). Thyroid function tests are frequently misleading, and sometimes uninterpretable in this situation. Many drugs alter levels of thyroid binding proteins (Chapter 38). Because of this free thyroxine measurements are superior to total thyroxine, as the latter is difficult to interpret when both thyroid disease and binding protein abnormalities are present. Many radiographic agents cause transient changes in thyroid function due to their iodine content. Testing should be deferred until a month after most contrast imaging studies, although effects may persist for months with some agents such as lipiodol. In patients given thyroid hormones, testing should be done before the patient takes medication on that day, since transient increases in thyroid hormone after ingestion may be misleading.

HYPERTHYROIDISM

Excess thyroid hormone (hyperthyroidism) often produces symptoms such as weakness, nervousness, weight loss, loose stools, heat intolerance, and palpitations. Patients may present with nonspecific findings, and occasionally are recognized because of cardiac arrhythmias, especially atrial fibrillation or flutter. Most commonly, hyperthyroidism is caused by Graves' disease, an autoimmune disease producing antibodies which stimulate TSH receptors. Less common causes include transient hyperthyroidism due to thyroid injury, functional thyroid tumors, and toxic nodular goiter.

Laboratory Approach to Diagnosis of Hyperthyroidism

Virtually all cases of hyperthyroidism are due to primary thyroid gland disease. The most sensitive test is for TSH level, which should be suppressed below the lower limits of detection of even a third generation assay. The time course of changes in TSH and free thyroid hormones is illustrated in Figure 13.8. It shows changes in total thyroid hormones generally parallel those in free hormones, but are less likely to be abnormal in early stages. If T_3RU is used along with total T_4, both will be increased, while if

T-uptake is performed, total T_4 will still be high but T-uptake will be normal or slightly decreased. Most hyperthyroid patients have elevations of both T_3 and T_4. In rare cases, only T_4 is elevated (T_4 toxicosis), due to factors inhibiting conversion of T_4 to T_3 (acute illness, β-adrenergic blockers, glucocorticosteroids, or high iodine intake). An algorithm for the evaluation of suspected hyperthyroidism is shown in Figure 13.9.

Graves' Disease

The most common cause of hyperthyroidism, Graves' disease, is due to autoantibodies to TSH receptors stimulating thyroid activity and diffuse thyroid enlargement. Hyperactivity is documented by high RAIU; in most cases, it is markedly elevated at both 6 and 24 hours, but very active glands have low uptake at 24 hours due to rapid hormone synthesis and release. In equivocal cases, demonstration of the presence of thyroid antibodies is helpful. Anti-TPO and TSH receptor antibodies are present in 85–95% of cases, but also in other forms of thyroiditis, while TSI is highly specific for Graves' disease.

Nodular Thyroid Diseases

Hyperthyroidism due to thyroid nodules is usually recognized by one or more nodules, with any increased RAIU limited to the nodules. Total RAIU is often normal or only slightly elevated. Both TSI and anti-TPO are negative, helpful when other features suggest Graves' disease.

Thyroiditis

Transient hyperthyroidism is often the initial clinical presentation of thyroiditis. The thyroid is usually only slightly enlarged, and in contrast to Graves' disease, RAIU is typically decreased, anti-TPO is transiently present in low to moderate titers, and TSI is never present. Most patients have mildly elevated free T_3 and T_4, in contrast to much greater elevations in Graves' disease. Hyperthyroidism often resolves after only one to two months, followed by hypothyroidism in many patients before thyroid function returns to normal (in 95% of cases).

HYPOTHYROIDISM

Thyroid hormone deficiency (hypothyroidism) is often recognized by clinical manifestations such as cold intolerance, weight gain, weakness, mental status changes, myxedema, and constipation. As with hyperthyroidism, clinical symptoms are less characteristic in elderly, who often present with dementia, heart failure, or nonspecific symptoms. In adults, hypothyroidism is most commonly due to destruction of the thyroid gland by Hashimoto's thyroiditis, atrophic autoimmune thyroid disease, or surgical removal of the gland. Hypothyroidism may also occur many years after radioiodine therapy for Graves' disease.

Laboratory Approach to Hypothyroidism in Adults

A flow chart for evaluating a patient for suspected hypothyroidism is presented in Figure 13.10. As with hyperthyroidism, most cases are due to primary thyroid disease, making TSH the best test. Levels typically are mildly (up to 4 times) elevated in early, asymptomatic (subclinical) stages, but TSH is typically 10–100 times normal by the

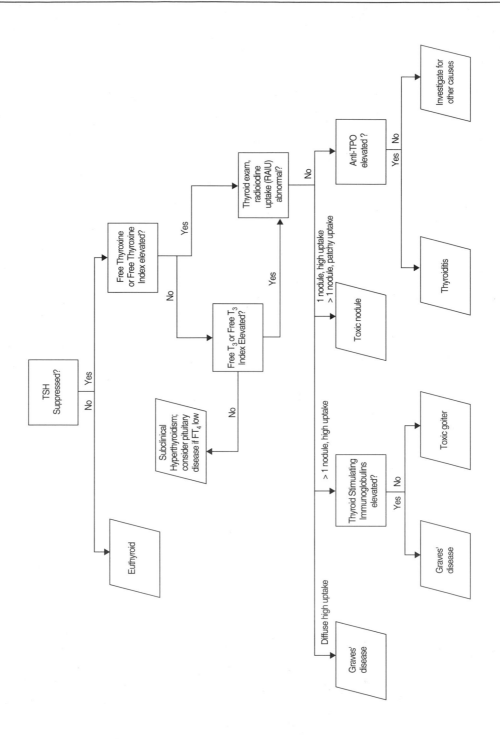

Figure 13.9. Approach to Suspected Hyperthyroidism. Since essentially all cases of hyperthyroidism are due to primary thyroid disease, TSH is the best initial diagnostic test. TSH suppressed below the lower limits of detection in a TSH assay with a lower limit of under 0.05 mU/L in a patient not taking thyroid hormone virtually always indicates thyroid hyperfunction, while a measurable TSH almost always rules out that diagnosis. Measurement or estimation of free T_4 and, if that is normal, T_3, will separate subclinically hyperthyroid patients. Many of these will develop symptomatic hyperthyroidism on follow-up. Elevation of either indicates thyroid hyperfunction. Thyroid examination and RAIU will correctly classify most patients. Graves' disease causes a diffusely enlarged thyroid gland with high RAIU, toxic adenomas produce solitary nodules with high uptake, toxic nodular goiter produces patchy uptake in a gland with many nodules, and thyroiditis produces low uptake. Patients with high uptake and multiple nodules may have coexisting Graves' disease and multinodular goiter; measurement of TSI will resolve this dilemma. A low uptake due to thyroiditis can be confirmed by measurement of anti-TPO, which should be positive in all forms of thyroiditis. Patients with thyroiditis usually have only transient hyperthyroidism, and often progress rapidly to hypothyroidism which then resolves. A negative anti-TPO suggests a rare cause of hyperthyroidism, such as ingestion of thyroid hormone, iodine induced hyperthyroidism, or ectopic thyroid tissue as may occur with ovarian teratomas (struma ovarii).

time symptoms develop. Total and free T_4 are low more often than T_3. Around 30–40% of hypothyroid patients have normal free and total T_3 (due to increased T_3 production when TSH is increased). Since low TBG levels are less common than high ones, total T_4 measurements are adequate, with T_3RU done only in equivocal cases. Thyrotropin alone misses many cases of secondary hypothyroidism, often in presenting finding pituitary disease. In the author's institution, about 2–3 cases of secondary hypothyroidism are detected each year out of 6000 thyroid function tests performed. In patients with symptoms and signs of hypothyroidism, TSH and free T_4 are done together.

Differential Diagnosis of Hypothyroidism in Adults

Most patients with hypothyroidism have markedly elevated TSH, indicating primary thyroid disease. In patients with a history of thyroid disease (previous Graves' disease, surgical thyroidectomy, or radioactive iodine treatment), further workup is not needed. In other hypothyroid patients, the most important question is whether thyroid dysfunction is likely to be transient or permanent. Patients with small thyroid glands usually have thyroid atrophy, associated with anti-TPO in 80% of cases. With normal or enlarged glands, the differential is between transient inflammation (subacute, postpartum, and lymphocytic thyroiditis) and Hashimoto's thyroiditis. Hypothyroidism is usually permanent in the latter, while typically transient in the former. Anti-TPO titer may help in the differential, with high titers characteristic of Hashimoto's thyroiditis. In equivocal cases, a repeat anti-TPO test three to six months after diagnosis may be helpful: if the antibodies disappear, Hashimoto's thyroiditis is unlikely and the return of normal thyroid function is likely. If TSH is not appropriately elevated, pituitary disease should be suspected. Most patients with pituitary disease have evidence of other endocrine abnormalities which can help establish the diagnosis (Chapter 15).

Laboratory Approach to Diagnosis of Hypothyroidism in Neonates

Congenital hypothyroidism is present in about 1 in 4000 births. Routine neonatal screening is performed in all states. The vast majority of cases are due to failure of thyroid development, causing very low total T_4 and markedly elevated TSH. In some cases, the thyroid is much smaller than normal, resulting in low normal T_4 and elevated TSH at birth. In 5–10% of cases, hypothalamic or pituitary disease causes hypothyroid-

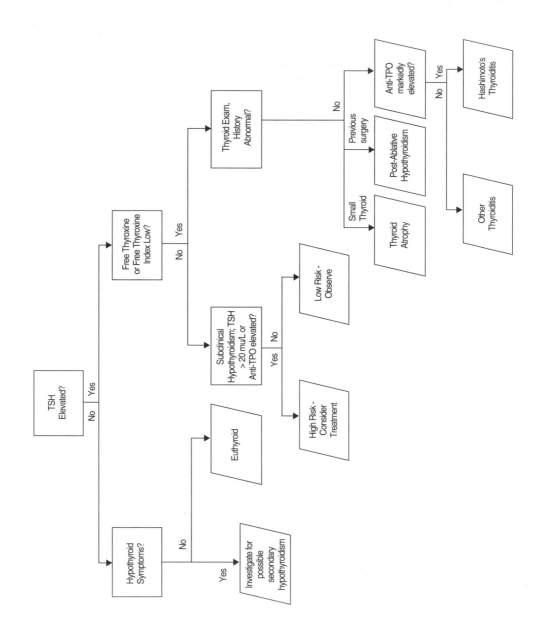

Figure 13.10. Approach to Suspected Hypothyroidism in Adults. The vast majority of cases of hypothyroidism in adults are primary in the thyroid gland, so that increased TSH is the earliest change seen. Patients with pituitary disease often have normal TSH; thus, any patient with symptoms of hypothyroidism should also have measurement of free T_4 or FTI. Normal results for both tests rule out hypothyroidism. If only TSH is elevated, the patient has subclinical hypothyroidism; a TSH greater than 20 mU/L or a positive anti-TPO indicates high risk of subsequent clinical hypothyroidism. Such patients should be closely followed or be started on replacement hormone. If free T_4 is decreased, the thyroid exam and clinical history will categorize most patients accurately. A previous history of thyroid surgery or presence of an atrophic thyroid strongly suggest postablative and atrophic hypothyroidism, respectively. A normal or enlarged thyroid in a hypothyroid patient is usually due to thyroiditis. Anti-TPO titers will help to separate the different forms, which is important for prognosis. Patients with Hashimoto's thyroiditis have high titers of anti-TPO, and typically have persistent hypothyroidism. Patients with subacute, lymphocytic, and postpartum thyroiditis usually have low to moderate titers of anti-TPO. In the majority of these cases, hypothyroidism is transient. If a low titer of anti-TPO is found, repeat testing may be done 3–6 months later. If the antibody is no longer detected, a trial of discontinuation of thyroid hormone will indicate whether thyroid function has returned to normal.

ism, with normal or low TSH. T_3 is normally very low in neonates, making its measurement of no use in screening. Because neither TSH nor T_4 by itself will detect 100% of cases, many recommend screening all neonates with both tests; in many states, T_4 is done first and TSH is run if T_4 is below a particular threshold. In some states, a second specimen is obtained several weeks after birth to detect infants with small thyroid glands.

Subclinical Hypothyroidism

This relatively common state refers to elevated TSH in patients with normal free T_4 and no clinical evidence of hypothyroidism. Its incidence rises with increasing age, and is more common in women than men. It may occur transiently in patients with varying forms of thyroiditis, such as painless, postpartum, and granulomatous thyroiditis. It may persist unchanged for many years, a relatively common event in patients with prior thyroid surgery. In many cases, it progresses over time to symptomatic hypothyroidism. The likelihood of progression is related to baseline TSH, previous history of thyroid surgery, and titer of anti-TPO. If baseline TSH is below 20 mU/L and anti-TPO is absent or present in low titers, there is little likelihood of progression. Most patients will develop symptoms of hypothyroidism if TSH is above 20 mU/L or high titer antibodies are present.

FOLLOWING THYROID HORMONE REPLACEMENT

Thyrotropin levels should be measured on a sample drawn before thyroid hormone is taken on the day of testing. In patients being treated for hypothyroidism, optimal therapy results in TSH within the reference range. In patients with thyroid carcinoma, TSH should be near the lower limits of detection on a third generation TSH assay to assure adequate suppression of TSH. Free and total T_4 are not routinely useful in following thyroid hormone replacement, and will be misleading in those patients receiving T_3. After adjusting the dose of thyroid hormone, it takes at least six weeks for TSH levels to stabilize; levels drawn earlier are misleading. In patients on stable doses and without symptoms, TSH should be measured every 6–12 months and dosage adjusted to maintain TSH at the appropriate levels.

LABORATORY ABNORMALITIES NOT INDICATING THYROID DISEASE

If TSH alone or TSH and free T_4 are used for thyroid function tests, practitioners will seldom encounter the abnormalities described below. In many hospitals, total thyroid hormone tests (total T_4, T_3RU, and total T_3) are performed routinely on many hospital inpatients. In hospitalized individuals, abnormal thyroid function tests occur frequently in patients with normal thyroid function. The most common causes are discussed below. Among the rare causes is resistance to thyroid hormone action, in which a congenital deficiency in tissue thyroid receptors requires more thyroid hormone to produce a euthyroid state. Antibodies to thyroid hormone occur in a small fraction of patients with thyroiditis, causing falsely elevated total T_4 and T_3 levels. In both situations, TSH is normal and symptoms of thyroid disease are absent.

Euthyroid Sick Syndrome or Nonthyroidal Illness

In persons with acute illness, the most consistent change is decreased T_3 due to decreased peripheral conversion of T_4 to T_3; decreased metabolism leads to accumulation of rT_3. This occurs with even minimal illness, and may also be produced by fasting. As patients become more severely ill, there is often decreased affinity of binding proteins for T_4, rT_3, and T_3, leading to decreases in plasma levels. The altered affinity affects many free T_4 tests, causing falsely low results in analogue assays. Changes in pituitary response lead to lowered TSH, and response to TRH is typically blunted. These results may suggest secondary hypothyroidism; during recovery from illness many patients have increased TSH, supporting transient pituitary suppression. There does not appear to be any benefit in treating acutely ill patients with thyroid hormone. If clinical findings suggest hypothyroidism, many endocrinologists suggest treatment and repeating the workup after recovery from illness.

Increased or Decreased TBG

Increased levels of TBG are induced by many drugs; among the most common are estrogens, oral contraceptives, phenothiazines, and opiates. Active liver injury (acute and chronic hepatitis) is often associated with increased TBG. Both TSH and free T_4 will be normal, although total T_4 is increased and T_3RU is decreased. Decreased TBG levels are common with protein losing states, chronic liver disease, and occasionally are due to congenital deficiency. Androgens and phenytoin also decrease TBG (phenytoin also decreases free T_4 and TSH). Again, free T_4 and TSH are normal, T_4 is low, and T_3RU is increased.

Familial Dysalbuminemic Hyperthyroxinemia

Inherited variants of albumin produce increased T_4 affinity. These patients are clinically euthyroid, and have normal free T_4 by equilibrium dialysis, normal T_3, normal T_3RU, and normal TSH. Biochemical features may suggest hyperthyroidism as total T_4 and free thyroxine index are increased. Immunoassays and analogue assays for free T_4 often show falsely increased results in this disorder, although the frequency of elevation varies from one assay to another. This is a relatively common laboratory abnormality, affecting about 3 in 2000 individuals.

CHAPTER 14

Laboratory Evaluation of Adrenal Function

D. ROBERT DUFOUR

The adrenal gland is unique among endocrine organs in that it functionally behaves as three relatively independent organs, each with its own regulatory mechanisms. These produce mineralocorticosteroids, catecholamines, and combined sex steroid and glucocorticosteroid.

THE HYPOTHALAMIC–PITUITARY–GLUCOCORTICOSTEROID AXIS

Regulation of glucocorticosteroid production is the most complex in the endocrine system (Fig. 14.1). Corticotropin-releasing hormone (CRH) and corticotropin (ACTH) are released in secretory pulses throughout the day, but most secretion occurs during the latter half of sleep. The pineal hormone **melatonin,** released in the dark, is at least partly responsible for diurnal variation. Persons who travel from one time zone to another, or who work irregular shifts, will take from days up to weeks to adjust melatonin synthesis patterns to match their new waking hours. Even after adjustment, they have different diurnal cortisol patterns than individuals working "normal" hours.

Direct Tests of the Hypothalamic–Pituitary–Adrenal Axis

Cortisol and ACTH are often difficult to interpret because of the effects of stress and diurnal variation.

Cortisol

Assays for total cortisol are not specific, since synthetic steroids may cross react (although dexamethasone does not). Almost all cortisol is bound to **cortisol binding globulin** (CBG). Changes in CBG will cause abnormal cortisol levels. Increased CBG occurs with estrogens and in pregnancy, while decreased CBG is seen in liver disease, malnutrition, and protein losing states. Plasma cortisol, which has less variation than ACTH, averages 13 μg/dL (390 nmol/L) at 8 AM, 6 μg/dL (170 nmol/L) in late afternoon, and 3 μg/dL (85 nmol/L) at 11 PM. With acute illness, cortisol increases, with a rough correlation to severity of illness, particularly inflammation. Critically ill patients may have 8 AM cortisol levels of over 100 μg/dL (2800 nmol/L).

Urine Free Cortisol

Most plasma cortisol is protein bound. Very little is excreted unchanged in urine before being metabolized in the liver. Urine free cortisol (UFC) measures the degree to which plasma cortisol exceeds protein binding capacity. Slight increases in average cortisol result in marked increases in UFC. Free cortisol excretion also correlates well with total cortisol production. The UFC reference range is 20–90 μg (5.6–25 μmol) per

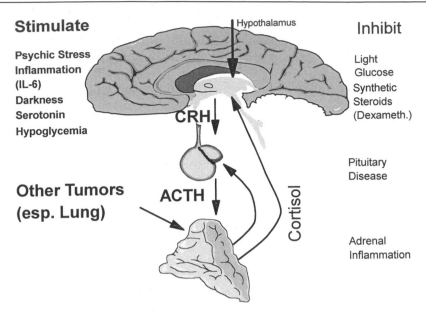

Figure 14.1. The Hypothalamic–Pituitary–Glucocorticosteroid Axis. Hypothalamic production of CRH is affected by such mediators as hypoglycemia, serotonin, melatonin, and various cytokines, especially inter-leukin-6. There is also a pronounced diurnal variation, with production highest during sleep. CRH stimulates pituitary production of POMC, which is cleaved to produce many smaller peptides, including ACTH. ACTH is the major stimulus to adrenal production of steroid hormones, mainly cortisol and sex steroids; ACTH also transiently increases aldosterone. Cortisol is the only adrenal product which inhibits CRH and ACTH production, although synthetic glucocorticosteroids and hyperglycemia are also inhibitory.

day in adults. Urine free cortisol can be used to monitor hydrocortisone replacement therapy in adrenal insufficiency, with results in the reference range the best indication of adequate replacement.

Corticosteroid Intermediates

Chemical assays for cortisol precursors are nonspecific, outmoded tests. Their only utility is in the evaluation of suspected congenital adrenal hyperplasia or adrenal carcinoma, where blocks in synthesis prevent formation of active compounds such as cortisol. **17-Hydroxysteroids** include cortisol, its immediate precursor, and their metabolites. **17-Ketosteroids** include most adrenal androgens, but not testosterone. A number of compounds interfere in both assays, resulting in falsely increased urine levels.

Adrenal Androgen Production

Dehydroepiandrosterone sulfate (DHEA-S) is the major androgen produced by the adrenal gland, and may be measured in either plasma or urine. More potent androgens, such as testosterone (Chapter 15) come primarily from gonads, while weak androgens come both from adrenal and gonad. These latter are less reliable measures of adrenal androgen production.

Corticotropin

Episodic bursts of ACTH release cause difficulty in interpreting a single ACTH level, unless cortisol is markedly abnormal. Current ACTH methods use two site immunoassays which are specific for ACTH; other pituitary pro-opiomelanocortin (POMC) metabolites do not react. Corticotropin in plasma is quite labile, mandating special collection and handling to prevent falsely low results. Assays show varying results in patients with ectopic ACTH production, since ACTH from other sites is often composed of different sized fragments of POMC than with pituitary production. Corticotropin is released from the pituitary into blood reaching the inferior petrosal sinus. Direct sinus sampling is increasingly used to determine both the pituitary origin and the side of the pituitary affected in patients with Cushing's syndrome. This technique requires highly skilled interventional radiologists to be able to successfully catheterize the sinus. Because of episodic bursts of release, single values widely separated in time from the two sinuses are not reliable indicators of lateralization of ACTH overproduction.

Dynamic Tests of the Hypothalamic–Pituitary–Adrenal Axis

Because single measurements of plasma or urine cortisol and ACTH are difficult to interpret, tests evaluating the response to physiologic factors are the most reliable means to evaluate the axis. By using agents having effects on different portions of the axis, it is usually possible to identify the source of the problem.

Dexamethasone Suppression Tests, or DST

Dexamethasone, a potent glucocorticosteroid inhibiting ACTH synthesis, does not cross-react in cortisol assays. By varying dexamethasone dose, it is possible to determine the responsiveness of the axis.

Overnight DST

A dose of dexamethasone (1 mg) slightly in excess of physiologic cortisol production is given at bedtime, just before most ACTH production occurs. This test is widely used to screen for Cushing's syndrome, with a normal response ruling out that diagnosis. Normally, plasma cortisol remains below 5 μg/dL (less than 140 nmol/L) at 8 AM (and throughout the day). Lack of suppression is common in hospitalized, acutely ill individuals, in states of stress, particularly depression, in obese individuals (due to lower plasma dexamethasone levels), with drugs that increase dexamethasone metabolism (dilantin, ethanol), and with poor dexamethasone absorption (renal failure).

"Low Dose" DST

A supraphysiologic dose of dexamethasone (0.5 mg every 6 hours for 2 days) should prevent pituitary ACTH production in normal individuals. Urine free cortisol should fall below the lower reference limit during the second day of dexamethasone administration. Failure to suppress cortisol has been considered diagnostic of Cushing's syndrome, but does not discriminate among various causes. However, more recent studies show a high false negative rate. Most causes of nonsuppression with the overnight test do not affect the low dose test.

"High Dose" DST

A greatly supraphysiologic dose of dexamethasone (2 mg every 6 hours for 2 days) will inhibit ACTH production by pituitary tumors, with UFC falling to below 20% of the basal level. In other causes of Cushing's syndrome, no change occurs in cortisol production. The test can also be done more simply by giving 8 mg of dexamethasone at bedtime. Here the morning cortisol level should be less than 50% of basal. Some patients with pituitary tumors may require 16 mg or 32 mg to show suppression. Occasional patients with adrenal tumors show cyclic production of cortisol, and may appear to show suppression if the UFC test is performed at the time of cyclic decrease.

Stimulatory Tests

Response of the axis to stimuli can localize the source of dysfunction. These tests are most commonly used in evaluation for adrenal insufficiency.

Cortrosyn Stimulation

A synthetic, bioactive ACTH fragment (cortrosyn, cosyntropin) tests adrenal cortisol producing ability. The short form is most commonly used. Classically, 250 μg of cortrosyn is administered by intravenous bolus, with plasma cortisol measured at 0, 30, and 60 minutes after injection. An increase of at least 7 μg/dL (195 nmol/L) in plasma cortisol with a peak cortisol over 18–20 μg/dL (500–560 nmol/L) is a normal response. More recently, 1 μg cortrosyn has been used as a more physiologic dose, since many patients with pituitary tumors or on long term steroids fail to respond to 1 μg despite a normal response to 250 μg. In patients with chronically suppressed adrenal glands (prolonged high dose steroids, long-standing hypopituitarism), normal response may require cortrosyn administration for several days; 250 μg cortrosyn is infused over 6 hours for two to five days. An increase in urine 17-hydroxysteroids of 2–5 fold over baseline indicates capacity for normal adrenal function. Cortrosyn stimulation is not needed if basal cortisol is over 18–20 μg/dL (500–560 nmol/L).

Metyrapone Test

Metyrapone (Metapyrone) inhibits the last step in cortisol synthesis, removing feedback inhibition on ACTH. The increased ACTH causes a rise in 11-deoxycortisol of more than 7 μg/dL (29 nmol/L). Metyrapone is no longer commercially available in North America, but may be obtained from the manufacturer for testing purposes. This test is dangerous with low basal cortisol, and may produce adrenal crisis if the patient is not pretreated with dexamethasone.

Insulin Hypoglycemia

Low glucose stimulates ACTH production. Insulin given intravenously (0.05–0.1 U/kg) can reduce glucose below 40 mg/dL (2.2 mmol/L) to provide adequate stimulation. Cortisol should increase by at least 7 μg/dL (195 nmol/L) with a peak over 18–20 μg/dL (500–560 nmol/L). Insulin hypoglycemia is the most sensitive test to document inadequate pituitary ACTH production.

Corticotropin-releasing Hormone Stimulation

Synthetic CRH, either human or ovine, tests pituitary response; however, it is not yet commercially available. After a 100 μg intravenous bolus, ACTH should rise 2–4 fold, and cortisol should increase by at least 7 μg/dL (195 nmol/L) with a peak over 18–20 μg/dL (500–560 nmol/L).

ABNORMALITIES OF GLUCOCORTICOSTEROID PRODUCTION

Suspected Cushing's Syndrome

Cushing's syndrome, a clinical disorder caused by excess glucocorticosteroids, commonly presents with obesity, hypertension, virilization, poor wound healing, and hyperglycemia. Hypokalemia and metabolic alkalosis may occur since cortisol activates aldosterone receptors. Other laboratory findings may also be present, including a low lymphocyte count. While Cushing's syndrome due to treatment with high dose steroids is relatively common, Cushing's syndrome due to disease is rare (1 per 1,000,000 population annually).

When Not to Test for Cushing's Syndrome

Exogenous steroids should be discontinued, since they may be measured in plasma and urine cortisol assays. Stress stimulates cortisol production, and severe stress may induce a state termed Pseudo-Cushing's Syndrome. This is particularly common in psychiatric disorders, especially depression, alcohol abuse, and in critically ill patients. Hospitalization for acute illness commonly doubles plasma cortisol, while critical illness may increase cortisol by over eightfold. Evaluation should be deferred during times of acute illness if at all possible.

Diagnosis of Cushing's Syndrome

Either urine free cortisol or the overnight DST are used to screen for Cushing's syndrome (Fig.14.2). While DST is easier to perform, it is subject to falsely abnormal results in a variety of situations. On the other hand, UFC has fewer false positive results, but requires accurate 24 hour urine collection. Many textbooks suggest loss of diurnal variation in cortisol as a good screening test, but many Cushing's patients still show diurnal variation in cortisol, while variation is lost with acute illness. Only 5–10% of Cushing's patients have normal cortisol at 11:00 PM; however, this test is less reliable than DST or UFC. Abnormal results of screening tests can be confirmed with the low dose DST, which has few false positive results. This should be used for initial screening if patients must be tested during acute illness.

Once diagnosis of Cushing's syndrome is established, laboratory tests are used to determine the cause. The three common causes of endogenous Cushing's syndrome are: pituitary ACTH producing tumors (**Cushing's disease,** 60–70%); benign and malignant adrenal tumors (15–20%); and ectopic ACTH production (small cell carcinoma or carcinoid tumor of lung most commonly, 15–20% of cases). Most patients with malignant tumors producing ACTH ectopically do not have full blown Cushing's syndrome, but metabolic abnormalities (metabolic alkalosis, hypokalemia, and hyperglycemia) are usually present. Most commonly, high dose DST is the initial test, although if skilled interventional radiologists are available, inferior petrosal sinus ACTH sampling is more reliable (a threefold gradient between two sides indicates Cushing's disease). Patients without Cushing's disease can usually be distinguished by ACTH levels seen with ectopic ACTH production.

Adrenal Insufficiency

Adrenal insufficiency is more frequent than Cushing's syndrome. Mineralocorticosteroid deficiency causes dehydration, hyponatremia, hyperkalemia, and non-anion gap

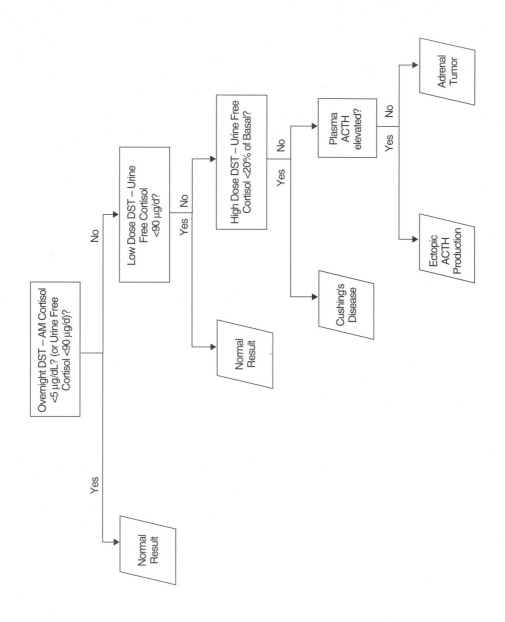

metabolic acidosis. Glucocorticosteroid deficiency produces weight loss, nausea, vomiting, weakness, and occasionally hypoglycemia. In primary insufficiency (**Addison's disease**), deficiency of both hormone classes is associated with increased pigmentation of skin and mucous membranes due to high POMC production (melanocyte stimulating hormone is a fragment of POMC). In secondary adrenal insufficiency (due to pituitary disease) or tertiary insufficiency (due to hypothalamic dysfunction), neither mineralocorticosteroid problems nor excess ACTH is present, and the diagnosis is often delayed because of the nonspecific symptoms of glucocorticosteroid deficiency. In secondary or tertiary disease, hypoglycemia is more common due to deficiencies of growth hormone and thyroid hormone. Hyponatremia may occur without hyperkalemia or metabolic acidosis in secondary insufficiency due to lack of cortisol inhibition of ADH production (Chapter 5). Electrolytes are usually normal in tertiary insufficiency.

When Not to Test for Adrenal Insufficiency

Some synthetic corticosteroids cross-react in cortisol assays, and all can suppress cortisol production; plasma cortisol should not be used to evaluate adrenal function in patients on glucocorticosteroids. If the patient has only recently been started on steroids, dexamethasone can be substituted and rapid cortrosyn stimulation testing can be used to determine adequacy of response. If steroids have been used for over one month, rapid stimulation testing is often abnormal; prolonged infusion may be needed to evaluate adrenal function. Rapid cortrosyn testing using 250 μg often gives normal results in patients with secondary adrenal insufficiency; 1 μg cortrosyn testing or insulin hypoglycemia should be used in such patients. If plasma cortisol is greater than 20 μg/dL (560 nmol/L), stimulation testing is not needed to rule out adrenal insufficiency.

Diagnosing Adrenal Insufficiency

If the patient is stable, plasma cortisol should be measured, with cortisol above 18–20 μg/dL (500–560 nmol/L) ruling out adrenal insufficiency. If the signs and symptoms suggest hypoadrenalism, treatment should start as soon as possible. A commonly suggested laboratory and therapeutic approach involves administration of dexamethasone to treat adrenal insufficiency after drawing basal cortisol and ACTH, followed by rapid cosyntropin testing to determine adrenal response. In our institution, we are giving 1 μg of cortrosyn initially (sampling at 0 and 30 minutes), waiting 90 minutes, then giving 250 μg (sampling at 0, 30, and 60 minutes). A normal response to low dose testing rules out adrenal insufficiency, an abnormal low dose response and a normal high dose response indicates impaired adrenal function usually due to pituitary disease, while abnormal responses to both tests suggests severe adrenal dysfunction and is more commonly seen with primary adrenal failure and long-standing pituitary failure. A corticotropin measurement is useful in equivocal cases; markedly elevated ACTH con-

Figure 14.2. Approach to Suspected Cushing's Syndrome. Testing for Cushing's syndrome should be deferred in acutely ill patients. Initial testing with overnight DST or UFC establishes the presence of inappropriate cortisol production. Positive results are usually confirmed by low dose DST, which eliminates most false positives. Abnormal results indicate Cushing's syndrome. Differential tests establish the etiology of Cushing's. Pituitary ACTH overproduction (Cushing's disease) is the most common cause; initial testing should distinguish this from rarer causes. Either high dose DST or petrosal sinus ACTH are used, with either a fall in cortisol production or high petrosal sinus ACTH establishing the presence of Cushing's disease. Adrenal tumor and ectopic ACTH production can be distinguished with ACTH levels (increased in the latter).

Table 14.1.
Enzymatic Steps in Steroid Synthesis and Congenital Adrenal Hyperplasia

Enzyme	Needed for Synthesis?			Compound Before Block	Clinical Findings in Deficiency
	Gluco-	Sex	Mineralo-		
17-Hydroxylase	Yes	Yes	No	Corticosterone	Hypoglycemia, hypertension, hypokalemia; males with female external genitalia
3-β-ol-dehydrogenase	Yes	Yes[a]	Yes		Addison's disease; males with female external genitalia in complete form, impotence and infertility in partial form
21-Hydroxylase	Yes	No	Yes	Pregnanetriol	Addison's disease in complete form, females with masculinized external genitalia; normal adrenal function, hirsutism, menstrual abnormalities in women with partial form
11-Hydroxylase	Yes	No	Yes[b]	17-OH Progesterone 11-deoxycortisol, deoxycorticosterone	Hypoglycemia, hypertension, hypokalemia; females with masculinized external genitalia

[a] Except for the weak androgen, dehydroepiandrosterone

[b] Except for the weak mineralocorticosteroid, deoxycorticosterone

firms primary adrenal failure, while low ACTH and low cortisol are seen in secondary adrenal insufficiency.

Congenital Adrenal Hyperplasia

Adrenal steroids are produced by a series of enzymatic steps which produce hormonally active and inactive intermediates (Table 14.1). Congenital adrenal hyperplasia (CAH) describes a group of genetic defects of these enzymes, producing a protein with either absent (complete) or reduced (partial) enzymatic activity. Lack of feedback from cortisol causes ACTH overproduction, leading to adrenal hyperplasia. Any adrenal steroids not requiring the deficient enzyme will be produced in excess, often producing a mixed picture of steroid excess (particularly androgens, causing adrenogenital syndrome described below) and steroid deficiency. Partial deficiency typically does not produce symptoms until adrenal androgen production increases shortly before puberty ("late onset" adrenal hyperplasia). The compound immediately before the block in synthesis (Table 14.1) tends to be most elevated, and is the best substance to measure to establish the diagnosis. Only the two most common forms are discussed here.

Adrenogenital Syndromes

While internal sex organs develop based on chromosomal sex, external genitalia develop as female unless androgens are present. In cases of a deficiency of enzymes needed to synthesize androgens, male fetuses have female external genitalia. In cases of a deficiency of enzymes not needed for androgen synthesis, excess androgens in female fetuses causes hypertrophy of the clitoris and partial fusion of the labia, resembling male external genitalia. Affected females with excess androgen are usually recognized at birth, while males with androgen deficiency or excess or females with androgen deficiency typically have no recognizable genital abnormalities at birth. With partial enzyme deficiency in females, excess androgen may cause menstrual irregularities and hirsutism after puberty.

21-Hydroxylase Deficiency

Deficiency of this enzyme is the most common form of CAH (95% of cases). Complete deficiency prevents cortisol and aldosterone production, causing adrenal insufficiency. Excess androgen synthesis causes masculinization of female fetuses, while male fetuses appear normal at birth. Diagnosis depends on demonstrating deficient cortisol with elevated 17-hydroxyprogesterone (17-OHP). Only cortisol should be measured in the first few days of life because other steroids interfere with measurement of 17-OHP. Partial deficiency is also common, presenting in teenage girls with hirsutism and menstrual irregularities. Cortisol and aldosterone are usually at the lower end of the reference range, while 17-OHP is usually high normal or minimally elevated. Cortrosyn stimulation testing with 250 μg causes a slight increase in cortisol but a marked increase in 17-OHP.

11-Hydroxylase Deficiency

Absence of 11-hydroxylase causes about 5% of cases of CAH, with most findings similar to 21-hydroxylase deficiency. One of the major metabolites, deoxycorticosterone (DOC), is a weak mineralocorticosteroid. Marked elevation of DOC causes hypokalemia, metabolic alkalosis, and hypertension. Adrenal androgens are also overproduced, causing physical findings of adrenogenital syndrome. Affected patients have low cortisol and aldosterone, high androgens, and markedly increased DOC and 11-deoxycortisol.

RENIN–ANGIOTENSIN–ALDOSTERONE AXIS

The renin–angiotensin–aldosterone axis is diagrammed in Figure 14.3. Adrenal production of aldosterone is only transiently affected by ACTH; cortrosyn stimulation testing causes a 2–5 fold increase, but levels fall to baseline within hours with continued ACTH administration. The main stimuli to aldosterone release are angiotensin II and hyperkalemia.

Tests of Renin and Aldosterone Status

Production of renin and aldosterone are highly dependent on volume status: plasma levels are lowest in morning and when supine, and highest in afternoon and when upright. Plasma potassium is directly related to rate of aldosterone production: hyperkalemia stimulates and hypokalemia inhibits aldosterone production. To evaluate the appropriateness of production, testing should always be performed with known volume status and normal plasma potassium. If hyperaldosteronism is suspected, testing with high sodium intake and in the supine position allows easy recognition that renin or aldosterone production is inappropriate; for suspected hypoaldosteronism, testing while upright after volume depletion can demonstrate inadequate production.

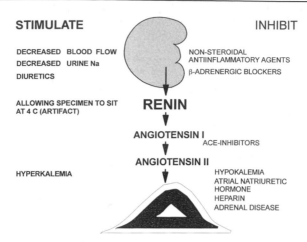

Figure 14.3. The Renin–Angiotensin–Aldosterone Axis. Renin production by the kidney is stimulated primarily by decreased renal blood flow or decreased distal tubular sodium. As shown, many drugs also affect renal responses to these stimuli, and must be controlled as much as possible prior to testing. Renin measurements are significantly affected by inappropriate sample handling; specimens must be kept at room temperature to prevent false increases. Hypokalemia inhibits aldosterone production, and should be corrected prior to testing aldosterone or renin levels.

Renin

Release of the active enzyme renin by kidney is stimulated by decreased renal blood flow or tubular sodium excretion. Other tissues produce an inactive proenzyme (**prorenin**) with blood prorenin to renin ratios of about 20. The conversion of prorenin to renin occurs in vitro at temperatures just above freezing. Samples for renin should be collected in lavender top tubes (EDTA inhibits conversion of prorenin) and kept at room temperature to prevent false increases in renin. Many laboratories still advise placing specimens in ice water, although this causes falsely high values. Assays measure enzymatic activity; changes in angiotensinogen (increased in pregnancy, Cushing's disease, and with estrogens or oral contraceptives; decreased with liver disease) will cause parallel changes in apparent renin.

Aldosterone

Either plasma or urine aldosterone can be measured, with normal values dependent on salt intake. Plasma aldosterone should be measured along with renin as the aldosterone to renin ratio improves the usefulness of measurements. A normal ratio of between 5:1 and 20:1 (when aldosterone is reported in ng/dL and renin is reported in ng/L per hr) is exceeded with primary hyperaldosteronism, lower levels are seen with adrenal insufficiency, and normal ratios with abnormal values occur with altered renin production.

When Not to Do Renin or Aldosterone Testing

Since renin and aldosterone must always be interpreted in light of volume status, random testing without patient preparation is never indicated. Acute illness impairs aldosterone production: testing should be deferred during acute illness. Testing for hyperaldosteronism is not indicated unless metabolic evidence of aldosterone effect (hypokalemia, increased urine potassium excretion) is documented. All drugs affecting renin or aldosterone production (Chapter 38) should be discontinued for at least 4–5 half-lives if possible before testing. If they can not, medications least likely to alter renin and aldosterone should be used. Among antihypertensive agents, the least problematic are centrally acting adrenergic antagonists and peripheral vasodilators. Calcium channel blockers alter aldosterone, but less so than other agents. β-Adrenergic antagonists, angiotensin converting enzyme inhibitors, and diuretics (especially spironolactone) have the greatest effects and should be discontinued if at all possible. Among other agents, nonsteroidal anti-inflammatory agents, estrogen, and heparin have the greatest chance of impairing test interpretation.

Primary Hyperaldosteronism

Approximately 1–2% of hypertension is due to primary hyperaldosteronism; some have reported the prevalence as high as 6%. Other factors increase the likelihood of hyperaldosteronism as a cause of hypertension: 5–10% of cases of refractory hypertension and 50% of cases with hypokalemia are due to aldosterone production. Hypokalemia, metabolic alkalosis, marked sodium retention (FE_{Na} less than 0.5%, even on a high salt diet), and excessive potassium excretion (urine K greater than 30 mmol/day, FE_K greater than 20%) all suggest aldosterone excess. The diagnostic approach to suspected hyperaldosteronism is outlined in Figure 14.4.

There are two common causes of primary hyperaldosteronism, adrenal adenoma and essential hyperaldosteronism, each responsible for about 50% of cases. This latter disorder is associated with increased sensitivity to the effects of angiotensin II, and seldom is cured by surgery. Table 14.2 outlines the differences in these two disorders. None of the tests is 100% accurate; a combination of tests is usually used to determine the correct diagnosis.

Secondary Hyperaldosteronism

Increased aldosterone caused by increased renin is termed secondary hyperaldosteronism. The most common cause is transient volume depletion, but the most important cause is renal artery stenosis, responsible for 2–3% of cases of hypertension. Clues to the presence of renal artery stenosis include abdominal bruits, hypokalemia, and metabolic alkalosis. In renal artery stenosis, renal vein renin helps determine the likelihood of revascularization being successful in controlling hypertension. With longstanding disease, renal damage maintains hypertension even if renin is normalized, but if renin activity is 1.5 to 2 times higher in the renal vein of the affected kidney, revascularization is likely to be of benefit. Secondary hyperaldosteronism occurs in accelerated hypertension; measurements should be repeated once blood pressure has been brought under control. Less likely causes include renin producing tumors and hyperplasia of the juxtaglomerular apparatus (Bartter's syndrome).

Hypoaldosteronism

Hypoaldosteronism should be suspected in patients with hyponatremia, hyperkalemia, decreased urinary potassium (fractional excretion less than 15%), increased urinary sodium (fractional excretion greater than 1%), non-anion gap metabolic acidosis, and hypotension. The most common cause is decreased renin production (**hyporeninemic hypoaldosteronism**) due to renal damage, especially in diabetics. A decreased glomeru-

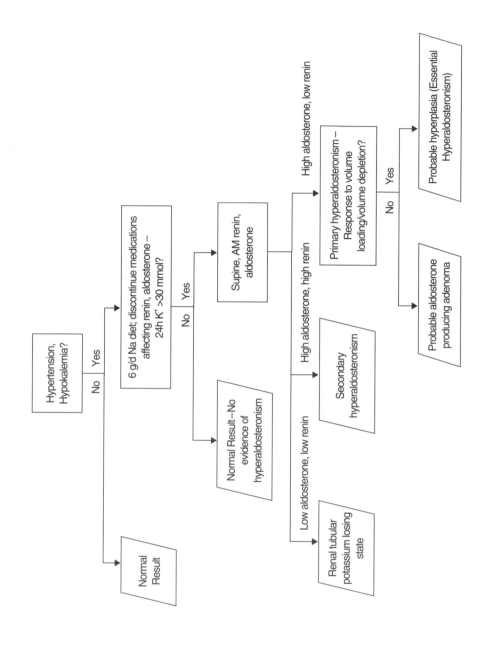

Table 14.2.
Differential Diagnosis of Causes of Primary Hyperaldosteronism

Aldosterone-Producing Adenoma	Essential Hyperaldosteronism (Hyperplasia)
Aldosterone > 40	Aldosterone < 40
Increased 18-OH corticosterone	Normal to slightly increased 18-OH corticosterone
Aldosterone/renin ratio > 100	Aldosterone/renin ratio 20–50
No response to volume loading	Decrease in aldosterone with volume loading
Paradoxical decrease in aldosterone with volume depletion	Increase in aldosterone with volume depletion
Mass on imaging studies in 80%	Mass rarely present
Marked increase in aldosterone from side of lesion when ACTH administered	No or minimal increase in aldosterone after ACTH; no difference between sides

lar filtration rate in diabetics makes hyponatremia uncommon. Patients with Addison's disease also have low aldosterone and high renin, but are usually easy to detect because of the severity of symptoms. Isolated deficiency of aldosterone is uncommon, but can occur with rare congenital enzyme deficiencies. Measurements of aldosterone and renin should be performed when expected to be high, during volume depletion. If the patient is hypotensive or dehydrated, further stimulation is not needed; if not, acute volume depletion is produced by administration of furosemide (80 mg intravenous push) followed by ambulating over a 4 hour period. Normally, renin will rise more than 5 ng/mL per hour, and aldosterone reaches at least 25 ng/dL (0.70 nmol/L).

ADRENAL MEDULLA

Normal Physiology

The adrenal medulla is a component of the sympathetic nervous system (Fig.14.5), synthesizing catecholamines, and is unaffected by hormones which affect adrenal cortex function. While dopamine and norepinephrine are produced in other sites, epinephrine is produced only in the adrenal medulla and the organ of Zuckercandl; this may be of help in localizing a catecholamine producing tumor. Catecholamines are metabolized by two enzymes, catecholamine-O-methyltransferase (COMT) and monoamine oxidase (MAO), to a variety of inactive metabolites, with a half-life of minutes.

Tests of Catecholamine Production

Measurement of catecholamines or their metabolites is most widely used for evaluating adrenal medulla function. However, since the adrenal is not the only source of their production, elevated catecholamine levels do not necessarily indicate adrenal medullary disease.

Figure 14.4. Approach to Suspected Hyperaldosteronism. Before performing testing, factors affecting renin or aldosterone production must be controlled. Medications such as β-adrenergic antagonists, diuretics, angiotensin converting enzyme inhibitors, and nonsteroidal anti-inflammatory agents should be stopped for at least five half-lives prior to evaluation. Salt intake should be increased prior to initial evaluation as well. If urine potassium excretion is greater than 30 mmol/day in the face of hypokalemia, further evaluation is warranted. A morning, supine specimen for renin and aldosterone will be adequate for initial evaluation.

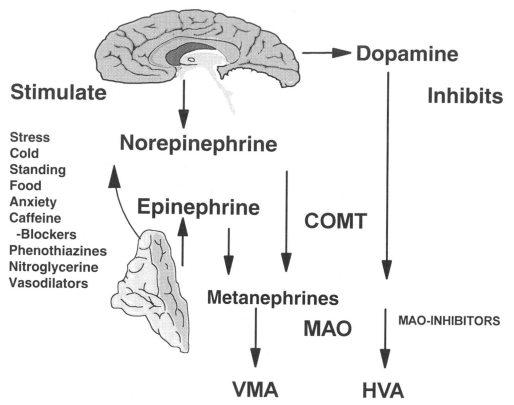

Figure 14.5. The CNS-Catecholamine Axis. The three major catecholamines are dopamine, norepinephrine, and epinephrine. Dopamine is primarily produced in the central nervous system, epinephrine is primarily produced by the adrenal, and norepinephrine is produced by both. Evaluation of catecholamine overproduction can be done by measuring daily excretion of catecholamines or their metabolites. The appropriate test depends on the clinical condition of the patient. For patients with signs and symptoms suggesting pheochromocytoma, fractionated urine catecholamines are the most sensitive test. In children with neuroblastoma, measurements of final metabolites VMA and HVA are preferred. In adults with asymptomatic adrenal tumors, either metanephrines or VMA may be the most helpful test, since some adrenal tumors do not release intact catecholamines.

Metanephrine

Measurement of this intermediate metabolic product is the most widely used chemical assay of catecholamine production. Assays usually measure total metanephrines, derived mainly from norepinephrine metabolism. Metanephrine and normetanephrine can be measured separately, increasing the sensitivity for detection of epinephrine producing tumors with normal normetanephrine but elevated metanephrine. Metanephrine measurements are falsely increased by α-methyldopa and by certain radiographic contrast agents, while propranolol causes falsely low results.

Vanillylmandelic Acid

Vanillylmandelic acid (VMA) is the final product of epinephrine and norepinephrine metabolism. Some VMA assays show cross-reactivity with many substances, among them substances found in bananas and citrus fruits. Some drugs block production of VMA, such as MAO inhibitors. Testing for VMA is the least sensitive method for detection of catecholamine excess.

Homovanillic Acid

Homovanillic acid (HVA) is the final metabolic product of dopamine. Many neuroblastomas produce only dopamine, not norepinephrine; HVA may be the only marker elevated in such tumors. Measurements of HVA and VMA are usually combined in initial evaluation and follow-up of neuroblastoma.

Urine Catecholamines

Most catecholamine excretion occurs as conjugated derivatives; as with cortisol, free catecholamines are a good indicator of catecholamine production. Each catecholamine is measured separately, so that central and adrenal sources can be distinguished in some cases. Normally, dopamine is present in the greatest amount, followed closely by norepinephrine, with only a small amount of epinephrine excreted normally. A small percentage of pheochromocytomas produce only epinephrine, which may not increase total catecholamines or their metabolites; such patients often have less dramatic symptoms than in classic pheochromocytoma. To detect these tumors, it is recommended that fractionated catecholamines or fractionated metanephrines be used instead of total metabolite assays.

Plasma Catecholamines

Levels of catecholamines in plasma react almost immediately to any form of stress. In one study, applying a tourniquet and cleaning the arm (as if to perform venipuncture) caused significant increases in catecholamine levels when blood was sampled through an indwelling catheter in the other arm. Catecholamines are highly labile once collected; specimens should be collected into chilled vacutainer tubes, placed on ice immediately after collection, and separated in refrigerated centrifuges before freezing plasma. In patients with widely separated episodes of hypertension due to pheochromocytoma, plasma catecholamines may be the only abnormal test. Patients needing plasma catecholamine measurements should have an indwelling catheter, should be relaxed, and preferably located in a quiet room isolated from loud noises.

Dynamic Testing

Clonidine is a centrally acting inhibitor of catecholamine release, and should decrease stress related overproduction of catecholamines, but not that due to adrenal tumors. Patients with minimal elevations of catecholamines show suppression into the normal range, regardless of the cause.

When Not to Test for Catecholamine Overproduction

In addition to assay interferences, any state or agent which increases catecholamine production increases plasma and urine catecholamines and their metabolites. Caffeine, other methylxanthines (theophylline), β-blockers, amphetamines, and other sympathomimetic agents (diet and allergy control products) also cause false increases. Acute stress increases catecholamine production, and most forms of acute illness, psychiatric disease, and anxiety may all increase test results. Testing should be delayed until after recovery from any of these states. Medications affecting catecholamines should be discontinued for at least five half-lives before testing. Caffeine intake should be limited to no more than 2–3 cups of coffee (or equivalent amounts of other beverages containing caffeine) for several days before testing. Since most screening tests are done in urine, renal insufficiency may be associated with falsely low results on urine tests due to decreased filtration, although this is not commonly of significance until late in the course of renal disease.

Approach to Suspected Pheochromocytoma

The classic pattern of pheochromocytoma (episodic hypertension, sweating, postural hypotension, headache) is present in only a minority of patients. Pheochromocytoma is a rare cause of hypertension (fewer than 1 in 1,000 cases) with an incidence of 3–4 per 1,000,000 population annually. Fractionated catecholamines or fractionated metanephrines is the best test for the low risk patient; patients do not require any special diet, since erroneous false positive results are rare. If any individual catecholamine result is elevated, repeat testing is performed after placing the patient on dietary restrictions (eliminating caffeine, over the counter medications, and discontinuing medications). Fractionated urine catecholamines detect more than 98% of cases, total metanephrines about 90%, and VMA 80–85%. Combining total metanephrines with fractionated catecholamines increases sensitivity to virtually 100%, and this is recommended if clinical findings strongly suggest pheochromocytoma. In patients with widely separated episodes of paroxysmal hypertension, plasma catecholamines should be measured if urine measurements are normal.

Testing in Neuroblastoma

This tumor of childhood is usually diagnosed from its mass effects, rather than from hormone production. Measurement of VMA and HVA is useful at baseline and for follow-up after treatment to detect residual or recurrent tumor. Both tests are recommended, since neither has high sensitivity because of individual differences in catecholamine production by the tumors.

THE INCIDENTAL ADRENAL MASS

With increased use of imaging studies, incidental adrenal masses have become a common problem; many autopsy studies have found incidental adrenal nodules in up to 5% of patients. Review of history and simple laboratory results (such as electrolytes) may suggest what, if any, workup should be initiated. Patients with signs or symptoms of overproduction of a particular hormone should be evaluated as discussed in the appropriate section of the chapter. In asymptomatic patients with normal electrolytes, a limited workup including overnight dexamethasone suppression test and 24 hour urine for metanephrines or fractionated catecholamines is appropriate for small tumors. Many patients will fail dexamethasone suppression ("subclinical Cushing's syndrome"); it is estimated that fewer than 1% will go on to develop clinical evidence of Cushing's syndrome if left untreated. Larger tumors, if derived from functional cells, probably are not producing an active hormone. In this situation, measurements should be aimed at detecting inactive metabolites such as VMA or 17-ketosteroids.

CHAPTER 15

Pituitary Function

D. ROBERT DUFOUR

NORMAL PITUITARY FUNCTION

The pituitary produces hormones in response to stimuli from the hypothalamus and, indirectly, the brain (Table 15.1). For most pituitary hormones, production is passive, that is, unless a hypothalamic hormone is present, virtually no hormone is produced. Prolactin production is inhibited by hypothalamic hormones; loss of this inhibition increases prolactin production. Antidiuretic hormone (ADH) is synthesized by the hypothalamus, stored in pituitary cells, and released by hypothalamic stimuli (Chapter 5).

PITUITARY DYSFUNCTION

Overproduction of pituitary hormones is usually due to a deficiency of the hormone regulated (e.g., high TSH in hypothyroidism) or inappropriate overproduction by a tumor. Symptoms related to increased prolactin, growth hormone, and ACTH are what brings many patients with pituitary tumors to seek medical attention. Underproduction of pituitary hormones has more varied causes. Isolated deficiency of one hormone is often due to hypothalamic injury, while deficiencies of more than one hormone may be due to hypothalamic damage, pituitary destruction, or pituitary stalk compression. Abnormalities of TSH, ACTH, gonadotropins, and ADH are discussed in Chapters 5, 13, 14, and 16, respectively.

Prolactin

A major pregnancy hormone, prolactin is responsible for proliferation of breast tissue and milk production, and also inhibiting GnRH pulses. Prolactin production is primarily under inhibitory control of dopamine (Fig. 15.1). Either dopamine antagonists or an interruption in blood flow from the hypothalamus will cause prolactin overproduction.

Laboratory Tests

Plasma prolactin varies considerably during the day (Fig. 15.2), although single samples are adequate to evaluate symptomatic patients. Thyrotropin-releasing hormone (TRH) stimulates prolactin production, but TRH stimulation adds nothing to differential diagnosis. Normal prolactin values are slightly higher in women (up to 20 ng/mL) than men (up to 12 ng/mL). Furthermore, they are slightly higher in women who have never been pregnant.

When Not to Do Prolactin Testing

Prolactin levels rise in response to stress; testing should not be done in acutely ill patients. A number of medications (Fig. 15.1) affect prolactin production, usually in-

Table 15.1.
Pituitary Hormone Action and Physiologic Regulation

Hormone	Action	Stimulated by	Inhibited by
Growth hormone (GH)	Increases growth of bones, other organs by production of somatomedin (IGF-I), increases serum glucose	Growth hormone releasing hormone (GHRH),* sleep, low glucose, meals, exercise	Somatostatin, high glucose, insulin-like growth factor-1 (IGF-1)
Prolactin	Increases secretion of milk by breast	Thyrotropin releasing hormone (TRH), ADH, sleep, nipple stimulation	Dopamine*
Thyrotropin (TSH)	Increases production of thyroid hormone	TRH*	Thyroid hormones,* dopamine, somatostatin
Corticotropin (ACTH) (proopiomelanocortin)	Increased production of cortisol	Corticotropin releasing hormone (CRH),* sleep, stress, cytokines	Cortisol
Follicle stimulating hormone (FSH)	Increased production of ova by ovaries and sperm by testes	Gonadotropin releasing hormone (GnRH)* when released in spikes	Inhibin (from testis and ovary), GnRH in high concentrations, dopamine, prolactin
Luteinizing hormone (LH)	Production of sex hormones; ovulation	GnRH* when released in spikes	High testosterone or estrogen; GnRH in high concentrations, dopamine, prolactin
Antidiuretic hormone (ADH)	Conservation of water	Increased osmolality of blood,* decreased blood pressure, nausea	Decreased osmolality of blood,* cortisol
Oxytocin	Onset of labor and release of milk by the breast	Unknown	Unknown

*Most important factor affecting production

creasing it, and these should be discontinued before testing if at all possible. Hypothyroidism increases prolactin, and may cause pituitary enlargement which simulates pituitary adenoma. If TSH is elevated, further workup should be delayed until hypothyroidism is corrected. Prolactin levels are markedly increased during pregnancy, however, prolactin producing lesions are not common in pregnant women.

Prolactin Excess

Overproduction of prolactin is the most common pituitary hormonal abnormality. In women, it causes milk production (**galactorrhea**) and often leads to cessation of menstrual periods (**amenorrhea**). In men, symptoms are less commonly present. Infertility and impotence are most common, and rarely breast enlargement (**gynecomastia**) develops. Prolactin levels greater than 200 ng/mL virtually always indicate prolactin-producing pituitary tumors, while prolactin levels from 100–200 ng/mL are usually due to tumors. Prolactin levels of 20–100 ng/mL are often due to diurnal variation, medications, stress, or pituitary stalk compression. Often patients with space occupying lesions

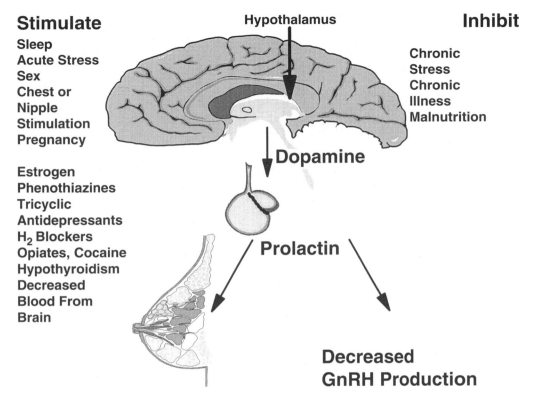

Stimulate

Sleep
Acute Stress
Sex
Chest or
Nipple
Stimulation
Pregnancy

Estrogen
Phenothiazines
Tricyclic
Antidepressants
H₂ Blockers
Opiates, Cocaine
Hypothyroidism
Decreased
Blood From
Brain

Hypothalamus

Inhibit

Chronic
Stress
Chronic
Illness
Malnutrition

Dopamine

Prolactin

Decreased
GnRH Production

Figure 15.1. Prolactin Regulation and Actions. Prolactin differs from most other pituitary hormones, being primarily under inhibitory control from dopamine. Other medications which block dopamine action will lead to increased prolactin production. Interruption of hypothalamic blood flow increases prolactin. The major effects of prolactin are stimulation of breast tissue, which leads to galactorrhea in women, and inhibition of GnRH production, causing hypogonadism (Chapter 16). Hypothyroidism also stimulates prolactin production, although the mechanism is not clear.

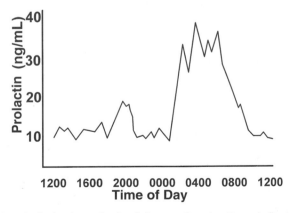

Figure 15.2. Prolactin Levels. Prolactin production follows a diurnal pattern similar to that of other pituitary hormones, with most production occurring during sleep. At other times, prolactin is released in episodic bursts, with individual results as much as 2–3 times basal levels. Mildly increased prolactin may be due to such diurnal variation, but values greater than 5 times normal are almost always pathologic.

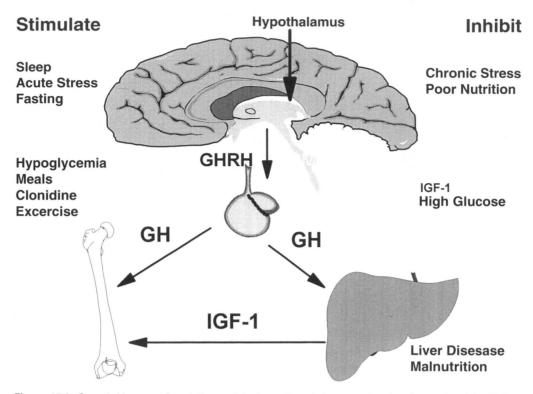

Figure 15.3. Growth Hormone Regulation and Actions. Growth hormone is primarily regulated by GHRH, modified by signals occurring through food ingestion, exercise, and stress. Growth hormone has direct effects on tissues, but most skeletal growth promotion is through the actions of IGF-1, produced by the liver in response to growth hormone. Insulin-like growth factor 1 also provides feedback inhibition on GH production, completing the loop. To properly interpret IGF-1 or GH levels, patients should be in a usual state of health and fasting, or have been exposed to an agent affecting GH production.

in the pituitary have mildly elevated prolactin. If patients are on medications increasing prolactin (Chapter 38 and Fig. 15.1), the medication should be discontinued for five half-lives (if possible) and prolactin repeated before performing imaging studies. Normal results on the repeat test establish the medication as the cause. Nonpregnant patients with continued prolactin elevation (or initial values over 200 ng/mL) should have pituitary imaging studies.

Growth Hormone (Fig. 15.3)

Growth hormone (GH) is unique among pituitary hormones in that most effects are mediated through another hormone, **insulin-like growth factor 1** (IGF-1, also called **somatomedin C**), produced in the liver and other tissues in response to GH. Both GH and IGF-1 are unusual among peptide hormones in that they circulate bound to transport proteins. The major IGF-1 binding protein, IGFBP-3, is produced primarily by the liver in response to GH. Protein binding gives IGF-1 a long half-life and little diurnal variation. Levels are low with liver disease and protein malnutrition.

Laboratory Tests

Evaluation of GH production is difficult because of marked diurnal variation (Fig. 15.4), variation in responsiveness to stimuli, effects of coexisting disease on GH and

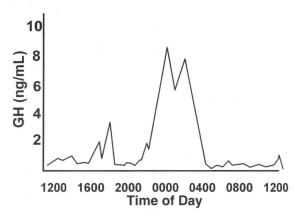

Figure 15.4. Growth Hormone Levels. Growth hormone is released in episodic spikes throughout the day, with the vast majority of secretions occurring during the first four hours of sleep. Single levels drawn during the day are difficult to interpret because of the marked difference between basal production and concentration during a spike.

IGF-1, and marked age-related variation in normal values. Several tests of GH status are often needed to reach a correct diagnosis.

Growth Hormone Levels

Single random measurements of GH are of little worth unless drawn at the maximum, (1 hour after onset of deep sleep), which requires hospitalization.

Response to Physiologic and Pharmacologic Changes

Among agents used to stimulate GH are exercise, insulin hypoglycemia, growth hormone releasing hormone (GHRH, 1 mg/kg), clonidine (4 mg/kg), l-dopa (0.5 g), and arginine (0.5 g/kg). Only 70–80% of normal persons respond to any one, with failure to respond to at least two the minimum criterion for GH deficiency. Administration of a glucose load should cause GH to fall to within the normal range.

IGF-1 and Binding Proteins

In most situations, IGF-1 levels are the best marker for evaluation of GH production. Normal values vary significantly with age; before age 5, levels are quite low and cannot be reliably used to recognize GH deficiency. Results must be evaluated with the appropriate reference range for age and sex. Liver disease, acute illness, and malnutrition inhibit production of IGF-1 and IGFBP-3, making interpretation difficult.

When Not to Test for Growth Hormone

Growth hormone, IGF-1, and IGFBP-3 are decreased by acute illness; testing should be deferred until recovery if at all possible. Malnourished patients should not be tested until nutritional state has returned to normal. A number of medications affect GH, most importantly corticosteroids, antiepileptics, some psychiatric medications, and nonsteroidal anti-inflammatory agents, with a complete listing found in Chapter 38.

Ideally, these medications should be discontinued for at least five half-lives before testing.

Growth Hormone Overproduction

The only common cause of excess GH is pituitary tumor. The major clinical manifestation is increased bone growth, causing **gigantism** in children and thickening of bones (**acromegaly**) in adults and children. Other GH effects include thickening, and increased sweating and oiliness of the skin, hypertension, joint pain, and hyperglycemia in 50% of cases. IGF-1 is the best screening test, although some prefer GH after glucose administration. Single random GH measurements are not useful. A normal result on either screening test effectively rules out GH overproduction. After therapy, IGF-1 is the most reliable test, the goal being to normalize results. Many GH producing tumors are associated with increased prolactin, and prolactin should be measured in any patient with acromegaly or gigantism.

Growth Hormone Deficiency

Symptoms of GH deficiency are usually absent except in infants or small children, where it causes growth retardation; severely deficient children develop hypoglycemia. A minority of children with short stature have GH deficiency. Diagnosis requires failure of GH to respond to at least two normal stimuli. Low IGF-1 is useful in older children, but is falsely low in liver disease or malnutrition states. Stress inhibits GH production; children should not be tested while ill or in severe psychological stress. Monitoring of therapy with GH is usually done by clinical criteria, rather than laboratory tests.

Panhypopituitarism (Pituitary Insufficiency)

Although the term panhypopituitarism (and its clinical synonym, pituitary insufficiency) implies underproduction of all pituitary hormones, in most cases not all hormones are decreased. Typically, symptoms of hormone underproduction do not develop simultaneously. The first hormone to show decreased production is usually growth hormone. Deficiency of GH is usually asymptomatic in adults. Decreased FSH and LH production also occur early. In men, impotence may result, and in premenopausal women, amenorrhea develops, but postmenopausal women and many men are asymptomatic. Sometimes years later, evidence of hypothyroidism develops and often brings older men and women to seek medical attention. In late stages, decreased ACTH production leads to secondary adrenal failure. Diabetes insipidus (Chapter 5) is not common with pituitary disorders, although it is frequent with pituitary stalk or hypothalamic damage. While most patients develop hormonal deficiency in the order shown, a particular deficiency may develop at any time in the course of disease. The most common cause for pituitary insufficiency is pituitary tumors; pituitary infarction due to peripartum hemorrhagic shock (**Sheehan's syndrome**) is now rare. Less frequently, other pituitary diseases (autoimmune inflammation [**lymphocytic hypophysitis**], granulomatous disease), damage to the pituitary stalk (tumors, trauma, or aneurysms), or hypothalamic disease may cause hypopituitarism.

When Not to Test for Hypopituitarism

Acute illness and malnutrition decrease production of most pituitary hormones; in critically ill patients, even response to stimuli may be lost. Since only deficiency of thyroid hormone and cortisol are life threatening, a reasonable approach to suspected pituitary insufficiency in critically ill patients is to measure cortisol and free thyroxine; if low, treatment can be given until illness resolves, when a full workup can be performed. Although a variety of factors affect one or a few pituitary hormones, they will not generally affect all of them.

Laboratory Approach to Suspected Hypopituitarism

Because tests of peripheral endocrine hormones are simpler, more rapidly available, and less expensive, they should be the initial tests performed. Normal menstrual periods rule out gonadotropin deficiency, as does a normal testosterone, normal free thyroxine rules out TSH deficiency, and normal cortisol rules out ACTH deficiency. If one or more of the screening tests are abnormal, measurement of pituitary hormone levels (FSH, LH, TSH) or response to normal stimuli (cortrosyn stimulation test) can be done to confirm hypopituitarism. Measurement of GH or IGF-1 is not usually needed in adults. Prolactin is often elevated in hypopituitarism due to interruption of inhibitory regulation, making its measurement not helpful.

CHAPTER 16

Gonadal Function

D. ROBERT DUFOUR

HYPOTHALAMIC–PITUITARY–GONADAL AXIS (GENERAL)

The interactions among the various components of this system are illustrated in Figure 16.1.

Hypothalamic Regulation

The hypothalamus makes a single releasing hormone, gonadotropin-releasing hormone (GnRH), sometimes called luteinizing hormone–releasing hormone (LHRH). The pattern of GnRH production determines the production of pituitary gonadotropins (follicle stimulating hormone (FSH), luteinizing hormone (LH)) by a single cell (gonadotrope). When produced in a pulsatile manner, GnRH stimulates production of FSH and LH, with frequent pulses favoring LH production, and less frequent pulses stimulating FSH more. Constant GnRH production inhibits both FSH and LH synthesis. Before puberty, little GnRH is produced and gonadal function is largely nonexistent in both boys and girls. At puberty, pulsatile GnRH release starts and sexual maturation begins.

Pituitary Regulation

Follicle stimulating hormone and LH are glycoprotein hormones, related to TSH and HCG, composed of a common α subunit and a β subunit unique to each hormone. In normal circumstances, virtually no free α or β subunits are released. Pituitary production of FSH and LH is modified by feedback signals from gonads. Constant, high concentration of all sex steroid hormones (androgens, estrogens, and progesterone) inhibits FSH and LH production. In women, when estrogen concentration is low but progressively rising, LH production occurs; a critical rate of change leads to a marked surge in LH and FSH production, inducing ovulation.

HYPOTHALAMIC–PITUITARY–GONADAL AXIS FEATURES UNIQUE TO EACH SEX

Normal Female Gonadal Function

Most sex hormones of importance are produced in the ovary; fat cells also synthesize hormones and may contribute significant amounts in certain situations (Fig. 16.2). A normal relative ratio and timing of gonadotropin production is necessary for normal hormone levels. Before puberty, little gonadotropin is produced and sex hormone levels are low. At puberty, cyclic production of gonadotropins begins and estrogen and progesterone are produced. Estrogens stimulate cell growth and proliferation in the endometrium and breast, while progesterone promotes cell maturation and secretion. Both estrogens and progesterone circulate primarily protein bound, with about 3%

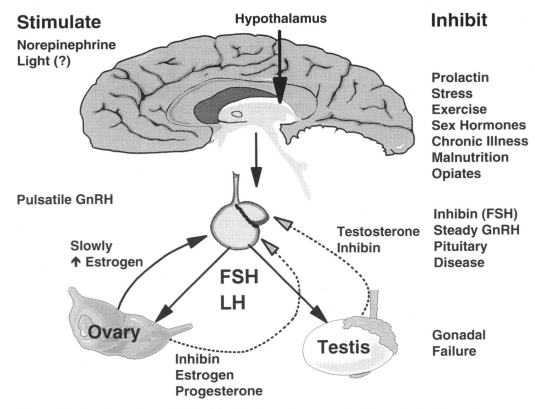

Figure 16.1. Regulation of Gonadal Function. The hypothalamus synthesizes a single releasing hormone, GnRH. Many factors lower GnRH production: feedback inhibition from sex steroids, prolactin, stress, weight loss, and malnutrition. When released in a pulsatile fashion, GnRH stimulates production of FSH and LH. In women, FSH stimulates development of follicles to prepare for ovulation. Luteinizing hormone stimulates steroid synthesis. Before ovulation, androgen production predominates, with androgens converted to estradiol under the influence of FSH. After ovulation, progesterone is the dominant hormone produced. In males, FSH (under the influence of testosterone) stimulates proliferation of germ cells to form sperm, while LH stimulates testosterone synthesis. Sex steroids inhibit FSH and LH production. Inhibin, produced by follicles and semeniferous tubules, also inhibits FSH production.

free. Sex hormone and gonadotropin levels fluctuate markedly during a normal menstrual cycle (Fig. 16.3). Before ovulation, ovarian follicles mature under the influence of FSH, termed the follicular phase; estradiol predominates during this period. After ovulation, LH stimulates progesterone production by theca lutein cells in ovarian corpus luteum. If fertilization occurs, human chorionic gonadotropin (HCG, Chapter 17) maintains hormone production.

Normal Male Gonadal Function

Before puberty, lack of gonadotropin secretion is associated with markedly low androgen levels. At puberty, increased LH and FSH secretion causes testicular development. Luteinizing hormone stimulates Leydig cells to produce androgens, mainly testosterone. Androgens are transported bound to protein. Only approximately 2% of testosterone is free and presumably bioactive. Free testosterone serves mainly as a prohormone, converted in peripheral tissues (by the enzyme 5-α-reductase) to **dihydrotestosterone,** which causes most androgen effects in males.

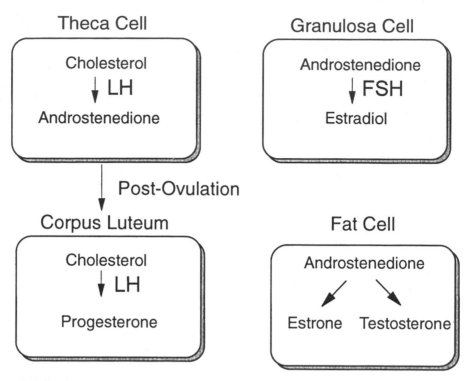

Figure 16.2. Sex Steroid Synthesis in Females. Luteinizing hormone stimulates the production of androgens, primarily androstenedione, in the theca cells before ovulation. Follicle stimulating hormone stimulates conversion of androstenedione to estradiol. The relative amounts of LH and FSH determine the relative production of androgen and estrogen. After ovulation, LH stimulates conversion of cholesterol to progesterone; if fertilization occurs, HCG continues progesterone production. Fat cells also perform endocrine functions, converting androstenedione to both estrone and testosterone.

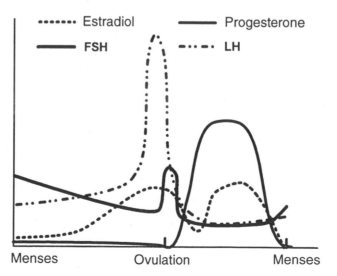

Figure 16.3. Cyclic Variation in Hormones in Females. Levels of gonadotropins and sex steroids must be interpreted in light of timing in the menstrual cycle. Before ovulation, estradiol dominates, while progesterone is the more important hormone after ovulation.

Transport of Sex Steroids in the Blood

Testosterone and estradiol are predominantly protein bound, mainly to **sex-hormone binding globulin** (SHBG). Rate of liver SHBG production is dependent on sex hormones: estrogens increase and androgens decrease production, with SHBG levels twice as high in women as in men. As estrogen production decreases, total hormone and free hormone decrease in parallel. When androgen production declines, increased SHBG initially causes total androgen to reach a plateau, while free hormone levels continue to decrease. Total testosterone levels may thus be inappropriately normal in early testicular disease. Liver disease and malnutrition also decrease SHBG.

NORMAL PROCESS OF FERTILIZATION

The main purpose of gonadal function is to provide gametes required for reproduction. In addition to gonads, an intact transport mechanism for sperm to reach the ovum, hormones to allow maturation of sperm and ova, and a normal endometrium to support the fertilized ovum are all needed for normal pregnancy. Interference with any phase of the process (Fig. 16.4) may cause infertility.

Normal Gamete Development

In the ovaries, germ cells divide during fetal life, reaching maximum numbers at about six months gestation. Germ cells begin the process of duplication of chromosomes,

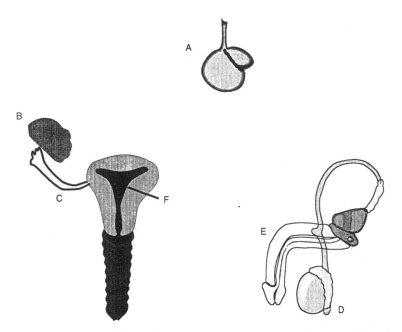

Figure 16.4. Factors Affecting Fertility. Normal fertility requires normal structure and function of many organs. Normal cyclic gonadotropin production, (**A**) with normal cyclic production, is critical for normal gonadal function. In women, the ovaries (**B**) must be able to respond to pituitary hormones. The fallopian tubes (**C**) are critical to fertility; scarring is a common factor in infertility. The testes and epididymis (**D**) must function properly to form, activate, and store sperm. Impotence due to penile erectile dysfunction (**E**) may prevent fertilization. Once an ovum is fertilized, the endometrium (**F**) requires a constant supply of progesterone to maintain the developing embryo.

termed meiosis, and enter a quiescent stage before completing the first meiotic division. They remain inactive until, at puberty, surrounding cells begin to develop follicles. Follicle maturation continues under the influence of FSH until the middle of a menstrual cycle when the LH surge stimulates ovulation. The shed oocyte then completes the first meiotic division. In the testes, germ cells are relatively quiescent until puberty, when FSH production stimulates germ cell proliferation and division. Mature sperm enter the epididymis, where they become activated by an obscure mechanism. They are stored there until ejaculation.

Fertilization

After sexual intercourse, semen coagulates in the vagina and eventually liquefies, releasing sperm. The sperm actively move through the cervix, the endometrial cavity, and reach the fallopian tubes. After ovulation, the ovum also enters the fallopian tube. Generally, sperm remain viable for 1–3 days. If an ovum is present, the sperm cell must penetrate the outer coat of the ovum (**zona pellucida**) for its chromosomes to enter the ovum. When this occurs, the second meiotic division of the ovum is then completed. Under the influence of LH, the corpus luteum produces estrogen and progesterone needed to prepare the endometrium for implantation. The fertilized ovum implants about five days after fertilization, by which time it has usually reached the endometrial cavity.

Support for the Developing Embryo

After implantation, the developing embryo receives nutrition from glucose stored in endometrial stromal cells. After 10–14 days, the early placenta produces HCG (Chapter 17), which maintains hormone production by the corpus luteum. Failure of corpus luteum or HCG production leads to spontaneous miscarriage.

EVALUATION OF SUSPECTED GONADAL DYSFUNCTION

Clinical Evaluation

Before laboratory tests are performed, physical examination and clinical testing can establish some types of normal and abnormal hormone production, particularly in women. Laboratory testing may then not be needed. In both men and women, measurement of arm span relative to height can establish defective estrogen or androgen production. Normally, this span is not more than 2 inches greater than height, while a deficiency of sex hormones delays closure of epiphyses and increases the ratio of arm span to height. Midline truncal hair, a male pattern of pubic hair, acne, and facial hair more than on the lip all indicate significant androgen production and response.

Clinical Evaluation of Female Gonadal Function

Normal breast development indicates normal estrogen production at puberty. Normal vaginal folds and lubrication indicate current estrogen production. Normal menstrual cycles indicate normal cyclic function of the entire axis. In women with irregular menses or anovulation, withdrawal bleeding after administration of progesterone for several days indicates adequate estrogen production. A rise in basal body temperature indicates ovulation and progesterone production; maintenance of elevated temperature indicates adequate progesterone production.

Clinical Evaluation of Male Gonadal Function

Clinical evaluation is less reliable in males than in females for determining current gonadal function, since most acquired diseases impair sperm development more than androgen production. Determination of arm span and body hair pattern can indicate long term deficiency of androgens, but current androgen production may be deficient without any physical findings. Acquired androgen deficiency should be associated with decreased libido and impotence, but often sexual function is reported as normal in men with low androgen levels. Loss of body hair is a late finding with acquired androgen deficiency. Small testes are often seen in hypogonadal states.

Sex Steroid Levels

Measurements of progesterone and testosterone are widely used in evaluation of female and male infertility, respectively. Testosterone levels are also used in evaluation of hirsutism in women. Estradiol levels are almost never required, since adequate estrogen production can be determined clinically in most cases.

Progesterone

In women, determination of progesterone is often used in evaluation of infertility. Progesterone levels are interpreted as normal or abnormal for the time in the menstrual cycle; laboratories often publish multiple reference ranges for different days post-ovulation. Since the time from ovulation to menstruation is relatively constant, the appropriateness of results can be determined retrospectively from the onset of subsequent menstruation. There is considerable overlap in progesterone levels between adequate and clinically inadequate values; levels must be clearly reduced on several measurements to diagnose inadequate progesterone production.

Testosterone

Testosterone levels are used in the evaluation of impotence and infertility in men. Most laboratories measure total testosterone, which remains normal early in gonadal failure while free testosterone falls. For this reason, some experts suggest routine use of free testosterone measurements; however, these assays are more expensive and require different specimen handling than total testosterone. We prefer to measure total testosterone first; if the results are markedly low or more than 10–15% above lower reference limits, free testosterone is not needed. A borderline low total testosterone level requires free testosterone for correct interpretation.

Gonadotropin Levels

Evaluation of gonadotropin production is necessary to determine the cause of gonadal dysfunction. A number of factors make evaluation of gonadotropin production much more difficult than for other pituitary hormones.

Selection of Sampling Method

As with growth hormone, gonadotropins are released in episodic spikes at infrequent intervals (Fig. 16.5), making use of single specimens for gonadotropin levels not recommended in men or in menstruating women. Single specimens are typically adequate

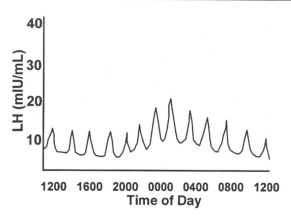

Figure 16.5. Diurnal Variation in Gonadotropin Levels in Men. There is a pronounced diurnal variation in levels of both LH and FSH (not shown, but similar to LH). Both gonadotropins are released in episodic bursts, approximately every two hours, with peak height slightly greater at night. Single specimens usually do not provide accurate information on gonadotropin production; use of three or more pooled specimens drawn 20–30 minutes apart is more reliable. In women, the peaks occur approximately each hour, with basal levels somewhat higher than in men, so that single specimens may occasionally be of benefit; however, most recommend use of pooled specimens.

for determination of gonadal failure, as occurs after menopause and in men with Kleinfelter's syndrome. In most situations, pooled samples (three to five specimens, each obtained 15–30 minutes apart) provide better information than single specimens. Even using this method, it is possible to miss a peak of LH production, particularly in men; testing should be confirmed by repeat pooled specimens if the findings suggest central hypogonadism.

Gonadotropin Subunits

Pituitary tumors commonly arise from gonadotrope cells; 20–25% produce either intact LH, the β-subunit of LH, or the α-subunit. In contrast to normal persons, those with pituitary gonadotrope tumors often show an increase in production of gonadotropins in response to TRH. In patients with clinically non-functioning pituitary tumors, measurement of α and β subunits before and after TRH may help to identify a tumor marker that can be monitored after therapy.

Stimulatory Testing

Theoretically, it should be possible to recognize early gonadal dysfunction and separate secondary (pituitary dysfunction) from tertiary (hypothalamic) causes of decreased gonadotropins by measuring response to pharmacologic stimulation of the pituitary. When a bolus of GnRH is given, there is typically a rapid rise in LH production, with plasma levels increasing 3–5 fold from baseline at 30 minutes. Follicle stimulating hormone rises little or not at all after GnRH administration. Reproducibility is poor, and most authors no longer recommend use of this or other, less effective stimuli such as clomiphene citrate.

Evaluation of Semen Production

Semen is the product of several organs in the male genital system; normal semen production is critical to normal fertility. Evaluation of semen is commonly performed early in evaluation of infertile couples.

Collection of Semen Specimens

Proper patient preparation and specimen handling are essential for correct interpretation of semen analysis. Sperm count varies with the time since the last ejaculation. Patients should be instructed to abstain from sex for 2–4 days, not longer or shorter, and the actual time should be recorded. Semen should be collected into a special collection container. If it is collected at home, the specimen must reach the laboratory within one hour of collection, and protected from heat or cold (preferably carried in an inside pocket to be near body temperature). The time of collection should be recorded.

Tests of Semen

A wide variety of tests have been proposed for the analysis of semen; most are only offered by specialized laboratories serving fertility specialists. Only the most common tests, offered by most laboratories, will be discussed. Patients with abnormal results for two or more tests likely have a male factor in infertility and should be evaluated by a fertility specialist to determine whether a reversible cause of semen production is present.

Physical Characteristics

Evaluation of sperm color, odor, pH, viscosity, liquefaction, and volume are the most common characteristics measured. Any abnormal results often provide clues to a male cause of infertility.

Microscopic Analysis

Routine microscopic examination includes evaluation of sperm count, motility, and morphology. Low or high sperm counts are often associated with infertility. Most sperm should show purposeful forward motion; the percent moving, the relative speed of motion, and the direction of motility (forward versus random) are all important in evaluating sperm function. Most sperm should be relatively uniform in size and normal in appearance; large, small, and abnormally shaped sperm in increased numbers are all associated with reduced fertility.

Postcoital Test

Examination of vaginal fluid after intercourse near the time of ovulation may help to identify a cause of infertility; however, not all authorities agree on the usefulness of this test. As with semen analysis, there should be a 2–4 day period of abstinence before intercourse near the expected time of ovulation. Between 6 and 24 hours after intercourse, a sample of cervical mucus is obtained and examined for the presence of motile sperm. If over 3–5 motile sperm are identified per high power field, adequate sperm are present to potentially fertilize an ovum. If the male has a normal semen analysis, an abnormal postcoital test implies the presence of a cervical factor (such as poor mucus production, infection, or antisperm antibodies) contributing to infertility.

When Not to Do Gonadal Function Testing

Marked changes in gonadotropin production occur with acute stress; gonadal function tests should not be performed during any acute illness. Malnutrition and strenuous

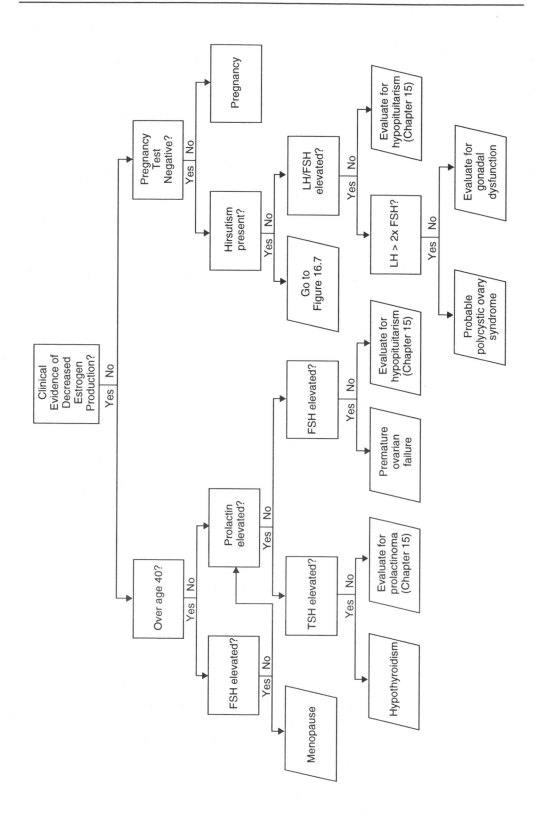

exercise commonly produce gonadal abnormalities; again, testing for intrinsic diseases should be deferred until after recovery is complete. In women who are menstruating normally, only progesterone levels are likely to be of use in evaluation of infertility, with other gonadal function tests will not producing useful information. Semen production is influenced by acute illnesses and stress. Testing should be deferred for 2–3 months after any acute illness requiring hospitalization, and should ideally be deferred even after a milder acute illness.

SPECIFIC PATTERNS OF GONADAL DYSFUNCTION

Amenorrhea

Absence of menses (Fig. 16.6) can be divided into primary (never had menses) and secondary (cessation of previously normal menses). Primary amenorrhea is often due to congenital disorders, and will not be discussed further here; more detailed information can be found in gynecology texts. Secondary amenorrhea is usually due to hormonal abnormalities. Laboratory testing is often of use in determining the cause. Polycystic ovary syndrome (discussed in more detail below) is the most common cause, followed by excess prolactin.

Hirsutism

Increased body hair (Fig. 16.7) in androgen-dependent areas (midline trunk, face), often accompanied by acne, is usually due to increased local or circulating androgens. Very high androgen levels cause further masculinization, such as enlargement of the clitoris, male hair pattern, and vocal changes, collectively termed virilization. In women of African or Mediterranean ancestry, hirsutism is often familial and not related to circulating hormonal abnormalities; a family history is often diagnostic. Hirsutism without other clinical findings (normal menstrual periods, no evidence of masculinization) is often not evaluated further by many practitioners. Androgen levels can help determine source of increased production: the most important are testosterone (primarily from the ovaries), and dehydroepiandrosterone sulfate (**DHEA-S**) (primarily from the adrenal).

Ovarian Androgen Overproduction

Approximately 75% of hirsutism is due to ovarian disorders. Testosterone levels over 100–150 ng/dL are commonly due to ovarian tumors. Workup of such patients should be more aggressive. Increased ovarian androgen production is most often caused by polycystic ovary syndrome, due to abnormal central regulation of steroid synthesis.

←——————————————————————————————————————

Figure 16.6. Approach to Amenorrhea. Initially, clinical evaluation should determine whether estrogen production appears adequate. With evidence of estrogen deficiency, FSH should be used initially in women over age 40; elevated levels indicate onset of menopause. In women younger than 40, prolactin should be the initial test, with TSH usually measured at the same time. If prolactin and TSH are not elevated, FSH should be determined to identify hypopituitarism. In women with adequate estrogen production, a pregnancy test should be performed initially; a positive test eliminates the need for further workup. If the pregnancy test is negative and hirsutism is present, consult Figure 16.7 for further guidance. In non-pregnant women who are not hirsute, LH and FSH are useful differential tests. Low FSH and LH suggest hypopituitarism. Elevated LH more than twice FSH strongly suggests polycystic ovary syndrome. Elevations of both FSH and LH, with similar FSH and LH, suggest ovarian dysfunction.

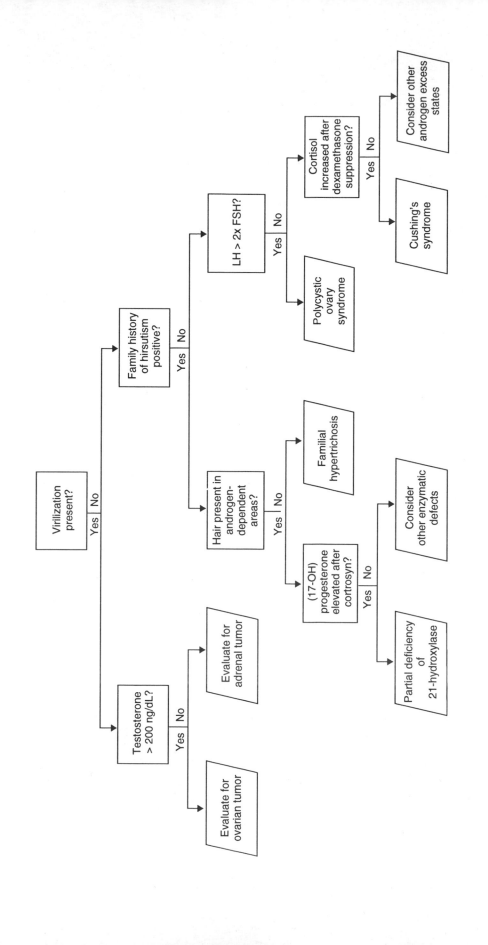

Affected individuals are often obese, with hirsutism and amenorrhea. Typically, FSH is decreased and LH increased, with a ratio of LH to FSH of greater than $2:1–3:1$.

Adrenal Androgen Production

The most common adrenal cause is partial ("**late onset**") congenital adrenal hyperplasia (Chapter 14). Serum cortisol is typically low normal and fails to rise normally after administration of ACTH. Very high DHEA-S levels are often due to androgen producing adrenal tumors. Cushing's syndrome is also responsible for a small percentage of cases.

Idiopathic Hirsutism

A relatively common cause of hirsutism is increased peripheral conversion of precursors to active androgens, termed idiopathic hirsutism. Affected women have normal testosterone and DHEA-S levels, normal menstrual periods, and excess hair in androgen dependent areas. Some have increased levels of advanced androgen metabolites such as 3-androstanediol glucuronide.

Male Impotence

Most cases of impotence are due to nonendocrine causes, but abnormal gonadal function causes 15–20% of cases. Testosterone and prolactin are adequate screening tests. Normal results here can rule out an endocrine cause. If testosterone is low or low normal and prolactin is normal, measurement of FSH and LH should distinguish primary gonadal failure (high values) from pituitary disease (low values); repeated measurement of LH is recommended because of significant day to day variation in results. With gonadal failure, both FSH and LH are usually increased; a discrepancy between FSH and LH increases the likelihood of a pituitary gonadotrope tumor.

Infertility

Infertility is thought to affect about 15% of couples desiring to become pregnant. In many cases, more than one factor appears to contribute to fertility problems. In a review of published studies on infertility, about 20% of couples had no identifiable factors causing infertility. The most common factors recognized include: mechanical problems with fertilization (previous pelvic inflammatory disease with tubal scarring, endometriosis), 25%; defective semen production (related to varicocele in 40% of cases), 25%; and hormonal factors affecting ovulation (such as increased prolactin and polycystic ovary syndrome), 30%. In many couples, more than one problem is often present. As might be expected from this list, history and physical examination often

---

Figure 16.7. Approach to Hirsutism. In women with hirsutism and evidence of virilization (clitoral enlargement, change in voice, male pattern of pubic hair distribution), an androgen producing tumor is likely; testosterone greater than 200 ng/dL suggests an ovarian tumor. In nonvirilized women, a family history of hirsutism suggests either familial hirsutism or a congenital steroid synthetic defect. The pattern of hair distribution is usually helpful in distinguishing these disorders. In the absence of family history, elevation of LH to more than twice FSH is characteristic of polycystic ovary syndrome. Lack of elevation of LH should lead to evaluation for Cushing's syndrome. Patients with normal hormone levels commonly have idiopathic hirsutism, with increased peripheral generation of androgens or increased androgen sensitivity.

identify one or more of these characteristics. Semen analysis and clinical examination and laboratory tests to detect abnormal androgen, estrogen, or progesterone production are initial tests performed in infertile couples, and may be performed easily by primary care practitioners. A postcoital test may be helpful if initial tests are unrewarding. A number of more sophisticated tests are available in specialized fertility testing laboratories, but not in most regular laboratories.

CHAPTER 17

Diagnosis and Monitoring of Pregnancy

D. ROBERT DUFOUR

PHYSIOLOGIC CHANGES DURING PREGNANCY

A number of factors significantly alter a woman's physiologic state during pregnancy, leading to corresponding changes in laboratory tests. While the most important are detailed below, additional information is found in Chapter 38.

Hormonal Changes

There are marked increases in several hormones, including estrogens, progesterone, human placental lactogen (HPL), human chorionic gonadotropin (HCG), and prolactin, during normal pregnancy. Human placental lactogen affects maternal metabolism in much the same way as growth hormone: it favors fatty acid use, inhibits glucose use, and stimulates gluconeogenesis, leading to increased plasma glucose. Estrogens stimulate marked increase in plasma lipids: total cholesterol, low density lipoprotein cholesterol, and high density lipoprotein cholesterol approximately double during pregnancy. Estrogen also stimulates production of some plasma proteins, notably ceruloplasmin, fibrinogen, and transferrin. Thyroid function is significantly altered during normal pregnancy. Total thyroid hormones increase approximately 15–20%, mainly due to increased thyroxine-binding globulin stimulated by estrogen. Free thyroxine transiently increases during early pregnancy, probably due to thyroid stimulation by HCG. In later pregnancy, however, free thyroxine is slightly lower than in nonpregnant women. Total cortisol increases due to increased cortisol binding globulin induced by estrogen.

Volume Changes

Blood volume increases by approximately 50% during normal pregnancy, gradually increasing during the first two trimesters to reach a plateau at about 32 weeks. Plasma volume increases more than red cell volume, causing hematocrit to fall by about 15%, though rarely below 33%, while plasma proteins decrease by 33%. Renin and aldosterone are markedly increased but plasma sodium falls, at least in part because the "normal" osmolality needed to prevent ADH production and thirst decreases.

Placental Products

In addition to HCG (discussed below), the placenta produces alkaline phosphatase, which approximately doubles by delivery. Creatine kinase BB isoenzyme is also produced. This increase may cause falsely elevated creatine kinase MB as measured by some methods (Chapter 12).

Renal Function Changes

During early pregnancy, glomerular filtration rate increases approximately 50%, causing decreased BUN and creatinine compared to prepregnancy results, with changes usually persisting until delivery. Urine glucose and protein excretion also increase, apparently due to increased filtration rate.

DIAGNOSIS OF PREGNANCY

Laboratory tests recognize presence of trophoblastic tissue, not pregnancy. Pregnancy tests detect HCG produced by syncytiotrophoblast cells in the placenta, hydatidiform mole, choriocarcinoma, and other germ cell tumors. Human chorionic gonadotropin is produced ectopically by tumors, particularly breast cancers and large cell carcinoma of the lung.

HCG Production During Normal Pregnancy

Human chorionic gonadotropin is a glycoprotein hormone, composed of α and β subunits, similar in structure and function to luteinizing hormone (LH). The HCG α subunit is identical to that in LH, FSH, and TSH, while its β subunit is similar to that of LH (although slightly longer). Production of HCG starts as soon as trophoblastic cells are formed. Blood levels typically rise after implantation (about 4–6 days after fertilization), and become detectably elevated 8–10 days after fertilization (about 3–$3\frac{1}{2}$ weeks after the last menstrual period). Human chorionic gonadotropin rises in geometric fashion during the first trimester of pregnancy (Fig. 17.1), producing different reference ranges for each week of gestation (Table 17.1). In a number of pregnancy abnormalities (such as Down's syndrome and hemolytic diseases), HCG levels are higher than in normal pregnancy.

HCG Tests

Assays for HCG typically use antibodies to the β subunit (termed β-HCG assays). In this chapter, these will be referred to as HCG assays. In normal women, only slight

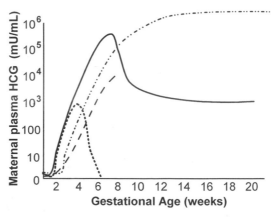

Figure 17.1. HCG Levels in Pregnancy. In normal pregnancy, HCG becomes elevated between one and two weeks after fertilization. Levels double approximately every two days until concentrations reach 2000 mU/mL, then rise more slowly to reach a peak at eight to ten weeks before falling to a plateau. In ectopic pregnancy (dashed line), HCG levels rise more slowly. With fetal death (dotted line), levels rise normally until death, then fall with a half-life of 24 hours. With trophoblastic tumors such as hydatidiform mole (dashed and dotted line), HCG rises more slowly at first, but continues to rise and reaches higher levels than with normal pregnancy.

Table 17.1.
Plasma HCG During Pregnancy

Duration of Pregnancy (from time of ovulation)	Plasma HCG (mU/mL)
1 week	5–50
2 weeks	50–500
3 weeks	100–10,000
4 weeks	1,000–30,000
5 weeks	3,500–115,000
6–8 weeks	12,000–270,000
8–12 weeks	15,000–220,000
20–40 weeks	3,000–15,000

amounts of HCG (less than 5 mU/mL) are present in plasma, although a small percentage of women (1–2%) have "elevated" HCG up to 25 mU/mL (possibly due to interferences from other hormones). The HCG level can be measured in either plasma or urine.

Urine HCG

Assays for HCG in urine are preferred to recognize normal pregnancy. Total urine HCG excretion closely parallels plasma concentration, although urine concentration is dependent both on plasma HCG and relative urine concentration. First morning specimens have less variability in relative concentration and generally higher levels, improving accuracy. Urine tests vary significantly in the amount of HCG needed to produce a positive result. Assays detecting 25 mU/mL recognize pregnancy with 95% sensitivity by one week after the first missed menstrual period. Urine HCG assays may be falsely negative with very dilute urine specimens, and falsely positive in the presence of proteinuria and urinary tract infection. Home pregnancy test kits perform well when tested in laboratory settings, but have high rates of false positive and false negative results when used by inexperienced individuals (the usual situation for these kits). Results should be confirmed in a laboratory if clinical findings are inconsistent with home test results.

Plasma HCG

Plasma HCG levels are used when quantitative information is needed (diagnosing ectopic pregnancy, monitoring trophoblastic tumors, and screening for fetal abnormalities). Plasma HCG levels do not provide additional information in diagnosing routine pregnancy, since they become positive less than one week before urine HCG.

When Not to Do HCG Tests

In general, plasma HCG tests are not needed to diagnose pregnancy. Assays for HCG should not be done before a woman has missed a menstrual period because of low sensitivity. Positive urine HCG may be erroneous in patients with proteinuria, and should be confirmed with plasma HCG, whereas negative results are reliable. Urine HCG should not be used when quantitative results are needed (suspected spontaneous abortion, ectopic pregnancy, or trophoblastic tumor).

HCG Production During Ectopic Pregnancy

Approximately 1.5% of pregnancies occur outside the uterus, usually in the fallopian tube, where they have a high tendency for severe hemorrhage due to spontaneous miscarriage or rupture. Ectopic pregnancy is more common in women with a history of sexually transmitted diseases or previous ectopic pregnancy. Placental tissue grows less well in ectopic sites; plasma HCG therefore rises more slowly than with uterine pregnancy. The rate of plasma HCG rise is used to confirm a clinical suspicion of ectopic pregnancy: before six weeks of gestation, HCG levels will fail to double in two days in 70% of ectopic pregnancies, but only 15% of normal pregnancies. By the time plasma HCG reaches 5000 mU/mL, an intrauterine gestation can be reliably recognized by ultrasound; HCG levels help in interpretation of negative ultrasound examination.

HCG Production During Spontaneous Abortion

An estimated 25% of pregnancies end in spontaneous abortion, many before the woman realizes she is pregnant. Spontaneous abortions are usually preceded by death of placental and fetal tissue, causing declining HCG. Plasma HCG is usually below the 95th percentile for gestational age and characteristically falls in measurements two days apart.

DIAGNOSIS OF FETAL ABNORMALITIES

A relatively small number of pregnancies are associated with major fetal abnormalities. The most important are Down's syndrome, neural tube defects, and hydatidiform mole (Chapter 21). In certain high risk populations, other inherited disorders may be particularly common, particularly in families with common genetic heritage or with previously affected offspring.

Normal Products of the Fetal-Placental Unit

The fetus and placenta produce several substances synthesized in only trace amounts by normal adults. These substances cross the placenta and increase maternal blood levels.

Free β Subunit of HCG

Only small amounts of free β subunit are present during normal pregnancy, with significant increases in abnormal gestations, particularly Down's syndrome. Free β subunit must be ordered specifically; standard HCG assays detect predominantly intact HCG and are insensitive to changes in β subunit levels. In some diseases, particularly hydatidiform mole and other trophoblastic tumors, a significant proportion of free β subunit is partially metabolized ("nicked HCG" and a smaller "β core" fragment). These metabolites are not detected in some HCG assays.

α-Fetoprotein

The fetal liver and yolk sac produce large amounts of α-fetoprotein (AFP), a small protein present in fetal plasma at levels approximately a million times those in adult plasma. A small proportion of AFP reaches amniotic fluid, crosses the placenta, and increases maternal AFP concentration (peak is 25 times normal at 25 weeks gestation;

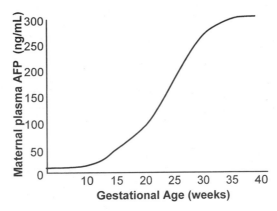

Figure 17.2. AFP Levels in Pregnancy. During normal pregnancy, AFP increases slowly during the first trimester, but then more rapidly, reaching a peak value 25 times normal. Maternal plasma levels are dependent on maternal blood volume, race, and presence of diabetes. Increased leakage into amniotic fluid from fetal skin or renal defects increases maternal levels, as does multiple pregnancy. Low levels occur with fetal abnormalities such as trisomy. With fetal death, levels are usually increased but may be decreased.

increases 4–6 fold at 16–20 weeks, a common time for testing) (Fig. 17.2). Fetal abnormalities causing increased leakage of fetal plasma into amniotic fluid (open neural tube defects, omphalocele, nephrotic syndrome) or reducing clearance from amniotic fluid (esophageal atresia) increase maternal AFP. Fetal production increases with fetal liver mass. Maternal levels are affected by gestational age and the number of infants present. Maternal levels are also affected by maternal blood volume (higher volume causes lower AFP), and are corrected for maternal weight. Finally, there are differences in AFP levels in persons of different ethnic backgrounds (higher in those of African ancestry, lower in those of Asian ancestry when compared to those of European ancestry) and in women with diabetes. Accurate data on all of these parameters must be supplied to the laboratory for proper interpretation of maternal AFP levels. Results are usually expressed as multiples of the median value (MoM) at a particular gestational age.

Estriol

During pregnancy, the most abundant estrogen is estriol, produced in the placenta from precursors synthesized in fetal adrenal and liver. Estriol levels rise gradually during the first two trimesters and more rapidly near term. For many years, estriol in maternal urine or plasma was used as a test of fetal well being, but has largely been abandoned as less reliable than clinical evaluation. Estriol is currently used in screening for fetal abnormalities, particularly chromosomal disorders such as Down's syndrome. The levels are lower than in normal infants. As with AFP, values must be corrected for gestational age.

When Not to Do Testing for Fetal Abnormalities

The main indication for fetal abnormality testing is to allow therapeutic abortion if an abnormality is detected. It follows that testing should not be done if the parents would not consider this as an option. All tests must be interpreted in light of maternal age, weight, race, and gestational age; testing should not be requested unless these values can be provided to the laboratory. α-Fetoprotein may be falsely elevated in women with chronic hepatitis; other tests should be used in this setting.

Specific Fetal Abnormalities and Their Detection

Laboratory tests can screen for common congenital defects and (in those at risk) determine the presence or absence of specific genetic abnormalities.

Neural Tube Defects

Approximately 1 in 1000 pregnancies is associated with defects in fusion of the neural tube, producing neurologic abnormalities such as spina bifida, meningomyelocele, and anencephaly. Risk factors (overt folate deficiency, previous infant with neural tube defect) are present in only a small minority of cases. With open defects, AFP leakage causes increased maternal plasma AFP. α-Fetoprotein screening is performed at 16–18 weeks gestation, with results corrected for maternal weight, race, and diabetes (if present). Values over 2.0 MoM are found in about 90% of open neural tube defects (anencephaly, meningomyelocele), which comprise the vast majority of neural tube defects. Abnormal values are usually followed by ultrasound or measurement of amniotic fluid AFP, both of which are more sensitive and more specific than maternal plasma AFP. Other causes of elevated AFP are discussed above.

Chromosomal Abnormalities

A high percentage of fertilizations result in chromosomally abnormal products. An overwhelming majority of these cause spontaneous abortion, often before the woman realizes she is pregnant. In a small percentage, usually trisomy (an extra copy of one chromosome), an infant with multiple congenital abnormalities is the result. The frequency of trisomy increases with parental age, reaching approximately 1% at age 40. However, 80% of infants with trisomy are born to mothers younger than 35. Chromosomally abnormal fetuses produce lower amounts of AFP and estriol, but higher amounts of free β HCG; measurement of these compounds is commonly used to screen for trisomy. The additional yield from estriol above the other two tests is only slight. An abnormal result on one or more tests detects 60% of chromosomally abnormal infants, with falsely abnormal results in 5–10% of normal pregnancies. Follow-up of abnormal results requires ultrasound and chromosomal analysis of fetal tissues to detect trisomy.

Genetic Diseases

A number of inherited diseases are associated with specific chromosomal or DNA markers. The number is increasing monthly, and a complete listing is far beyond the scope of this book. Inherited defects are usually classified as recessive (disease occurs only if both copies of the gene are abnormal) or dominant (disease occurs if one copy of the gene is abnormal). In recessive diseases, both parents must possess the gene ("carrier state"), but have no clinical evidence of disease. Most dominant diseases occur due to spontaneous mutations or inheritance from an affected parent; fetal testing is usually done only in the latter case.

Testing for genetic disorders is indicated if there is a family history of the disorder, parents are members of an ethnic group with a high incidence of the disease, or a previous infant was affected with the disease. For many recessive diseases, tests on the parents can determine the presence of a carrier state. Hemoglobin electrophoresis or sickle cell preparation detects hemoglobin S (which causes sickle cell disease); plasma hexosaminidase A detects Tay-Sachs disease carriers; and the presence of an abnormal gene can be used for many important disorders, such as cystic fibrosis. If the carrier state is present in both parents, genetic testing of the infant is done by culturing cells from fetal or placental tissue and examining chromosomes or DNA. Cells can be obtained from amniotic fluid at about 16–18 weeks, or by chroionic villus sampling at about 10 weeks. The risk of fetal loss is slightly higher with chorionic villus sampling, and the success rate may be slightly lower.

EVALUATION OF FETAL LUNG MATURITY

A major cause for neonatal mortality is **respiratory distress syndrome (RDS)** of the newborn, often called hyaline membrane disease. This disorder is caused by immaturity of fetal alveolar cells producing surfactant. Without surfactant, the lungs collapse during expiration, preventing normal gas exchange. Production of surfactant indicates fetal lung maturity and correlates strongly with likelihood of survival after birth.

Normal Surfactant Production

Surfactant is a complex mixture of phospholipids and protein. Surfactant is not released to alveoli before about 34–36 weeks of gestation, but can be stimulated by cortisol at earlier ages. The major lipids in surfactant are lecithin (L) and phosphatidylglycerol (PG); other tissues (including other lung cells) produce a relatively constant amount of another lipid, sphingomyelin (S). Before surfactant is produced, the relative amounts of L and S are approximately equal, but the ratio rises rapidly once surfactant is produced, with a value of more than 2:1 indicating lung maturity. While L is the most abundant lipid in surfactant, PG appears more important to surfactant function; in infants of diabetic mothers, RDS often develops in infants with L:S ratio greater than 2:1 but deficient in PG.

Tests for Surfactant Production

Fetuses "breathe" amniotic fluid, so that amniotic fluid reflects alveolar fluid contents. Examination of amniotic fluid lipids or physical properties associated with surfactant are widely used to determine fetal lung maturity. Not all tests produce equivalent results; it is important for the practitioner to understand the relative value of each test. Blood and meconium contain various surfactant lipids. Their presence causes erroneous results in most tests.

Physical Tests for Surfactant Production

The most common bedside screening tests for surfactant use the foam stability test. Ethanol prevents bubbles (foam) from forming in fluid samples, while surfactant allows foam formation. A simple test takes equal volumes of 95% ethanol and amniotic fluid; after mixing by shaking, the presence of foam indicates surfactant presence. Sensitivity for detecting lung maturity is less than with other tests, but falsely mature results are uncommon in uncontaminated specimens (except in infants of diabetic mothers). Contamination with meconium, blood, or vaginal fluid causes falsely mature results. Precise measurement of volumes of ethanol and amniotic fluid are essential, since a lower percentage of ethanol causes falsely mature results while a high percentage causes falsely immature results.

Lecithin/Sphingomyelin Ratio

The L/S ratio is the most widely used laboratory test for determining fetal lung maturity. Phospholipids are separated on a chromatographic plate and the relative amounts of L and S are measured, with L/S ratio reported. As with foam tests, blood and meconium usually cause falsely mature results in immature infants, but rarely produce falsely immature results. Infants of diabetic mothers may also have falsely mature L/S ratios. The test is relatively insensitive for detecting surfactant production; a significant number of infants do not develop RDS despite having low L/S ratio.

Phosphatidylglycerol

Phosphatidylglycerol is produced almost exclusively in surfactant, making it the most sensitive and specific test for fetal lung maturity. Most commonly, PG is identified by chromatography along with L/S ratio. Phosphatidylglycerol can also be determined by a slide immunoassay, which is slightly less sensitive than chromatography but much easier to perform. Levels of PG are not affected by blood or meconium, and produce reliable results in infants of diabetic mothers. As with the L/S ratio, many infants without evidence of respiratory distress syndrome have a falsely immature PG.

When Not to Do Tests of Surfactant Production

Meconium and blood produce falsely mature results for most tests; pigmented fluids should only be tested for PG. Both PG and the L/S ratio are relatively reliable in the presence of vaginal fluid. Foam stability tests should not be used if there is a clinical suspicion of rupture of the membranes. The L/S ratio and foam tests are falsely mature in infants of diabetic mothers; PG should be used in diabetic women.

EVALUATION OF POSSIBLE HEMOLYTIC DISEASE OF THE NEWBORN

Half of all antigens in a fetus come from the father, potentially able to stimulate maternal immune response that may damage fetal tissues. The most common immune damage occurs with antibodies to fetal red blood cells, causing hemolytic disease of the newborn (HDN). In severe cases, this produces severe fetal anemia and congestive heart failure, termed **erythroblastosis (hydrops) fetalis.** With milder damage, anemia is present at birth, and continued hemolysis after birth causes increased unconjugated bilirubin. At high levels, bilirubin may accumulate in the brain and cause damage (**kernicterus**). Hemolytic disease of the newborn occurs when the mother lacks an antigen present in the fetus. Fetal red cells then trigger an immune response when they reach the mother's circulation. Large numbers of fetal red cells cross the placenta at delivery, while smaller numbers reach maternal blood earlier in pregnancy, especially if uterine bleeding occurs. Antibodies usually form after delivery, and typically affect second and subsequent pregnancies, rarely causing a problem for the first infant. Less commonly, women develop antibodies when exposed to antigens by previous abortion, blood transfusions, or natural exposure (as with A and B antigens). In these situations, even a first-born infant may be affected. IgM antibodies do not cross the placenta, and so cannot cause HDN. IgG antibodies cross the placenta and may cause HDN if the infant's red cells contain the antigen. Determining the likelihood of fetal antigen expression is usually based on determining the father's phenotype. If the father is homozygous (has two copies) of the antigen, the infant will always possess the antigen and HDN is likely; if he is heterozygous (has one copy), the risk of an affected infant is 50%. For some antigens, detection of antigen presence can be made by chorionic villus sampling, especially for the D (Rh) antigen. In questionable cases, fetal blood can be obtained from the umbilical vein under ultrasound guidance. This approach also allows determination of fetal hematocrit and can detect direct evidence of severity of HDN.

Screening for Risk of HDN

Screening does not detect the most common cause of HDN, IgG antibodies to A and B blood group antigens occurring in group O women. ABO HDN is usually mild and rarely requires treatment. The most important type of antibody is anti-D (Rh), occurring in Rh negative women; development of anti-D can be prevented in most cases (see below). Less commonly, antibodies develop to other red cell antigens. The most common method to screen for risk of HDN is a maternal antibody screen at the time of initial visit. If the initial screen is negative, it is usually repeated at 24–28 weeks. If the initial screen is positive, repeat testing is done at 12 and 20 weeks; if the antibody titer is low (less than 1:16) and remains stable, the likelihood of HDN is low and many practitioners do not perform further testing. A high or rising titer strongly suggests HDN is present.

Management of Increasing or High Titer IgG Antibodies

If maternal antibody titers indicate high risk of HDN, monitoring for hemolysis is usually begun at 20–24 weeks by measuring amniotic fluid bilirubin. (Direct sampling of fetal blood is used in only a few centers and is not discussed further.) During normal pregnancy, bilirubin gradually decreases in amniotic fluid; increases are usually due to hemolysis. Amniotic fluid bilirubin cannot be measured in the same way as in plasma, rather, absorbance of light at 450 nm (Δ OD_{450}) is used to estimate concentration. Because meconium (fetal stool) and hemoglobin also absorb light at 450 nm, these may give erroneous results. Results are interpreted based on a nomogram developed by Liley (Fig. 17.3).

Management of Antibody-Negative Rh Negative Women

If an antibody screen is negative at 24–28 weeks, an injection of 300 mg of anti-D antibody (RhoGam) is given to the mother to prevent antibody development. This injection is repeated at delivery if the baby is Rh positive, with the amount increased based on number of fetal red cells in the mother's circulation. These can be identified by treating a blood sample with acid, which elutes most hemoglobin (but not fetal hemoglobin). This method has sometimes been called the **Kleihauer-Betke test.** If the volume of fetal red cells is over 15 mL, an extra 300 mg of anti-D is used for each fraction of 15 mL above this amount. Additional anti-D should be given to the mother at the time of amniocentesis or whenever there is uterine bleeding.

Detection and Monitoring of HDN at Birth

At delivery, fetal red cells from umbilical cord blood are tested for surface antibody by the **direct antiglobulin (Coombs') test (DAT).** Anti-human IgG is incubated with the

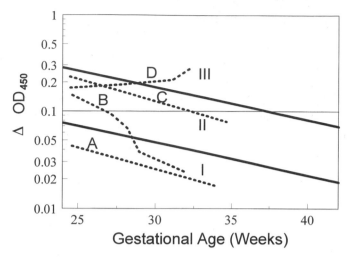

Figure 17.3. Amniotic Fluid Bilirubin for HDN. Bilirubin is measured by measuring light absorbance (ΔOD_{450}); results normally decline during pregnancy. The lower solid line indicates normal values (Zone I); the upper solid line distinguishes moderately (Zone II) from severely (Zone III) affected infants. Curve **A** represents results from an unaffected infant. Curve **B** indicates initially high bilirubin, but with a subsequent fall; HDN is not likely to be present. Curve **C** represents a moderately affected infant who may need treatment after birth. The increasing values in Curve **D** indicate a severely affected infant who requires treatment. Very immature infants receive intrauterine transfusions, while mature infants may be delivered and are treated after birth as indicated.

infant's red cells, with cell agglutination indicating an antibody coating. If DAT is negative, there is no evidence of HDN. A positive DAT is followed by an eluate test, in which antibody is removed from red cells and tested to determine which antigen it is attacking. Infants with positive DAT are usually monitored by frequent measurement of plasma bilirubin and hematocrit to detect significance of hemolysis and need for treatment; details of therapy are beyond the scope of this book. Total bilirubin over 9 mg/dL (154 μmol/L) in premature infants or over 18 mg/dL (310 μmol/L) in term infants is usually used as an indication for treatment. Over 90% of cases of ABO HDN require no treatment; a much higher percentage of HDN due to other antibodies requires therapy. Infants with other antibodies are usually followed more carefully than ABO HDN infants.

CHAPTER 18

Principles of Therapeutic Drug Monitoring

D. ROBERT DUFOUR

THERAPEUTIC DRUG MONITORING

Measurement and interpretation of body fluid levels of therapeutic drugs, termed therapeutic drug monitoring (TDM), is performed to assure adequacy of treatment and prevent toxicity. This assumes a direct linear relationship between drug concentration and drug effects (both therapeutic and toxic), an assumption which is not always correct. Several factors affect interpretation of drug levels.

Free Versus Total Drug Levels

Most assays measure total drug concentration, both free and protein bound (Table 18.1). The major proteins binding drugs are albumin and orosomucoid; the factors affecting these proteins' levels are discussed in Chapter 9. For most drugs, only the free fraction binds to receptors and produces effects. With low amounts of binding proteins, the total drug level drops while free drug concentration increases. Total drug assays must be interpreted with caution in patients with abnormal amounts of binding proteins. In some laboratories, assays for free drug are available. Salivary drug concentration is essentially equal to plasma free drug concentration, and no venipuncture is required (a particular advantage in children).

Dose-Response Curves

For most drugs, therapeutic effect is related to drug concentration over a limited range (Fig. 18.1). Concentrations below a threshold value are ineffective, while high concentrations produce no additional effect. Rarely, as with some antidepressants, the effect increases up to a certain point, after which further increases in concentration cause a lesser response. With such drugs, determination of concentration is essential for evaluating patients with poor drug effects.

Other Factors Altering Drug Effects

Some drugs alter metabolism to exert their effect, which is then related to cumulative drug effects rather than to concentration. Warfarin inhibits a vitamin K dependent enzyme, altering calcium binding by coagulation factors and inhibiting clot formation. Clotting proteins have varying half-lives, causing delay in onset of warfarin's effect, while anticoagulation persists after warfarin is discontinued. Digoxin's effect is related to plasma potassium and magnesium concentrations; a level producing therapeutic effects in a normal patient may be toxic with hypokalemia or ineffective with hyperka-

Table 18.1.
Protein Binding of Various Drugs

Highly bound (>75%):
  Carbamazepine, cyclosporine, phenytoin, quinidine, salicylate, valproic acid
Moderately bound (25–75%)
  Acetaminophen, caffeine, digoxin, lidocaine, phenobarbital, theophylline, vancomycin
Essentially unbound (<25%)
  Amikacin, gentamycin, lithium, procainamide, tobramycin, tricyclic antidepressants

lemia. Valproic acid alters γ-aminobutyric acid levels in the brain, delaying onset of drug action.

Drug Metabolites

For many drugs, some metabolites contribute to therapeutic effects which may be greater, lesser, or different than with the parent drug. Therapeutic monitoring should measure all active metabolites, but no inactive ones. The antiepileptic drug mysoline is metabolized to phenobarbital, another antiepileptic drug with differing therapeutic effects. Procainamide is metabolized to N-acetyl procainamide; while both are antiarrhythmics, their mechanism of action and potency differ. Cyclosporine has multiple metabolites; assays using a polyclonal antibody (measuring parent drug and several metabolites) show better correlation with in vitro immunosuppressant activity than those which measure cyclosporine alone. Digoxin is metabolized to a number of inactive products which cross-react in many assays.

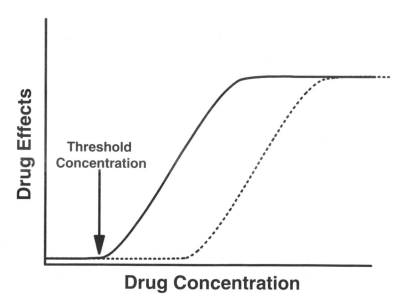

Figure 18.1. Relationship of Drug Concentration to Drug Effects. At low concentration, many drugs have no effects. Once the level increases above a threshold, therapeutic effects (solid line) increase up to a given concentration, when any further increase in level produces no additional therapeutic effect. Toxic effects (dotted line) also illustrate the same threshold and plateau as the therapeutic effects. The ratio of average toxic to average therapeutic effect is termed the therapeutic index.

Drug Toxicity

Adverse reactions to drugs are relatively common, and occur from two basic mechanisms.

Dose Related Toxicity

For most drugs, toxic effects are directly related to drug concentration. The therapeutic index is the ratio of average toxic dose to average therapeutic dose. For drugs with a large therapeutic index, drug monitoring is not needed to prevent toxicity, and therapeutic monitoring is seldom performed. Most drugs discussed in this chapter have a low therapeutic index.

Idiosyncratic Reactions

With some drugs, adverse effects develop from an immunologic reaction to the drug, abnormal metabolic pathways, or interaction between two different medications. In such cases, drug levels may provide no clue to toxicity. Monitoring the status of organs affected allows detection of toxicity, such as measurement of AST or ALT to detect early isoniazid (INH) toxicity.

PHARMACOKINETICS

Study of drug handling and excretion underlies the use of drug levels to adjust therapy. While standard references recommend drug dosages and frequency of administration, these represent average values and may lead to overdosage or undertreatment with individual variation in two key parameters, volume of distribution and clearance. Use of individual pharmacokinetic information helps optimize patient therapy, as will be discussed later in the chapter.

Absorption and Distribution

After a drug is ingested, it must reach the bloodstream to have an effect. For oral drugs, a variable fraction is absorbed (bioavailability). After absorption, the drug reaches an equilibrium with tissue receptors or cells (distribution). For most drugs, distribution occurs in a few minutes; however, for some drugs, such as digoxin, it is not complete for 6–8 hours (even after intravenous administration). A sample of blood obtained before distribution is complete has a higher drug concentration than at equilibrium. With digoxin, 98% of the drug is receptor-bound at equilibrium. Samples drawn too soon after ingestion are the most common cause of "toxic" digoxin levels.

Volume of Distribution

The apparent volume in which drug is dissolved when distribution is complete is termed the volume of distribution (V_d). For some drugs, V_d corresponds to an actual fluid compartment, such as total body water, plasma, or extracellular fluid. Lipid soluble or receptor bound drugs have a very large V_d. Most textbooks assume V_d is nearly constant between individuals, although in practice, V_d is quite variable. V_d can be calculated by measuring the concentration (C) of the drug before an intravenous dose and again after distribution is complete (Eq. 18.1).

$$V_d = \frac{Dose}{C_{after} - C_{before}} \qquad (1)$$

Clearance

The rate at which a drug is removed by renal excretion and/or liver metabolism is termed clearance (Chapter 6). Most drugs are cleared by first order kinetics, with the rate of drug removal directly related to drug concentration. A rate constant (K_d) describes the fractional clearance of drug per unit time (Eq. 18.2)

$$C_t = C_0 \times e^{-K_d \times t} \qquad (2a)$$

$$\frac{C_t}{C_0} = e^{-K_d \times t} \qquad (2b)$$

(C_0: drug concentration at its maximum (time 0), C_t: drug concentration at time t after administration).

With first order kinetics, concentration falls by a constant fraction (fractional clearance) in a given time, t. If C_t is one-half of C_0, the time interval t is termed the half-life (symbolized $T_{1/2}$). By using this equation, it is possible to predict the fraction that drug concentration will fall in any specific time interval. For drugs that are metabolized or secreted, processes become saturated and a maximum rate of clearance occurs (zero order kinetics); at this point, a specific amount of drug is cleared in a given time. Any drug administered above this amount accumulates, leading to progressively increasing concentrations and frequent toxicity. Zero order kinetics are commonly observed for phenytoin, salicylates, ethanol, and occasionally for theophylline. With first order kinetics, it is possible to predict changes in drug levels with changes in therapy; with zero order kinetics, it is impossible to make such predictions, and changes in therapy often lead to toxicity or undertreatment.

Steady State

At steady state, drug levels are the same after every dose. Concentrations are at 88% of steady state at three half-lives and 98% of steady state after five half-lives. Levels are reasonably accurate after three to five half-lives. It is important to note that steady state is based on the number of half-lives that have passed, not doses. Many drugs are administered at intervals other than one half-life. If the aim of treatment is to maintain stable levels, small doses are given at intervals shorter than $T_{1/2}$. When the recovery of cells is needed (antibiotics, antineoplastic agents), large doses are administered at intervals greater than $T_{1/2}$, giving markedly different levels just after drug distribution is complete (peak) and just before the next dose (trough).

USE OF DRUG LEVELS TO SELECT OR ADJUST DOSAGE

Using pharmacokinetic principles, treatment can be modified based on measured levels. Figure 18.2 illustrates the effects of dosing interval and route of administration on drug levels. For drugs administered as a sustained release oral preparation, by continuous intravenous infusion, or at intervals very short relative to the drug's $T_{1/2}$, timing of collection is not critical since levels fluctuate little. For drugs administered at intervals near $T_{1/2}$, levels are drawn just before the next scheduled dose. This may either represent the lowest level (trough) or an average value, depending on the route

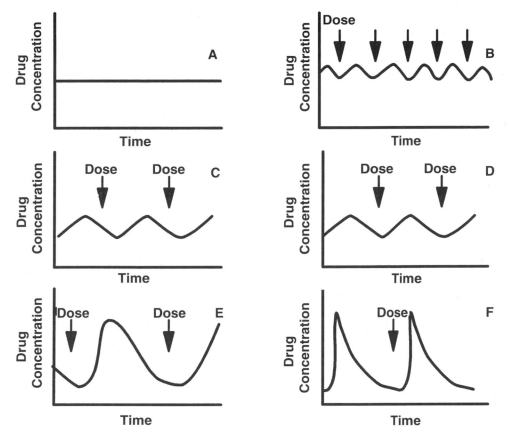

Figure 18.2. Effects of Route of Administration, Rate of Absorption, and Relation to $T_{1/2}$ on Drug Levels. (**A**) Continuous infusion or sustained release oral preparations show stable levels: sampling at any time provides equal results. (**B**) Short dosing interval compared to $T_{1/2}$ (e.g., thyroid hormone): levels rise slightly after a dose but show little fluctuation between doses. (**C**) Interval equal to $T_{1/2}$, slow absorption: levels fall for a short period after drug ingestion before rising, specimens obtained just before dose are average for dosing interval. (**D**) Interval equal to $T_{1/2}$, fast absorption: Similar to (**C**), but levels are near minimum just before the next dose. (**E**) Interval greater than $T_{1/2}$, slow absorption: drugs administered orally or intramuscularly may be absorbed slowly, with "trough" levels occurring some time after the drug is administered. (**F**) Interval greater than $T_{1/2}$, fast absorption: for drugs such as antibiotics given intravenously, there are marked differences between peak and trough levels, although the peak and trough occur when expected.

of administration and rate of absorption. For drugs administered at intervals greater than $T_{1/2}$, it is common to obtain both peak and trough levels.

Selecting Initial Dosage and Interval

Using data for the average volume of distribution in Table 18.2, the initial dosage needed to produce a therapeutic level can be estimated using Equation 18.3.

$$Dose = \frac{V_d \times Weight}{Desired\ Concentration} \qquad (3)$$

The interval between doses is adjusted for known differences in renal or hepatic function. While it is usually not possible to predict directly how liver metabolic functions

Table 18.2.
Average Pharmacokinetic Data for Commonly Monitored Drugs

Drug	Protein Binding (%)	Distribution Volume (L/kg)	Half-life (hrs)	Route of Clearance
Amikacin	<25	0.25	2–3	Renal
Caffeine	50	0.5	3–6; 48 in premature infants	Hepatic
Carbamazepine	75	0.8–1	10–30	Hepatic
Cyclosporine	90	4		Hepatic
Digoxin	25	7	36	Renal
Gentamicin, Tobramycin	<25	0.25	2.5	Renal
Lidocaine	50–60	0.5	1.5	Hepatic
Lithium	0	0.8	24	Renal
Methotrexate	35–45	0.75	8	Renal
Phenobarbital	50	0.7	50–150	Hepatic
Phenytoin	90	0.7	20	Hepatic
Primidone	<25	0.8	8–14	Hepatic[a]
Procainamide	0	2	2.5–5	Renal, Hepatic[b]
Quinidine	75	2–3	6–7	Hepatic, Renal
Salicylates	80–90	0.15–0.2	2–3	Hepatic, Renal
Theophylline	50	0.5	3–10	Hepatic
Tricyclics	15–25	10–30	24–48	Hepatic
Valproic acid	90	0.25	10–12	Hepatic
Vancomycin	50	0.75–1	3–4	Renal

[a] Metabolized to phenobarbital, which should also be measured

[b] Metabolized to N-acetylprocainamide (NAPA), which should also be measured

are affected by liver disease, the most important abnormality affecting drug clearance is blood flow. Patients with portal hypertension usually have retarded metabolism and prolonged half-lives of liver metabolized drugs. Renal clearance can be estimated readily for most drugs using estimated creatinine clearance (Eq. 18.4).

$$Estimated \ C_{Cr} = \frac{(140 - Age \ (yrs)) \times Wt \ (kg)}{72 \times Serum \ Creatinine \ (mg/dL)} \tag{4}$$

For adult women, the estimated clearance is multiplied by 0.85.

The dosing interval should be adjusted using estimated clearance (Eq. 18.5).

$$Interval = Normal \ Interval \times \frac{125}{Estimated \ Clearance} \tag{5}$$

Monitoring Therapy

Once a drug is begun, levels should be checked after three to five half-lives (estimated as discussed above). If the values are within the therapeutic range, dosage and interval are continued. If the function of organs involved in clearance changes, repeat drug levels should be obtained. Any change in volume status or clinical evidence of under-treatment or toxicity is cause for repeating drug levels. If the patient is clinically stable, there is no need to repeat drug levels frequently.

Modifying Therapy with Single Levels

As mentioned above, for drugs given at intervals equal to or less than $T_{1/2}$, single levels can be used to adjust therapy. The change in dosage is based on the percentage change

Table 18.3.
Effects of Change in Dose and Interval on Pharmacokinetic Parameters

Dose	Interval	Peak	Trough	Increment	Fractional Clearance
↑	same	↑	↑ by less than peak	↑	same
↓	same	↓	↓ by less than peak	↓	same
same	↑	↓	↓ by same amt. as peak	same	↑
same	↓	↑	↑ by same amt. as peak	same	↓
↑	↑	↑	↓	↑	↑
↑	↓	↑	↑ by less than peak	↑	↓
↓	↑	↓	↓ by less than peak	↓	↑
↓	↓	↓	↑	↓	↓

needed to reach therapeutic levels. For example, if the level is 50% of the desired therapeutic concentration, then the dosage is doubled, and as a result the concentration should also double. Levels can be verified after three to five half-lives on the new dosage. For drugs subject to zero order kinetics, changes in dosage should be checked sooner. At one half-life after changing the dose, the drug level should be 50% of the difference between old and target concentrations. For example, if the phenytoin level was 10 mg/L on 200 mg per day, an increase in dosage to 300 mg per day should increase levels to 15 mg/L. Normal phenytoin $T_{1/2}$ is one day; levels one day after a change in dose should be approximately 12.5 mg/L. Significantly higher levels indicate zero order kinetics, and the dose should be reduced to initial therapy. Unfortunately, levels cannot be used to calculate dosage when zero order kinetics are present.

Modifying Therapy with Peak and Trough Levels

When a drug is given at intervals much greater than $T_{1/2}$, it is often necessary to adjust both the dose and the interval to achieve therapeutic levels for both peak and trough. Table 18.3 illustrates, in general, effects that changing the dose or interval have on peak, trough, increment, and fractional clearance of a drug. Pharmacokinetic rules predict the proper dose and frequency needed to achieve therapeutic concentrations (Fig. 18.3).

MONITORING OF SPECIFIC DRUGS

Drugs for which therapeutic monitoring is commonly performed are listed in Table 18.2. In addition to pharmacokinetics, some drugs require special consideration. These are discussed in this section.

Salicylates (Aspirin)

Though the most widely used nonsteroidal anti-inflammatory agents, use of salicylates has decreased as other nonsteroidal anti-inflammatory agents have decreased in cost. Renal salicylate clearance by tubular secretion is affected by urine pH (increased by alkaline urine), and is subject to saturation at plasma levels slightly above therapeutic range, producing zero order kinetics. Toxicity is relatively common with high dose therapy. The therapeutic range is 15–30 mg/dL. Mild toxic symptoms (tinnitus, dizziness, sweating, nausea, and vomiting) begin at concentrations greater than 30 mg/dL, with severe toxicity (central nervous system effects ranging from irrationality and

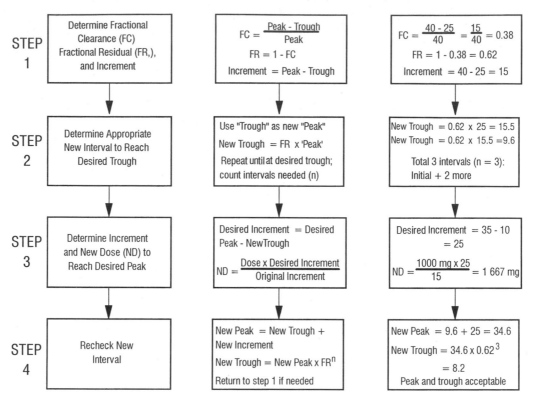

Figure 18.3. Using Peak and Trough Levels to Modify Treatment. The first column indicates the parameters which must be calculated, the second column lists the formulas, and the third column illustrates with an example from a patient receiving 1000 mg vancomycin every 12 hours. The therapeutic peak is typically 30–40 mg/mL, and the therapeutic trough is 5–10 mg/mL. Using pharmacokinetic principles, the increment predicts constant rises expected after each equal dosage. Fractional clearance predicts the fraction of drug removed in each equal interval. Using these parameters, it is possible to quickly calculate the appropriate dosage and interval needed to achieve therapeutic levels. While the calculation indicates precise values, it is usually adequate to approximate. For example, the fractional clearance is approximately 0.4, the trough is approximately 10, etc. Use of this approach simplifies changes in therapy.

confusion to convulsions and coma) occurring at concentrations above 50 mg/dL. Salicylates increase respiratory rate, causing respiratory alkalosis and, at high levels, increased anion gap metabolic acidosis. In children younger than four years, metabolic acidosis usually predominates, but in adults respiratory alkalosis or a mixed picture is present. The degree of salicylate toxicity correlates with peak concentration and rate of decline.

Digoxin

Cardiac glycosides such as digoxin are widely used in treatment of congestive heart failure and cardiac arrhythmias. It is difficult to establish a therapeutic range for digoxin, as its response is increased by hypokalemia and hypomagnesemia, and decreased by increased concentrations of these electrolytes. Distribution to tissues occurs slowly over 6–8 hours, even after intravenous dosage, with most digoxin (98%) bound to cardiac and skeletal muscle receptors at equilibrium. Levels drawn before equilibrium will be falsely elevated. To prevent misleading results, many hospitals administer digoxin at bed time (levels are usually drawn in mornings). Several other factors affect digoxin levels and effects. Quinidine displaces digoxin from receptors in skeletal muscle and retards digoxin clearance, increasing plasma levels 2–3 fold. Digoxin metabolites or naturally occurring digoxin-like substances (DLIF, digoxin-like immunoreactive factors) cross-react in digoxin assays. These inactive products are increased in the serum of patients with renal or hepatic insufficiency, in pregnancy, and in newborn infants, causing falsely increased levels. Digibind (antidigoxin Fab fragments) is used to treat digoxin toxicity by binding digoxin and displacing it from cell receptors. After digibind, total plasma digoxin is very high, but free and receptor bound digoxin are low and digoxin effects are reversed. Most digoxin assays are unreliable in patients given digibind, sometimes giving markedly elevated levels and sometimes reporting undetectable digoxin. The average $T_{1/2}$ for clearance of digibind–digoxin complexes is about 18 hours with normal renal function; however, clearance is markedly retarded in renal insufficiency.

Lidocaine

The therapeutic range for lidocaine is 1.5–5.0 mg/L with toxic symptoms (neurologic dysfunction, seizures, and bradycardia) occurring with concentrations above 9.0 mg/L. Lidocaine is significantly bound to orosomucoid. The increased orosomucoid in acute inflammation causes higher plasma levels but lowers the therapeutic effect. Liver clearance is highly dependent on hepatic blood flow; hypotension significantly retards clearance and produces rapid increases in concentration. Frequent monitoring of lidocaine levels in patients with shock is needed to prevent toxicity.

Theophylline

Use of theophylline and other methylxanthines for treatment of obstructive lung disease has declined recently. Liver clearance is accelerated by tobacco, while cirrhosis decreases clearance. Zero order kinetics occasionally are observed at concentrations in the mildly toxic range. Distribution is not complete for approximately 30 minutes after an intravenous bolus. Oral doses are absorbed slowly, and peak levels occur 2–4 hours after ingestion. Levels should be drawn just before the next dose, whether oral or intravenous. Caffeine is used in neonatal apnea; in neonates, about 25% of theophylline is converted to caffeine. Therapeutic values are similar to those for theophylline, with a usual upper therapeutic limit of 25 mg/L. Zero order kinetics may develop at concentrations near the upper limit of the therapeutic range.

Phenytoin

The pharmacokinetics of phenytoin depend on the formulation. With the Dilantin brand, absorption is gradual over approximately 24 hours, but many generic forms and oral suspensions have rapid absorption, causing fluctuating plasma levels. Drugs which stimulate or compete with microsomal enzymes lower or raise the $T_{1/2}$, respectively. Phenytoin is commonly associated with toxicity because zero order kinetics may occur at therapeutic levels. Plasma levels can be measured anytime after steady-state is reached, 4–6 days after starting oral therapy and 0.5–4 hours after intravenous therapy begins. If a change in dosage is begun, checking levels after 24 h, as outlined above, is useful for detection of zero order kinetics.

Primidone

A member of the barbiturate family, primidone is commonly used as an antiepileptic drug, particularly in children. Primidone is metabolized in the liver to phenobarbital, responsible for at least some antiepileptic activity. Phenobarbital's $T_{1/2}$ is 50–150 hours, much longer than that of primidone (8–14 hours). Other drugs increase conversion of primidone to phenobarbital, most notably phenobarbital itself, phenytoin, and carbamazepine. In monitoring patients, measuring levels of both active drugs is important, and may provide a clue to compliance with medication: normal primidone concentration but low phenobarbital concentration is indicative of recent resumption of therapy after a long period of nonuse.

Methotrexate

The potent folic acid antagonist methotrexate is used in treatment of malignant tumors, serious autoimmune diseases, and psoriasis. Other organic acids such as salicylate interfere with renal excretion and lead to delayed clearance and increased levels. After high dose therapy with leucovorin rescue, methotrexate levels greater than 5 μmol/L at 24 h, 0.5 μmol/L at 48 h, or 0.05 μmol/L at 72 h indicate toxicity is likely unless additional leucovorin is administered.

Cyclosporine

The immunosuppressant cyclosporine is used after organ transplantation and in a growing number of other diseases. Cyclosporine is metabolized by the liver to multiple breakdown products, most of which are eventually extracted into bile but some of which are excreted in urine. Cyclosporine is found in both red cells and in plasma in roughly equal proportions at body temperatures. However, as sample temperature falls, cyclosporine tends to shift into red cells, so most laboratories measure whole blood cyclosporine to minimize these artifacts. The major factor limiting cyclosporine use is renal tubular damage, but liver and CNS toxicity may also occur. Drugs increasing clearance include those inducing microsomal enzymes such as phenytoin. It is difficult to determine which metabolites are important in monitoring efficacy and toxicity. As mentioned earlier, polyclonal immunoassays may correlate better with immunosuppressive effect than assays which measure cyclosporine only. Assays measuring cyclosporine and metabolites have therapeutic trough levels of 250–800 ng/mL, while assays specific for cyclosporine have therapeutic ranges of 100–150 ng/mL. Different therapeutic ranges are used for different organ transplants and different times following transplantation.

CHAPTER 19

Toxicology

D. ROBERT DUFOUR

LABORATORY EVALUATION OF SUSPECTED TOXICITY

A wide variety of compounds cause damage (toxicity) to various organ systems when present in excess. For many compounds, even small amounts produce injury: these are termed classic toxins or poisons. Many laboratory assays measure only their presence or absence, although an assessment of severity of toxicity requires quantitative levels. For other compounds, there is a therapeutic effect at low concentrations, while toxicity occurs at higher concentrations. These agents are more fully discussed in Chapter 18. For therapeutic agents, laboratory tests must measure concentration to determine whether symptoms are due to drug toxicity, since qualitative tests (only determining drug presence) could indicate therapeutic as well as toxic amounts of drug. A third major class is that of illegal and abused drugs, where drug presence is considered abnormal. For these agents, quantitative assays are not needed. A number of important points must be considered when testing patients suspected of drug toxicity.

"Complete Drug Screens" Do Not Exist

In many laboratories, a "drug screen" or "comprehensive drug screen" is available. These screens typically test for the presence of organic compounds often associated with overdosage or toxicity, such as therapeutic drugs and drugs of abuse. A number of important toxins are not detected in such drug screens, including heavy metals, iron, carbon monoxide, cyanide, ethylene glycol, and organophosphates. In addition, since these tests detect only the presence of compounds, they are not useful in searching for overdosage of therapeutic drugs prescribed to or taken by a patient (and, in fact, some important therapeutic drugs are not detected with standard drug screens, including digoxin, lithium, and oral hypoglycemic agents). Careful communication between the practitioner and the laboratory is essential to assure that proper testing is performed. Practitioners should also become familiar with the types of drugs routinely detected (or not detected) by the laboratory's "drug screen."

Type of Fluid to Test

The proper type of fluid for testing depends on a number of factors. Timing of ingestion relative to testing affects the ability to detect drug ingestion. In the first few hours after ingestion, gastric fluid is the most reliable source for determining the presence of a potentially toxic substance. For many compounds (e.g. heroin, cocaine), blood levels are elevated for only a short period of time; urine testing is better if ingestion occurred more than a few hours before presentation. For other compounds (e.g. lead, carbon monoxide), urine excretion is minimal, and blood is most appropriate for testing. When quantitative results are needed, especially with therapeutic drugs, blood is the only suitable fluid.

Table 19.1.
Patterns of Toxicity with Poisoning

Clinical Pattern	Symptoms	Typical Toxins
Sedative-hypnotic	Lethargy/coma, decreased reflexes, hypotension, depressed respiration	Barbiturates, benzodiazepines, ethanol and other alcohols, chloral hydrate
Anticholinergic	Dry skin, fever, thirst, dilated pupils, difficulty swallowing, urinary retention	Phenothiazines, tricyclic antidepressants, antihistamines, jimsonweed
Cholinergic	Sweating, lacrimation, salivation, diarrhea, constricted pupils, productive cough, vomiting	Organophosphates, pilocarpine
Sympathomimetic	Agitation, tremor, tachycardia, hypertension, sweating, dilated pupils	Amphetamines, cocaine, phencyclidine, LSD, theophylline, nonprescription sympathomimetics (ephedrine, phenylpropanolamine)
Narcotic	CNS depression, bradycardia, seizures, pulmonary edema, pinpoint pupils	Opiates, propoxyphene, pentazocine

Reliability of Drug Screens in Detecting Unsuspected Drug Ingestion

Many practitioners routinely order drug screens to evaluate patients with neurological symptoms such as confusion, coma, or delirium. Numerous studies have shown that drug screens are almost never positive in patients who do not have a defined history of exposure to these agents, with the exception of illegal drugs. As already mentioned, generic "drug screens" would provide no useful information when searching for an overdosage of a drug prescribed for the patient, such as tricyclic antidepressants. In such situations, it is much more important to request quantitative blood levels of the drug most likely to cause the clinical findings than to perform urine drug screens.

CLINICAL PATTERNS OF TOXICITY

A limited number of patterns of clinical findings occur with many types of drug overdoses (Table 19.1). Recognition of these patterns can serve to narrow the scope of drug screening and direct quantitative plasma levels when needed.

SPECIFIC TOXIC AGENTS OF IMPORTANCE

This section discusses the most important drugs associated with clinical toxicity in alphabetical order. Toxicity due to salicylates and to therapeutic drugs is discussed in Chapter 18.

Acetaminophen

While widely used safely, acetaminophen produces toxicity when taken in amounts that exceed liver metabolic capacity (Fig. 19.1). Details on the pattern of liver toxicity are discussed in Chapter 11. Renal toxicity is also common, producing acute tubular necrosis. It is important to recognize toxic plasma acetaminophen levels to detect patients who may benefit from acetylcysteine treatment. Levels should ideally be drawn 4 hours after ingestion; values greater than 150 μg/mL (993 μmol/L) indicate likely toxicity if untreated. Levels can be interpreted from the Rumack nomogram (Fig.

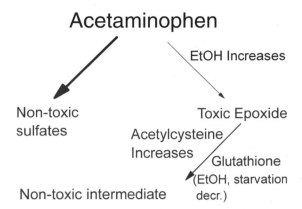

Figure 19.1. Metabolism of Acetaminophen. Normally, most acetaminophen is conjugated to water soluble compounds and excreted in urine. A small fraction is metabolized to a toxic intermediate which is inactivated by glutathione. Alcohol and starvation deplete glutathione stores, while alcohol increases the rate of production of the toxic intermediate. In normal individuals, the average toxic dose is 15 grams, while in starvation and alcohol abuse toxicity may be seen with less than 4 grams. Acetylcysteine regenerates glutathione and is the major antidote to acetaminophen toxicity.

19.2) at any time in the first 24 hours. Patients who have ingested sustained release acetaminophen should have levels measured several times in the first few hours of observation, since peak levels may not occur at the same times as with standard preparations.

Alcohols

Ethanol Abuse

Ethanol is the most common compound producing toxicity, with the linkage between alcohol abuse and various types of accidents and organ damage is well known. Blood alcohol values correlate with patterns of toxicity (Table 19.2), although values are much higher in alcohol addicts for any given clinical pattern. Alcohol metabolic capacity is limited, and usually follows zero order kinetics (Chapter 18), with alcohol concentration falling by about 18 mg/dL per hour.

Detection of Chronic Ethanol Abuse

Laboratory tests to detect chronic ethanol abuse have, in general, not been very successful. The most widely touted are γ-glutamyl transferase (GGT) and mean corpuscular volume (MCV) of red cells, where high levels are associated with abuse. Most studies have shown these tests to detect only about 60–70% of patients with ethanol abuse, while specificity is relatively poor. A number of more esoteric tests correlate more closely with ethanol ingestion; the most reliable is carbohydrate-deficient transferrin (CDT). This test is not widely available in North America.

Ingestion of Other Alcohols

Other alcohols are less commonly used, but typically are intentionally ingested as overdoses; fatality in untreated cases is high. A useful screen for ingestion of ethylene glycol

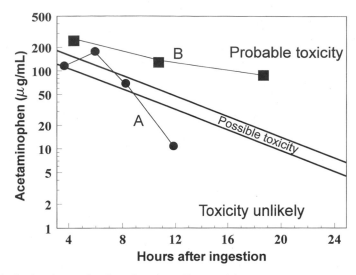

Figure 19.2. Monitoring Acetaminophen Overdose. The need for treatment is based on acetaminophen levels interpreted using the Rumack nomogram. Another way to interpret results is to estimate $T_{1/2}$ by measuring levels 4 hours apart. Normally, $T_{1/2}$ is less than 4 hours. If the acetaminophen level fails to fall by half in this time, toxicity is likely. Care must be taken in evaluating levels in patients who have taken sustained release forms of acetaminophen (curve **A**), where peaks occur later and do not have the same significance. In curve **B,** very delayed clearance is observed and the patient developed hepatic injury (peak AST 25,000 U/L).

(found in antifreeze), isopropanol (rubbing alcohol), or methanol (wood alcohol, brake fluids) is to measure osmolality and calculate the osmotic gap (Chapter 4). Ethylene glycol and methanol are metabolized to more toxic acid byproducts, producing metabolic acidosis with increased anion gap. Isopropanol is metabolized to acetone, which causes ketosis but not acidosis. In addition to being useful for detecting the presence of these toxins, osmotic gap can be used to monitor treatment; the aim is to reduce levels to zero, which would eliminate the osmotic gap. Osmotic gap can be converted to concentration in mg/dL by multiplying by the appropriate factor (methanol 3.2, ethylene glycol 6.4, isopropyl alcohol 6.0).

Aluminum

Although aluminum is seldom a cause of toxicity in the general population, it is a major concern in patients with chronic renal failure. Aluminum is widely found in

Table 19.2.
Correlation Between Blood Alcohol Level and Clinical Effects in Acute Overdosage

Blood Alcohol (mg/dL [mmol/L] for %, divide mg/dL by 1000)	Clinical Effects
0–50 [0–10.9]	Usually none
50–100 [10.9–20.7]	Mild euphoria, decreased inhibitions
100–250 [20.7–54.4]	Impaired judgment, incoordination, excitement
150–300 [32.6–65.2]	Disorientation, exaggerated emotions, double vision
250–400 [54.4–87.0]	Stupor, vomiting, severe incoordination
350–450 [76.1–97.8]	Coma, decreased reflexes, hypothermia
>450 [97.8]	Death

drinking water, where aluminum salts are used to clear water at water purification plants. Dialysis patients may be inadvertently exposed to large amounts of aluminum in this fashion. Aluminum antacids have been used to prevent elevated serum phosphate in renal failure patients. Aluminum accumulates in bone, contributing to bone weakness in renal failure. Cerebral aluminum accumulation may cause dementia. Normal levels of aluminum are less than 5–10 μg/L (0.18–0.37 μmol/L), although concentrations up to about 50 μg/L (1.85 μmol/L) are typically asymptomatic. Because of the extremely low concentrations, contamination of specimens during collection and transportation is a major concern. Rubber stoppers in collection tubes commonly have large amounts of aluminum, and many plastics and glass also contain aluminum. It is essential to collect specimens in specially prepared tubes to prevent contamination, which may produce aluminum concentrations up to 500 μg/L (18.5 μmol/L).

Carbon Monoxide

This odorless, colorless gas produced from incomplete combustion of hydrocarbons causes over 50% of deaths from poisoning in the United States; approximately 1/3 of these are accidental. Carbon monoxide produces toxicity by binding tightly to hemoglobin, preventing oxygen transport. It also binds to myoglobin in muscle, so that exercise intolerance is a common early finding. The major method used to detect carbon monoxide overdosage is to measure carboxyhemoglobin in a blood gas laboratory. Symptoms are generally related to the relative carboxyhemoglobin level with acute carbon monoxide exposure (Table 19.3), but vary depending on whether oxygen has been given before blood is drawn (lowering carboxyhemoglobin concentration). Symptoms occur at lower concentrations in those with advanced cerebral or cardiac vascular disease and in children. In chronic poisoning, acute symptoms may be replaced by neurologic and psychiatric findings. Carbon monoxide may also produce lactic acidosis, and any patient with unexplained symptoms and lactic acidosis should have carboxyhemoglobin determined.

Iron

Accidental ingestion of iron is the most common cause of fatal poison ingestion in children, usually from ingestion of prenatal iron supplements. Initially, high iron concentration in the intestine causes mucosal injury, often leading to vomiting, gastrointestinal bleeding, and abdominal pain. If the amount of iron absorbed exceeds the binding capacity of transferrin, free iron causes damage to many cells, producing shock and lactic acidosis between 6 and 24 hours after ingestion; once this stage is reached, fatality

Table 19.3.
Symptoms in Acute Carbon Monoxide Poisoning Related to Levels

Carboxyhemoglobin%	Symptoms
0–2.5	Normal result; no symptoms
2.5–10	No symptoms in acute exposure; may have mild weakness with chronic exposure
10–20	Exercise intolerance, mild headache
20–30	Severe headache, irritation, fatigue; simulates viral illness
30–40	Confusion, weakness, dizziness, nausea/vomiting
40–50	Syncope, tachycardia, tachypnea
50–60	Coma, convulsions, may be fatal

rate is high. Measurement of iron and iron binding capacity is critical in detecting dangerous overdosage. Levels are ideally drawn at 2–4 hours after ingestion, when peak concentrations occur. Toxicity is unlikely if serum iron is less than 300 μg/dL (53.7 μmol/L), while severe toxicity is common with levels over 1000 μg/dL (179 μmol/L) unless treatment is instituted. Chelation is recommended for levels over 500 μg/dL (89.5 μmol/L).

Lead

This heavy metal is a common cause of poisoning in children.

Sources of Lead

The major source of lead exposure is from interior house paints. Lead was widely used in the United States until it was outlawed from house paints in 1972 (although it is still in paints used on metals and in art). Old paint which becomes exposed and flakes off of walls, or that is removed by heavy sanding, can be ingested by children as it contaminates their hands while playing on the floor. Less commonly, lead exposure comes from aerosolized lead. This is most commonly seen in those working to dismantle lead containing structures such as metal frames on buildings, as instructors on firing ranges, or from burning automobile batteries. Rarely, lead is ingested in liquids, such as from lead solder in pipes or leached from glazes on pottery by acid products (such as orange juice).

Correlation of Lead Levels with Toxic Symptoms

In children, chronic exposure to low levels of lead causes developmental impairment which may become permanent. Common findings are lowered intelligence and delay in developmental milestones. In children less than 6 years of age, such toxic symptoms may occur at levels over 10 μg/dL (0.48 μmol/L). In older children, developmental abnormalities may occur with levels greater than 25 μg/dL (1.21 μmol/L). Classic symptoms of heavy metal poisoning such as abdominal pain, neuropathy, and anemia typically start with lead levels over 40 μg/dL (1.93 μmol/L), although anemia is rare unless levels are significantly elevated. With remote lead poisoning, evidence of chronic lead toxicity such as renal tubular injury and peripheral neuropathy may occur with normal blood lead levels.

Laboratory Tests for Poisoning

The most reliable test for acute lead poisoning is whole blood lead concentration. As is done with aluminum, specimens should be collected in special tubes to prevent contamination. Historically, screening programs used the measurement of zinc ("free erythrocyte") protoporphyrin, which accumulates because lead inhibits the incorporation of iron into heme. Although this test is extremely easy to perform and relatively sensitive in detecting lead levels over 40 μg/dL (1.93 μmol/L), it is unable to detect more than 25% of children with lead levels over 25 μg/dL (1.21 μmol/L) and virtually none with 10 μg/dL (0.48 μmol/L). It should be used only in screening for more severe forms of lead poisoning which may require hospitalization. With remote lead exposure, blood lead levels are typically normal while total body lead is greatly increased. In such cases, urine lead excretion should be measured after intramuscular administration of a chelating agent such as EDTA (50 mg/kg up to 1000 mg); a ratio of greater than 1 μg lead/mg EDTA excreted in 24 hours confirms a high body lead.

Organophosphates

In agricultural areas, organophosphate insecticides are a relatively common cause of poisoning. These agents inhibit acetylcholinesterase, producing a cholinergic picture described in Table 19.1. Levels are too low to detect in urine and blood, but effects on circulating cholinesterases can be readily determined. In blood, two forms of cholinesterase exist: true cholinesterase (red blood cells), and plasma cholinesterase, or pseudocholinesterase (liver). Plasma cholinesterase is usually the first to decrease with acute poisoning, with toxicity common when levels are below 50% of normal. In suspected chronic poisoning, plasma cholinesterase returns to normal more quickly than red cell cholinesterase. Plasma cholinesterase is also decreased by liver disease, pregnancy, or malnutrition. In patients with any of these conditions, red cell cholinesterase should be used.

Tricyclic (and Related) Antidepressants

Because they are prescribed for patients who are prone to suicide attempts, tricyclic antidepressants (TCAs) are among the most commonly encountered toxic agents. Chemically, many of the newer antidepressants are not tricyclic compounds, although their mechanism of action and toxicity are similar. With overdosage, an anticholinergic pattern is seen, and cardiac arrhythmias are the most dangerous complication. Toxic levels vary for each drug; however, for the TCAs themselves, levels over 500 ng/mL are often toxic and levels over 1000 ng/mL have a high rate of cardiac toxicity, with levels above 3000 ng/mL commonly fatal. As mentioned earlier, qualitative urine tests cannot distinguish therapeutic and toxic levels; plasma levels must be obtained. In many hospitals, quantitative TCA levels are sent to a reference facility and may not be available for many hours. Some laboratories offer a plasma tricyclic screen which is positive only in the presence of toxic levels of TCAs, but this assay will not detect antidepressants which are not chemically tricyclics.

DRUG OF ABUSE TESTING

Screening for use of illegal drugs is done by many companies to detect employee drug abuse. Drug of abuse screens are also widely used in psychiatric and medical settings to determine if unreported drug use could be causing clinical symptoms. It is essential for the practitioner to be aware of the factors which affect results. Knowledge of interferences is widespread among drug users and is used to "cheat" on drug tests, producing falsely negative results.

Methodology for Drug of Abuse Testing

Typically, urine is tested using immunoassays against drugs (or drug metabolites). With employee drug testing, most laboratories then confirm any positive results using a more specific method, often gas chromatography with mass spectrometry (GC-MS) (considered 100% reliable). These assays report positive results when drug **concentration** is above a particular level (**detection limit**); urine concentration is dependent on drug dosage, time since last ingestion, and overall urine concentration. For any amount of drug ingested, concentration is more likely to be below detection limits in very

Table 19.4.
Duration of Positivity of Drug of Abuse Screens

Drug Class	Average Duration of Positive Results
Amphetamines	2–3 days
Barbiturates	Varies markedly depending on type used; with phenobarbital, may be positive for several weeks
Benzodiazepines	Varies markedly depending on type used; most common agents detectable for 2–3 days
Cannabinoids (marijuana)	100 ng/mL cutoff: 2–3 days in single use, 1–2 weeks for chronic users 20 ng/mL cutoff: 5–7 days in single use, 2–3 months in chronic users
Cocaine	8–12 hours after single use, 2–3 days in chronic users
Methadone	2–3 days
Opiates	1–2 days after single dose, 2–4 days in chronic users
Phencyclidine (PCP)	5–7 days after single dose, 1–2 weeks in chronic users

dilute urine or with a long delay between ingestion and testing. Using the most widely employed methods, drug use can be detected for several days since last ingestion (Table 19.4).

Causes of False Positive Results

Immunoassays detect chemicals with specific structures; false positive drug tests occur with compounds chemically similar to the abused drug. Poppy seeds contain chemically inactive opiates; positive urine opiates may occur for 2–3 days after ingestion of poppy seed bagels, cookies, or pastries. Coca tea, commonly used in South America, contains less active forms of cocaine and can produce a positive urine cocaine for 1–2 days. Many over the counter sympathomimetic agents (found in cold tablets, weight loss pills, and antihistamines) are chemically similar to amphetamines and may cause false positive results in certain screening tests; unrelated compounds such as ranitidine also have been reported to cause false positives for amphetamines. In addition, any prescribed drugs of the same chemical class can also produce positive screens for "drugs of abuse." Common examples are barbiturates used to control seizures or migraine headaches, codeine (opiates) in cough suppressants or pain relievers, and amphetamines for attention deficit disorder.

Causes of False Negative Results

Drug users employ a number of approaches to produce falsely negative drug screens. The simplest is submitting a urine specimen from another individual; military programs and drug abuse clinics commonly observe collection to prevent this problem. Urine temperature measurements (often with liquid crystal thermometers in the container) can determine if urine was not within the bladder; normal freshly voided urine should be 36–38 C. Water may be ingested by the drug user or added to the container after collection to dilute the urine. This may cause false negative results when urine concentration is near the lower detection limit. Immunoassays depend on normal urine pH, so that compounds may be ingested or added to change urine pH (such as liquid soap). Many laboratories routinely test urine specific gravity and pH to detect altered specimens. Finally, agents which denature protein may be added to urine after collection to mask positive results. Chlorine bleaches have been most widely used, but can be detected by their odor. Recently, glutaraldehyde has been marketed in underground newspapers as a specific product to cause undetectable false negative results. Glutaraldehyde will not be discovered by usual laboratory methods.

CHAPTER 20

Body Fluids

D. ROBERT DUFOUR

CEREBROSPINAL FLUID

Cerebrospinal fluid (CSF) provides nutrients for the meninges covering the brain and serves as a shock absorber to prevent brain injury. It is formed primarily by filtration of serum in the choroid plexus of the lateral ventricles, producing a fluid largely devoid of protein. Total volume in an adult is approximately 150 mL, with 500 mL produced daily. Absorption of CSF occurs from pressure differences between CSF and dural venous sinuses over the superior portions of the brain. Cerebrospinal fluid pressure depends on normal CSF circulation and normal pressure gradients. Increased CSF pressure occurs with blocks in circulation (by tumor, hemorrhage, or edema), inflammatory damage to arachnoid granulations (site of CSF absorption), or increased venous pressure.

Laboratory Tests of CSF Composition

Protein

As an ultrafiltrate of plasma, CSF has very low protein concentration (15–40 mg/dL in adults, less than 1% of plasma protein concentration). Most CSF protein is albumin, with very little immunoglobulin or other large proteins. Increased protein usually indicates damage to the blood-brain barrier by inflammation, tumor, or degenerative disease, but may be due to traumatic taps. Methods for recognizing a traumatic tap are discussed below under red blood cells. When protein is truly elevated, electrophoresis may be helpful in determining the pattern of abnormality causing protein leakage. In inflammatory disorders, small proteins such as albumin leak in increased amounts, preserving a relatively normal pattern. With immunologic disorders (such as multiple sclerosis), immunoglobulins are disproportionately increased. This can also be estimated by determining the relative rate of entry of albumin and IgG into CSF, using the "IgG synthesis rate" (Eq. 20.1) or "IgG index" (Eq. 20.2).

$$IgG\ Synthesis = 5 \times \left[\left\{ IgG_{CSF} - \frac{IgG_{plasma}}{369} \right\} - \left\{ \left(Alb_{CSF} - \frac{Alb_{plasma}}{230} \right) \right. \right. \tag{1}$$
$$\left. \left. \times \frac{0.43 \times IgG_{plasma}}{Alb_{plasma}} \right\} \right]$$

$$IgG\ Index = \frac{IgG_{CSF} \times Alb_{plasma}}{Alb_{CSF} \times IgG_{plasma}} \tag{2}$$

In these equations, concentration of proteins is expressed in mg/dL, requiring conversion of plasma concentrations (usually reported as g/dL) by multiplying by 1000. An IgG synthesis rate greater than 8 mg/day or an IgG index greater than 0.7 indicates increased production of IgG in the CNS.

Immunoglobulin synthesis in the CNS is often in response to particular antigens,

245

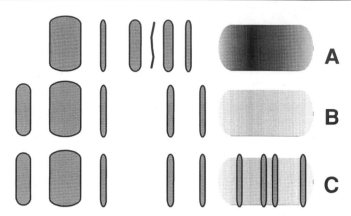

Figure 20.1. CSF Electrophoresis. Normally, CSF protein can only be detected on electrophoresis after concentration of specimens or with use of sensitive silver stains. Normal CSF protein (**B**) differs from serum (**A**) in having lower α_2-globulins, low complement, and an extra transferrin band; immunoglobulins are much lower than in serum, while prealbumin represents about 5% of total CSF protein. With disorders with an immune reaction taking place in the CNS, such as multiple sclerosis, there are typically multiple discrete immunoglobulin bands, a pattern termed oligoclonal bands (**C**). The pattern of oligoclonal bands differs from patient to patient, and has no correlation with disease activity.

producing discrete immunoglobulin **oligoclonal bands** (Fig. 20.1). This pattern is seen in the majority of patients with multiple sclerosis, and is also commonly found in Guillain-Barre syndrome and chronic CNS infectious diseases such as syphilis, Lyme disease, HIV, and subacute sclerosing panencephalitis (SSPE).

Glucose

In CSF, glucose enters both by filtration and active transport, with CSF levels approximately 60–70% of the average plasma glucose concentration over the past 4–6 hours. Once plasma glucose reaches approximately 300 mg/dL, CSF transport reaches its maximum values, and further increases in plasma glucose do not produce the same increment in CSF glucose as at lower levels. Levels of CSF glucose must be interpreted cautiously in patients with diabetes. When the metabolic rate is increased by increased numbers of cells in contact with CSF (acute inflammation, meningeal carcinoma), CSF glucose falls to less than 50% of plasma glucose.

Inflammatory Cells

Normal CSF in adults has few white blood cells (fewer than 5 per mm^3), and no neutrophils. In neonates, normal cell counts are up to 30 per mm^3, and neutrophils are a normal finding. Increased white blood cells indicate the presence of inflammation. Neutrophils predominate in bacterial meningitis, in very early stages of viral meningitis, and after acute cerebral hemorrhage; lymphocytes predominate in viral infections, immunologic disorders such as multiple sclerosis, and in recovery from bacterial meningitis; monocytes often predominate in tuberculous meningitis. Mixtures of different inflammatory cells are common during treatment of bacterial meningitis, with brain abscesses, and in other infectious diseases affecting the brain.

Red Blood Cells

Normally, red blood cells (RBC) are absent from CSF; their presence indicates bleeding. Because blood vessels may be damaged during lumbar puncture, leakage of blood during sampling must always be ruled out before diagnosing cerebral hemorrhage. The two major methods for distinguishing traumatic tap from cerebral hemorrhage are examination for xanthochromia and differential red cell counts. **Xanthochromia** refers to the presence of any color in CSF, which is normally as colorless as water. The CSF sample is centrifuged within 1 hour of collection (to prevent breakdown of any red cells currently present) and the supernatant is compared to water. Xanthochromia is most commonly due to hemoglobin, indicating the presence of bleeding prior to the time of collection. It may also be due to bilirubin (when serum direct bilirubin is greater than 5 mg/dL, 85 μmol/L) or protein (greater than 150 mg/dL, 1.5 g/L) and contamination by colored antiseptics during CSF collection. **Differential red cell counts** in the first and last tubes collected are also helpful in distinguishing traumatic tap from cerebral hemorrhage: if the first tube has a significantly higher cell count than the last, traumatic hemorrhage can be recognized.

Lactate

The product of anaerobic glycolysis, lactate accumulates in CSF when there are increased numbers of cells, particularly tumor cells, bacteria, or granulocytes. It is often used along with other tests to recognize the presence of bacterial meningitis or tumor involvement of the meninges.

Myelin Basic Protein

Myelin, the insulating sheath around nerve fibers, is composed of phospholipids and proteins, including myelin basic protein (MBP). With damage to oligodendroglia (the cells producing myelin) or myelin in the brain, MBP is released and enters CSF. Myelin basic protein is elevated only transiently with demyelination, so its presence confirms active damage to myelin at the time of sampling. It is used as a marker of disease activity in multiple sclerosis, but can be elevated in any other demyelinating state.

Tests for CNS Infections

When CNS infection is suspected by tests such as WBC and glucose, treatment must be started quickly. Laboratory tests that identify the specific infectious agent may not be available rapidly enough to allow specific therapy. Tests to identify specific types of agents should be based on pattern of laboratory tests (Tables 20.1 and 20.2).

Direct Stains

A CSF gram stain is positive in 80–90% of cases of meningitis overall, but is often negative with *Listeria* or gram negative bacilli. A false positive gram stain can occur

Table 20.1.
Prevalent Causes of Bacterial Meningitis, by Age of Patient

Neonate: Group B *streptococci, E. coli*
Infant–5: *Hemophilus influenzae* (if not vaccinated)
5–30: *Neisseria meningitidis, Streptococcus pneumoniae*
Over 30: *Streptococcus pneumoniae*
Immunosuppression: *Listeria monocytogenes, Streptococcus pneumoniae*, gram negatives

Table 20.2.
Patterns of Abnormality with CNS Disorders

Disorder	Cell Count (0–5/mm³, 100% lymphocytes)	Protein (10–45)	Glucose (60–90)	Other
Traumatic tap	↑ RBC in early tubes, ↓ in later tubes	↑ (>100)	Nl	No xanthochromia
Subarachnoid hemorrhage	↑ RBC in early and late tubes	↑ (>100)	Nl	Xanthochromia present except in first 1–2 hours
Bacterial meningitis	↑ WBC (usually >500/mm³), predominantly neutrophils	↑ (100–400)	↓	Gram stain + in most cases of gram positive infection
Viral meningitis	↑ WBC (usually <500/mm³), predominantly lymphocytes; neutrophils may predominate in first 24 hours	sl ↑ (<100)	Nl	
Cryptococcal meningitis	Nl–↑ (usually <500/mm³)	↑ (100–200)	Nl–↓	Cryptococcal antigen; india ink + in 30–50%
Tuberculous meningitis	↑ (200–500/mm³); mixed cells or monocyte predominance	↑ (100–250)	Nl–↓	
Neurosyphilis	Nl–sl ↑	sl ↑ (<100)	Nl	VDRL + in 50%; FTA-ABS positive in most but often falsely high; oligoclonal bands on protein electrophoresis
Multiple sclerosis	Nl–sl ↑	Nl–sl ↑ (<100)	Nl	Oligoclonal bands on protein electrophoresis; myelin basic protein elevated during active stages of disease

with contamination of fluids or, rarely, when nonviable bacteria remain in tubes used for CSF collection. When meningitis has been partially treated, gram stain has a sensitivity of less than 30%. India ink preparation, which highlights the nonstaining encapsulated fungi such as *cryptococcus neoformans*, has a sensitivity of less than 50% overall, but is higher in patients with AIDS.

Antigen Tests

Rapid assays to identify particular bacteria are widely available for *streptococci, neisseria meningitidis,* and *hemophilus influenzae,* as well as for *cryptococcus neoformans.* The sensitivity of these assays is usually over 85%. In suspected neurosyphilis, CSF tests should only be performed if plasma tests are positive. Positive CSF VDRL is specific for neurosyphilis, but is positive in only 30–60% of cases. Additionally, as it does in plasma, VDRL remains positive after successful treatment. The FTA-ABS test is more sensitive, but is falsely positive with meningitis or traumatic tap.

Culture

Bacterial cultures are considered most sensitive for detecting meningitis, but are not positive until 18–24 hours after collection. With brain abscess, anaerobic organisms are often the cause, which are often missed by routine cultures. If brain abscess is suspected, the practitioner should alert the laboratory to perform an anaerobic culture. Fungal and AFB cultures require large amounts of CSF, and take from several days to weeks to become positive. Viral cultures have a low yield in CSF; in herpes encephalitis, fewer than 10% have positive culture.

When to Perform CSF Tests

Examination of CSF is most useful in evaluation for CNS infections or neurologic symptoms which could indicate inflammation, bleeding, or demyelination in the CNS.

How to Collect CSF

Cerebrospinal fluid should be collected in several numbered clear plastic tubes, with the first CSF collected in tube 1. Most kits for performing lumbar puncture contain 3 or 4 numbered tubes. Cell counts are normally performed on a tube other than 1, unless there is suspicion of traumatic tap, in which case counts should be performed on both tube 1 and tube 4. Tube 1 should never be used for gram stain or bacterial tests, since it is the most likely to be contaminated. Certain tests (cultures for fungi and AFB, protein electrophoresis) require up to 5 mL of CSF; tubes used for these tests should contain at least that volume. Cell counts, routine bacterial culture, and tests for protein, glucose, and lactate require only a small amount of CSF, and tubes for these tests require no more than 1 mL each.

Selection of CSF Tests to Request

In patients with suspected infections, cell count, glucose, and tests for infections are most useful, with lactate of possible benefit when other tests are equivocal. Elevated protein is a useful nonspecific indication of damage to the blood-brain barrier, and should be obtained in all cases. Protein is elevated in most infections but seldom of use in their diagnosis; however, normal CSF protein virtually rules out CNS infection. Glucose provides useful information only with meningeal involvement by carcinoma or infections. It should not be ordered unless these are suspected. The most useful tests for other neurologic problems are cell count, protein and protein electrophoresis, and MBP. With suspected CNS bleeding, red cell counts in the first and last tubes and examination for xanthochromia are most useful in distinguishing CNS hemorrhage from traumatic tap.

PLEURAL AND PERITONEAL FLUID

Normal fluid in these cavities is minimal, composed of an ultrafiltrate of plasma with approximately 4 g/dL (40 g/L) of protein, mainly albumin. It forms in the same manner as interstitial fluid (Chapter 5).

Mechanisms of Pleural and Peritoneal (Ascitic) Fluid Accumulation

Two fundamental mechanisms cause fluid accumulation: **transudation** and **exudation.**

Transudation

Alteration of pressure differences between the cavity and plasma causes fluid accumulation by transudation, most commonly due to increased venous hydrostatic pressure in congestive heart failure or, in the peritoneum, portal venous hypertension (usually due to cirrhosis). Less frequently, decreased plasma oncotic pressure (decreased plasma proteins) in nephrotic syndrome or malnutrition is responsible. Transudation causes accumulation of an ultrafiltrate of plasma, producing a fluid (transudate) in which normal fluid protein concentration is diluted. Characteristically, transudates have low concentrations of albumin and other proteins and low specific gravity.

Exudation

Alteration in vascular permeability to protein and, often, cells causes fluid exudation, most commonly due to cytokines in inflammation or leaky vessels in malignant tumors. Exudates typically have protein concentration and specific gravity higher than normal fluid, in most cases associated with inflammatory cells. When exudates are present for a long time (loculation of fluid), inflammatory cells degenerate and cell membrane lipids cause cloudy fluid, termed a **pseudochylous** effusion, grossly resembling chlyous effusions described below. Cell walls contain large amounts of cholesterol but no triglyceride.

Chylous Effusions

Rarely, an obstruction of lymphatic drainage allows leakage of lymphatic fluid into pleural or peritoneal space. Lymphatic fluid contains large amounts of chylomicrons rich in triglyceride, producing a cloudy to almost white fluid which can be recognized grossly.

Tests to Distinguish Type of Effusion

Protein (or Albumin)

Protein content is most reliable in distinguishing transudates (low protein content) from exudates (high protein content). In pleural fluid, total protein greater than 3.0 g/dL (30 g/L) or greater than 50% of plasma protein indicates exudate. In ascitic fluid, total protein is unreliable in differential diagnosis; however, a difference in albumin between plasma and ascitic fluid (A-a gradient) of more than 1.1 g/dL (11 g/L) indicates transudate. Specific gravity has been used as a surrogate marker of total protein, but is affected by concentrations of other compounds as well and is not as accurate.

LDH

Lactate dehydrogenase does not freely pass into transudates or exudates because of its large size. A high cellular concentration causes LDH elevation in most exudates. Fluid LDH greater than 60% of plasma LDH is considered evidence of an exudate. Because of LDH abundance in red cells, hemolyzed plasma specimens or traumatic taps can invalidate LDH as a diagnostic test.

Cholesterol and Triglyceride

Most plasma cholesterol is bound to large low density lipoprotein; even with exudates, little LDL is lost into fluid. Cells (often present in exudates) contain cholesterol in membranes and may release it. Fluid cholesterol greater than 60 mg/dL (1.55 mmol/L) or more than 30% of plasma cholesterol indicates an exudate. Lymphatic fluid contains large amounts of chylomicrons, with a ratio of triglyceride to cholesterol approximately 10:1 (with concentration expressed in mg/dL); chylous effusions have similarly high ratio. With longstanding exudates, cholesterol and cell debris may give fluid a cloudy appearance similar to that of chylous effusion; however, the triglyceride to cholesterol ratio will typically be less than 1.

Tests Useful in Evaluating Exudates

As transudates are due to alterations in pressure differences, further laboratory testing of transudates is not indicated. Exudates should have further testing to determine the cause of altered vascular permeability.

Cell Count and Differential

The most useful differential test is determination of the number and type of inflammatory cells present. Many laboratories perform a count of total nucleated cells and report it as "WBC count." This number includes mesothelial and tumor cells, and may be much higher than true WBC count. It is important for practitioners to know which approach is used by the laboratory they use. In pleural fluid, a true WBC count greater than 1000 per mm^3 indicates inflammation, while in peritoneal fluid a neutrophil count (true WBC count times fraction of neutrophils) above 250 per mm^3 is considered diagnostic. Increases in lymphocytes and monocytes are typical in tuberculosis, viral infections, malignancies, and autoimmune diseases. Red blood cell count is used to detect evidence of hemorrhage into pleural or peritoneal cavities.

Cytology

Examination of pleural or peritoneal fluid for cytology is often done to recognize malignancy as a cause of effusion; sensitivity is considerably less than 100%.

pH

Normally, pH of pleural and peritoneal fluid is near or above blood pH. A low pH in either fluid indicates a high likelihood of infection. In pleural fluid, pH under 7.3 indicates a high likelihood of infection requiring pleural drainage. In peritoneal fluid, pH less than 7.32 strongly suggests bacterial peritonitis. Low pH in both pleural and peritoneal fluid is also seen in tuberculosis and malignancies.

Amylase

Amylase is a small enzyme which can freely enter pleural or peritoneal fluid; normally, amylase is similar in plasma and body fluids. If pleural or peritoneal fluid amylase is more than 1.5 times plasma amylase, pancreatitis is typically the cause of the effusion present. With damage to the pancreatic duct, peritoneal fluid amylase may be more than 1000 times plasma concentration. Occasionally, levels like this may cause errors in measurement, producing markedly low results. If an amylase result is very low, the laboratory should be contacted to recheck the result after diluting the specimen.

Distinguishing Urine from Other Fluids

Occasionally, particularly in the case of ascites, it may be difficult to determine whether the fluid obtained is actually peritoneal fluid or urine. Measurement of urea or creatinine in the fluid is the best test to make this distinction. Both substances are markedly elevated in urine compared to levels in fluids, which are similar to those in plasma.

Glucose

In normal body fluids, glucose concentration is similar to plasma. A markedly low glucose concentration commonly occurs with severe infections, malignant effusions, and in rheumatoid arthritis.

Tests for Infection

In bacterial infection, gram stain is positive in less than 75% of pleural infections but in fewer than 30% of peritoneal cases; culture is preferred. Pleural infections are usually diagnosed by culture, but cultures are less reliable in peritoneal fluid (probably less than 50% of cases), where the total neutrophil count is considered more reliable. In tuberculous infections, AFB stains are positive in less than 10% of cases. A diagnosis usually requires culture and AFB stain of a pleural biopsy. **Adenosine deaminase** is elevated in most cases of tuberculosis involving pleura or peritoneum, but the test is offered only in research laboratories and is not commercially available.

SYNOVIAL FLUID

Normally, only a small volume of synovial fluid is present within a joint space to provide lubrication and nutrition to cartilage cells. It is similar in composition to an ultrafiltrate of plasma except for high concentrations of hyaluronic acid, which produces fluid with the high viscosity needed for lubrication. Normal synovial fluid contains few cells (normal nucleated cell count is less than 150 per mm^3).

Causes of Joint Effusion

Increased volume of synovial fluid is usually due to joint damage from one of several causes. Trauma, including degenerative joint disease, is the most common cause of joint effusions. Tests are usually performed to distinguish traumatic effusions from inflammatory causes with specific pathogenesis and therapy: infection, crystals, and immunologic diseases.

Laboratory Tests of Use in Differential Diagnosis of Joint Effusions

Cell Count

Total nucleated cell count (as with pleural and peritoneal fluid, often reported as WBC count) is the most reliable test to distinguish trauma from inflammatory arthritis. Total cell count is usually under 3,000 per mm^3 in traumatic arthritis, with higher results in inflammation. Counts above 50,000 are often due to infection. Differential counts are also helpful in determining the likelihood of infection. In traumatic arthritis, neutrophils are usually fewer than 30% of cells, while values above 75% are found in about 75% of infections, but rarely in other forms of arthritis.

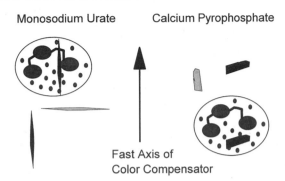

Figure 20.2. Synovial Fluid Crystals. Crystals are absent from normal synovial fluid. In gout, monosodium urate (MSU) crystals are found, while calcium pyrophosphate (CaPP) crystals are responsible for pseudogout. Crystals can be differentiated both by their appearance and their color when examined by polarized light using a color compensator. A color compensator separates light into perpendicular fast (blue) and slow (yellow) axes. In the figure, blue is indicated by the stippled crystals and yellow by the solid crystals. MSU crystals are elongated needles which are "negatively birefringent," behaving opposite of the color compensator; in the color compensator, they appear blue when perpendicular to the fast axis and yellow when parallel to the fast axis. CaPP crystals are generally shorter and wider, with blunted ends. CaPP is positively birefringent; crystals appear blue when parallel to the fast axis. The colors remain the same whether the crystals are free or within neutrophils. Between attacks, most crystals are free, while with acute attacks crystals are both free and within white cells.

Crystal Examination

Most crystals causing arthritis can be identified easily by examining synovial fluid microscopically using polarized light (Fig. 20.2). Crystals are normally absent from synovial fluid, but may be found when plasma concentrations are elevated. Crystals are considered significant as a cause of arthritis when found within neutrophils.

Gram Stain and Culture

Septic arthritis is most commonly due to gram positive cocci, particularly *Staphylococcus aureus*, and *Neisseria gonorrheae*. Gram stain is positive in the majority of patients with gram positive infections, but in less than one-quarter with gonorrhea. Culture of both blood and synovial fluid is usually necessary for maximum diagnostic yield. Fluid cultures are positive in most patients with joint infections, but in only one-third to one-half of patients with gonorrhea.

CHAPTER 21

The GI Tract and Pancreas

D. ROBERT DUFOUR

GASTRIC FUNCTION

The stomach produces three important components needed for nutrient digestion: acid, intrinsic factor, and pepsinogen. Hydrochloric acid (HCl), secreted by parietal cells, begins breakdown of dietary components and converts pepsinogen to pepsin. Production of HCl is stimulated by food ingestion, vagal nerve induced release of histamine, and gastrin (discussed in more detail below). Intrinsic factor, also secreted by parietal cells, is needed for absorption of vitamin B_{12} in the ileum. Pepsinogen (produced by chief cells) is converted by HCl to pepsin, a protease producing small polypeptides acted upon by pancreatic enzymes. Pepsinogen production is stimulated by the same factors stimulating HCl production. Gastrin is the primary gastric hormone, produced by G-cells in the gastric and duodenal mucosa and in pancreatic islets. Normally, most gastrin is produced by the stomach. Gastrin production is stimulated by dietary protein and by low gastric acidity (high pH).

Tests of Gastric Function and Status

Rarely, tests of gastric function (other than gastrin levels) are needed to evaluate gastric functioning. Tests of vitamin B_{12} status are discussed in Chapter 22.

Gastrin

Measurement of plasma gastrin is often used in patients with recurrent ulcers or ulcers in unusual locations. Although gastrin exists in many forms, immunoassays detect most forms equally well. Gastrin response to stimuli can also be evaluated. For instance, tumors producing gastrin often show an exaggerated increase in gastrin level in response to administration of calcium or secretin, or after food ingestion.

Acid Production

After meals, gastric pH falls to less than 2.0 in normal individuals. Determination of gastric pH is the simplest way to determine if acid is being produced. A pH greater than 6.0 after stimulation is termed achlorhydria, or the lack of HCl production. Rarely, especially when gastrin producing tumors are suspected, measurement of total acid production is needed. After insertion of a nasogastric tube, gastric fluid is aspirated and collected in four 15 minute aliquots to determine the **basal acid output** (BAO) (normally less than 6 mmol/hr). Histamine, one of its analogues, or pentagastrin is then administered and an additional four 15 minute aliquots are collected. The amount produced is totaled to determine the **maximal acid output** (MAO) (normally less than 40 mmol/hr). Finally, the highest two consecutive 15 minute aliquots are added to determine the **peak acid output** (PAO).

Helicobacter pylori

Helicobacter pylori colonizes the protective mucous layer of the stomach and duodenum. This bacterium appears to damage mucosal cells, causing gastritis, and markedly increases the likelihood of development of peptic ulcers. It is thought to be responsible for almost 100% of duodenal and 80% of gastric ulcers. The most common way to detect *H. pylori* infection is by measurement of antibodies to the organism. Definitive diagnosis by identification of organisms in a gastric biopsy or demonstration of bacterial urease activity in gastric aspirates is seldom needed. With successful therapy, there is typically at least a fourfold reduction in titers (e.g., from 1:64 to 1:16).

When Not to Perform Tests of Gastric Function

Tests of acid production are seldom needed in patients with initial presentation of gastric disease, and should not be performed routinely. Gastrin levels show pronounced variation after meals, and should always be obtained in the fasting state unless stimulatory testing is being performed. Many medications used to treat ulcers increase gastrin, particularly H_2 antagonists, antacids, and proton pump inhibitors such as omeprazole. Ideally, gastrin levels should be obtained before treatment is started or after treatment is discontinued. Caffeine ingestion and tobacco also increase gastrin production. The use of these should be limited before measurement of gastrin.

Gastric Diseases

Peptic Ulcer

Ulceration of gastric or duodenal mucosa by acid and pepsin occurs when there is an imbalance between acid production and mucosal defense mechanisms. The most important factor in most cases is *H. pylori* infection. Although antibodies to *H. pylori* are common in North America (with a prevalence approximately equal to patient age), the presence of antibodies in association with dyspepsia is considered evidence of need for antibacterial treatment.

Atrophic Gastritis

Atrophy of gastric mucosa is common in older individuals. The more important type A gastritis, due to autoimmune damage to parietal cells, is often associated with antibodies to parietal cells and intrinsic factor. Antiparietal cell antibodies are more sensitive, but are relatively nonspecific. Anti-intrinsic factor antibodies occur in 50–70% of cases of autoimmune atrophic gastritis and are quite specific. The more common type B gastritis is usually caused by *H. pylori*.

Gastric Bleeding

In severe cases, vomiting of blood can be recognized grossly. With lesser bleeding, vomited blood is converted to black heme-derived pigments (producing "coffee ground" emesis). In such cases, confirmation of heme presence depends on laboratory tests. Standard tests used for fecal or urine occult blood testing are often falsely negative at low pH or in the presence of cimetidine. A specific test for gastric occult blood testing is available and should be used routinely for suspected gastric bleeding.

Zollinger-Ellison Syndrome

Tumors producing gastrin are a rare cause of recurrent gastric ulcer and, in some cases, diarrhea. Most commonly, gastrin secreting tumors are malignant and arise from pancreatic islets. Such tumors characteristically produce markedly elevated gastrin, causing marked acid overproduction. Before further workup of very high gastrin, gastric pH should be measured; values above 6.0 indicate atrophic gastritis. With borderline high gastrin levels, determination of gastric acid secretion or gastrin response to stimuli are needed. While G-cell gastrin production does not increase in response to secretin, pancreatic islet gastrin production does. Secretin stimulation is the best differential test in patients with elevated gastrin and increased acid production.

EXOCRINE PANCREATIC FUNCTION

The exocrine pancreas produces a large volume of fluid with high concentrations of degradative enzymes and bicarbonate (needed to neutralize gastric acid and allow activation of pancreatic enzymes). The major pancreatic enzymes are amylase, needed to cleave polysaccharides to simple sugars; lipase, needed to convert triglycerides to free fatty acids; and proteases (including trypsin and chymotrypsin), needed to release amino acids from polypeptides. Absence of pancreatic enzymes prevents complete digestion of food and causes nutrient malabsorption.

Tests of Pancreatic Function

Plasma Enzyme Levels

Normally, trace amounts of pancreatic enzymes reach the circulation, in rough proportion to pancreatic mass. With pancreatic damage, increased amounts reach the circulation.

Amylase

Amylase is produced by several types of cells, primarily by the pancreas and salivary gland, with each producing a distinct isoenzyme, although only a few laboratories measure amylase isoenzymes. The salivary isoenzyme of amylase is also produced by the fallopian tube, with trace amounts in lung and ovary. Amylase is a small enzyme, filtered by glomeruli and reabsorbed by renal tubules, with renal disorders also affecting plasma amylase, showing low values with tubular injury and high levels in renal failure. Renal clearance contributes to the short half-life of amylase (3–4 hours) in blood. Intestinal injury allows pancreatic amylase absorption, raising blood levels. For obscure reasons, diabetic ketoacidosis also increases plasma amylase. As with creatine kinase (Chapter 12), autoantibodies to amylase occur, termed **macroamylase,** commonly associated with high plasma amylase but low urine amylase. Macroamylase is relatively common in patients with AIDS. Amylase activity is inhibited by very high triglycerides.

Lipase

True lipase is produced primarily by the pancreas, but other enzymes similar to lipase in activity may also be measured as part of "lipase" in laboratories. Lipase is also produced by lingual glands, stomach, and intestinal cells. Lipase, like amylase, is a small enzyme, although normally tubular absorption is complete. Renal disease may affect lipase in the same fashion as amylase. Intestinal injury also increases absorption of lipase and causes increased plasma lipase activity. In general, however, the magnitude of lipase elevation with intestinal injury is less than that of amylase. Lipase is cleared more slowly than amylase because of lower renal clearance.

Trypsin and Chymotrypsin

As with amylase and lipase, these enzymes normally reach plasma in only trace amounts. Immunoassays for trypsin are available in some laboratories, and are primarily used in children to detect pancreatic injury from cystic fibrosis. In adults, most trypsin in stool is digested by intestinal bacteria, making stool trypsin an inaccurate test of pancreatic function. Chymotrypsin is more resistant to bacterial cleavage; stool chymotrypsin can be used to estimate pancreatic enzyme synthesis.

Bentiromide

This synthetic compound contains a small peptide and *p*-amino benzoic acid (PABA). Pancreatic enzymes release PABA, which is absorbed and subsequently metabolized by the liver to hippuric acid (and other related compounds), and subsequently excreted in urine. The amount of hippuric acid excreted is directly related to pancreatic enzyme production. Intestinal disease, severe liver damage, and renal insufficiency all cause falsely low results.

Secretin Test

Normally produced by duodenal cells, secretin stimulates pancreatic secretion of bicarbonate-rich fluid. Performance of this test requires duodenal intubation to allow fluid collection. After parenteral administration of 1 unit of secretin per kilogram, fluid is collected by continuous aspiration into 10 minute aliquots. A normal response is to produce more than 15–30 mmol bicarbonate in 30 minutes. The test is not commonly used currently, with pancreatic duct cannulation more widely used.

When Not to Do Tests of Pancreatic Function

Plasma enzyme levels are useful in the diagnosis of acute pancreatitis, but are not generally helpful for the diagnosis of pancreatic insufficiency. They should not be used when this diagnosis is considered. Tests of function such as bentiromide and secretin are relatively insensitive, and should not be used unless patients have clinical symptoms suggesting pancreatic insufficiency. Amylase and lipase need not be measured more than once per day in patients with pancreatitis. Since amylase will return to normal earlier, it is a better test for monitoring disease activity. While some authorities suggest the use of fractional excretion (see Chapter 6) of amylase, this is neither more sensitive nor more specific than plasma amylase for pancreatitis and should not be used.

Pancreatic Diseases

Acute Pancreatitis

The most common pancreatic disease, acute pancreatitis, is most commonly due to alcohol or gall stones. Pancreatitis may be difficult to diagnose clinically, as other causes of abdominal pain may produce similar signs and symptoms. Measurement of plasma enzymes is typically used for diagnosis. In general, lipase is both more sensitive and

Table 21.1.
Ransom Laboratory Criteria for Severity in Acute Pancreatitis

At time of admission:
- WBC > 16 × 10³/μL (16 × 10⁹/L)
- Glucose > 200 mg/dL (11.1 mmol/L)
- LDH > 400 U/L or AST > 250 U/L

During first 48 hours:
- Hematocrit fall > 10%
- Calcium < 8 mg/dL (2 mmol/L)
- BUN increase by >5 mg/dL (1.8 mmol/L)
- Albumin < 3.2 g/dL (32 g/L)

specific than amylase for pancreatitis. Elevations of both more than three times normal markedly increase the likelihood of pancreatitis. Once a diagnosis is made, other laboratory tests detect severity (Table 21.1). The presence of two or more of the Ransom criteria is associated with high mortality. Amylase generally remains elevated for 2–4 days after an episode of pancreatitis, while lipase may be elevated for 5–7 days.

Pancreatic Pseudocyst

After episodes of pancreatitis, there is often a residual area in which tissue has been dissolved by pancreatic enzymes, forming a pseudocyst. While this cannot be diagnosed by laboratory tests, persistent elevation of amylase and lipase suggest its presence.

Chronic Pancreatitis

In many patients, chronic or recurrent pancreatic injury results in destruction of pancreatic tissue and, in late stages, malabsorption due to insufficiency of pancreatic enzymes. In many patients, plasma amylase and lipase are in the low end of normal or frankly low. In patients with symptoms of malabsorption, bentiromide or secretin tests may be done if necessary to confirm the diagnosis. Tests to distinguish pancreatic from intestinal causes of malabsorption are discussed later in the chapter.

INTESTINAL FUNCTION

The major function of the intestinal tract is to allow absorption of nutrients; other endocrine functions will not be discussed in this chapter. Food digestion and absorption is a complicated process (Fig. 21.1). Failure of any of the organs involved in normal food digestion may cause a clinical picture of malabsorption, in which weight loss (or, in children, lack of weight gain) is often associated with loose, foul smelling stools.

Tests of Intestinal Function

Fecal Fat

The absorption of lipid is most prone to failure, which is characterized by bulky stools which appear oily and float. Normally, the small amount of fat reaching stool comes from desquamated cells and waste lipids. Increased stool fat (**steatorrhea**) is the most common manifestation of maldigestion or malabsorption. To recognize steatorrhea, patients must be on a normal oral diet; for quantitative determination, fat intake must

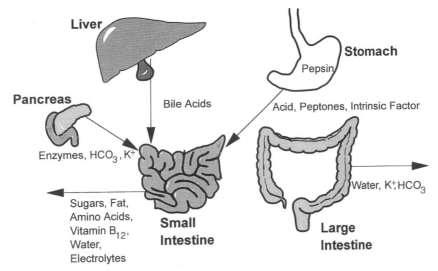

Figure 21.1. Normal Food Digestion and Absorption. Digestion begins with acid and pepsin in the stomach, along with the action of salivary amylases. Within a few hours, this partially digested food reaches the small intestine. Acid and food stimulate cholecystokinin and secretin production, leading to release of bile (with bile acids) from the gall bladder and digestive enzymes, bicarbonate, and electrolytes from the pancreas. Pancreatic amylases release glucose and other simple sugars from food starches, pancreatic proteases (such as trypsin) release amino acids from peptones produced in the stomach, and pancreatic lipase converts triglycerides to free fatty acids and glycerol. Lipase activity is maximal only in the presence of bile acids. Sugars and amino acids can be absorbed directly by the small bowel, while free fatty acids and glycerol are reassembled in intestinal cells and converted to chylomicrons for transport into blood. Water and electrolytes are absorbed without need for pancreatic enzymes. Vitamin B_{12} absorption occurs in the last portion of the small bowel, the ileum, only when complexed to intrinsic factor made by parietal cells in the stomach. The colon absorbs the remaining water and electrolytes, mainly potassium and bicarbonate.

be known with reasonable accuracy. The simplest test examines stool for fat droplets using a fat stain (Sudan or Oil Red O). In normal stool, few fat droplets of small size (usually less than 5 droplets per high power field, smaller than normal red cells) are present. With malabsorption, large numbers of larger droplets (usually more than 20 droplets per high power field, with most many times the size of a red cell) are visible. In equivocal cases, quantitative stool fat can be measured, although because of day to day variation, accurate results require collection of stool for 72 hours. This is often difficult for patients and, in the hospital, nursing staff. Patients should be on approximately 100 grams of fat daily; excretion of more than 7 g/day describes steatorrhea.

Examination for Meat Fibers

With lack of pancreatic enzymes, dietary proteins cannot be broken down and will not be absorbed. Meat, being mostly protein, requires digestion for absorption. Examination of stained stool can identify residual meat fibers and provide suggestive evidence of pancreatic insufficiency.

D-Xylose Absorption

Xylose is a simple sugar which is readily absorbed across intact intestinal epithelium; its absorption is not dependent on pancreatic function. A dose of 25 grams of xylose is given orally, urine is collected for 5 hours after ingestion, and blood is drawn at 2 hours. In normal persons, over 5 g of xylose is excreted in 5 hours, and peak blood levels are greater than 25 mg/dL (1.66 mmol/L). In patients with renal insufficiency, urine collection adds little to plasma levels and need not be done.

Carotene

In persons on a normal diet, carotene (found in green and yellow vegetables) is readily absorbed; it is not stored in the body to any extent. Plasma carotene levels are a reasonable measure of fat absorption from the intestine in patients on a normal diet. For measurement of plasma carotene to be useful, it is important to determine that patients have had normal intake of vegetables; for this reason, many prefer stool fat examination. Carotene is also unstable if exposed to light; specimens should be wrapped in aluminum foil after collection.

Other Tests of Intestinal Status

Stool Electrolytes and Osmolality

In patients with watery diarrhea, stool electrolyte measurements are most useful in guiding fluid replacement therapy. If the cause of diarrhea is unknown, adding osmolality may help to clarify the cause. Watery diarrhea may be due to damage to intestinal mucosa; sodium and potassium (along with associated anions) make up almost all of the solute in stool (**secretory diarrhea**). In some cases, nonabsorbable solutes (unabsorbed nutrients in malabsorption, magnesium salts or other nonabsorbable laxatives) are responsible (**osmotic diarrhea**). If there is a difference between measured osmolality and calculated osmolality (Eq. 21.1) of greater than 50 mosm/kg, osmotic diarrhea is diagnosed. Stool magnesium measurement is helpful in determining the cause.

$$Calculated\ stool\ osmolality = 2 \times (Na^+ + K^+) \qquad (21.1)$$

Occult Blood

Normally, only a small amount of blood enters stool each day. Increased stool blood loss is common with tumors, ulcers, ischemia, inflammation, anal fissures, and hemorrhoids. Measurement of stool blood is most commonly done by measuring peroxidase activity of the heme (in hemoglobin) using guaiac or other indicators. False positive results may occur with heme from myoglobin (in dietary meat) or from iron. False negative results may occur with breakdown of heme in the intestine (upper intestinal bleeding) or with inhibitors (high concentrations of ascorbic acid). In addition, stool which has dried on a card may not react with reagents. More sensitive tests, including those in which rehydration is used, and immunoassays for hemoglobin (such as Heme-Select) tend to give fewer false negative results but more false positive results.

When Not to Do Tests of Intestinal Function

Tests for fat malabsorption (including carotene) should not be performed unless patients are ingesting a normal diet. Stool electrolytes and osmolality are not useful unless patients have watery diarrhea; in fact, they cannot be measured in solid or semisolid stools. Specimens for occult blood should ideally be rehydrated (if based on guaiac or other heme detection methods) to increase sensitivity. Ideally, tests should not be done

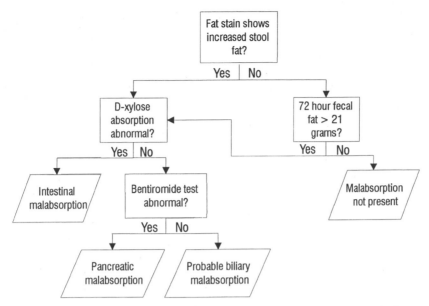

Figure 21.2. Approach to Suspected Malabsorption. Patients with malabsorption typically present with weight loss and loose, malodorous stools which often appear oily. All forms of malabsorption usually cause increased stool fat. Fat stains are a qualitative screen for malabsorption. They are fairly specific, so that increased fat confirms malabsorption; normal or equivocal results should be confirmed with a 72 hour fecal fat measurement. D-Xylose is a simple sugar absorbed without digestion. Abnormal absorption of xylose confirms intestinal disease. Pancreatic insufficiency is likely in patients with nonintestinal malabsorption. While no test is perfect, a bentiromide test is abnormal in most patients with pancreatic insufficiency. A normal result suggests possible biliary malabsorption; further invasive procedures such as endoscopic examination of the bile and pancreatic ducts or secretin test are often needed to establish the correct diagnosis.

when patients are on iron or while ingesting meat. However, since it is difficult for many people to totally abstain from meat and fish, patients with high meat intake could be retested using a hemoglobin immunoassay to eliminate this cause of false positive results.

Evaluation of Malabsorption

The determination of the cause of malabsorption is summarized in Figure 21.2.

CHAPTER 22

Evaluation of Nutrition

D. ROBERT DUFOUR

FREQUENCY OF NUTRITIONAL PROBLEMS

While gross nutritional deficiency states such as kwashiorkor and marasmus are rare in Europe and North America, nutritional problems are common in ill patients. Nutritional deficiency leads to poor wound healing, longer hospital stays, and increased morbidity and mortality. In a study done in the mid 1970s, almost 75% of patients hospitalized more than two weeks showed clinical or laboratory evidence of nutritional deficiency, which in many patients as still present at discharge. Many studies have demonstrated nutritional problems in half of acutely ill hospital patients on admission. Eating disorders are common among adolescent and young adult women. Anorexia nervosa is found in about 5 out of 100,000 women between the ages of 10 and 30, while classic bulimia nervosa occurs in 1–2% of women in this age group.

LABORATORY EVALUATION OF GENERAL NUTRITIONAL STATUS

A number of laboratory tests correlate with nutritional status, allowing recognition of nutritional problems and monitoring of the response to nutritional therapy. Many of these tests are discussed in other chapters, with only those aspects related to nutrition discussed here.

Laboratory Evaluation of Protein Nutrition

Albumin

Plasma albumin has been the most widely used, since it is routinely measured in many hospitals. Because albumin has a normal half-life of 20 days, there is a delay between the onset of nutritional problems (or their resolution) and changes in plasma albumin. Albumin levels are affected by other disorders, notably liver disease, protein losing states, inflammation, and corticosteroid therapy, all of which cause lowered results. Albumin levels between 2.8 and 3.5 g/dL (28–35 g/L) are considered mildly decreased, values of 2.1–2.8 g/dL (21–28 g/L) are moderately lowered, while those less than 2.1 g/dL (21 g/L) are markedly decreased. If chronically low results due to cirrhosis can be ruled out, markedly low albumin indicates a high risk for nutrition-related complications.

Transferrin

Transferrin (TF) has a shorter half-life than albumin (approximately 8 days), and is also widely available in hospitals, either by direct measurement or by calculation from total iron binding capacity (TIBC) using the formula TF (in mg/dL) = [0.8 × TIBC (in μg/dL)] − 44. Transferrin will be 150–175 mg/dL (1.5–1.75 g/L) in mild protein deficiency, 100–150 mg/dL (1.0–1.5 g/L) with moderate deficiency, and less than 100 mg/dL (1.0 g/L) with severe deficiency. In addition to nutritional problems, transferrin is lowered by all of factors described for albumin, and is increased by iron deficiency.

Transthyretin (Prealbumin)

This trace protein is theoretically better than albumin or transferrin because it has a much shorter half-life of 1–2 days, allowing it to detect changes in protein nutrition in a much shorter period than the other two proteins. As with the other proteins, low levels occur with liver disease, protein losing states, and inflammation; however, transthyretin levels are increased by corticosteroids.

Urine Urea Nitrogen

In nutritional balance, rate of nitrogen loss equals rate of nitrogen intake in food. In normal individuals, urine represents only one of three sources of nitrogen loss from the body; the others are skin and feces. In patients receiving parenteral nutrition, fecal losses of nitrogen and skin losses are quantitatively small compared to urine losses, which are often used to evaluate nitrogen balance. In urine, the major form of nitrogen is urea (representing 80% of urine nitrogen losses). Multiplying urine urea nitrogen (UUN) by 1.25 gives a rough approximation of total urine nitrogen losses. Protein nitrogen intake must exceed losses to improve nutritional status.

Total Lymphocyte Count

In nutritional deficiency states, immunodeficiency is a common complication. Total lymphocyte count, either directly measured (by many current cell counters) or calculated from the percentage of lymphocytes and total white blood cell count, correlates reasonably well with nutritional status, with counts less than $1.2 \times 10^3/\mu L$ ($1.2 \times 10^9/L$) considered evidence of malnutrition. As with serum proteins, however, total lymphocyte counts are decreased with inflammation and with corticosteroids. In addition, values are typically markedly decreased in patients with AIDS, in malignancies, and with other immunosuppressive drugs.

Laboratory Evaluation of Mineral and Electrolyte Metabolism

While protein malnutrition is usually the most apparent feature of malnutrition in ill patients, mineral abnormalities commonly accompany nutritional disorders. Refeeding of malnourished patients often causes profound shifts in minerals and electrolytes which may be clinically important.

Magnesium

Deficiency of magnesium is most commonly due to increased losses, rather than to malnutrition, and is discussed more fully in Chapter 10. Magnesium deficiency due to dietary problems is relatively common in alcoholics.

Potassium

As with magnesium, potassium deficiency (discussed more fully in Chapter 5) is not commonly due to malnutrition, although since potassium losses occur each day, hypokalemia is a common finding in malnourished individuals. Low insulin production in malnutrition often masks the extent of potassium deficiency; with refeeding, increased insulin causes potassium to enter cells and further lowers plasma potassium. Potassium should be monitored at least every 6 hours when nutritional replacement is begun after a period of prolonged malnutrition.

Phosphate

Deficiency of phosphate is extremely common in malnourished patients, particularly those with deficient carbohydrate intake and in alcohol abuse. An inability to perform glycolysis leads to loss of phosphate from the body, although plasma phosphate levels remain relatively normal. In patients using fatty acids for energy, phosphate may even be elevated due to the release of phosphate salts from bone to serve as buffers. With refeeding, phosphate enters cells for glycolysis, leading to a rapid fall in plasma phosphate concentration. If levels fall below 1.0 mg/dL (0.32 mmol/L), glycolysis may be inhibited, causing the dysfunction of cells preferentially using glucose (muscle, red cells, brain). Phosphate should be monitored at least every 6 hours when nutritional replacement therapy is begun after prolonged malnutrition, and more frequently if levels fall below 1.5 mg/dL (0.5 mmol/L).

Zinc

Zinc is a cofactor for many essential enzymes, and thus is essential for protein and nucleic acid synthesis. Zinc deficiency is common in nutritional diseases, although in most cases it is mild and produces no specific symptoms. Severe deficiency may produce poor wound healing, dry skin, diminished taste, and hypogonadism. Plasma zinc levels are commonly used to evaluate zinc status, but are difficult to interpret in malnourished patients as 85% of zinc is protein bound; a low zinc level may reflect normal levels of physiologically active free zinc. Contamination of specimens by zinc in rubber stoppers is a significant problem; special collection containers must be used. With severe deficiency, serum alkaline phosphatase activity in serum is reduced, providing an indirect measure of zinc status.

Laboratory Evaluation of Vitamin Status

In most parts of the world, isolated nutritional deficiency of most vitamins is rare in the general population because of vitamin supplementation of processed foods. In these countries, vitamin deficiency is usually seen only as part of generalized malnutrition. Deficiency of certain vitamins occurs in specific situations; for example, folate deficiency during times of increased demand (pregnancy), vitamin B_{12} deficiency in pernicious anemia, and vitamin D deficiency with renal disease. Only the most important vitamins are discussed in this chapter.

Vitamin A (Retinol) and Carotene

Vitamin A, a fat soluble vitamin found predominantly in animal livers, is essential for night vision and serves as an antioxidant, stabilizing cell membranes. It is stored in the liver, with body stores typically lasting for months. Carotene, a precursor of vitamin A found in yellow vegetables, is the major dietary source of Vitamin A. It is not appreciably stored, and blood levels reflect recent intake and intestinal absorption (Chapter 21). Vitamin A deficiency may cause night blindness, corneal degeneration (**keratomala-**

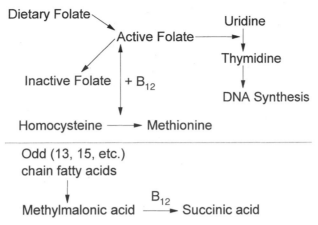

Figure 22.1. Metabolic Activity of Vitamin B_{12} and Folate. Interrelationships in folate and B_{12} metabolism are shown in the top half of the figure. Both folate and B_{12} are needed for normal DNA synthesis and the conversion of homocysteine to methionine. Deficiency of either vitamin increases plasma and urine homocysteine concentration. High levels of dietary folate in B_{12} deficiency can generate enough active folate to allow adequate DNA synthesis, but will cause increased homocysteine. B_{12} is also needed to metabolize fatty acids with an odd number of carbon atoms. In the absence of B_{12}, methylmalonic acid will accumulate in plasma and urine. In patients with borderline B_{12} levels, elevation of plasma methylmalonic acid and homocysteine confirms biochemically a deficiency of B_{12} at the tissue level and indicates the need for B_{12} replacement therapy.

cia), and dry, rough skin. Vitamin A toxicity may also occur; long term complications include increased intracranial pressure, bone pain, and hypercalcemia.

Vitamin B_1 (Thiamine)

Thiamine, a water soluble vitamin found primarily in whole grains, is needed as a cofactor for the enzyme transketolase (an enzyme in the pentose phosphate pathway needed to keep cells stable), and to generate acetyl-CoA for entry into the Krebs cycle and for cholesterol synthesis. Most laboratories do not actually measure thiamine, rather measuring the activity of transketolase both before and after thiamine addition to the sample. It is important for practitioners to know that this method is used, since plasma thiamine levels respond rapidly to thiamine administration while transketolase does not return to normal for up to two weeks. In most countries, thiamine deficiency is usually due to alcohol abuse, where nutritional deficiency is accompanied by defects in thiamine absorption and storage. Thiamine deficiency is classically associated with **beriberi,** affecting primarily muscles (including cardiomyopathy and congestive heart failure) and the nervous system (peripheral neuropathy, Wernicke's encephalopathy, and Korsakoff's psychosis).

Vitamin B_{12} (Cyanocobalamin)

Vitamin B_{12} is a water soluble vitamin found mainly in meat, eggs, and dairy products. Body stores of B_{12} last for several years on a normal diet; most B_{12} deficiency is due to malabsorption. It serves as a cofactor for methyl transfer enzymes (Fig. 22.1), important in the synthesis of nucleic acids and in metabolism of fatty acids. B_{12} deficiency may lead to megaloblastic anemia (Chapter 24). However, in persons with high intake of folic acid (common in Europe and North America), anemia may not occur with B_{12}

deficieny (at least one-third of B_{12} deficient persons do not have anemia or increased MCV).

Absorption and Transport of Vitamin B_{12}

B_{12} absorption is a complicated process, requiring gastric acid and pancreatic enzymes to separate B_{12} from food proteins and nonspecific binders, intrinsic factor (Chapter 21) to bind liberated B_{12}, and undamaged ileal mucosa to absorb the intrinsic factor–B_{12} complex. In plasma, B_{12} is almost exclusively protein bound to either **transcobalamin II,** a physiologic transport protein which delivers B_{12} to tissues, or to other transcobalamins (also called cobalophillins) which have no physiologic role in B_{12} delivery or metabolism. Cobalophillins are produced in many tissues, including granulocytes, and are often markedly increased with malignancies, granulocytosis, and myeloproliferative diseases, causing marked increases in plasma B_{12}. This dual binding system results in a broad overlap of B_{12} levels between normal and deficient individuals: B_{12} levels less than 100 ng/mL are almost always associated with evidence of deficiency, levels between 100 and 200 ng/mL indicate deficiency in about two-thirds of cases, levels of 200 to 300 ng/mL correlate with deficiency in about one-third of cases, and levels greater than 300 ng/mL are rarely found in B_{12} deficient individuals.

Evaluation of B_{12} Absorption

The most common cause of true B_{12} deficiency is pernicious anemia, caused by type A atrophic gastritis (Chapter 21). Less commonly, low B_{12} may be due to pancreatic insufficiency, ileal disease, bacterial overgrowth of the small bowel, or the fish tapeworm *diphyllobothrium latum*. Antibodies to parietal cells are present in most patients with pernicious anemia, but are found in many other individuals and are not usually used for diagnosis. Antibodies to intrinsic factor are found in about 50–70% of patients with pernicious anemia, and are highly specific. B_{12} absorption can be evaluated directly using the Schilling test. Initially, an intramuscular dose of B_{12} is given to saturate all B_{12} binding proteins. A dose of radioactively labeled B_{12} is given orally, and urine is collected for 24 hours; normally, over 7% of radioactivity is excreted in urine in 24 hours. If this initial stage is abnormal, a second dose is given accompanied by intrinsic factor; normalization is usually considered to confirm pernicious anemia. Some patients with pernicious anemia may have normal B_{12} absorption in the first stage, but will show abnormal results if B_{12} is given along with food. Normalization in the second stage may also occur with pancreatic insufficiency. Rarely, a third stage involves repeating the first stage after administration of nonabsorbable antibiotics.

Biochemical Evidence of B_{12} Deficiency

As shown in Figure 22.1, methylmalonic acid and homocysteine will accumulate in patients with biochemical B_{12} deficiency. Measurement of these two compounds can confirm that a low or borderline B_{12} indicates true tissue deficiency of B_{12}, although as these tests are relatively expensive, this is typically used only in patients with neurologic findings strongly suggestive of deficiency. Homocysteine is also increased with congenital disorders of homocysteine metabolism and in folate deficiency, and both are increased by renal failure.

Folic Acid

Folic acid, a water soluble vitamin found mainly as polyglutamates in green leafy vegetables, is released by enzymes found in intestinal mucosa and readily absorbed. Body stores of folate only last for a few months. As with thiamine, plasma levels reflect recent intake, and can be normalized by ingestion of folate. Red blood cell folate levels return to normal much more slowly.

Vitamin D

"Vitamin" D, a fat soluble vitamin, can either be ingested from the diet or produced in the skin by sunlight. It actually is a prohormone, converted in the liver and kidneys to its active form, 1,25-dihydroxyvitamin D. Its metabolism and effects are discussed more fully in Chapter 10.

Vitamin E (Tocopherol)

A fat soluble vitamin, Vitamin E is found mainly in vegetables and vegetable oils. Its main function is to prevent oxidation of cell membrane fatty acids. After absorption from the intestine, Vitamin E is transported to tissues primarily by low density lipoprotein (LDL), where it is stored in fat cells. Vitamin E deficiency is especially common in premature infants, where it may produce hemolytic anemia due to cell membrane defects. In adults, deficiency usually occurs with malabsorption or, rarely, with LDL deficiency, and often presents with peripheral neuropathy.

Clinical Use of Nutritional Tests

There is no uniform opinion on routine evaluation of nutrition in patients admitted to hospitals. Several studies have shown a correlation between decreased albumin and increased mortality, and most authorities recommend albumin measurement to evaluate nutritional status. Addition of other tests increases the frequency of nutritional problems identified, but also increases the cost. Measurement of plasma potassium and phosphate during nutritional therapy is essential to prevent dangerous hypophosphatemia. Transthyrctin can be used to determine the adequacy of nutritional replacement, especially if a baseline value is available. These levels should normalize within 3–4 days once adequate protein is administered.

CHAPTER 23

Tumor Markers

D. ROBERT DUFOUR

LABORATORY MARKERS OF MALIGNANT TUMORS

Tumor cells differ from normal cells in many ways. This has led to a continual search for laboratory tests which would allow diagnosis and monitoring of patients with tumors in a noninvasive fashion. An ideal tumor marker would have the characteristics shown in Table 23.1. Unfortunately, none of the tumor markers yet identified meets the majority of these characteristics. A large number of markers are useful for follow-up of patients who have undergone treatment of primary tumors. Few tumor markers allow early detection of a tumor while still curable. Most plasma substances are not produced by tumors only, although a few genetic markers appear to be highly tumor specific. With few exceptions, most tumor markers are produced by a variety of tumors, and are not helpful in differential diagnosis. Most tumor markers are produced in proportion to tumor mass, but because there is a limited amount of tumor when malignancies are localized, virtually no tumor markers lead to early detection of curable tumors. A few genetic markers have shown promise of predicting aggressive tumors.

Chemical Nature of Tumor Markers

A variety of substances are useful in diagnosis and monitoring of patients with malignant tumors, summarized in Table 23.2. Tumor markers generally are classified into one of two major categories: normal cell products synthesized in excess by tumor cells, or "ectopic" proteins produced by different cell lines. Normal cell products include cell surface proteins (typically glycoproteins and mucins, often called cancer antigens, or CAs), secretory products (hormones, enzymes), and oncofetal antigens (made by fetal and tumor cells). "Ectopic" proteins are produced normally by one type of cells (e.g., pituitary ACTH production), but synthesized in other neoplastic cells (ACTH production by small cell lung carcinoma). In most cases, a limited number of tumor types reproducibly make particular "ectopic" products (ACTH and ADH in small cell carcinoma, PTH-related peptide in squamous carcinomas and breast carcinoma, erythropoietin in cerebellar hemangioblastoma, IGF-2 in leiomyosarcoma). However, normal, benign cells of the same type usually also produce the product in trace amounts.

Oncogenes

A variety of genes direct production of proteins regulating normal cell proliferation (Fig. 23.1). Mutations involving these genes are found in many types of tumors and have been termed oncogenes. The normal cell analogues of these genes are termed proto-oncogenes.

Activation of Oncogenes by Mutation

The type of mutation causing oncogene activation varies. In some cases, typically involving the *ras* oncogene, a single point mutation causes production of protein with mark-

268

Table 23.1.
Characteristics of Ideal Tumor Markers

- Produced only by tumor, or differs from normal product in some fashion
- High gradient between tumor and serum allows early detection while still in curable stage
- Produced by only a single type of tumor to allow specific diagnosis
- Levels should differ by stage
- Should separate aggressive from nonaggressive tumors
- Levels should be related to tumor mass to allow monitoring of effects of treatment
- After successful treatment, levels should allow detection of early tumor recurrence

edly increased activity. In other cases, the gene is **translocated** to a different location in the DNA, adjacent to another gene which is normally expressed. Common examples of this form of activation include the *myc* oncogene translocation to the region of the heavy chain gene in Burkitt's lymphoma, and the *abl* oncogene translocation to the *bcr* region in chronic myelogenous leukemia. In other malignancies, multiple copies of the gene are present (**gene amplification**), such as the N-*myc* oncogene in neuroblas-

Table 23.2.
Characteristics of Various Classes of Tumor Markers

Type of Marker	General Features	Other Causes of Elevation	Examples
Cell surface glycoproteins and mucins	• Found on normal and tumor cells • Requires increased production or damage to tissue to produce increased levels • Often cleared by liver	• Benign damage to normal tissues (inflammation, infarction, smoking) • Liver disease	• CA-125 • CA 19-9 (CA 50) • CA 15-3 (CA 27,29)
Oncofetal antigens	• Produced in large amounts by specific cells during fetal life, in only trace amounts by adult cells • May be expressed again with proliferation of cells (after cell injury, with tumors)	• Benign causes of cell proliferation	• α-Fetoprotein • CEA • Human chorionic gonadotropin • Placental alkaline phosphatase
Normal cell products	• Produced by normal cells and in excessive amounts by tumors of those cells • Typically produced by a limited number of cell types	• Benign proliferation of normal cells	• Monoclonal immunoglobulin • Hormones • Enzymes (PSA, acid phosphatase, alkaline phosphatase, LDH)
Genetic markers	• Usually present in tumor cells; not typically found in circulation (may be identified by PCR) • Often due to mutations, so differ from form found in normal cells • Some specific to tumor type • Some relate to prognosis	• May be abnormal in premalignant states or in families with predisposition to tumor	• Oncogenes • Chromosomal translocations • Chromosomal mutations • Oncogene products in future
Markers of host response to tumor or altered cell metabolism	• Nonspecific markers of tissue injury • With enzymes, may indicate organ involved (which may be site of primary tumor or metastases)	• Other causes of inflammation or damage to organs	• Acute phase reactant proteins (tumor necrosis factor, α₁-acidic glycoprotein) • Tissue enzymes (alkaline phosphatase, LDH) • Products of metabolism (uric acid, polyamines)
Cellular markers related to prognosis	• Found only within cells, not in circulation • Can be used only when tissue sampled (biopsy, cytology for some tumors) • Often labile, require rapid transport to laboratory and immediate freezing	• None reported	• Steroid hormone receptors • DNA ploidy • S-phase analysis (% of cells synthesizing DNA) • Cathepsin D

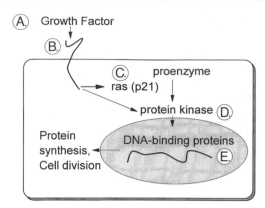

Figure 23.1. Actions of Oncogene Products. Oncogenes are analogous to normal cell genes; their products are involved in regulation of cell growth. Oncogene products may code for growth factors (**A**), such as epidermal growth factor, or growth factor receptors (**B**). Other oncogene products, such as that of the *ras* gene, serve as activators of protein kinases (**C**), while others have protein kinase activity (**D**). The final product of these steps is typically a DNA binding protein (**E**), such as the *myc* oncogene product, which stimulates DNA synthesis and, typically, protein synthesis. Other oncogenes code for proteins which inhibit cell replication, such as the *Rb* and p53 genes.

toma and the c-*erb*-2 oncogene in breast cancer. In several types of tumors, amplification of genes is associated with a poor prognosis or a more aggressive clinical course.

Tumor Suppressor Genes

A number of genes are involved in inhibiting cell replication through a variety of mechanisms. The most commonly affected gene of this type is the p53 gene, which controls processes leading to cell death (**apoptosis**). Mutations in this gene often lead to accumulation of an abnormal product in the cytoplasm which fails to prevent cell replication. Other tumor suppressor genes include the retinoblastoma (*Rb*) and breast cancer (*BrCa*) genes. Mutations in these genes are common in many types of malignancies.

Detection of Oncogene Products

Recently, a number of tests for detection of the products of certain oncogenes in plasma have been developed, although they are not yet widely available; they have mostly been used in research studies. There is hope that these will be useful as tumor markers, but most studies to date have not shown them to meet all or most of the criteria of ideal tumor markers.

Chromosome Abnormalities

A common feature of many types of malignant tumors is an alteration in the number of chromosomes (aneuploidy), with the number often varying from cell to cell. This has been used to detect tumors by examination of the cells shed from surfaces or in tissue biopsies using flow cytometry; for instance, aneuploidy in urine cytology is used for detection of recurrent bladder cancer. In many cancers, aneuploidy is associated with a poorer prognosis, while tumors with a normal chromosome number often follow a more benign course.

Demonstration of Monoclonality

As with immunoglobulins in serum, immunoglobulin gene structure is quite heterogeneous in normal B lymphocytes and plasma cells. It is necessary to delete and rearrange large amounts of DNA to produce an active immunoglobulin gene, so that early in differentiation B lymphocytes can be distinguished from all other cells. In addition, since each B lymphocyte responds to only one antigen, each has a different immunoglobulin gene structure. In a similar fashion, rearrangements in the T-cell receptor gene determine the monoclonality of T cell proliferation. Detection of rearranged immunoglobulin or T receptor genes can be accomplished by Southern blots or polymerase chain reaction; identification of a monoclonal cell proliferation can be used to diagnose lymphoma and lymphocytic leukemias.

SPECIFIC TUMOR MARKERS

A number of tumor markers have come into use for diagnosis, prognosis, and monitoring of patients with a variety of malignancies (Table 23.3).

Cell Surface Glycoproteins and Mucins

Nomenclature of these normal cell surface compounds, overexpressed in cancer cells, is based on the specific monoclonal cell line which produces an antibody against the cancer antigen. It bears no relation to the actual structure or function of the protein. With overproduction by tumors, injury to tissues, and increased cell turnover, these markers may be increased in plasma. All glycoprotein markers are cleared by the liver, with levels increased in liver disease (particularly cirrhosis or obstructive jaundice). Carcinoembryonic antigen (CEA), while a cell surface glycoprotein, is usually classified with oncofetal markers.

CA 125

This glycoprotein antigen was isolated from ovarian cancer cell lines, but is also produced by normal mesothelial cells of the peritoneum, pleura, and pericardium. CA 125 is produced by most ovarian epithelial carcinomas (except mucinous carcinomas); it is increased in 80% of patients with metastatic (Stage III) ovarian cancer, but in fewer than 50% of localized ovarian carcinomas (in some studies, in as few as 10% of cases). CA 125 is also elevated in other malignancies, notably lung, pancreatic, endometrial, and endocervical carcinomas, and in benign peritoneal disorders including endometriosis, pelvic inflammatory disease, and peritonitis. CA 125 is not recommended for use as a screening test in the general population, but may be helpful in patients with a family history of ovarian carcinoma or in evaluation of patients with ovarian masses (although sensitivity is low).

CA 19-9 (CA 50)

This mucin is a modified form of Lewis blood group antigens, originally isolated from pancreatic carcinoma. It is also increased in other GI tract malignancies, hepatocellular carcinoma, ovarian carcinoma, and in a minority of patients with lung carcinoma, particularly adenocarcinomas. Because some patients lack the Lewis gene, they will not synthesize CA 19-9 (another antibody, CA 50, detects the protein in patients lacking

Table 23.3.
Characteristics of Tumor Markers in Current Use

Marker	Tumors Producing	Tumor Specific?	Early Detection?	Related to Stage?	Related to Prognosis?	Change with Tumor Mass?	Detection of Recurrence?	Interferences, Limitations?
α-Fetoprotein (AFP)	Liver, germ cell tumors	Increased in chronic liver injury	Yes in Asia, probably not in Europe, North America	Rough correlation for germ cell tumor, not for liver	No	Yes	Yes	Falsely elevated with liver injury
β$_2$-Microglobulin	Multiple myeloma, B-cell lymphoma	Increased with renal failure, inflammation, AIDS; low with renal tubular injury	No	Rough correlation	No	Yes	Yes	Affected by renal disease
CA-125	Ovary (surface epithelial tumors)	Increased in benign peritoneal diseases (endometriosis, PID, pregnancy, ascites), liver disease	<50% of localized tumors have increased levels	Rough correlation	No	Yes unless ascites present	Yes	Falsely elevated with liver disease, ascites
CA-19-9	Pancreas, colon, stomach, lung	Increased with liver disease, particularly obstructive jaundice	<50% with pancreatic tumors <4 cm in diameter	Rough correlation	No	Yes	Yes	Falsely elevated with obstructive jaundice
CA 15-3 (27.29)	Breast	Increased with liver disease	No	No	No	Yes	Yes	Falsely elevated with liver disease
Carcinoembryonic antigen (CEA)	GI tract, pancreas, lung, breast, uterus	Increased with liver disease, smoking	<50% with localized tumors, <25% with breast	Rough correlation	No	Yes	Yes	Falsely elevated with liver disease
Cathepsin D	Breast	No	No	No	Yes	No	No	Requires tissue biopsy

Estrogen and progesterone receptors	Breast	Found in normal cells, benign tumors	No	No	No	Receptor-positive tumors have better prognosis, respond to hormone manipulation	No	Can only be detected on tumor tissue, not in blood; markers labile, require prompt specimen handling
Human chorionic gonadotropin (HCG)	Chorionic tumors (gestational trophoblastic neoplasia, germ cell tumors), breast, rarely with other tumors	Produced in normal pregnancy	No	No	No	High correlation with residual tumor mass	Yes	Some tumors produce predominantly HCG fragments or "nicked" HCG, which may cause falsely low results.
Monoclonal gammopathy	Multiple myeloma, chronic lymphocytic leukemia, B-cell lymphomas, mycosis fungoides	Produced with benign proliferation of plasma cells (monoclonal gammopathy of undetermined significance)	No	No	No	Yes; half-life of three weeks causes lag in response to treatment	Yes	Cannot separate from other causes of monoclonal gammopathy by laboratory tests alone
Prostate specific antigen (PSA)	Prostate cancer; small amounts in renal, breast cancer	Increased with benign prostate, hyperplasia prostate infarcts, acute prostatitis	About 60% of localized tumors	Rough correlation; rarely <10 ng/mL with stage D tumors	Not generally; lack of fall with androgen deprivation therapy predicts poor prognosis	Yes; half-life of three days. More rapid fall with androgen deprivation therapy than radiation therapy	Yes	Transiently elevated after biopsy, not generally affected by rectal exam unless baseline elevated. Most assays measure total PSA; percent free lower with cancer than with benign disease

the Lewis gene). CA 19-9 is elevated in 40% of small, localized pancreatic carcinomas and 90% of patients with larger tumors.

CA 15-3 (CA 27.29)

This glycoprotein antigen is found in breast milk globules; it is also produced by carcinomas of the lung, ovary, and GI tract (including the pancreas). Approximately 80–90% of patients with metastatic breast carcinoma have increased CA 15-3, but only about 25% of patients with localized breast carcinoma have elevated levels at time of diagnosis.

Oncofetal Antigens

This class of tumor markers is produced by normal cells of the fetus or placenta, with levels in the mother or baby markedly higher than the trace levels found in adults. With activation of cells normally producing these markers, levels increase, although almost never to levels encountered during fetal life. This class of markers is also increased with benign proliferation of cells in the organs normally manufacturing these proteins.

Carcinoembryonic Antigen

The first widely used tumor marker, CEA is a cell surface glycoprotein expressed in large amounts on many fetal cells. Only small amounts of CEA are produced by normal adult cells. CEA is a family of related proteins detected by immunoassays; this heterogeneity can lead to different CEA results when measured by different laboratory tests. Practitioners should use the same laboratory for CEA measurements on a single patient; if a switch is needed, a sample should be assayed using both old and new methods for comparison. Carcinoembryonic antigen is elevated in carcinomas of the GI tract, lung, breast, bladder, ovary, and uterus. It is also increased with inflammatory bowel disease, lung infections, and smoking. Like other glycoproteins, it is cleared by the liver and increased with liver disease, particularly cirrhosis. In healthy persons, CEA is rarely greater than 3 ng/mL, but may be 5–10 ng/mL in benign disease and as high as 10–20 ng/mL in smokers. In cancer patients, CEA is elevated in less than 25% of patients with localized disease, but in about 60–80% (depending on tumor type) with distant metastases. Poorly differentiated tumors typically do not produce CEA. Measurement of CEA is most useful in follow-up after therapy. Rising levels will indicate likely tumor recurrence several months before clinical evidence of recurrent disease. Large studies indicate few patients detected by elevated CEA actually benefit from earlier diagnosis of recurrence, however.

α-Fetoprotein

During fetal life, α-fetoprotein (AFP) is a major serum protein synthesized primarily in the liver and rudimentary yolk sac, with small amounts made in the fetal GI tract and kidney. The average plasma concentration peaks at 1–3 mg/mL (1,000,000–3,000,000 ng/mL) near three months gestation. Levels reach 50 μg/mL (50,000 ng/mL) at birth and average adult levels of 0–10 ng/mL by one to two years of age. In adults, increased AFP is usually due to chronic hepatitis, hepatocellular carcinoma, or germ cell tumors. Approximately 30% of patients with chronic hepatitis have increased AFP, usually less than 10 times normal but occasionally up to 25 times normal. Elevated AFP occurs in 80–90% of patients with hepatocellular carcinoma, with 50–70% having levels more than 100 times normal. In areas where hepatocellular carcinoma is usually due to chronic hepatitis B infection without cirrhosis, screening programs using AFP and ultrasound have improved survival in patients with tumor, but in countries where most cases occur in association with cirrhosis, AFP seldom detects curable hepatocellular carcinoma. In germ cell tumors, AFP is increased in about 40% of patients, primarily in those with embryonal carcinoma or yolk sac tumors. After tumor treatment, AFP half-life is about 5–7 days; to detect significant falls, levels should not be performed more frequently than once a month.

Human Chorionic Gonadotropin

Aside from pregnancy, human chorionic gonadotropin (HCG) (Chapter 17) is typically produced by trophoblastic tumors. In normal pregnancy, HCG is rarely over 1,000,000 mU/mL, with values above this suggesting trophoblastic neoplasia. In plasma, HCG has a half-life of approximately one day, and markedly elevated levels may require 2–3 weeks to return to normal. About 10% of patients with germ cell tumors of the ovary or testis also have elevated HCG. Human chorionic gonadotropin is also increased in some patients with large cell carcinoma of the lung, lymphoma, gastric carcinoma, and breast carcinoma.

Normal Cell Products

This class represents the largest group of tumor markers. Some of the markers are produced by one principal cell type (prostate specific antigen (PSA), monoclonal immunoglobulins, β_2-microglobulin, hormones) and are highly specific for proliferation of that cell, whether benign or malignant. Other markers are found in many cells (enzymes such as LDH, alkaline phosphatase, acid phosphatase) and may help to detect many types of tumors, although specificity for tumor or type of tumor is low. Hormone production by tumors is discussed in Chapters 10, 13, 14, and 15.

Prostate Specific Antigen

Prostate specific antigen is an enzyme produced predominantly in the prostate, with trace amounts synthesized in other organs including kidneys and breast. It is a protease, involved in liquefaction of semen after ejaculation. Prostate specific antigen production is stimulated by sex steroids, particularly dihydrotestosterone. Levels of PSA increase slowly with increasing age, and plasma levels are directly related to prostate mass; upper reference limits are usually set at 4 ng/mL. Benign prostatic hyperplasia (BPH) is associated with increased PSA in about 33% of cases. In most, PSA is slightly elevated, with values greater then 10 ng/mL in only 5% of cases. Acute inflammation or infarction of the prostate and acute renal failure produce transient increases in PSA which may exceed 20 ng/mL, while chronic prostatitis does not cause increased PSA. Prostate specific antigen is transiently increased (for about one month) by prostate biopsy, but not by rectal examination if patients have normal PSA. For reasons that are not clear, PSA is approximately 25% lower during hospitalization; PSA testing should ideally be performed on outpatients. A number of approaches have been suggested for separating mild (4–10 ng/mL) PSA elevations due to BPH from those due to prostate cancer. In plasma, PSA is largely bound to antiproteases, with the free PSA fraction higher in BPH than in prostate cancer. Free PSA of less than 15% of an elevated total PSA strongly suggests prostate cancer. The PSA "density" (PSA divided by prostate volume as determined by ultrasound) is higher with prostate cancer than with BPH. A PSA density greater than 0.15 indicates an 80% likelihood of prostate cancer. The PSA velocity, the rate of increase in PSA over time, is higher with prostate cancer than with BPH. The level of PSA starts to increase an average of 5 years before clinical diagnosis of prostate cancer and increases, on average, more than 0.75 ng/mL per year in measurements performed at least 6 months apart, with an increase in three consecutive specimens confirming a trend.

As with other tumor markers, PSA is less sensitive in detecting localized disease, with only about 60% of Stage A and B prostate cancers associated with increased PSA, and only 20% having PSA greater than 10 ng/mL. A few studies have suggested that PSA is more likely to be elevated in aggressive cancers than in those that will progress slowly. Only about 1% of prostate cancers do not appear to produce PSA. Following radical prostatectomy, PSA should fall to undetectable levels by three months after surgery. After radiation therapy, PSA falls gradually, usually to within the reference range, by six months after completion of radiation. A rising PSA after treatment almost always indicates recurrent cancer, with increases occurring an average of 1–2 years before clinical evidence of recurrence. Measurement of PSA is useful for evaluating the response to chemotherapy; even though antiandrogens can decrease PSA production in the absence of decreased tumor mass, normalization of PSA levels with antiandrogens is associated with a better prognosis and prolonged survival compared to those without at least an 80% fall in PSA.

β_2-Microglobulin (Chapter 9)

This HLA antigen associated protein is increased with malignant neoplasms of B lymphocytes (particularly lymphoma and multiple myeloma). Levels are related to tumor mass, but are also affected by impaired renal tubular function (common after chemotherapy and in light chain nephropathy); falsely low levels occur due to increased urinary losses. Falsely elevated levels occur in renal failure. Nonspecific stimulation of the immune system in infection (particularly in HIV infection) also increases β_2-microglobulin levels.

5-Hydroxyindole Acetic Acid

Serotonin is produced by tumors derived from cells of the diffuse neuroendocrine system, particularly carcinoid tumors of the intestine. 5-Hydroxyindole acetic acid is a major liver metabolite of serotonin and is excreted in the urine. Increased 5-HIAA is often used to recognize and monitor patients with carcinoid tumors. Many foods, particularly nuts and many fruits, also give rise to 5-HIAA; dietary intake must be controlled before collection to avoid variation in results that are not due to tumor.

Enzymes

Increases in enzymes due to cell or tissue damage are common in tumors, and are discussed below. A number of tumors make enzymes which are not commonly found in plasma; these may be used as tumor markers. Germ cell tumors such as seminoma or dysgerminoma and renal cell carcinoma produce primarily LDH isoenzyme 1; prostate and small cell lung cancers synthesize CK BB isoenzyme; some germ cell tumors manufacture placental isoenzyme of alkaline phosphatase; and a number of tumors synthesize an unusual alkaline phosphatase termed the Regan isoenzyme.

Genetic Markers

Since the mid-1980s, oncogenes have been recognized to play a pivotal role in development of cancer. To date, oncogenes have not been widely used as tumor markers in clinical practice. Typically, tumor cells have mutations involving several oncogenes; common alterations involve the *ras* and *myc* oncogenes and the p53 tumor suppressor gene. The genes themselves can only be detected in tumor cells, which usually requires tissue biopsy or examination of cells shed into body fluids. In research laboratories, amplification techniques such as PCR have detected mutated oncogenes in circulating tumor cells in patients with metastatic cancer, however, specific mutations occur in a relatively small percentage of tumors of a given type. One application which has proven useful is the *bcr-abl* fusion gene found in chronic myelogenous leukemia. Detection of the abnormal gene has proven to be the most sensitive means for detecting residual leukemia. In many cases, oncogene mutations occur in premalignant conditions (such as p53 mutations in colon polyps and *ras* oncogene mutations in bladder carcinoma-in-situ), which conceivably could lead to prevention of invasive cancer. In some cases, oncogene products differ from normal cell products and can be detected in blood or body fluids. Rarely, hereditary mutation in a tumor suppressor gene (such as *BrCa* and *Rb* genes) can be found in all cell lines; presence of the mutant gene predicts high likelihood of cancer development. It is likely that the use of oncogenes in tumor diagnosis will continue to expand in the future.

Markers of Host Response to Tumor or Altered Cell Metabolism

A number of changes take place in an individual with cancer which may lead to an alteration in laboratory test results. These types of tumor markers are typically elevated only with advanced tumors and are commonly affected by benign disease. In some tumors, they may be the only biochemical marker that allows monitoring of the effects of treatment.

Nonspecific Response to Tumors

Tumors typically trigger the production of cytokines, causing increased production of acute phase reactant proteins (Chapter 9). Tumors commonly metastasize to liver and bone, causing increased production of alkaline phosphatase. Tumor cells often turn over at a faster rate than normal cells, producing increases in plasma levels of cell contents such as uric acid (from breakdown of purines in DNA and ATP) and lactate dehydrogenase (LDH).

Tumor Lysis Syndrome

When tumor cells are destroyed rapidly, either by high spontaneous turnover or therapy, most commonly in leukemia, lymphoma, and small cell carcinoma of lung, the release of cell contents increases blood levels of LDH, K^+, and PO_4. Hyperkalemia and hyperphosphatemia may become symptomatic, with the latter inducing hypocalcemia or metastatic calcification. Uric acid (formed from purines) may cause renal failure which further worsens hyperkalemia and hyperphosphatemia, while lactic acidosis is often present as well.

Abnormal Amine Accumulation

Many tumors have abnormal metabolism, causing accumulation of amines such as putrescine and spermidine. In brain and bladder tumors, concentrations are markedly increased in CSF and urine, respectively, and relate to tumor mass.

Cellular Markers Related to Prognosis

In certain types of cancers, a variety of cell markers predict prognosis or guide treatment in patients with localized tumors. These markers have been most widely used in breast cancer, although they have been studied in other types of tumors. Cellular markers can only be studied when tumor cells can be sampled, either through biopsy or, for tumors on mucosal surfaces, by exfoliative cytology. Although a number of markers belong to this category, only the most important are discussed in detail.

Steroid Receptors

In hormone responsive cells, steroid hormones exert their effects by binding to cytoplasmic or nuclear receptors which ultimately alter DNA synthesis. In normal breast tissue, estrogen receptors trigger production of nuclear progesterone receptors which exert hormonal effects. Breast tumors which have either estrogen or estrogen plus progesterone receptors tend to have a slightly better prognosis, and typically respond to hormonal manipulation (estrogen deprivation or antiestrogens such as tamoxifen). Steroid receptors are highly labile, and tissue must be promptly frozen after removal.

DNA Ploidy

Normal cells have 46 chromosomes, while many tumor cells have a different chromosome number. In some tumors, the chromosome number differs markedly from 46 (aneuploidy). In bladder cancers, tumor recurrence can often be detected by performing DNA analysis of cells shed in urine using flow cytometry. In some other tumors, aneuploidy is associated with poor prognosis.

Cathepsin D

Normal cells produce a variety of proteases; cathepsin D is normally found in lysosomes. In breast cancer, overproduction of cathepsin D has been associated with poor prognosis. As with steroid hormone receptors, rapid handling and freezing of tissue is needed to prevent loss of activity.

USES OF TUMOR MARKERS IN PATIENTS WITH CANCER

Tumor markers could conceivably be used to predict individuals likely to develop cancer, to detect cancers early while they are still curable, to stage tumors, and to monitor the effects of treatment. Most tumor markers function poorly in all areas except monitoring therapy.

When Not to Measure Tumor Markers

In addition to limitations discussed below under each category of use, a number of situations affect levels of tumor markers independent of changes in tumor status. In most tumors, marker levels are much higher within the tumor than in plasma; levels should not be measured for at least one month after surgery or biopsy of a tumor. Most tumor markers are measured by immunoassays, using monoclonal antibodies raised in mouse cell lines; exposure to mouse proteins (as may occur with use of mono-clonal antibodies in imaging or treating tumors) can cause false elevations of tumor markers. If a patient has been treated with monoclonal antibodies, the laboratory should be notified to attempt to limit interference in measuring the tumor marker. Random variation in tumor marker levels is much greater than for most other sub-stances. In general, a change of 25% or less is usually due to random variation in levels, and changes in therapy should be based on greater changes documented in three consecutive measurements. Tumor marker levels are often affected by diseases in or-gans involved in clearance of the tumor marker. Acute liver disease leads to increased levels of markers cleared by liver (CEA, CAs) and, often, to increased production of AFP. Acute renal failure often causes increased PSA and β_2-microglobulin. Injury to benign cells producing tumor markers can cause increased marker levels: CA 125 is often increased with ascites and peritonitis, CA 19-9 may be increased with pancreatitis, AFP is increased in chronic hepatitis, PSA is increased with acute prostatitis or prostate infarcts, and β_2-microglobulin is increased with acute inflammation. Tumor markers should not be measured in states of damage to organs clearing or producing the marker.

Tumor Markers in Cancer Screening

Ideally, tumor markers should allow early detection of tumors to permit early diagnosis and cure. Because of the nonspecific nature of most tumor markers and low sensitivity in localized disease, almost all tumor markers have failed to be useful in cancer screen-ing. Two major exceptions are PSA and AFP. As discussed in Chapter 3, biases may be introduced by screening which appear to produce a benefit when none actually exists. It is known that many prostate cancers are slowly progressive and would produce no ill effects if not diagnosed. Because of this, many authorities have questioned the wisdom of screening for prostate cancer until firm evidence supports a benefit from screening. Others have looked at the large number of deaths from prostate cancer and have advocated universal screening. It is clear that PSA will detect approximately 60% of localized prostate cancers, with specificity increased by using such measurements as PSA density and free PSA fraction.

Screening for hepatocellular carcinoma has proven successful in detecting resect-able carcinomas in high risk populations in Asia, but not in Europe or North America. The poor performance in these populations relates to the high prevalence of elevated AFP in patients with chronic hepatitis, the major risk factor for development of hepato-cellular carcinoma.

Tumor Markers in Cancer Staging

Most tumor markers show a relationship between levels and extent of tumor, although in general, overlap in values between stages does not allow accurate staging (Fig. 23.2). Over 80% of patients with distant metastases of prostate cancer have PSA greater than 10 ng/mL. A PSA below this value has been used in deciding not to perform bone scan. For many other tumor markers, marked elevations in the tumor marker suggest widespread metastases and a need for evaluation for metastases before attempting surgical resection for cure of the tumor.

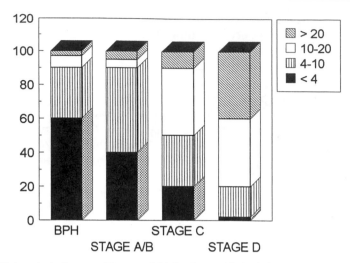

Figure 23.2. PSA Levels in Prostate Disease. PSA is elevated in both benign and malignant diseases of prostate. In most assays, normal PSA is less than 4 ng/mL. In patients with benign prostatic hyperplasia (BPH), PSA is increased in about 40% of cases, but is greater than 10 ng/mL in only about 10% of cases. In localized prostate cancer, while PSA is increased in 60% of patients, it is above 10 ng/mL in a similar 10% of cases, making PSA a poor test for differentiating localized prostatic cancer from BPH. With advancing stage, most patients have PSA greater than 10 ng/mL. Other tumor markers show similar overlap in values between localized cancer and benign diseases, performing well only with advanced cancer.

Tumor Markers in Cancer Follow-up

Monitoring the effects of treatment is the most widely accepted indication for measuring tumor markers. Changes in tumor mass are generally reflected in changes in marker levels. It is important for practitioners to be aware of whenever a laboratory changes its method for measuring a tumor marker (or whenever tests are sent to a different laboratory); tumor marker levels are generally not interchangeable between methods or laboratories. If a change in laboratory testing is needed, it is important to measure the marker level with both the new and old methods to check for differences in patient results; if the level using the old method was unchanged from earlier results, the result from the new method is accepted as a baseline. After successful tumor treatment, marker levels should fall (if previously elevated) to within reference limits. This may take several months, depending on the initial marker level and the rate of marker clearance. For example, in trophoblastic neoplasia, HCG levels may be 1,000,000 mU/mL or higher at diagnosis, with reference limits of 5 mU/mL; with a half-life of 24 hours, it takes almost 3 weeks for HCG to fall within reference limits. Many tumor markers have a much longer half-life, so that one or two months are needed for levels to reach their lowest point. A common approach after surgical tumor resection checks marker levels one to three months after surgery; failure to normalize suggests residual tumor. For many tumors, such as breast and colon cancer, tumor markers are not elevated at initial diagnosis, but rise with tumor recurrence. In these cases a normal initial tumor marker level does not rule out its use for following therapy. Once marker levels are within the reference range, repeat testing is generally done every 3 months for 1–2 years and every 6 months thereafter. An increase of more than 25% in marker level should be confirmed by a repeat level in about one month; a further increase strongly suggests tumor recurrence. In general, markers become elevated several months to (in the case of PSA) years before clinical evidence proves tumor recurrence. Because of high specificity, rising PSA and HCG are used to begin chemotherapy in patients with prostate cancer and trophoblastic neoplasia, respectively. For other tumors, it is usually considered necessary to confirm tumor recurrence by biopsy or cytology before therapy is begun. Once therapy is given, successful treatment should again cause marker levels to fall within reference limits.

SECTION III.

HEMATOLOGIC PATHOLOGY

CHAPTER 24

Red Blood Cell Disorders

D. ROBERT DUFOUR

PHYSIOLOGY OF RED BLOOD CELL PRODUCTION AND DESTRUCTION

Red blood cells (RBCs) are the most numerous blood cells, with an average adult having 4.5–6.0 trillion RBCs per liter of blood. RBCs are nondividing and contain predominantly hemoglobin, needed for the delivery of oxygen to tissue. Continual bone marrow production of RBCs is necessary to replace the approximately 1% of cells destroyed each day at the end of their useful lifespan.

Production of Red Blood Cells

Red blood cell production occurs predominantly in bone marrow (Fig. 24.1). Each of the four key elements must be present in proper balance for maintenance of normal RBC production.

Bone Marrow Stem Cells

Through unclear mechanisms, uncommitted marrow stem cells transform to early RBC precursors, capable of reproducing in bursts of activity (**B**urst **F**orming **U**nits-**E**rythroid, or BFU-E). As these mature, they become more committed stem cells (**C**olony **F**orming **U**nits-**E**rythroid, or CFU-E), capable of establishing colonies of hemoglobin synthesizing erythroblasts. The CFU-E contain many erythropoietin (EPO) receptors, and EPO promotes survival of these cells.

Erythrocyte Maturation

Once stimulated by EPO, CFU-E divide to produce pronormoblasts, accompanied by a reduction in size of the nucleus and the synthesis of hemoglobin (discussed below), structural proteins such as spectrin and ankyrin (necessary for normal cell fluidity), red blood cell antigens, and enzymes (needed to maintain cell integrity). Cell multiplication and division occurs rapidly, and requires Vitamin B_{12} and tetrahydrofolate (Chapter 22) for normal maturation. As cells mature, they acquire more hemoglobin while becoming gradually smaller, ultimately losing the ability to divide; the nuclei then condense. Eventually, precursors lose their nuclei, precluding further RNA synthesis, However, RNA persists for several more days, allowing additional enzyme synthesis. The RNA gives young RBCs a purplish tint when stained with Wright's stain (**polychromatophilic RBCs**) and cells containing RNA (**reticulocytes**) can be identified as dots and lines of staining with dyes such as New Methylene Blue. Once released from the bone marrow, reticulocytes generally lose their RNA within about 24 hours.

Erythropoietin

Production of EPO occurs in response to tissue hypoxia. Interstitial cells of the renal cortex make 95% of EPO in adults, but the liver makes most EPO in fetuses and about

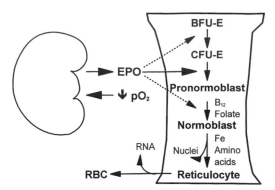

Figure 24.1. Regulation of RBC Production. Erythropoietin is produced by the kidney in response to decreased oxygen delivery. EPO stimulates division of CFU-E and production of early committed RBC precursors, pronormoblasts. Initially, DNA synthesis is rapid in these early cells, requiring folic acid and vitamin B_{12}. As cells mature further, they require amino acids and iron for synthesis of hemoglobin, which constitutes 95% of RBC protein. In the late stages of maturation, the nuclei involute and are eventually lost, usually before cells are released from the marrow. RNA persists in released cells, usually for a period of one day; RNA containing cells are called reticulocytes. After losing their RNA, RBCs survive for approximately 4 months in the circulation; thus, about 1% of cells are replaced each day by reticulocytes.

5% in adults. EPO has a half-life of about 4–12 hours, with most of the hormone apparently removed by metabolism.

Hemoglobin

This oxygen carrying protein comprises about 95% of red cell protein; the size and color of red cells is thus dependent on relative amount of hemoglobin present. To produce hemoglobin, it is necessary to synthesize the protein globin chains, a porphyrin ring (protoporphyrin), and incorporate iron (converting protoporphyrin to heme) (Fig. 24.2).

Globin Chain Synthesis

Hemoglobin consists of four globin chains, arranged in two pairs. Normally, there are two α chains and two chains of another type. It is the additional chains that give rise to different forms of hemoglobin. In adults, the predominant form is hemoglobin A ($\alpha_2\beta_2$), with a small percentage (less than 2.5%) of hemoglobin A_2 ($\alpha_2\delta_2$). During fetal life, the predominant form, hemoglobin F ($\alpha_2\gamma_2$), has a much higher affinity for oxygen, facilitating transport from mother to baby across the placenta. There are two pairs of genes on chromosome 16 controlling the synthesis of α chains, and on chromosome 11 a single pair of genes each for synthesis of β, γ, and δ chains. Genes for these latter three globin chains are located adjacent to each other.

Porphyrin Synthesis

Porphyrins, the precursors to heme, are synthesized by a complicated pathway illustrated in Figure 24.2. A similar pathway is employed in the liver, but there are different isoenzymes, causing some deficiencies to affect red cell formation while others do not. Deficiencies in porphyrin synthesis may give rise to neuropsychiatric symptoms, skin blisters associated with sensitivity to light, and hemolytic anemia. The most common

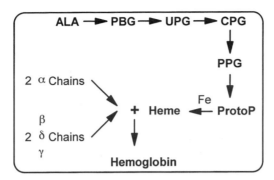

Figure 24.2. Production of Hemoglobin. Heme, the iron containing compound which binds oxygen, is synthesized from succinyl-CoA by a complicated series of enzymatic steps. δ-Aminolevulinic acid (ALA) is converted to a single ring structure, porpholinogen (PBG), by ALA dehydratase. Many drugs, including ethanol and barbiturates, increase activity of this enzyme. PBG is converted to uroporphyrinogen (UPG), a four ring structure, by porphobilinogen deaminase; this enzyme is deficient in acute intermittent porphyria. UPG is converted to coproporphyrinogen (CPG) by UPG decarboxylase; this enzyme is deficient in porphyria cutanea tarda. CPG is converted to protoporphyrinogen (PPG) and then to protoporphyrin (Proto-P). The enzyme ferrochelatase adds iron, producing heme; this enzyme is inhibited by lead poisoning or iron deficiency, producing the alternate chelated compound zinc protoporphyrin. Globin chains are synthesized by two types of genes, producing α chains and either β, δ, or γ chains. Two of each type combine with heme to produce the oxygen carrying protein hemoglobin.

disorders of porphyrin synthesis, enzymes affected, products accumulating, and clinical manifestations are listed in Table 24.1.

Iron Metabolism

The normal absorption, storage, and delivery of iron to tissue is illustrated in Figure 24.3. Dietary iron requires liberation from food and normal gastric acid production to allow its absorption. In the duodenum, iron uptake is dependent on the proportion

Table 24.1
Patterns of Common Porphyrias

Disorder	Enzyme Deficient	Product(s) Accumulating	Clinical Features
Acute intermittent porphyria (AIP)	Porphobilinogen deaminase	Porphobilinogen, aminolevulinic acid	Abdominal pain, neuropathy, SIADH, weakness, psychiatric symptoms—often precipitated by drugs
Porphyria cutanea tarda (PCT)	Uroporphyrinogen decarboxylase	Uroporphyrin	Skin blisters, particularly after sun exposure, onset in adulthood, skin fragility and abnormal pigmentation, increased and decreased hair
Variegate porphyria	Protoporphyrinogen oxidase	Protoporphyrinogen	Features of both AIP and PCT often present, but those of AIP more dominant
Erythropoietic protoporphyria	Ferrochelatase	Protoporphyrin	Skin burning, erythema, itching, edema after light exposure, usually occurring in children, gallstones

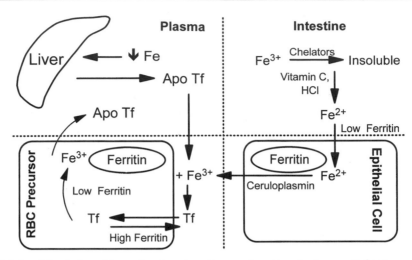

Figure 24.3. Iron Metabolism. Dietary iron is reduced by gastric acid to the ferrous (Fe^{2+}) ion and is subsequently absorbed in the duodenum. Iron equilibrates with ferritin in mucosal cells, and some iron is oxidized by ceruloplasmin to ferric (Fe^{3+}) ion, allowing it to bind to molecules of apotransferrin synthesized by the liver. Transferrin (Tf) delivers iron to many tissues, most importantly to RBC precursors, which have Tf receptors. Inside cells, Tf releases iron in inverse proportion to cellular ferritin iron stores; high ferritin favors release of Tf back to plasma, while low ferritin favors iron release and release of apotransferrin into plasma. The released iron is then available for incorporation into heme.

in the free Fe^{++} state: complexing agents such as oxalate decrease absorption, while reducing agents (like vitamin C) convert more iron to Fe^{++} and allow its absorption. The amount of iron in the duodenal mucosal cells also affects absorption: low iron content favors absorption, while high content slightly inhibits iron uptake. However, the amount of available Fe^{++} in the intestines is the most important factor affecting absorption. Transferrin, the iron transport protein, is synthesized by the liver (Chapter 9) in inverse proportion to iron stores in the body. In the intestine, transferrin takes up two molecules of iron from the mucosal cell as it is oxidized to Fe^{+++} by ceruloplasmin (Chapter 9). In the bone marrow (and in many other body cells), red cell precursors have transferrin receptors which lead to the uptake of transferrin, removal of iron and its incorporation into heme, and the release of transferrin back to the circulation. Heme inhibits release of iron from transferrin. Excess iron accumulates as part of the soluble storage protein **ferritin.** Excess ferritin may lose some of its protein and become converted to **hemosiderin,** an insoluble form of storage iron. While large hemosiderin aggregates may be visible as golden brown deposits in tissue, both hemosiderin and ferritin are best identified in tissue using iron stains.

Red Cell Destruction

Since RBCs cannot replicate, they have a finite lifespan in the circulation (average 120 days). The use of the term "half-life" is not accurate with RBCs, as few fail to survive for 100 days, but then die rapidly after this time. As RBCs age, they lose some enzymes and surface membrane, making the cells less able to traverse the narrow passages through the spleen. Eventually, cells are trapped in the spleen and destroyed. Liberated hemoglobin is metabolized to heme and protein. The protein is converted to amino acids while the heme is broken down to bilirubin and free iron. Some of the iron is released to transferrin, while some may accumulate as ferritin. When red cell death occurs in the circulation, hemoglobin combines with haptoglobin (Chapter 9). The hemoglobin-haptoglobin complex is removed from the circulation within minutes.

LABORATORY TESTS OF RBCS AND RBC COMPONENTS

While patients with severe anemia (deficiency of RBCs) can be recognized by pallor on clinical examination, laboratory testing is usually needed to determine the severity of anemia and detect its presence in milder cases, as well as to determine the pathogenesis of anemia and monitor its treatment. Laboratory tests are also useful in the diagnosis and determination of the etiology of polycythemia (increased RBCs).

Complete Blood Count

The most common test used to evaluate circulating blood cells is the complete blood count (CBC). In most laboratories, automated instruments perform quantitation of RBCs, white blood cells (WBCs), and platelets, as well as evaluation of the size and shape of RBCs (WBCs and platelets are discussed in subsequent chapters). While there are manual methods available for measurement of the three key RBC measurements (hemoglobin, hematocrit, and RBC number) and manual calculation of most so-called RBC indices, they are seldom employed except for hematocrit measurements. Specimens for CBC are collected in a lavender top tube, containing the anticoagulant and calcium chelator EDTA, usually in liquid form. The most common cause of problems with improper collection is a failure to mix the tube completely, causing blood clotting. Large clots will be readily detected and the specimen will be rejected, but smaller clots may cause underestimation of true values. Inadequate filling of the tubes will also cause falsely low results due to dilution by the anticoagulant. As discussed in Chapter 1, hemoconcentration increases concentration of proteins and cells; drawing blood in persons who have been standing, or with prolonged use of tourniquets, may cause an average 5–8% increase in RBC concentration. Because supine posture causes movement of fluid back into the vessels, it is common for patients admitted to hospitals to show an average 5-8% fall in RBCs due to fluid movement. Such collection and patient preparation variables must always be kept in mind when evaluating CBC results.

Hematocrit

The percentage of blood volume occupied by red cells is termed the hematocrit. In automated instruments, hematocrit is calculated from the RBC count times the average cell size (**M**ean **C**ell **V**olume, MCV). The calculated hematocrit is also affected by factors which interfere with measurement of RBC count or MCV, as discussed below. Hematocrit can also be measured after centrifuging a capillary tube containing blood and determining the height of the RBC column compared to the total height of the blood column. In general, the spun hematocrit is slightly (2–3%) higher because a small amount of plasma is trapped between RBCs. With abnormal RBC shapes, the difference between "spun" and machine hematocrit increases. Practitioners should keep this difference in mind if using both types of measurements on the same patient.

Hemoglobin

The amount of hemoglobin is measured directly by its ability to absorb light. To prevent differences in the relative amounts of oxyhemoglobin and other forms of hemoglobin from affecting results, all hemoglobin is converted to cyanmethemoglobin before measurement. Hemoglobin measurements are, in general, the most reliable in the CBC; when there is a discrepancy between the hemoglobin and the hematocrit or RBC count, the hemoglobin is almost always correct. One exception to this rule occurs when there are other substances in plasma which absorb or scatter light, particularly triglycerides. In such cases, the hemoglobin is falsely increased.

RBC Count

The number of circulating RBCs is determined by counting cells as they pass through a sizing chamber or a laser beam. This also allows determination of the size of the cells. Red blood cell counts may be falsely low in patients who have cold agglutinins (common following mycoplasma infections) or in whom RBCs are abnormally stacked (with increased immunoglobulins). This will also cause falsely high MCV.

RBC Indices

A number of ways of determining RBC size and hemoglobin content have been used for many years. Of these, the most useful is the MCV, a measure of the average size of RBCs. Although usually measured directly, it can also be calculated using the formula in Equation 24.1.

$$MCV \ (fL) = \frac{Hematocrit \ (in \ \%)}{RBC \ Count \ (in \ millions/\mu L)} \times 10 \tag{1}$$

The MCV is of help in determining the cause of anemia as will be discussed later: small RBCs are almost always due to decreased hemoglobin production, while large RBCs usually indicate a defect in cell maturation. As an average, MCV may be affected by the presence of two divergent problems, so that a combination of small and large cells may produce a normal MCV. The instrument is set to include only sizes tradition-ally associated with RBCs in its calculation. Sometimes, the instrument may include large platelets (smaller than a normal RBC) in its MCV calculations, causing falsely decreased results. Red blood cell clumps which falsely decrease the RBC count will falsely increase the MCV. The other two indices, MCH (Eq. 24.2)

$$MCH \ (pg) = \frac{Hemoglobin \ (in \ g/dL)}{RBC \ Count \ (in \ millions/\mu L)} \times 10 \tag{2}$$

and MCHC (Eq. 24.3),

$$MCHC \ (g/dL) = \frac{Hemoglobin \ (in \ g/dL)}{Hematocrit \ (in \ \%)} \times 100 \tag{3}$$

seldom provide additional information to the MCV because, as mentioned earlier, most of the size of the RBC in normal individuals is due to its concentration of hemoglobin.

Red Cell Distribution Width

The red cell distribution width (RDW), the standard deviation of the MCV, is a measure of the degree of uniformity in size of RBCs. It is of most use in evaluation of patients with microcytosis: thalassemia is expected to produce uniformly sized cells and a nor-mal RDW, while iron deficiency would cause a gradual reduction in cell size and a high RDW. In practice, the sensitivity of the RDW for iron deficiency is relatively high, but about 40–50% of patients with other causes of anemia (including thalassemia) also have high RDW. Thus, a normal RDW is helpful in excluding iron deficiency, but a high RDW has little utility in differential diagnosis because most types of anemia are associated with increased RDW.

Reticulocyte Count

The number of red blood cells containing RNA is a marker of the rate of release of cells from the bone marrow. With increased EPO levels, production of new RBCs should increase, producing a rise in reticulocyte count. The number of reticulocytes is the most reliable measure of rate of RBC production. Many laboratories, however, still report reticulocyte *percentage* of total RBCs. If there are fewer RBCs than normal, this percentage can increase slightly. For proper interpretation, the reticulocyte number should always be used. Many laboratories still use manual reticulocyte counts, which show high variability from one measurement to the next. Automated instrument methods are used by many laboratories and are both more accurate and highly reproducible. It is important for clinicians to be aware of the method used by the laboratory in interpreting reticulocyte counts.

Peripheral Blood Smear

Although many practitioners have come to rely on MCV in initial evaluation of patients with anemia, there are a number of abnormalities in RBC size and shape that can only be appreciated by examination of the peripheral smear. Figure 24.4 illustrates the most common RBC abnormalities. Although it does not allow diagnosis of any disorders directly, the information obtained from peripheral smear review often suggests the correct diagnosis and helps in guiding further diagnostic tests. It should be performed in all patients in whom the etiology of anemia is not clear from the initial evaluation, before extensive laboratory tests are ordered. When examining the peripheral smear, the area where cells are just touching each other should be examined; cell appearance is often altered in thinner and thicker parts of the smear. Cell clumps are also common at the edges of the smear, and do not have the same significance in that location. True morphologic changes will appear uniformly throughout the thin part of the smear, while artifacts will be present occasionally.

Tests of Iron Metabolism

Iron deficiency is the most common cause of microcytic anemia and occurs in up to 8% of children and menstruating women. Iron overload (hemochromatosis) is the most common congenital disorder in persons of European ancestry. Tests of iron status are commonly ordered to identify both iron deficiency and overload.

Serum Iron

Serum iron concentration usually measures iron bound to transferrin, and provides an indirect measure of the rate of delivery to tissue. In iron deficiency, iron is rapidly taken off of transferrin and serum iron will be low, while high levels occur with iron overload at least partly due to delayed clearance. Serum iron is a relatively simple test, but must be collected appropriately to allow proper interpretation. Red blood cells contain many times the iron content of plasma. Hemolysis falsely elevates iron concentration, and serum iron is transiently elevated (usually for less than 24 hours) following

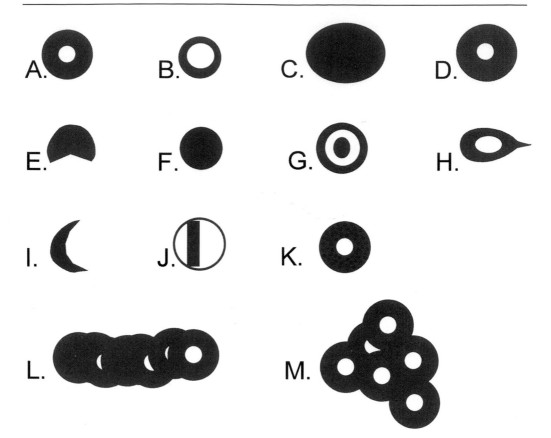

Figure 24.4. Common RBC Abnormalities. Normal RBCs (**A**) are usually similar in size to the nucleus of a normal small lymphocyte, and have a small central zone of pale staining. With deficient hemoglobin synthesis, cells become smaller (microcytic) and lighter stained, with a larger unstained area (hypochromic) (**B**). Defective maturation of RBCs, usually due to folate deficiency, causes larger RBCs (macrocytes), often oval in shape rather than round (**C**). Other causes of macrocytosis usually produce round, larger cells. Young red cells (**D**) have a somewhat bluer stain than normal RBCs (polychromatophilia), due to their higher RNA content. With mechanical fragmentation, cells are sliced to abnormal shapes, often forming "helmet cells" (**E**) or smaller fragments, collectively called schistocytes. With deficient cell membrane, cells become darker stained, slightly smaller, and have a reduced zone of pallor, forming spherocytes (**F**). When there is excess membrane, cells form target cells (**G**), most commonly seen in thalassemia, liver disease, or hemoglobinopathies. Tear drop cells or dacrocytes (**H**) occur with bone marrow replacement. Homozygous mutations in hemoglobin can cause gelation of hemoglobin, forming sickled cells (**I**) or crystals of hemoglobin C (**J**). Basophilic stippling (**K**) can occur with many causes of anemia, but large, coarse granules are more commonly seen with lead poisoning. Clumps of RBCs fall into two major types: linear stacks (**L**), termed rouleaux, usually seen with increased globulins (particularly in multiple myeloma or Waldenstrom's macroglobulinemia), or cell clumps with irregular clusters of cells (**M**), usually due to cold agglutinins.

blood transfusion. Iron levels are up to 40% higher in the morning than later in the day. Serum iron concentration is also affected by menstrual bleeding, being significantly lower in women during the time of menstrual bleeding. Absorption of dietary iron (or iron in multivitamins) may cause transient elevation in serum iron concentration; patients should be told not to take iron containing medications on the morning when serum iron is to be measured. Because transferrin levels fall with acute inflammation, liver disease, and nephrotic syndrome, serum iron will be low in all of these situations.

Evaluation of Transferrin Concentration

Transferrin concentration can either be measured directly or estimated as **T**otal **I**ron **B**inding **C**apacity, or TIBC, using the formula in Chapter 9. In general, transferrin production is inversely related to body iron stores: low stores are associated with high transferrin, while high stores cause low transferrin. As discussed earlier, however, transferrin levels are also affected by inflammation, protein loss, nutritional status, and liver disease.

Transferrin Saturation

The ratio of serum iron to iron binding capacity is termed transferrin saturation. Iron deficiency is typically associated with low saturation (below 15%), while iron overload usually causes high saturation (greater than 50% in women, greater than 62% in men). High saturation is common with many of the situations listed above under iron, and in many patients with other forms of anemia.

Serum Ferritin

In normal individuals, the amount of ferritin in serum is directly related to total body iron stores, making it a good marker of iron deficiency. Because ferritin is widely distributed in tissues, many forms of tissue damage cause falsely elevated ferritin: this includes inflammatory disorders, malignancy, and particularly hepatitis. In acutely or chronically ill patients, ferritin may not be a useful test. Additionally, administration of iron supplements causes an increase in serum ferritin. In children, this occurs quickly, while in adults the increase takes 2–3 weeks after oral supplements but occurs within 24 hours with parenteral iron. Ferritin does not appear to be affected by blood transfusion.

Zinc ("Free Erythrocyte") Protoporphyrin

The last step in the synthesis of heme is incorporation of iron into protoporphyrin, producing heme. When incorporation of iron is not possible, zinc is added instead. Zinc protoporphyrin has a different pattern of fluorescence than heme, and can be readily detected with simple fluorescence readers. Any other disorder impairing the addition of iron to protoporphyrin, including lead poisoning and anemia of chronic disease, will also cause increased zinc protoporphyrin. Because the test can be performed using capillary blood, it is often used to screen for iron deficiency and lead poisoning in children.

Bone Marrow Iron Stain

The most definitive way to recognize iron deficiency is by documenting reduced bone marrow iron stores using an iron stain. Iron stores are best identified using the Prussian Blue reaction, where iron in macrophages and in red cell precursors stains deep blue. Iron stores in macrophages are usually reliable indicators of total body iron content; however, marrow iron may be transiently increased following blood transfusion, and may be falsely low in patients with myeloproliferative disorders.

Identification of Congenital RBC Defects

A number of congenital RBC defects may cause anemia or, rarely, polycythemia. Defects in RBC metabolism, structure, and hemoglobin composition may all be detected by screening tests and confirmed by more definitive testing.

RBC Enzyme Deficiencies

A number of enzymes are important for normal RBC function; congenital deficiency often causes hemolysis. Deficiency of enzymes in glucose metabolism, such as pyruvate kinase, impairs production of ATP necessary to maintain RBC shape. Glucose-6-phosphate dehydrogenase (G6PD) is an enzyme of the hexose monophosphate shunt, the defense mechanism of the red cell against free radicals. Measurement of red cell activity of these enzymes can be used to detect deficiency.

RBC Structural Variants

A number of rare inherited defects cause abnormal formation of RBC structural proteins such as spectrin or ankyrin, causing abnormal RBC shape and decreased RBC survival. The most common are spherocytosis, elliptocytosis, and pyropoikilocytosis. Because of a reduced surface area to volume ratio, cells are more sensitive to lysis in low ionic strength solutions than normal cells. This can be detected using osmotic fragility, in which cells are incubated with varying concentrations of saline and the fraction of cells lysing is measured.

Hemoglobin Variants

Mutations in genes producing globin chains are relatively common, usually associated with single amino acid changes in globin chains. Such mutations may be clinically insignificant, but the more important ones cause hemolysis or alter oxygen affinity. Other mutations involve deletion or impaired expression of globin chains, causing decreased production of structurally normal hemoglobins.

Hemoglobin Electrophoresis

Many hemoglobin variants have single amino acid substitutions in one of the α or, more commonly, β chains, altering hemoglobin charge and producing different migration of the variant from hemoglobin A on an electrophoretic gel (Figure 24.5). Because the charge on a given amino acid varies with pH, some variants cannot be separated from hemoglobin A or each other at one pH, but may be separated if electrophoresis is performed at another pH. Because of this, laboratories often perform electrophoresis for hemoglobin variants at pH 8.6 and pH 6.0 to allow identification of most common variants. With many hemoglobin variants, production of the abnormal globin chain is somewhat impaired compared to the normal chain. Persons who are heterozygous for a β chain variant, producing one normal globin chain and one abnormal chain, will generally have about 55–60% hemoglobin A and 40–45% of the variant; with an α-chain variant, single gene mutations cause about 20–25% variant and the remainder hemoglobin A. Persons homozygous for a β chain variant have no normal hemoglobin A.

Solubility Tests

A few hemoglobin variants, especially hemoglobin S, are unstable in the deoxyhemoglobin form; exposure of blood to reducing agents causes precipitation. In test tubes, this causes a solution of hemoglobin to become cloudy, best seen by holding the tube in front of newspaper or lined paper and noting distortion or an inability to see the

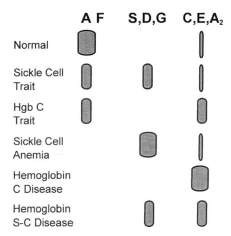

Figure 24.5. Hemoglobin Electrophoresis. At pH 8.6, the most common hemoglobin variants migrate in groups, as illustrated here. Hemoglobin C, S, and G are relatively common in persons of African ancestry, while hemoglobin E is common in individuals from the Indochinese peninsula. Hemoglobin D and O are rarely seen in North America. While presumptive diagnosis of hemoglobinopathies can be made based on the patterns illustrated, most laboratories also perform electrophoresis at a second pH to allow separation of these variants when there is any question as to the correct type of hemoglobin present. Quantitation of hemoglobins A_2 and F can not be reliably determined from electrophoresis. The positions of less common hemoglobin variants are not illustrated in this figure.

normal markings. On a slide, deoxyhemoglobin will precipitate and cause deformity of cells (sickle cells) which can be seen under the microscope.

Quantitation of Hemoglobin A_2 and F

Low levels of hemoglobin A_2 and F, and migration of hemoglobin F close to hemoglobin A, preclude accurate quantitation of these variants by electrophoresis. In situations where quantitative levels are needed, such as in diagnosis of thalassemia, different methods are used. Hemoglobin A_2 can be quantified using column chromatography. Hemoglobin F is resistant to denaturation in alkali, and can be quantified as residual hemoglobin after alkali is added. Additionally, hemoglobin F is not eluted from cells on exposure to acid, a feature used in the Kleihauer-Betke test described in Chapter 17.

Oxygen Affinity

Some hemoglobin variants have mutations in the region of the globin chain that binds heme, altering their affinity for oxygen. Variants with high oxygen affinity produce polycythemia, while variants with low affinity produce anemia (due to the effects of altered oxygen delivery on EPO production). Standard measures of oxygen saturation, such as pulse oximeters and estimation of saturation from blood gases, are inadequate to demonstrate altered oxygen affinity. Measurement of the pO_2 at which hemoglobin is half-saturated (P_{50}) is the best screening test for documenting such variants.

Evaluation of RBC Turnover

Uncommonly, anemia is due to decreased survival of cells. When this occurs, RBC contents are released, producing a number of biochemical changes that allow detection of hemolysis.

Increased Reticulocyte Count

In response to anemia, normal bone marrow increases RBC production, increasing the reticulocyte count. This simple test is often overlooked in the initial evaluation of patients with anemia. Deficiency of factors needed to make red cells or damage to bone marrow prevents reticulocyte response; thus, a high count is helpful in suggesting increased turnover as a cause of anemia, but a normal or low count does not rule it out.

Increased Plasma Levels of RBC Contents

When RBC turnover occurs, there will be increased plasma levels of substances present in high concentration in RBCs, but in low concentration in plasma. The most common markers of this type are hemoglobin, LDH, and indirect bilirubin. Plasma free hemoglobin is elevated only with severe, intravascular hemolysis, making it an insensitive test; moreover, hemolysis due to specimen collection is extremely common. LDH is more sensitive than hemoglobin, but elevation of LDH can occur in many other disorders and from hemolysis during specimen collection. An increase in unconjugated (indirect) bilirubin is seen with moderate to severe hemolysis, but also occurs in the relatively common Gilbert's syndrome (Chapter 11). Comparison of current bilirubin results to previous ones is more helpful than the absolute level, as Gilbert's syndrome causes a relatively stable elevation of unconjugated bilirubin.

Decreased Plasma Haptoglobin

Haptoglobin, discussed more fully in Chapter 9, binds free hemoglobin with a rapid clearance of the resulting complex; hemolysis causes low haptoglobin levels. Because of the frequent presence of a congenital absence of haptoglobin and increases in haptoglobin that occur with inflammation, a change in haptoglobin is more helpful than an isolated level. If possible, specimens from before the episode of a fall in hematocrit should be used to document a decrease in haptoglobin concentration which would confirm hemolysis. Demonstration of increases in haptoglobin after resolution of anemia can also confirm hemolysis.

Urine Hemosiderin

Excess free hemoglobin (above the binding capacity of haptoglobin) passes through the glomerulus into urine. Tubular cells reabsorb some hemoglobin and degrade it, releasing iron which ultimately forms hemosiderin. As tubular cells are replaced, the shed cells can be stained with the Prussian Blue reaction to reveal the iron. Hemosiderin will appear in urine about 2–3 days after an episode of hemolysis.

Direct Antiglobulin (Coombs') Test

In some cases, hemolysis is caused by antibodies to red blood cell antigens. The antiglobulin (Coombs') reagent is an animal antibody to human immunoglobulin; most current antiglobulin reagents detect only IgG, but some detect other immunoglobulins or complement. In the direct antiglobulin test (DAT), the antiglobulin reagent is directly mixed with a patient's red cells; agglutination of red cells indicates antibody present on the red cell surface. A positive DAT is typically present with autoimmune hemolytic anemias and with some drug induced hemolytic anemias. Positive DAT also occurs with hemolytic transfusion reactions and in hemolytic disease of the newborn.

Tests of Porphyrin Metabolism

Congenital defects in the production of porphyrins may present as hemolytic anemias, although the most common porphyrias do not produce hemolysis. Tests of porphyrin metabolism are relatively rarely used, and many textbooks refer to older, relatively insensitive tests for detection of porphyrin disorders. Only the most important porphyrin tests are discussed here; older tests such as the bedside light exposure screen and Watson-Schwartz test are very insensitive and are not recommended for diagnostic purposes.

Quantitative Porphyrins

Increased urine excretion of porphyrins or their precursors is found in virtually all inherited and acquired disorders of porphyrin metabolism. Various porphyrins and precursors can be separated by chromatography and quantified. This test is the recommended screening test for porphyrias and should be done in a 24 hour urine. Since porphyrins are unstable at acidic pH and on exposure to light, the collection container should be opaque, and should have sodium carbonate added to it before collection begins to prevent deterioration.

Cell Enzyme Levels

The most common neurologic porphyria, acute intermittent porphyria, is caused by a heterozygous deficiency of the enzyme porphobilinogen deaminase. This enzyme can be measured in blood cells in a few reference laboratories.

Bone Marrow Examination

Although the cause of anemia and polycythemia can be determined without examination of bone marrow in many cases, bone marrow aspirate and biopsy remain the test of choice to document many disorders, particularly defects in precursors (aplastic anemia), myelodysplastic syndromes (Chapter 25), bone marrow replacement, and to confirm the diagnosis in anemias of chronic disease and megaloblastic anemias. Bone marrow aspirate is usually adequate to evaluate most RBC production disorders, but will not allow recognition of a number of important diseases with a nonuniform distribution of disease. For this reason, an actual biopsy of bone marrow is usually performed simultaneously. In the case of RBC disorders, the major factors evaluated in bone marrow are the relative number of RBC precursors, the overall cellularity of the bone marrow, the maturation of RBC precursors, and the amount of iron stores. Special procedures such as chromosomal analysis are usually not needed for RBC disorders unless myelodysplastic syndrome is suspected. Normal bone marrow has a ratio of myeloid to erythroid precursors (M:E ratio) of between 2:1 and 5:1; low ratios occur with normal bone marrow response to anemia. The overall ratio of hematologic cells to fat decreases with age, from about 3:1 in children, to about 2:1 in young to middle aged adults, down to about 1:1.5 in older adults (in marrow taken from the iliac crest, the most common site of bone marrow biopsy). Iron stain can be used to semiquantitatively identify storage iron in macrophages, as well as determine the rate of incorporation of iron in RBC precursors into heme. In normal individuals, iron staining can be

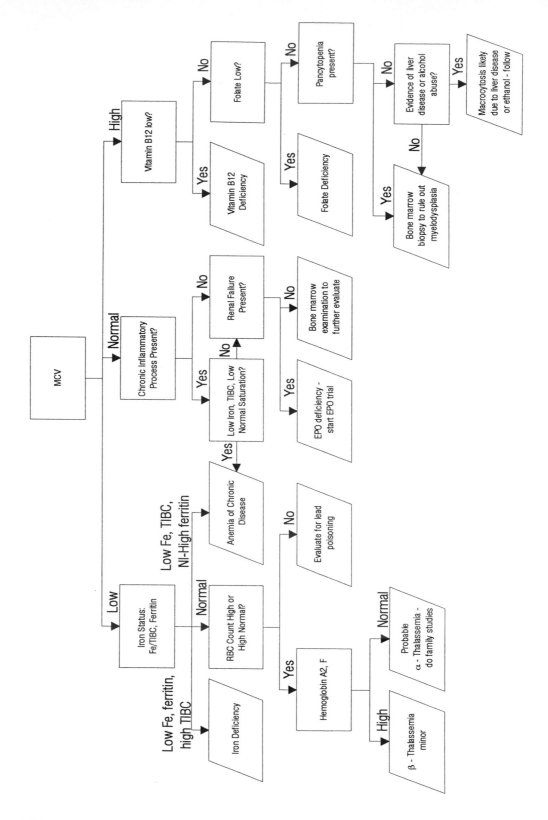

Table 24.2
Initial Evaluation of Anemic Patients

- Evaluate for evidence of bleeding (orthostatic hypotension, positive guaiac in stool or NG aspirate)
- Evaluate past and family history for clues to congenital causes of anemia
- If negative, evaluate MCV for clues to pathogenesis
- Use high reticulocyte count to recognize increased turnover
- In questionable cases, use markers of cell turnover (haptoglobin, urine hemosiderin, and nonspecific markers such as LDH, total bilirubin) to recognize hemolysis

seen in about $\frac{1}{4}$ to $\frac{1}{2}$ of RBC precursors (termed **sideroblasts**), usually as isolated granules of iron. With impaired iron incorporation, as in chronic disease anemia, the number of sideroblasts increases. In some myelodysplastic disorders, not only the number of sideroblasts but also the amount of iron in sideroblasts increases, producing extensive iron in mitochondria forming a circle around the nucleus (**ringed sideroblasts**).

ANEMIA

A decrease in the amount of hemoglobin is usually used as the definition of anemia. As discussed earlier, a relative fall in the number of RBCs and in hemoglobin occurs in most patients following admission to the hospital. It should also be remembered that pathologic changes in plasma volume, as occur with dehydration or overhydration, can also affect RBC count and hemoglobin level, either masking or falsely creating anemia, respectively. Anemia is far and away the most common red cell disorder, and is one of the most common coexisting conditions in hospitalized patients.

Pathogenesis of Anemia

Two major mechanisms are responsible for development of anemia: decreased RBC production and decreased RBC survival. Initial evaluation of patients with anemia (Table 24.2) should identify which mechanism is responsible for anemia. Some disorders (notably thalassemia major and vitamin B_{12} or folate deficiency) produce a mixed picture. Decreased survival may be caused by acute blood loss (usually readily apparent from history and physical examination), or to hemolysis. Hemolytic anemia can be suspected from an increased reticulocyte count, and confirmed by the presence of markers of hemolysis that were discussed earlier. Decreased production, recognized by anemia without increased reticulocyte response, accounts for approximately 90% of cases. An approach to decreased production anemias is outlined in Figure 24.6.

◀——

Figure 24.6. Approach to Anemia Due to Decreased Production. Before proceeding further, patients should be evaluated for evidence of blood loss (hypotension, positive guaiac tests) or increased turnover (increased reticulocyte count); the causes illustrated here represent about 90% of evaluations for anemia in nonbleeding patients. Initial classification is best based on cell size, which suggests general pathogenetic mechanisms. Small cells are usually due to impaired hemoglobin synthesis in iron deficiency, thalassemia, or rarely from chronic disease. Large cells are usually due to B_{12} or folate deficiency. Tests to identify the cause of these variants should be based on the pattern of cell size observed. Patients with normal cell size usually have either impaired EPO (renal failure, due to underproduction; chronic disease, due to impaired response) or bone marrow failure. Bone marrow examination is most commonly used to evaluate patients with normocytic anemias to determine the cause for marrow failure.

Microcytic Anemia

Decreased RBC size usually indicates defective synthesis of hemoglobin. On a peripheral smear, microcytosis is typically accompanied by hypochromia due to decreased hemoglobin, but MCHC is not always low in microcytic anemias. An increased MCHC should suggest the presence of spherocytosis (discussed under hemolytic anemias), although only 50% of patients with spherocytosis have high MCHC. The two most common causes of microcytic anemia are iron deficiency anemia and thalassemia; in young children, lead toxicity is an important cause. In some cases of anemia of chronic disease (discussed under normocytic anemia), microcytosis may occur, but MCV is typically not as low as in other causes. As discussed earlier, RDW may be helpful in patients with microcytic anemia: a normal result virtually rules out iron deficiency or lead poisoning, while making thalassemia the likely diagnosis; elevated results may occur in up to half of patients with thalassemia.

Iron Deficiency

The most common cause of anemia overall, iron deficiency may result from decreased iron intake (the most common cause in children) or increased loss of iron due to chronic blood loss (the most common cause in adults). In adult men and postmenopausal women, the diagnosis of iron deficiency requires documentation of the cause of blood loss. Early in iron deficiency, bone marrow and other cellular iron stores are depleted, without any effect on hemoglobin synthesis. After iron stores are depleted, serum ferritin levels fall. Decreased marrow iron stimulates production of transferrin, and also increases the rate of removal of iron from transferrin. This produces a decreased serum iron, increased TIBC, and low transferrin saturation (under 10%). As iron becomes deficient, zinc protoporphyrin accumulates. In otherwise healthy adults, ferritin is the best test for diagnosis of iron deficiency, however, in ill patients false increases in ferritin due to tissue injury often produce normal or increased serum ferritin in patients with iron deficiency. Because bone marrow aspiration is relatively invasive, in such cases serum iron and transferrin saturation are usually used to document iron deficiency (even though they are less sensitive than bone marrow iron stains).

Thalassemia

Defined as an inherited defect in the genes controlling globin chain synthesis (most commonly gene deletion), thalassemia is a common genetic defect in certain ethnic groups (Southeast Asians, Africans—α-thalassemia; Mediterranean, African—β-thalassemia). The type of thalassemia is determined by which genes are defective (α-thalassemia, defective α-chain genes, etc.). Because of differences in the number of genes for globin chains, the clinical manifestations of α-thalassemia and β-thalassemia differ somewhat. In addition, in the case of β-thalassemia, the defect may involve mutations in the gene controlling synthesis that reduces the rate of globin synthesized (β^+-thalassemia), rather than complete gene deletion (β^0-thalassemia). Hemoglobin E, a mutation common in southeast Asia, causes a clinical picture similar to thalassemia minor.

General Features of Thalassemia

Characteristically, thalassemia produces very small RBCs, often smaller than those in iron deficiency, while zinc protoporphyrin is typically normal. In milder forms, (thalassemia trait), anemia is often mild or absent, and the RBC count is characteristically high normal or elevated. Target cells are commonly seen on a peripheral smear; they are rare in iron deficiency. A number of indices have been proposed to help differentiate thalassemia trait from iron deficiency based on RBC parameters; the most widely used is given in Equation 24.4.

$$Index = MCV - 5 \times Hgb - RBC - 3.4 \qquad (4)$$

A positive number suggests iron deficiency, while a negative number suggests thalassemia. The index is helpful in otherwise healthy patients, but is affected by other factors altering RBC production which are commonly present in acutely ill patients.

In more severe forms of thalassemia, the imbalance between synthesis of α and β chains results in decreased red cell survival. In β-thalassemia, excess free α-chains precipitate, causing destruction of RBC precursors in the bone marrow (**ineffective erythropoiesis**). In α-thalassemia, β-chain tetramers (**hemoglobin H**) are unstable, precipitate as cells age, and result in decreased RBC survival.

α-Thalassemia

In North America, α-thalassemia is common in persons of African ancestry; approximately 25% have deletion of one gene, and 2–5% have deletion of two genes. Because α chains are needed for synthesis of all normal hemoglobins (A, A_2, F), the relative proportions of each are normal; thus, hemoglobin electrophoresis is not useful for diagnosis. In persons who also have a β-chain variant such as hemoglobin S trait, the relative percentage of S hemoglobin has been found to be helpful in recognizing the coexistence of α-thalassemia. In patients with normal α-chain genes Hgb S averages 42% of total hemoglobin, with one α-chain gene deletion the average Hgb S is 35%, and with deletion of two α-chain genes the average Hgb S is only 28%. Deletion of three α-chain genes causes excess Hgb H production and hemolytic anemia. Deletion of all four α-chain genes prevents production of hemoglobin F, causing severe fetal anemia, congestive heart failure (hydrops fetalis), and usually intrauterine death.

β-Thalassemia

Deletion or reduction in expression of one β-chain gene produces β-thalassemia minor, producing mainly decreased hemoglobin synthesis and microcytosis. The relative proportion of hemoglobin A_2 is increased in most cases, and hemoglobin F is increased in the majority of cases. With homozygous deficiency, no normal Hgb A is produced in β^0-thalassemia, although a small amount is present in homozygous β^+-thalassemia. At birth, infants appear relatively normal since Hgb F is the major hemoglobin during fetal life; symptoms of anemia generally develop by a few months of age.

Lead Poisoning

In children, severe lead poisoning (Chapter 19) may produce microcytic anemia. On a peripheral smear, coarse basophilic stippling in RBCs should suggest the diagnosis, which can be confirmed with blood lead levels. Zinc protoporphyrin is almost always increased in anemia due to lead poisoning, but is also high in iron deficiency.

Macrocytic Anemia

High MCV usually indicates defects in cell maturation, most commonly due to a deficiency of vitamins needed for DNA synthesis (folate, B_{12}), or myelodysplastic disorders.

High MCV with or without anemia is often present with alcohol abuse and liver disease; target cells are often present in patients with alcohol abuse. Initial evaluation of patients with high MCV should include a peripheral smear examination. Abnormal maturation due to a deficiency of B_{12} or folate typically produces oval macrocytes, and often is associated with an increased number of nuclear lobes in WBC (**hypersegmentation**); more than 5% of cells with five lobes, and any cells with six lobes strongly suggests this diagnosis. Laboratory testing for B_{12} and folate deficiency is discussed in Chapter 22. Vitamin deficiency may also be associated with ineffective erythropoiesis, producing laboratory evidence of hemolysis. In severe cases, decreased WBC and platelets are also present. In patients with documented vitamin deficiency, a trial of vitamin replacement should be given. A failure of cell counts to respond quickly to replacement of the deficient vitamin should cause re-evaluation and consideration of bone marrow biopsy.

Normocytic Anemia Due to Decreased Production

Failure of marrow production of RBCs in response to anemia is a common pathogenetic mechanism, especially in patients with a variety of chronic illnesses. In many cases, the pathogenesis can be determined from simple laboratory tests in the presence of a compatible clinical picture. Many patients with this pattern of anemia will require bone marrow examination to completely determine the pathogenesis of anemia.

Anemia in Renal Failure

Defective production of EPO is characteristically present in patients with renal disease. The degree of EPO underproduction is related to progression of disease; patients with end stage renal failure will produce virtually no EPO. Measurement of EPO is usually not necessary in such patients. Monitoring patients on EPO therapy should include regular measurement of serum iron and transferrin saturation to detect a need to treat these patients with iron supplements.

Anemia of Chronic Disease

Chronic inflammation, as occurs with chronic infections, inflammatory disorders such as autoimmune diseases, or in malignancies, is often associated with anemia. Although the exact pathogenesis of anemia is not known, there is typically relative resistance to the actions of EPO and defects in mobilization of iron from macrophages to transferrin. Serum iron and iron binding capacity or transferrin are typically both low, with low normal to normal saturation. Serum ferritin is typically normal or increased. Erythropoietin levels are often useful in determining likelihood of response to EPO therapy; patients with EPO concentration over 10–15 times normal seldom respond to EPO, while those with lower levels often respond to exogenous EPO even though plasma levels are already high. If a bone marrow aspirate is performed, iron stains typically demonstrate increased storage iron in macrophages but decreased numbers of sideroblasts, confirming a decreased ability to deliver iron to RBC precursors.

Bone Marrow Replacement

Any disorder in which a large percentage of the bone marrow is replaced by abnormal cells will cause anemia. Common causes include multiple myeloma, metastatic carcinoma, and myeloproliferative disorders. In many of these cases, the peripheral smear will show tear-drop shaped RBCs (dacrocytes), thought to be due to difficulty in RBCs escaping the damaged bone marrow. Immature RBCs (nucleated RBCs) and WBCs are often seen in peripheral blood smears. Bone marrow biopsy is usually needed to establish the diagnosis, since aspirates are often difficult or impossible to obtain in such cases. In patients with malignancies involving the bone marrow, tumor cells are often not present in the aspirate.

Aplastic Anemia

Failure of bone marrow is a rare cause of anemia due to decreased production. Anemia is often accompanied by low WBCs and platelets (pancytopenia). As with bone marrow replacement, bone marrow biopsy is typically needed to establish this diagnosis.

Low Affinity Hemoglobin Variants

Extremely rarely, normocytic anemia is due to congenital hemoglobin variants which release oxygen to tissues more readily than normal hemoglobin. While some of these variants can be identified using hemoglobin electrophoresis, the most reliable way to identify their presence is by measuring P_{50}.

Normocytic Anemia Due to Hemolysis

Approximately 10% of anemia is due to decreased RBC survival, suspected by increased reticulocyte count and confirmed in equivocal cases by the markers of hemolysis listed earlier. The MCV is usually normal or slightly increased, reflecting a higher percentage of younger cells. Hemolysis is usually divided into intrinsic RBC abnormalities, most of which are congenital and occur predominantly in children (such as hemoglobinopathies, enzyme deficiencies, and abnormal cell shapes due to structural protein deficiencies), and extrinsic RBC abnormalities, in which RBCs are damaged by factors external to the RBC that are almost always acquired and which occur predominantly in adults (such as autoimmune hemolysis and mechanical fragmentation). Examination of peripheral smears is especially helpful in hemolytic anemias; many hemolytic anemias can be presumptively identified from the peripheral smear.

Hemoglobinopathies

Several hemoglobin variants, most notably Hgb S and C, are associated with decreased RBC survival. Sickle cell anemia, due to homozygosity for a mutation on the β chain which allows stacking of deoxyhemoglobin causing changes in RBC shape, occurs in about 1 in 500 persons of African ancestry in North America. Hemoglobin C, found in about 1 in 5000 persons of African ancestry in North America, produces crystals of oxyhemoglobin. Both homozygous disorders can often be recognized on the peripheral smear. Patients heterozygous for either disorder typically have no clinical manifestations and do not have hemolysis or anemia. Persons inheriting one abnormal copy of each of these two abnormal hemoglobins (hemoglobin S-C disease) usually have mild anemia, but may develop vascular occlusions.

Glucose-6-Phosphate Dehydrogenase Deficiency

As an enzyme of the hexose monophosphate shunt, glucose-6-phosphate dehydrogenase (G6PD) plays an important role in the defense against oxidant stresses on the red cells. Deficiency of G6PD is common in persons of Mediterranean and African ancestry.

Exposure of deficient RBCs to infections or oxidant drugs, particularly sulfonamides, primaquine, pyridium, and nitrofurantoin, will cause hemolysis. In the most common form of G6PD deficiency (seen in persons of African ancestry), enzyme activity is relatively normal in young cells but decreases in older cells; activity may thus be normal following an episode of hemolysis. Because G6PD is an X-linked enzyme, it may be difficult to document deficiency in women who have a heterozygous deficiency.

Hereditary Spherocytosis and Related Disorders

As discussed earlier, defects in the synthesis of structural proteins produce RBCs that are more rigid than normal. Such cells are morphologically normal at the time of release from the bone marrow, but gradually become deformed from a loss of cell membrane to develop into spherocytes or elliptocytes. The abnormal cell shape eventually prevents these RBCs from passing through the spleen and causes premature cell lysis. Diagnosis can usually be suspected from examination of peripheral blood and recognizing the characteristic cell shapes. MCHC is increased in about half of cases, but MCV and MCH are usually normal. In equivocal cases, demonstration of increased osmotic fragility can establish the presence of abnormal cell surface area.

Autoimmune Hemolytic Anemia

Either as an isolated phenomenon, as part of an autoimmune disease such as systemic lupus, or due to drugs which attach to RBC membranes, IgG antibodies may develop against red cells, causing decreased RBC survival. Antigen–antibody complexes are partially removed, along with portions of membrane, in the spleen, producing spherocytic cells that have a shortened survival. Rarely, hemolysis is caused by IgM antibodies (cold agglutinins), which react best at low temperatures. In most cases, these antibodies only cause agglutination of cells after collection, causing a falsely low RBC and falsely high MCV. When present in high titers, they may produce hemolysis, particularly when patients are exposed to cold. Cold agglutinins often follow infection with *Mycoplasma pneumoniae* or infectious mononucleosis. In all types of autoimmune hemolysis, a peripheral smear often demonstrates increased numbers of spherocytes. The definitive test to diagnose this abnormality is the direct antiglobulin test (DAT). Because many patients have circulating antibody, cross-matching of blood for transfusion is typically incompatible. Generally, as long as the patient's serum is no more "incompatible" with the blood to be transfused than with the patient's own blood, there will be no risks to transfusion.

Hemolytic Disease of the Newborn

IgG antibodies are capable of crossing the placenta. Maternal antibodies against red cell antigens present on fetal RBCs will cause hemolysis of the baby's blood both before and after birth, as discussed in Chapter 17.

Microangiopathic Hemolytic Anemia

In patients with disseminated blood clotting or mechanical heart valves, RBCs may be sliced passing over strands of fibrin or valve surfaces. The resulting fragmented cells are termed **schistocytes,** often taking the shape of helmets or irregularly shaped cell fragments; they can be readily detected on peripheral smear. The most common causes

Table 24.3
Causes of Increased Erythropoietin and Secondary Polycythemia

Appropriate Response to Decreased O_2
- Smoking or other carbon monoxide exposure
- Chronic lung disease
- Right to left shunting of blood (including cirrhosis)
- High affinity hemoglobin variants
- High altitude

Inappropriate Production
- Renal cell carcinoma and renal cysts
- Hepatocellular carcinoma
- Leiomyoma
- Cerebellar hemangioblastoma

of microangiopathic hemolysis are disseminated intravascular coagulation, metastatic carcinomas, and thrombotic thrombocytopenic purpura.

POLYCYTHEMIA

An increase in RBC mass over normal is termed polycythemia. As an increased plasma volume may produce transient "anemia," dehydration or hemoconcentration can also cause a relative increase in RBC concentration without increased RBC mass. While the definition implies that RBC mass must be measured (which may be accomplished by using radioactive chromium to label a patient's red cells, then injecting them back and resampling to determine the degree of dilution of the label and, by inference, the volume of RBCs), polycythemia is usually recognized by increased hemoglobin and hematocrit if hemoconcentration can be excluded. Polycythemia is much less common than anemia.

Secondary Polycythemia

Increased RBC mass due to overproduction of EPO is termed secondary polycythemia. Causes of excess EPO production are outlined in Table 24.3. Because it is simple and noninvasive, determination of oxygen saturation should be the initial test in evaluation of polycythemia, with low saturation (as often occurs in cyanotic congenital heart disease, in smokers, and in chronic lung disease) providing an explanation for polycythemia. Measurement of EPO should be done if oxygen saturation is normal. Before searching for an EPO producing tumor, measurement of P_{50} should be done to rule out congenital hemoglobin variants with a high affinity for oxygen.

Polycythemia Vera

Inappropriate overproduction of RBCs as part of a myeloproliferative disorder is termed polycythemia vera (P. vera), an uncommon disorder, usually of older adults, due to mutations that cause BFU-E to proliferate in the absence (or reduced amounts) of EPO. Erythropoietin levels should be decreased in P. vera, but low levels are difficult to quantify in most laboratories. Chromosome analysis is normal in most patients at diagnosis, although the frequency of chromosomal abnormalities increases with duration of disease. P. vera is usually associated with an increased platelet count, often causing arterial or venous thrombosis. White blood cells are also increased in the majority of patients, often with increased basophils. Diagnosis of P. vera is made in patients with polycythemia and normal oxygen saturation if the patient has splenomegaly or two of the following features: thrombocytosis, leukocytosis, high leukocyte alkaline phosphatase score, or high vitamin B_{12}.

IRON OVERLOAD (HEMOCHROMATOSIS)

Increased accumulation of iron in the body often leads to damage to many organs, particularly the liver, heart, pancreatic islets, joints, and endocrine organs; the clinical picture is termed hemochromatosis. Iron excess may occur with heavy intake of iron, either orally (seen in South African Bantus who brew beer in iron pots) or in patients with chronic anemia following many years of blood transfusions. More commonly, however, hemochromatosis is due to a genetic defect in the regulation of iron absorption. The defective gene, located on chromosome 6 close to the HLA antigens (often linked to HLA-A3), is the most common genetic defect in persons of European ancestry. In the United States, the frequency of carriers of the gene is estimated to be 1 in 8, with homozygous individuals representing 1 in 200–300. This has led some groups, such as the College of American Pathologists, to recommend routine screening for this disorder. Because of excess iron accumulation, serum iron is typically elevated, while transferrin is decreased, producing high transferrin saturation. Proposed decision levels are saturation over 50% in women or over 62% in men. In younger adults, ferritin may be normal, but in older adults ferritin levels are often 10–20 times normal or even higher. Therapy usually consists of regular phlebotomy (either once or twice monthly) until MCV begins to fall, indicating iron deficiency; serum ferritin is then usually used to indicate the need for further phlebotomy. Iron removal often improves certain complications, particularly cardiac and liver disease, but does not improve many of the complications such as diabetes, arthritis, or hypogonadism, and may not lower the risk of hepatocellular carcinoma.

CHAPTER 25

White Cells and Related Disorders

SCOTT GRAHAM

NORMAL WHITE BLOOD CELL STRUCTURE AND PHYSIOLOGY

Granulocyte Physiology

Neutrophils are produced in the bone marrow, arising from a common neutrophil-monocyte progenitor cell, under the influence of various hematopoietic growth factors. Granulocyte, monocyte colony-stimulating factor (GM-CSF) is the primary factor involved in neutrophil maturation, and is produced by activated T lymphocytes, monocytes, endothelium, and fibroblasts. Other factors influencing neutrophil maturation include granulocyte colony-stimulating factor (G-CSF), interleukins 1, 3, and 6 (IL-1, IL-3, and IL-6).

Morphologically recognizable maturation begins with the myeloblast, and proceeds through promyelocyte and myelocyte within the mitotic pool. The postmitotic pool includes the metamyelocyte, band, and segmented neutrophil, and also constitutes the maturation-storage pool. Complete maturation requires about 12 days. Increased demand results in increased mitotic divisions and decreased maturation time.

Neutrophils spend only about eight hours within the peripheral circulation. Neutrophils in the vascular compartment are found either within the circulating pool or marginated pool. Marginated neutrophils move slowly along the endothelium of small vessels. Once neutrophils enter the tissues, they never return to circulation.

Migration of neutrophils to areas of infection or inflammation is mediated by chemotactic substances including the C5a complement fragment, platelet activating factor, and bacterial polypeptides. Neutrophils have IgG Fc receptors, which enhance the phagocytosis of bacteria opsonized by immunoglobulin.

Cytoplasmic components are responsible for bacteriocidal activity. The primary azurophilic granule develops at the promyelocyte stage and contains peroxidase and other enzymes specifically intended to kill and digest microorganisms. Secondary granules develop at the myelocyte stage and do not contain peroxidase, but do have a variety of other enzymes. Secondary granules can fuse with the cell membrane to export inflammatory mediators.

Eosinophils are produced in the bone marrow by division and maturation of a progenitor cell different from that of the neutrophil. Eosinophil colony-stimulating factor and IL-5 serve as eosinophil growth factors.

Eosinophils are attracted to areas of tissue invasion by parasites and allergic reactions. Chemotactic factors released by tissue mast cells may be responsible for eosinophil localization. Activated eosinophils release the contents of their cytoplasmic granules which contain major basic protein and eosinophil myeloperoxidase. These inflammatory substances damage parasites and often result in damage to adjacent native tissues.

Basophils are produced in the bone marrow. Once they reach the circulation, basophils enter the tissues within several hours. Little is known about the tissue phase, although they appear to function in hypersensitivity reactions. Basophils have surface receptors for IgE Fc. Binding of IgE Fc or specific antigen causes degranulation of the cytoplasm and the release of histamine, heparin, and a slow-reacting substance of anaphylaxis. There is no evidence to support the transformation of basophils to tissue mast cells.

Monocyte Physiology

Monocytes are produced in the bone marrow from a common neutrophil-monocyte progenitor. The maturation sequence starts at the monoblast stage, proceeds to promonocyte, and then to monocyte, which takes about four days. There is no bone marrow storage pool for monocytes. Monocyte maturation is influenced by a variety of growth factors, many of which are produced by monocytes in a positive feedback manner, and include GM-CSF, monocyte-CSF, IL-1, and tumor necrosis factor. Monocytes spend an average of three days in the peripheral circulation prior to entering the tissues, where they may become tissue macrophages or any number of specialized cells of the mononuclear phagocyte system, including Kupffer cells, alveolar macrophages, Langerhans cells, and microglia. Monocytes never return to peripheral circulation. Tissue monocyte-macrophages have the ability to proliferate, and are therefore not dependent on the bone marrow for replenishment.

In their role as phagocytes, mononuclear cells remove old red blood cells and denatured proteins from circulation. Mononuclear phagocytes have surface receptors for the Fc portion of IgG and complement components which enhance adherence and ingestion of microorganisms. The cytoplasm contains granules packed with a multitude of enzymes. Subsequent killing of microbes is enhanced by interaction with activated T lymphocytes. Numerous mediators of inflammation are secreted by mononuclear phagocytes, including IL-1, complement components, proteases, and lysozyme.

Mononuclear phagocytes play a vital role in cell mediated and humoral immunity by processing and presenting antigens to both T and B lymphocytes.

Lymphocyte Physiology

The lymphocyte stem cell pool is in the bone marrow. B and T lymphocytes undergo differentiation and maturation in the bone marrow and thymus respectively. After maturation, T and B cells migrate to occupy peripheral lymphoid tissues, including lymph nodes, spleen, tonsilar tissue, and mucosal associated sites. Both B and T lymphocytes move freely between circulation and tissues, and are indistinguishable morphologically. T cells account for about 70–80% of peripheral blood lymphocytes. B cells make up nearly all of the rest, save for a few natural killer cells.

Lymphocytes have a long life, and are responsible for the immune system's ability of self and nonself recognition, and immune memory. Lymphocytes are capable of proliferation when activated.

T cells are divided into two broad groups based on function and immunophenotype. T-helper cells are CD4 positive, assist in the production of antibodies by B cells, activate macrophages, and induce cytotoxic properties of other T cells. T-cytotoxic/suppressor cells are CD8 positive, are capable of antigen dependent lysis of virally infected cells, and modulate immune reactions. Natural killer (NK) cells may or may not share T-cell markers, and are able to cause cell lysis without prior antigen exposure, either directly or by antibody-dependent cell mediated cytotoxicity.

B cells function to differentiate into antibody producing plasma cells. B-cell differentiation involves interaction with antigen presenting T-helper cells.

TESTS FOR EVALUATION OF WHITE BLOOD CELL ABNORMALITIES

Specimen Acceptability and Anticoagulants

The most common specimen is venous blood, although free flowing capillary blood from skin punctures can be used in extremely young patients and in those with difficult venous access.

Potassium EDTA (ethylenediaminetetraacetic acid) is the standard anticoagulant used for cell counts and morphologic examinations of blood specimens. Although morphologic changes begin to occur in as soon as one hour after exposure to EDTA, acceptable smears and cell counts can be performed up to 24 hours if the specimen has been stored at 4 C. Heparin is primarily used for special red cell studies and is acceptable for spun hematocrits. It is unacceptable for leukocyte counts and morphologic examinations, as it causes white blood cell (WBC) and platelet clumping, and causes a blue background on prepared blood smears.

Difficult or traumatic venipuncture causes activation of the coagulation cascade, resulting in the formation of fibrin strands which trap leukocytes and platelets, producing artifactually low measurements.

Anticoagulant dependent or platelet specific agglutinins cause platelet clumps which may be counted as WBCs by some automated instruments, and cause artifactually low platelet counts.

Total WBC Counts

Automated Total WBC Counting

Automated instruments determine total WBC concentrations (after dilution and lysing of red cells) by either an electrical impedance method or by light scattering characteristics. Falsely elevated WBC measurements can be caused by the presence of nucleated RBCs, platelet clumps, giant platelets, incompletely lysed RBCs, or bloodborn parasites. Falsely diminished WBC measurements can be seen in situations of WBC fragility (as in some leukemias) or if the plasma contains paraproteins (as in multiple myeloma).

Differential Counts

Manual WBC Differential Counts

The manual WBC differential count is performed by examining a Wright's stained smear at $500\times$ or $1000\times$ magnification and classifying a minimum of 100 consecutive cells based on cytologic characteristics. The number of each cell type is expressed as a percentage of the total number of cells evaluated. If nucleated red blood cells (NRBCs) are present, they are expressed as the number counted per 100 WBCs; the total WBC concentration is corrected for NRBCs (Eq. 25.1).

$$\text{WBC (corrected)} = \frac{\text{uncorrected} \times 100}{100 + \text{\# of NRBCs}} \tag{1}$$

As compared to automated methods (discussed in the next section), manual differential counts are limited statistically by the number of cells which can be classified within a reasonable time period. At least 1000 cells would have to be classified to approach the precision of automated instruments.

Table 25.1.
Indications for Manual Peripheral Smear Review

Verify suspected erroneous results
Evaluate for morphologic WBC abnormalities
Look for suspected undetected low concentrations of abnormal cells:
    immature granulocytes, rare blast cells, and rare atypical cells as seen in hairy cell leukemia and peripher-
        alized lymphoma
Evaluate for suspected circulating parasites or other microorganisms

Automated WBC Differential Counts

Modern automated instruments classify thousands of cells, and allow analysis of about
100 samples/hour, dramatically faster than the manual procedure. Instruments use a
variety of technologies that provides either a three part (granulocytes, lymphocytes,
monocytes) or a five part (neutrophils, lymphocytes, monocytes, eosinophils, basophils)
differential. Automated differentials are superior for routine WBC evaluation, so that
manual differentials are seldom required. Manual differentials do allow identification
of abnormal cell types and non-WBC abnormalities. Situations where manual review
should be requested are shown in Table 25.1.

Interpreting WBC Differential Data

Modern automated instruments report total WBCs, relative percentages, and absolute
numbers of each cell type expressed as a concentration. When only percentages are
available, the absolute concentration can be calculated by multiplying the total WBC
count by the relative percent of the cell type of interest. When evaluating a sample for
disease, only absolute concentrations should be considered, as percentages are relative
and may be misleading. Normal absolute cell counts (concentration) are illustrated in
Table 25.2. Figure 25.1 illustrates the typical morphology of the common peripheral
blood WBCs.

Cytochemical Reactions

Sudan black B, myeloperoxidase, and chloroacetate esterase stains are used to demon-
    strate myelocytic (granulocytic) differentiation. The order listed is from most sensi-
    tive to most specific. AML M1, M2, M3, and M4 are positive for one or more of
    these stains.
Nonspecific esterases (α-naphthyl acetate esterase and α-naphthyl butyrate esterase)
    are used to demonstrate monocytic differentiation. AML M4 and M5 are positive
    for one or both stains.

Table 25.2.
Recommended Peripheral Blood Reference Ranges

Segmented neutrophils	1.8–7.80
Band neutrophils	0–0.70
Lymphocytes	1.0–4.80
Monocytes	0–0.80
Eosinophils	0–0.45
Basophils	0–0.20

absolute differential counts $\times$ 10^9/L ($\times$10^3/μL)

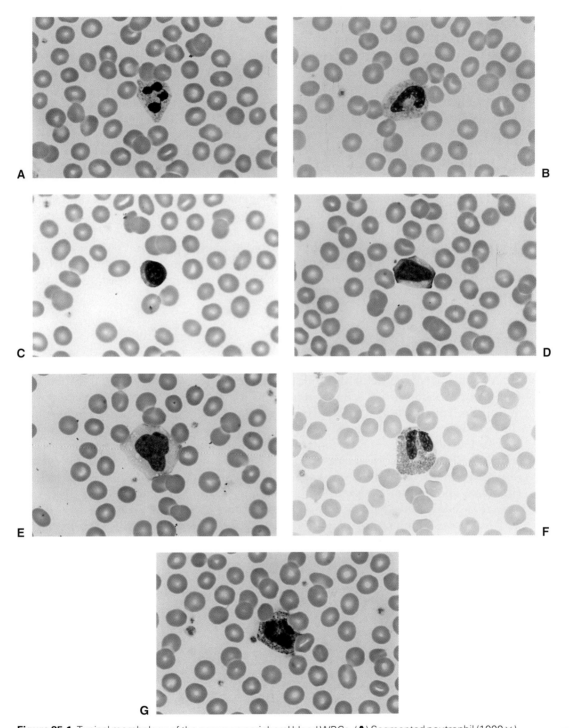

Figure 25.1. Typical morphology of the common peripheral blood WBCs. (**A**) Segmented neutrophil (1000×). (**B**) Band neutrophil (1000×). (**C**) Small lymphocyte (1000×). (**D**) Reactive lymphocyte (ATL) (1000×) (**E**) Monocyte (1000×). (**F**) Eosinophil (1000×). (**G**) Basophil (1000×).

Periodic Acid Schiff (PAS) stains glycogen in hematopoietic cells. Myeloblasts will have
   a finely granular cytoplasmic pattern, while lymphoblasts and erythroid precursors
   in AML M6 (erythroleukemia) will have large blocks of positivity.

Terminal deoxynucleotidyl transferase (Tdt) is a nuclear stain positive in almost all
   precursor ALLs, and is almost always negative in AMLs and ALL L3.

Leukocyte alkaline phosphatase (LAP) activity helps differentiate cases of chronic myelogenous leukemia (CML) from other chronic myeloproliferative disorders and
   leukemoid reactions. LAP activity is limited principally to granulocytes. LAP activity is expressed objectively as an "LAP score." Normal scores are in the range of
   20–200, and vary slightly between laboratories. Low LAP scores are observed in
   most cases of typical CML, and may be observed in non-neoplastic disorders such
   as infectious mononucleosis, sickle cell anemia, and paroxysmal nocturnal hemo-
   globinuria. Polycythemia rubra vera, pyogenic infections, pregnancy, and steroid
   therapy are characterized by elevated LAP scores. LAP scores tend to normalize
   in blast crisis of CML.

Acid phosphatase is present in all nonerythroid human blood cells. Of the seven isoenzymes, only isoenzyme 5 is resistant to tartrate inhibition, is present in the neoplastic cells of hairy cell leukemia, and is the basis for the tartrate resistant acid phosphatase (TRAP) reaction.

Flow Cytometry

Flow cytometry is used to rapidly evaluate hematopoietic cell populations. Peripheral
blood, bone marrow, other body fluids (i.e. pleural or peritoneal), and cell suspensions
from lymph nodes are all suitable specimens for analysis. Flow cytometry begins by
defining cell populations according to size and internal complexity via laser light scatter
characteristics. The population of interest can then be evaluated for the presence of
specific leukocyte surface and cytoplasmic differentiation antigens with specific fluorescent tagged antibodies. In practice, a logical panel of antibodies are used in the evaluation, providing a pattern of reactivity which provides lineage and differentiation specific data, allowing for the rapid differentiation of lymphoid and myeloid processes,
as well as subdividing lymphoid proliferations into B-cell and T-cell lineages. Table
25.3 lists uses and limitations of flow cytometry for evaluating hematologic cell popula-

Table 25.3.
Uses and Limitations of Flow Cytometric Immunophenotyping

Uses
Classify a lymphoid population as B-cell or T-cell
Identify clonal (neoplastic) B-cell populations
Subtype many chronic B-cell leukemias by unique phenotypic profile
Classify acute leukemias as lymphoblastic or myeloblastic
Classify acute lymphoblastic leukemia as T-cell or B-cell lineage
Provide prognostically important phenotypic data for B-cell lineage acute lymphoblastic leukemia
Provide prognostic information for patients with immunodeficiencies

Limitations
Data must be correlated with cellular morphology
Clonal T-lymphocyte populations are usually not easily identified
Acute myelogenous leukemias are not readily subtyped, except for acute megakaryoblastic leukemia

Table 25.4.
Leukocyte Differentiation Antigens

T-Lymphocytes	B-Lymphocytes	Natural Killer Cells
CD2	CD19	CD16
CD3	CD20	CD56
CD4 (helper)	CD21	CD57
CD5	CD22	
CD7	CD23	
CD8 (suppressor)	κ, λ Light chains	

Myeloid Cells	Miscellaneous Markers
CD13 (granulocytes, monocytes)	CD10 (common ALL antigen)
CD14 (granulocytes, monocytes)	CD25 (IL-2)
CD33 (granulocytes, monocytes)	CD34 (hematopoietic progenitors)
CD36 (monocytes)	CD45 (leukocyte common antigen)
CD41 (megakaryocytes, platelets)	
CD61 (megakaryocytes, platelets)	

ALL = acute lymphoblastic leukemia

tions, and Table 25.4 outlines the most commonly used lineage and differentiation specific antigens to distinguish different types of hematopoietic cells.

Bone Marrow Examination

Bone marrow procurement in adults can usually be accomplished using local anesthesia, while children ordinarily require sedation. The procedure is performed aseptically, often at the bedside or in the clinic. Preferred sample sites are the posterior or anterior iliac crest. Other sites are occasionally used in children and infants, including vertebral spinous processes (age greater than 2 years) or tibia (birth to 1 year). Sternal aspirates are performed when other sites are unavailable.

Maximum yield is achieved by evaluating both aspirate and biopsy specimens. The aspirate consists of marrow particles removed by syringe suction. Particles are smeared on a glass slide, stained, and examined microscopically. Bone marrow differential cell counts are performed, qualitative abnormalities of hematopoiesis are identified, and abnormal cells such as metastatic tumor or granulomata are searched for. Staining for iron is routine; cytochemical stains are applied if the specimen is leukemic. Heparinized bone marrow aspirate material is often collected for adjuvant studies, such as flow cytometry, cytogenetics, molecular studies, and microbial cultures. Occasionally, aspirate material is unobtainable, resulting in a "dry tap." This situation occurs when marrow fibrosis is present, or when the marrow is "packed" with tumor cells or other infiltrative processes. In the event of a "dry tap," touch preparations of the biopsy are made and stained similarly to aspirate smears.

The bone marrow biopsy consists of a cylindrical portion of medullary bone with intervening bone marrow. Examination of biopsy material is particularly useful in evaluating marrow cellularity and identifying infiltrative processes which may be focal, such as granulomata, plasma cell dyscrasias, involvement by malignant lymphoma, and metastatic tumors. Stromal components are also evaluable for vasculitis and metabolic bone disease.

Table 25.5.
Indications for Bone Marrow Examination

Unexplained anemia, leukopenia, or thrombocytopenia
Unexplained polycythemia, leukocytosis, or thrombocytosis
Suspected leukemia
Staging for solid tumors, lymphomas, and Hodgkin's disease
Diagnosis of suspected plasma cell dyscrasias
To obtain culture material for suspected chronic infections
To support the diagnosis of various anemias

Indications for bone marrow examination are listed in Table 25.5. Situations in which bone marrow examination is unlikely to provide diagnostic information include metastatic tumor searches without hematologic evidence of marrow involvement, and in patients with constitutional symptoms of unknown etiology.

WHITE BLOOD CELL DISORDERS

Specific Morphologic Abnormalities of WBCs

Pelger-Huet anomaly is an autosomal dominant condition resulting in bilobed and unsegmented neutrophil nuclei. Neutrophil function is normal. There is also an acquired Pelger-Huet anomaly (also known as pelgeroid or pseudo-Pelger-Huet) with bilobed or unsegmented neutrophils seen as a manifestation of myelodysplasia or myeloid leukemia. Toxic granulation refers to the presence of red-purple granules in the cytoplasm of neutrophils, and Dohle bodies are light blue cytoplasmic inclusions consisting of RNA remnants or rough endoplasmic reticulum. Both are nonspecific, but often observed in infections, other inflammatory conditions, and in patients receiving antineoplastic medications. **Neutrophil hypersegmentation** is defined as more than 5% of neutrophils having five nuclear lobes, or any having six lobes. It is commonly seen in megaloblastic anemia and chronic myelogenous leukemia.

General Abnormalities of WBC Number

Neutropenia

Absolute neutropenia is defined as less than 1.8×10^9 neutrophils/L. Infections caused by bacteria, viruses, rickettsiae, and protozoans may all be associated with neutropenia. While infection associated neutropenia can be observed in persons without predisposing conditions, patients who have been exposed to myelotoxic medications, have nutritional deficiencies, or are otherwise debilitated, are more likely to manifest neutropenia, particularly when overwhelming bacterial infections are involved. Viral agents such as hepatitis B and human parvovirus B19 have a well known association with aplastic anemia. Toxic chemical and physical agents which are known to be myelotoxic can produce neutropenia via bone marrow suppression in previously healthy individuals. Many medications produce neutropenia; the more common ones are listed in Chapter 38.

Neutropenia is regularly a manifestation of myelodysplasia (due to ineffective granulopoiesis) and acute leukemia. Other processes in which bone marrow infiltration is

Table 25.6.
Conditions Associated with Neutropenia

Infections	Toxins
Salmonella typhi	Ionizing radiation
Influenza	Benzene
Rubeola	Urethane
Viral hepatitis A	Antineoplastic medications
Varicella	
Rubella	
HIV	
Rocky Mountain Spotted fever	
Malaria	
Trypanosomiasis	
Human parvovirus B19	

Immune Mediated	Other
Felty's syndrome	Myelodysplasia
Systemic lupus erythematosus	Acute leukemias
	Some chronic leukemias
	Granulomatous disease
	Metastatic tumor
	Myelofibrosis

extensive may limit granulopoiesis by reducing the volume of active hematopoietic tissue. Such processes include granulomatous disease, metastatic tumors, myelofibrosis, and some chronic leukemias. Table 25.6 lists conditions associated with neutropenia.

Neutrophilia

Neutrophilia is defined as more than 7.8×10^9 neutrophils per L. Conditions associated with neutrophilia are extremely varied, and are listed in Table 25.7.

The clinical utility of relative and absolute neutrophilic band counts has been the subject of some debate. Studies involving neonates, children, and adults have demon-

Table 25.7.
Causes of Neutrophilia

Acute bacterial, fungal, and parasitic infection
Noninfectious inflammatory conditions
Tissue damage, destruction, or necrosis
Collagen vascular diseases
Acute hemorrhage or hemolysis
Solid tumors
Metabolic disorders
Diabetic ketoacidosis
Uremia
Eclampsia
Toxins and venoms
Physiologic
Exercise
Epinephrine
Steroids
Seizures

Table 25.8.
Neutrophilic Leukemoid Reaction vs. Chronic Myelogenous Leukemia

	Leukomoid	CML
Cell population	Predominantly PMNs/bands. Occasional metamyelocytes and myelocytes.	Entire spectrum of maturation present. Neutrophils and myelocytes predominate. Blasts may represent up to 3% of cells.
Basophilia	Absent	Present
Eosinophilia	Absent	Present
LAP score	Increased	Decreased to absent
Nucleated RBCs	Rare	Occasional

LAP = leukocyte alkaline phosphatase

strated that the absolute band count is no better at selecting at risk patients and provides no better prognostic data than the total WBC count. Band counts also tend to lack a high degree of precision and reliability due primarily to well documented interobserver variability.

Distinguishing between neoplastic neutrophilia as seen in chronic myelogenous leukemia (CML) and a benign neutrophilic leukemoid reaction is often difficult. Table 25.8 provides some useful distinguishing features.

Lymphocytosis

Absolute lymphocytosis is defined as greater than 4.0×10^9 lymphocytes per L. The term lymphocytosis refers to increased mature forms (reactive or neoplastic) and excludes lymphoblasts.

Lymphocytosis in children and young adults is almost always non-neoplastic. Lymphocyte morphology can vary from small round forms to large lymphocytes with irregular nuclei, visible nucleoli, and abundant clear to basophilic cytoplasm (cells commonly referred to as "atypical lymphocytes" or "ATLs") (Fig. 25.1 **C** and **D**).

Since the incidence of neoplastic lymphocytosis increases with age, such disorders must be excluded in older adults when an infectious etiology is not apparent. If lymphocyte morphologic evaluation reveals small round mature forms, then one must be suspicious of chronic lymphocytic leukemia, the most common leukemia of mature lymphocytes in adults. When lymphocytosis in adults consists of ATLs, the process is likely to be reactive, although some of the less common chronic lymphoid leukemias must be considered. Table 25.9 outlines the most common causes of lymphocytosis along with the associated lymphocyte morphology.

Both adults and children presenting with acute lymphoblastic leukemia (ALL) may

Table 25.9.
Causes of Lymphocytosis

Small Lymphocytes	"Atypical" Lymphocytes
Pertussis	Infectious mononucleosis
Acute Infectious lymphocytosis	Cytomegalovirus
Adenovirus	Infectious hepatitis
Coxsackle A, B6	Toxoplasmosis
Echovirus	Brucellosis
Chronic lymphocytic leukemia	Other chronic lymphoid leukemias

Table 25.10.
Conditions Associated with Lymphocytopenia

Acute pyogenic infections
Congestive heart failure
Carcinoma
Hodgkin's disease
Collagen vascular disease
Congenital and acquired immunodeficiency
Adrenal cortical steroid administration
Antineoplastic medications

have relative or absolute lymphocytosis consisting of small benign appearing lymphocytes or atypical forms. The key to recognizing ALL is examination of the peripheral blood for characteristic blast cells, which may be few in number. Careful examination of the peripheral smear is required if there is accompanying unexplained anemia or thrombocytopenia.

Peripheral blood flow cytometric immunophenotyping can help distinguish reactive from neoplastic lymphocytoses by identifying unique phenotypes and light chain restrictions characteristic of the chronic lymphoid leukemias.

Lymphocytopenia

Lymphocytopenia is defined as less than 1.5×10^9 lymphocytes per L. A variety of infections, immune disorders, and medications are associated with lymphocytopenia. Table 25.10 lists the most common associations. In patients with HIV infection, peripheral blood T-helper (CD4) lymphocyte concentration is used to monitor disease progression. The minimum normal CD4 level is 0.6×10^9 per L; concentrations less than 0.2×10^9 per L indicate advanced deficiency. Table 25.11 provides recommended peripheral blood lymphocyte subset reference ranges.

Monocyte Disorders

Absolute monocytosis is defined as more than 0.95×10^9 monocytes per L. In most circumstances, monocytosis is reactive. Neoplastic monocytosis, in which the monocytes are part of the malignant clone, occurs as a component of myeloproliferative and

Table 25.11.
Recommended Peripheral Blood Lymphocyte
Subsets Reference Ranges

Total lymphocytes	1.0–4.80
CD2	0.95–2.60
CD3	0.90–2.40
CD4	0.60–1.50
CD8	0.20–0.70
CD19	0.05–0.50
CD4/CD8 ratio	0.8–3.4

absolute differential counts $\times 10^9$/L ($\times 10^3/\mu$L)

Table 25.12.
Causes of Monocytosis

Infectious Monocytosis	Noninfectious Nonneoplastic Monocytosis	Neoplastic Monocytosis
Tuberculosis	Hodgkin's disease	Chronic myelogenous leukemia
Subacute bacterial	Non-Hodgkin's lymphoma	and other chronic
endocarditis	Multiple myeloma	myeloproliferative disorders
Syphilis	Inherited storage diseases	Acute myelogenous leukemia
Brucellosis	Carcinoma, melanoma	with monocytic differentiation
Malaria	Collagen vascular diseases	(AML-M4, AML-M5)
Leishmaniasis	Sarcoidosis	Chronic myelomonocytic
Trypanosomiasis	Idiopathic inflammatory bowel	leukemia
Typhus	disease	
Rocky Mountain Spotted		
Fever		

myelodysplastic disorders. Table 25.12 lists causes of monocytosis. The most notable association of monocytopenia is with hairy cell leukemia.

Eosinophil Disorders

Absolute eosinophilia is defined as greater than 0.7×10^9 eosinophils per L. Relative eosinophilia of greater than 5% is seen in some otherwise normal individuals and is not related to disease. In most instances, eosinophilia is related to allergic conditions or parasitic infestations. Eosinophilia associated with hematopoietic and other neoplasms is well documented. Table 25.13 lists the most frequent causes of eosinophilia.

Idiopathic hypereosinophilia is the appropriate designation for sustained eosinophilia, of six or more months duration, without a discoverable etiology. Hypereosinophilia is not a benign condition, as it is known to result in endocardial and myocardial fibrosis. Occasionally, hypereosinophilia may proceed the development of a myeloid leukemia. Absolute eosinopenia is most often associated with acute inflammatory or stress conditions resulting in neutrophilia. Corticosteroids also decrease eosinophils.

Basophilia

Absolute basophilia is defined as more than 0.15×10^9 cells per L. Conditions associated with basophilia are varied, and are listed in Table 25.14.

Table 25.13.
Causes of Eosinophilia

Allergic conditions
Drug reactions
Parasitic infections
Chronic myelogenous leukemia and other chronic
    myeloproliferative disorders
Hodgkin's disease
Solid tumors
Cigarette smoking
L-Tryptophan ingestion
Autoimmune disorders
Adrenal insufficiency

Table 25.14.
Causes of Basophilia

Chronic myelogenous leukemia and other chronic
   myeloproliferative disorders
Ulcerative colitis
Chronic sinusitis
Iron deficiency
Smallpox, varicella infections
Hodgkin's disease

Leukemias

Leukemias are unregulated proliferations of hematopoietic cells which involve the bone marrow, have peripheral blood manifestations, and often infiltrate other organs. Leukemias are described as either acute or chronic. Acute leukemias are characterized by the proliferation of immature or precursor cells and have a rapid clinical course if untreated. Chronic leukemias are proliferations of mature cells and have a longer clinical course than untreated acute leukemias. Both acute and chronic leukemias are subdivided into lymphoid and myeloid lineages.

Acute Leukemia

Patients who present with acute leukemia are ill, but complaints are usually nonspecific. Fatigue and fever are common complaints. Infection or bleeding may occur because of neutropenia and thrombocytopenia. Peripheral blood findings are variable. Most patients will have a normocytic normochromic anemia and thrombocytopenia. Total WBCs are quite variable, ranging from leukopenia to marked leukocytosis (cells greater than 100×10^9 per L). The peripheral blood may contain large numbers of blast cells, very few, or occasionally none (aleukemic leukemia). Blast cells must number 30% or more of all nucleated marrow cells to establish the diagnosis of acute leukemia. Acute leukemias are subtyped based on French-American-British (FAB) Cooperative Group criteria (Tables 25.15 and 25.16).

    Acute lymphoblastic leukemia commonly infiltrates organs to produce lymphadenopathy and hepatosplenomegaly. Meningeal infiltration occurs frequently, producing meningeal signs and symptoms. Cerebrospinal fluid is routinely evaluated for the presence of blast cells. Most acute myelogenous leukemias do not produce significant lymphadenopathy or hepatosplenomegaly, unless there is monocytic differentiation. The presence of Auer rods within the observed blast cells is strong evidence that one is dealing with an AML.

Table 25.15.
Features of Acute Lymphoblastic Leukemia

Immunologic Classification	FAB Morphology	Immunophenotype
T-Cell ALL	L2 or L1	Tdt, CD2, CD3, CD5, CD7
Early pre-B-cell ALL	L1 or L2	Tdt, HLA-DR, CD10, CD19
Pre-B-cell ALL	L1 or L2	Tdt, HLA-DR, CD10, CD19, CD20, cytoplasmic Ig
B-Cell ALL	L3	HLA-DR, CD10, CD19, CD20, surface Ig

Tdt = terminal deoxynucleotidyl transferase

Ig = immunoglobulin

Table 25.16.
Features of Acute Myelogenous Leukemia

FAB Subtype	Classification	% of AMLs	Most Frequent Cytogenetics	Prognosis	Unique Features
M0	Minimally differentiated	5–10		Poor	
M1	Myeloblastic without differentiation	10–20	t(9;22)	Intermediate	
M2	Myeloblastic with differentiation	30–45	t(8;21)	Intermediate to poor	
M3	Hypergranular promyelocytic	4–8	t(15;17)	Favorable	M3 and M3v: Disseminated intravascular coagulation. Respond to All-*trans*-retinoic acid.
M3v	Microgranular/hypogranular promyelocytic	1–2	t(15;17)	Favorable	
M4	Myelomonocytic	10–20		Intermediate	M4 and M4eos: gingival hyperplasia, leukemia cutis, and elevated serum lysozyme.
M4eos	Myelomonocytic with eosinophilia	3–5	Inv(16) or t(16;16)	Favorable	
M5a	Monoblastic, poorly differentiated	5–8	t(9;11)	Intermediate	M5a and M5b: extramedullary tumor masses, gingival hyperplasia.
M5b	Monoblastic, differentiated	3–6		Intermediate	M5b tends to occur in younger patients (median 16 years)
M6	Erythroleukemia	5	Partial 5q or 7q deletions	Poor	Occurs in older patients (median 54 years)
M7	Megakaryoblastic	8–10		Poor	May have peripheral thrombocytosis with abnormal forms. "Dry tap" often seen due to marrow reticulin fibrosis.

The evaluation of patients with suspected acute leukemia is laboratory intensive. The goals are to:

Establish the diagnosis of acute leukemia.
Subtype the leukemia into morphologic and lineage specific groups for treatment and prognosis.
Perform cytogenetic studies for prognosis.
Perform molecular genetic studies if requested.
Examine extramedullary tissues and fluids for involvement.
Evaluate the effectiveness of therapy.

With these goals in mind, the following studies are routinely performed:

Peripheral blood smear morphologic evaluation.
Bone marrow aspirate and biopsy for morphologic and cytochemical evaluation.
Bone marrow and/or peripheral blood for flow cytometric immunophenotyping.
Bone marrow or peripheral blood for cytogenetic studies.

Acute Lymphoblastic Leukemia

Acute lymphoblastic leukemia is predominantly a disorder of children, although no age group is exempt. Classic morphologic classification divided ALLs into three groups (L1, L2, and L3) (Fig. 25.2, **A** and **B**). The morphologic and phenotypic features of the different subtypes of ALL are listed in Table 25.15.

Prognosis in ALL has been correlated with a number of parameters. Favorable features include age 2–10 years, female gender, WBC count less than 10×10^9 per L, CD10 positive early pre–B-cell phenotype, and hyperdiploid cytogenetics with more

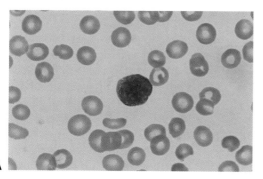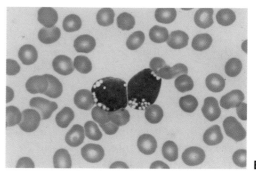

A   B

Figure 25.2. (A) Acute lymphoblastic leukemia L1 (1000×). L1 cells are small with homogeneous nuclear chromatin, inconspicuous nucleoli, and scant cytoplasm. L1 morphology tends to occur in children and corresponds to early pre B-cell ALL (common ALL). L2 cells (not shown) are larger, have irregular nuclear chromatin, conspicuous nucleoli, and more abundant cytoplasm. L2 morphology is seen more often in adults, and is frequently of T-cell phenotype. **(B)** Acute lymphoblastic leukemia L3 (1000×). L3 morphology is the least common at any age, is characterized by deeply basophilic vacuolated cytoplasm, corresponds to B-cell ALL, and has identical morphology, immunologic, and genetic markers as Burkitt's lymphoma.

than 50 chromosomes. There are some specific cytogenetic findings which correlate particularly well with prognosis. Structural abnormalities associated with a poor prognosis include t(9;22), t(1;9), t(11;14), and t(4;11). An intermediate prognosis is associated with normal chromosomes and hyperdiploid with 47–50 chromosomes. Hypodiploid karyotypes are usually associated with structural abnormalities and are considered intermediate to poor risk.

Acute Myelogenous Leukemia

Acute myelogenous leukemia (AML) is predominantly a disease of middle aged and older adults, although it is the most common acute leukemia in newborns and infants.

Acute myelogenous leukemias are subtyped based on their tendency toward differentiation as demonstrated by morphology and cytochemical reactions. Table 25.16 outlines the subtypes of AML, associated cytogenetic findings, and other characteristics. Figure 25.3 **A** and **B** illustrates AML M1 and M3 morphology.

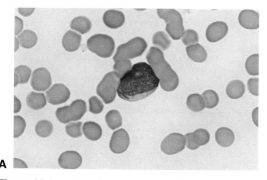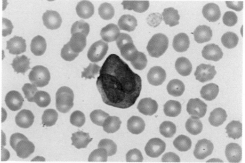

A   B

Figure 25.3. (A) Acute myelogenous leukemia M1, with Auer rod (1000×). M1 cells have large nuclei and multiple nucleoli. The nuclear chromatin is finely distributed. The Auer rod in the cytoplasm is indicative of AML. **(B)** Acute myelogenous leukemia M3 (1000×). M3 cells have lobed nuclei and abundant coarse red cytoplasmic granules.

Chronic Leukemias

Chronic leukemias are diseases of adults, although there is significant variation among the different diseases. Likewise, clinical presentations are variable. Certain chronic leukemias are associated with signs and symptoms which bring the patient to medical attention, while others are just as likely to be discovered incidentally upon evaluation for an unrelated complaint.

Peripheral blood findings range from pancytopenia to marked leukocytosis. In addition to morphologic evaluation of peripheral blood and bone marrow, flow cytometric immunophenotypic is playing an increasingly important role in the accurate classification of chronic leukemias, particularly those of B-lymphocyte lineage. Immunophenotype data for chronic lymphoid leukemias is presented in Table 25.17.

When morphology and immunologic methods fail to distinguish reactive from neoplastic proliferations, as may occur when evaluating T-cell lymphoproliferative disorders, clonality may be established by molecular techniques such as B-cell immunoglobulin and T-cell receptor gene rearrangement studies by Southern blot analysis, discussed more fully in Chapter 36.

Chronic Myelogenous Leukemia

Chronic myelogenous leukemia (CML) is a disease primarily affecting adults, with a median age of about 50 years, although a small percent of cases occur in children and younger adults. Males slightly outnumber females.

Clinical symptoms are usually nonspecific, and include fatigue, weight loss, anorexia, and headache. Most patients develop splenomegaly. Lymphadenopathy is unusual at presentation. About half of affected patients are asymptomatic.

Peripheral blood findings are highly suggestive of the diagnosis. Neutrophilic leukocytosis with a "left shift" (to less mature forms such as bands, metamyelocytes, etc.) is invariable. Total WBC counts are typically greater than 25×10^9 per L and in at least half of cases the WBCs number more than 100×10^9 per L. All stages of granulocytic maturation are present, with myelocytes and neutrophils predominating. From 3–10% myeloblasts are present. Eosinophilia and basophilia are typical; monocytosis is some-

Table 25.17.
Chronic Lymphoid Leukemias: Immunophenotype Data

	CD2	CD3	CD4	CD5	CD7	CD8	CD19	CD20	CD11c	CD25	sIg
B-CLL				+			+	+(dim)			+(dim)
B-PLL				±			+	+			+
HCL							+	+	+	+	+
T-PLL		+	+(70%)	+	+	+(10%)					
HTLV1 L/L	+	+	+	+	±					+	
MF/SS	+	+	+	+						±	

B-CLL = B-cell chronic lymphocytic leukemia

B-PLL = B-cell prolymphocytic leukemia

HCL = hairy cell leukemia

T-PLL = T-cell prolymphocytic leukemia

HTLV1 L/L = human T-cell leukemia virus-1 associated leukemia/lymphoma

MF/SS = mycosis fungoides/Sezary syndrome

sIg = surface immunoglobulin

dim = diminished

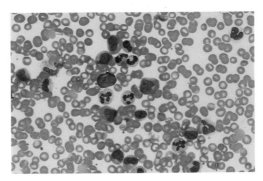

Figure 25.4. CML, peripheral blood (400×). The entire spectrum of granulocytic maturation is seen in the peripheral blood.

times present. More than half of patients have thrombocytosis. Most patients will have a mild to moderate normocytic, normochromic anemia. Circulating nucleated RBCs are often observed in small numbers. Figure 25.4 illustrates the typical CML peripheral blood appearance.

The LAP score provides initial diagnostic evidence, being typically low or absent. Additionally, elevated serum vitamin B_{12} and B_{12} binding proteins are also present.

Cytogenetic analysis demonstrates the Philadelphia chromosome (Ph1) (t(9; 22)(q34;q11)) in about 90% of cases resembling CML. Of the remaining 10%, about 5% will have a demonstrable bcr-abl molecular genetic equivalent. The remaining cases will have atypical clinical and pathologic features and may represent a different disease.

After the initial chronic phase, which lasts an average of 3–4 years, most patients develop what is termed "accelerated phase" or "blast crisis." Diagnostic criteria for accelerated phase include a peripheral blood or bone marrow blast count of 15–29% of nucleated elements. Blast crisis is recognized when the peripheral blood or marrow blast count meets or exceeds 30%. The LAP score may normalize, and cytogenetic studies usually demonstrate additional abnormalities, including a second Ph1. Cytochemical and immunophenotypic analysis of the blasts demonstrate myeloid differentiation in about 70% of cases. In approximately 30%, blast crisis is lymphoblastic, with FAB L1 or L2 morphology, and a Tdt positive, CALLA+, precursor B-cell phenotype. The median survival after development of blast crisis is 2–6 months. Blast crisis of CML is resistant to acute leukemia chemotherapy.

Chronic Lymphocytic Leukemia

Chronic lymphocytic leukemia (CLL) is the most common adulthood leukemia. The median age at diagnosis is 55 years, and males outnumber females by 2.5:1. The disease results in the accumulation of small round lymphocytes in the blood, bone marrow, and parenchymal organs. CLL is an indolent disorder, with a variety of late stage complications. Minimal diagnostic criteria according to the National Cancer Institute–Sponsored Working Group include:

At least 5×10^9 per L small mature appearing lymphocytes in the peripheral blood.
At least 30% of all nucleated cells in the bone marrow are lymphocytes.
Most peripheral blood lymphocytes should be CD19, CD20, or CD24 positive B-cells with coexpression of CD5, and low intensity surface immunoglobulin, with κ or λ restriction.

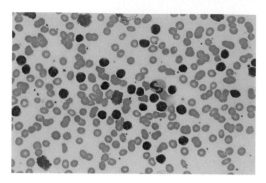

Figure 25.5. CLL, peripheral blood (400×). Small lymphocytes predominate; scattered "smudge" cells are present, with degenerated, pale staining nuclei (center of field, lower left corner).

The total WBC count ranges from the minimal numeric criteria for diagnosis up to 600×10^9 per L or more. Many patients are discovered incidentally.

Most peripheral blood WBCs will be small lymphocytes with condensed, blocky chromatin, absent to inconspicuous nucleoli, and scant cytoplasm. Peripheral blood smears often contain numerous "smudge" or "basket" cells which are a technical artifact. Figure 25.5 illustrates the typical CLL peripheral blood appearance. Up to 10% of circulating lymphocytes may be classified as prolymphocytes, with more abundant cytoplasm, nuclei with more open chromatin, and a single prominent nucleolus. The designation prolymphocytic transformation of CLL (CLL/PLL) is appropriate when prolymphocytes account for 11–55% of lymphocytes. If more than 55% of lymphocytes are prolymphocytes, then de novo prolymphocytic leukemia should be considered.

About 50% of CLL patients present with mild anemia, and 25% will have both anemia and thrombocytopenia. Anemia may be due to bone marrow infiltration or autoimmune hemolytic anemia. Neutropenia is not usually a feature at presentation, but develops as bone marrow infiltrates become more extensive. Almost all patients develop lymphadenopathy and splenomegaly.

Bone marrow infiltration is evaluated on biopsy sections; a diffuse pattern portends a more aggressive clinical course.

Evidence of immune dysregulation is present in most CLL patients. About half will have hypogammaglobulinemia and half will have a small amount of monoclonal immunoglobulin. There is also an increased incidence of secondary malignancies in CLL patients, including melanomas, carcinomas of the gastrointestinal tract and lung, and sarcomas. Cytogenetic studies demonstrate abnormalities in almost 50% of cases. Trisomy 12 is the most frequent abnormality reported, followed by numerous chromosome 14 anomalies, including 14q+, which has been associated with a poorer prognosis.

Staging in CLL has been shown to be of prognostic significance. The Rai and Binet systems are the most frequently utilized. The Rai system uses five categories which divide patients into low-risk (stage 0), intermediate risk (stages I and II), and high risk (stages III and IV) groups. The Binet system uses three categories and includes the enumeration of involved lymphoid areas. Table 25.18 lists the staging criteria for both systems.

About 40% of CLL patients will have cytologic transformation to a more aggressive morphology that is associated with a more rapid clinical course.

Table 25.18.
Staging of Chronic Lymphocytic Leukemia

Rai System		Binet System	
Stage 0	Lymphocytosis	Stage A	No anemia No thrombocytopenia Involvement of < 3 lymphoid areas
Stage I	Lymphocytosis and lymphadenopathy	Stage B	No anemia No thrombocytopenia Involvement of 3 lymphoid areas
Stage II	Lymphocytosis with hepatomegaly or splenomegaly		
Stage III	Lymphocytosis with anemia (Hgb < 11 g/dL)	Stage C	Anemia (Hgb < 10 g/dL), or Thrombocytopenia (platelets < 100×10^9/L)
Stage IV	Lymphocytosis with thrombocytopenia (platelets < 100×10^9/L)		

Lymphoid areas are defined as cervical, axillary, and inguinal lymph nodes.

Hairy Cell Leukemia

Hairy cell leukemia (HCL) is a relatively rare disorder of middle aged adults, although it is occasionally seen in persons under 30 years of age. Patients most often present with symptoms related to pancytopenia, such as easy bruising, infection, or fatigue. Splenomegaly may be so significant that abdominal discomfort becomes the primary complaint. Some patients present with splenic rupture after relatively minor abdominal trauma.

Physical examination reveals splenomegaly in most patients, and hepatomegaly in about half. Lymphadenopathy is unusual. Peripheral blood findings include moderate normocytic, normochromic anemia and thrombocytopenia. Absolute neutropenia and monocytopenia is common. Hairy cells are usually present in small numbers. Because the number of hairy cells in the peripheral blood is so low, buffy coat smears are often made for morphologic evaluation and to demonstrate tartrate resistant acid phosphatase (TRAP) activity, which is present in greater than 95% of cases at presentation. True leukemic presentation with greater than 5×10^9 hairy cells per L is uncommon, but may be seen after splenectomy. Figure 25.6 illustrates the typical hairy cell morphology.

Bone marrow evaluation is hindered by markedly increased reticulum fibrosis, resulting in a "dry tap" in most cases. Histologic sections of bone marrow biopsies reveal characteristic histology which is distinct enough to establish the diagnosis in most cases. The typical immunophenotyping for HCL is presented in Table 25.17. Cytogenetic analysis has demonstrated several nonrandom translocations, including t(14;18), t(9:14), and t(14;22).

T cells morphologically similar to hairy cells have been described in association with HTLV-II.

Mycosis Fungoides and Sezary Syndrome

Mycosis fungoides (MF) is a relatively uncommon disease of adults. It is classified as a cutaneous T-cell lymphoproliferative disorder which infiltrates the skin resulting in the development of scaly pruritic and erythematous patches, plaques, and tumor nodules. Sezary syndrome (SS) is considered to be a systemic manifestation of MF, with

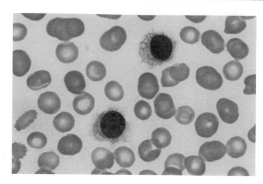

Figure 25.6. HCL, peripheral blood (1000×). Hairy cell morphology is unique but not specific. The cells are slightly larger than circulating small lymphocytes, have round to oval central or slightly eccentric nuclei, evenly distributed lacy chromatin, and one or two inconspicuous nucleoli. The abundant cytoplasm is pale gray-blue with ruffled or "hairy" borders.

patients presenting with diffuse erythroderma and numerous atypical convoluted lymphocytes present in the peripheral blood. The diagnosis of MF is made upon examination of skin biopsy material.

Sezary cells rarely number more than 20×10^9 per L in the peripheral blood. Two types of circulating Sezary cells have been characterized. The small cell variant is similar in size to normal small lymphocytes, except for its internally convoluted nucleus and coarsely clumped chromatin. The large variant has a nuclear diameter $2-3 \times$ larger than a small lymphocyte, has clefts or folds, more open chromatin, occasional small nucleoli, and more abundant cytoplasm. Twenty percent or more of peripheral blood lymphocytes, morphologically consistent with either large or small Sezary cells, are adequate to consider the peripheral blood positive for involvement. Bone marrow lesions are seen in up to 20% of cases at diagnosis.

The typical immunophenotypic pattern is shown in Table 25.17. Proof of clonality is best demonstrated by Southern blot DNA analysis, identifying the clonal T-cell receptor gene rearrangement.

Adult T-Cell Leukemia/Lymphoma

Adult T-cell leukemia/lymphoma (ATLL) was first described in southwest Japan in 1977. Epidemiologic studies have implicated HTLV-1, a single stranded RNA retrovirus which infects human T-helper lymphocytes. Endemic areas now include the Caribbean islands, the southeastern United States, parts of southern Italy, South America, and Africa. Seropositivity for HTLV-1 in these endemic areas is reported as high as 37%.

ATLL affects adults, with a wide age range (27–82 years of age) with a median age of about 55 years. Males outnumber females by 1.5:1.

Characteristic clinical manifestations include skin rash, lymphadenopathy, hepatosplenomegaly, and hypercalcemia. Peripheral adenopathy is present in about 70% of patients at diagnosis. Fifty percent of cases have skin infiltrates at presentation.

Sixty to seventy percent of patients present with peripheral blood involvement. Total WBC counts are quite variable, ranging from normal up to $> 500 \times 10^9$ per L. The characteristic leukemic cells are somewhat larger than small lymphocytes, with nuclei demonstrating marked irregularities, some having easily recognized "flower" or "propeller" morphology while others demonstrate two or more deep nuclear folds. The chromatin is coarse, with inconspicuous nucleoli. Cytoplasm is variably abundant and basophilic, occasionally vacuolated.

Bone marrow involvement is reported to occur in over 50% of cases. Patients with hypercalcemia have increased osteoclastic activity.

Immunophenotyping patterns are provided in Table 25.17. Cytogenetic studies have shown no consistent pattern, however reports of trisomy 3, trisomy 7, and chromosome 6 abnormalities are most common. Molecular genetic studies demonstrate a clonal rearrangement of the T-cell receptor genes.

Chronic Myeloproliferative Disorders

The chronic myeloproliferative disorders include CML, polycythemia vera, essential thrombocythemia, and myelofibrosis with myeloid metaplasia (MMM). These proliferative disorders have a common pathogenesis involving a myeloid stem cell clonal abnormality. MMM is discussed here as the others are covered elsewhere.

MMM is primarily seen in middle aged to elderly adults, although rare cases are reported in children. Massive splenomegaly brings most patients to evaluation. Other complaints are nonspecific, and include weight loss, fatigue, and bruising. Hepatomegaly may be found in half of patients.

Peripheral blood evaluation reveals normocytic normochromic anemia of varying degree. There is pronounced anisocytosis and poikilocytosis with frequent dacrocytes, target cells, elliptocytes, basophilic stippling, and polychromasia. Nucleated red cells are observed in most cases. Neutrophilic leukocytosis including immature forms, occasional myeloblasts, and basophilia are commonly present. Platelet counts may be elevated early in the disease, but usually fall to normal or decreased levels with disease progression. Abnormal hypogranular platelets are present. Circulating micromegakaryocytes are rather unique to MMM. Bone marrow aspirates are usually not obtainable. The appearance of bone marrow biopsy material varies with disease evolution, becoming increasingly fibrotic.

Extramedullary hematopoiesis (EMH) is invariably present in the spleen, almost always in the liver, and often within other organs as well. Involved organs do not appear to suffer functional deficits as a result of EMH, although mass effects are a recognized complication. It is known that EMH in adults is largely ineffective.

Cytogenetic studies reveal no Ph1, but slightly less than half of MMM patients demonstrate nonrandom chromosome anomalies, including trisomy 8, 9, or monosomy 7.

Median survival from diagnosis is approximately five years. The most frequent terminal events include infection, hemorrhage, leukemic transformation, and cardiac failure.

Myelodysplastic Syndromes

Myelodysplastic syndromes (MDS) are considered clonal disorders of hematopoietic stem cells. Affected patients are usually older than 50 years, and present with anemia and variable neutropenia and thrombocytopenia. The diseases are characterized by morphologically abnormal maturation of bone marrow cells. Peripheral blood examination demonstrates red cell changes (oval macrocytes, coarse basophilic stippling, dacrocytes, dimorphic anisocytosis), granulocyte changes (pseudo-Pelger-Huet forms and hypogranularity), and platelet abnormalities (giant and abnormally shaped hypogranular forms). Bone marrow examination is required for classification, based on the percent blasts and the presence of ringed sideroblasts. The most common MDS are **refractory anemia, refractory anemia with ringed sideroblasts, refractory anemia with excess blasts, refractory anemia with excess blasts in transformation,** and **chronic myelomonocytic leukemia.**

The diagnosis of MDS is made after the exclusion of conditions and exposures that are known to cause dyshematopoiesis, such as heavy metals, toxins, antineoplastic medications, and vitamin B_{12} or folate deficiency.

The prognosis for MDS patients is variable. Approximately 10–40% will develop acute leukemia, and 20–40% will succumb to bleeding or infection. Secondary MDS is known to follow exposure to alkylating chemotherapeutic agents, usually by three or more years.

CHAPTER 26

Evaluation and Diagnosis of Plasma Cell Dyscrasias

JAMES T. RECTOR

The term plasma cell dyscrasia (Table 26.1), refers to a group of disorders having in common the abnormal proliferation of plasma cells or lymphocytes, usually associated with production of a monoclonal immunoglobulin. Levels of other immunoglobulins are frequently decreased. The type of monoclonal protein along with other clinical and laboratory features can further classify plasma cell dyscrasias.

PLASMA CELL MYELOMA (MULTIPLE MYELOMA)

The most common of these disorders is multiple myeloma, a monoclonal proliferation of plasma cells producing monoclonal immunoglobulin. The bone marrow is the site of origin of almost all myelomas but other organs may be secondarily involved.

Incidence and Clinical Features

The incidence of myeloma in the U.S. in 1989 was 3.9 cases per 100,000. Males are more commonly affected than females by a ratio of about 3:2 and black Americans are affected more often than whites. Myeloma is not found in children and is rare before age 35. The incidence increases with age and is highest in the ninth decade.

Back or lower extremity pain due to lytic bone lesions is the most common presenting symptom, and fractures or severe osteopenia may be seen in advanced cases. Weakness or fatigue due to anemia are also common. Symptoms of renal failure or hypercalcemia may be the first manifestations in some patients. Mass disease, particularly in the head and neck region due to extramedullary plasmacytomas, can be a presenting symptom in a few patients. Organomegaly, lymphadenopathy, or hyperviscosity are also found in rare cases.

Laboratory Evaluation

Any of the above signs or symptoms in a middle aged or elderly adult should be followed up with appropriate tests. In patients with low suspicion of myeloma, normal CBC and normal serum globulins virtually rule out the diagnosis. In patients with anemia, bone pain, hypercalcemia, or other strongly suggestive symptoms, both serum and urine protein electrophoresis (and immunofixation if a monoclonal band is identified) should be performed. Radiographic skeletal survey and bone marrow examination are usually required to confirm the diagnosis. The requirements for diagnosis are increased abnormal bone marrow plasma cells (or a plasmacytoma) together with a monoclonal gammopathy in the serum or urine or lytic bone lesions recognized by radiographic studies (Table 26.2). At least 10% bone marrow plasma cells with 3 g/dL of monoclonal serum protein or more than 1 g/day of κ or λ light chains in the urine are considered diagnostic. In some cases, less than 10% plasma cells are identified, but

Table 26.1.
Plasma Cell Dyscrasias and Related Disorders

Plasma cell myeloma
Monoclonal gammopathy of undetermined significance
Macroglobulinemia (lymphoplasmacytic lymphoma)
Heavy chain disease
Primary amyloidosis

there is marked cytologic atypia or clustering of plasma cells. Rarely, some reactive conditions have greater than 10% plasma cells but will not have morphologic abnormalities or demonstrate monoclonality. Patients with myeloma should also be monitored with tests (CBC, serum calcium, albumin, BUN, creatinine, and uric acid) to detect common complications. For example, hypercalcemia is present in one-sixth of cases, BUN and creatinine are elevated in one-third, and hyperuricemia is found in one-half and indicates renal damage. Hypoalbuminemia is often observed in advanced cases and forecasts a poor prognosis.

A monoclonal protein is found in serum in the majority of cases, most commonly IgG or IgA of either light chain type. In a few cases IgD is the abnormal protein and, very rarely, IgE is produced. In some cases two monoclonal proteins are produced. The total immunoglobulin is commonly increased due to the presence of the monoclonal protein, but normal polyclonal immunoglobulins are decreased. Serum immunoglobulin levels can reach greater than 10 g/dL. In approximately 10% of patients, light chains without accompanying heavy chains are identified. This is referred to as light chain disease. Because of their small size, light chains are usually found only in urine (unless there is renal failure); for this reason it is important to assess both serum and urine when evaluating a patient for multiple myeloma. In some cases of suspected myeloma, a monoclonal serum band is found but a heavy chain cannot be found. In these cases immunofixation for IgD or IgE should be performed.

Radiologic Studies

Radiologic abnormalities (lytic bone lesions, pathologic fractures, or generalized osteoporosis) are seen in about 75% of cases. The vertebrae, pelvis, skull, ribs, femurs, and proximal humeri are most often affected. Skeletal surveys, rather than nuclear bone scans, are preferred because increased osteoblastic activity (detected by bone scans) is not usually present in myeloma. CT and MRI are useful for detecting small bone lesions and extramedullary plasmacytomas.

Table 26.2.
Clinical-Pathologic Criteria for the Diagnosis of Myeloma

  I.   Increased abnormal, atypical, or immature plasma cells in the bone marrow
 II.   Plasmacytoma
III.   Monoclonal gammopathy in serum or urine
 IV.   Radiologic bone lesions consistent with myeloma
Requirement for diagnosis:
I and either III or IV
II and either III or IV

Blood and Bone Marrow Findings

The CBC will demonstrate a normochromic normocytic anemia in most cases. Leukopenia and thrombocytopenia are not present at diagnosis but may evolve, reflecting marrow replacement by neoplastic cells. The most striking feature of the blood smear is rouleaux formation (Chapter 24), usually accompanied by a blue or purplish tinge of the background; both are directly related to immunoglobulin level. Circulating plasma cells may be found in low numbers in about 15% of cases but may be increased in advanced cases. In rare cases (plasma cell leukemia), plasma cells are greater than 20% of the white cell count, and 30×10^3 per μl ($\times 10^9$/L) or more can be found.

Bone marrow examination is essential for the diagnosis of myeloma. The diagnosis can be made from the bone marrow alone when there is extensive marrow replacement, abnormal clustering of plasma cells, or marked cytologic atypia of plasma cells. Bone marrow is almost always required to confirm radiologic and immunologic evidence of myeloma. An aspirate and core biopsy should be obtained for adequate evaluation. Because myeloma can focally involve the marrow, we perform bilateral bone marrow biopsies to maximize sampling. However, other institutions may perform only unilateral bone marrow biopsy and if the bone marrow findings are nondiagnostic, follow the patient with serial protein electrophoresis and repeat the bone marrow biopsy when increasing levels of monoclonal protein are demonstrated.

The core biopsy is particularly useful because immunostaining for immunoglobulins can differentiate a monoclonal or polyclonal pattern of immunoglobulin expression in the plasma cells, which distinguishes neoplastic from reactive plasmacytosis. It can also detect monoclonality in cases where plasma cells are dispersed in the bone marrow and difficult to identify on routine hematoxylin and eosin stains.

Ancillary Tests and Prognostic Considerations

Cytogenetic analysis is generally not performed, however, several cytogenetic abnormalities are associated with myeloma and can support the diagnosis in difficult cases. Rearrangements of chromosome 1 are most frequent, with abnormalities of chromosome 14q32 also frequent, most commonly as t(11;14). Abnormalities of chromosomes 5, 9, 11, and 12 are also seen.

β-2 microglobulin and *plasma cell labeling index* are used to assess prognosis in myeloma. β-2 microglobulin (Chapter 9) increases with increasing tumor burden and correlates with tumor cell mass. The level of β-2 microglobulin is used to assess prognosis and response to therapy; levels greater than 6.0 μg/mL reflect poor prognosis or inadequate response to therapy. Although not available at many institutions, the plasma cell labeling index (determined by incubating bone marrow cells with tritiated thymidine) is considered the gold standard in assessment of patient prognosis. Slides are subjected to autoradiography and Wright's staining, reporting the percentage of plasma cells labeled. A plasma cell labeling index greater than 3% is associated with a survival of less than 6 months, compared to a labeling index of less than 1% which is associated with a 30 month median survival. Unfortunately, the complexity of the test, the requirement for live cells, and the use of radioactivity limit its widespread use.

The presence of circulating plasma cells in the peripheral blood, hypercalcemia, or hypoalbuminemia reflect more extensive disease and indicate a poor prognosis.

Myeloma Variants

Plasma cell leukemia is diagnosed on the basis of greater than 20% circulating plasma cells or an absolute count of greater than 2×10^3 cells per μl. Plasma cell leukemia may be primary and present at time of diagnosis, or secondary and evolving during the course of disease. Most cases represent advanced stage disease; however, rare cases of primary plasma cell leukemia occur. Primary plasma cell leukemia has a different clinical presentation: most patients are younger and present with organomegaly, adenopathy, renal failure, and fewer bony lesions. It follows an aggressive course with short survival.

Smoldering myeloma is a rare clinical variant where all the diagnostic criteria for myeloma are present, but the disease shows no clinical progression for 5 years or more without any therapeutic intervention. Clinically, it is similar to monoclonal gammopathy of undetermined significance (MGUS, see below).

Solitary plasmacytoma of bone refers to a localized plasma cell tumor involving bone with the absence of a plasma cell infiltrate in marrow biopsies and no evidence of other bone lesions. There is generally no detectable monoclonal gammopathy. About 5% of patients with myeloma present with solitary plasmacytoma. In most patients there is eventual evolution to multiple myeloma within 2–10 years.

Solitary extraosseous (extramedullary) plasmacytomas are most common in the mucous membranes of the upper air passages. These patients may also progress to multiple myeloma but at a lower frequency (10–20% of cases). However, plasmacytomas arising in cutaneous sites demonstrate a high risk of developing multiple myeloma.

Osteosclerotic myeloma is a component of a very rare syndrome that includes **P**olyneuropathy, **O**rganomegaly, **E**ndocrine abnormalities, **M**onoclonal gammopathy, and **S**kin lesions (POEMS syndrome). There may be single or multiple sclerotic bone lesions (contrasted with typical lytic lesions of multiple myeloma). λ light chain monoclonal protein is identified in most cases, and bone marrow contains less than 5% plasma cells.

Aspects of Myeloma Treatment

Asymptomatic patients with myeloma often require no treatment. The decision to treat is based on the development of symptoms or increasing serum or urine monoclonal protein, both reflecting increased tumor cell burden. Patients can be effectively monitored by periodic evaluation of levels of monoclonal protein in serum or urine and by serial β-2 microglobulin measurements. Specialized laboratories may measure the plasma cell labeling index to guide treatment decisions. Once treatment is initiated, the patients are monitored monthly for serum monoclonal protein level, CBC, creatinine, and calcium to adjust therapy to maximize therapeutic effect and minimize myelosuppression.

MONOCLONAL GAMMOPATHY OF UNDETERMINED SIGNIFICANCE

Monoclonal gammopathy of undetermined significance, or MGUS, refers to a monoclonal spike in serum or urine without other evidence of myeloma, amyloidosis, or other lymphoproliferative disorders known to produce monoclonal proteins.

Incidence and Clinical Features

Monoclonal gammopathy of undetermined significance is found in at least 3% of individuals over age 70. It has a higher incidence in blacks than in whites and is often discovered during the work-up of other unrelated health problems in the elderly. There are no specific symptoms or physical findings. In the majority of cases, the monoclonal protein is stable with time. From 20–25% progress to myeloma, amyloidosis, or malignant lymphoproliferative disease. The progression can be gradual or abrupt.

Laboratory Evaluation

A monoclonal spike of variable size is identified on SPEP in most cases, ranging from 0.3 g/dL to more than 3.0 g/dL, with the majority less than 3.0 g/dL. IgG κ is most often identified. The blood findings are nonspecific, and the bone marrow has less than 10% mature plasma cells. The majority of cases have a polyclonal staining pattern with antibodies to light chains.

Diagnostic Considerations

Application of diagnostic criteria (Table 9.4) separates MGUS from myeloma in most cases. Patients with an increasing monoclonal spike, a relatively high percentage of plasma cells, immature features of the plasma cells, or monoclonality may be suspected to be evolving toward myeloma. Distinction from multiple myeloma and other malignant gammopathies requires serial measurement of monoclonal protein levels: patients with MGUS have stable levels of monoclonal protein, but multiple myeloma patients demonstrate increasing levels over time.

WALDENSTRÖM'S MACROGLOBULINEMIA (LYMPHOPLASMACYTOID LYMPHOMA)

Monoclonal gammopathies occur in lymphoproliferative disorders, most commonly lymphoplasmacytoid lymphomas and small lymphocytic lymphomas. The monoclonal protein can be IgM, IgG, or IgA and may be an incidental finding. However in some patients with IgM gammopathy, the monoclonal protein is a major factor in the pathophysiology and the clinicopathologic syndrome is referred to as Waldenström's macroglobulinemia. In most patients the lymphoma is disseminated and high IgM causes hyperviscosity syndrome, manifested by headache, CNS impairment, hypervolemia, congestive heart failure, and bleeding.

Incidence and Clinical Features

The actual incidence of Waldenström's macroglobulinemia is not known but estimated to be about 17% of IgM monoclonal gammopathies. It is a disease of the older adult, with an average age of 60 years, and two-thirds are males. Symptoms include weakness, fatigue, and bleeding problems. Neurologic symptoms secondary to hyperviscosity may occur at presentation. Raynaud syndrome may be seen in patients with a serum cryoglobulin (Chapter 37). Unlike myeloma, lymphadenopathy and organomegaly are prominent physical findings. The fundus of the eye may show congestion and hemorrhage of retinal vessels.

Laboratory Evaluation

SPEP usually demonstrates a monoclonal γ-globulin, identified as IgM by immunofixation or other techniques. Serum viscosity is increased in 90% of patients; cryoglobulins are detected in a small percentage of patients. Bleeding time and platelet aggregation tests are abnormal in most patients with significantly elevated IgM. Serum creatinine is elevated in approximately one-third of cases. Hypercalcemia and skeletal lesions are rare.

Blood and Bone Marrow Findings

Anemia is common and rouleaux is marked on the peripheral smear. Circulating mature or lymphoplasmacytoid lymphocytes may be identified and can give rise to a leukemic blood picture. The bone marrow findings are variable but most demonstrate involvement with a lymphoproliferative process. The morphology of the infiltrates is typical of small lymphocytic proliferations. Intranuclear inclusions (Dutcher bodies) are commonly observed in lymphocytes. Plasma cells and histiocytes may also be increased. Some cases may transform to a large cell lymphoma.

Ancillary Studies

Immunologic Findings

By flow cytometry, the neoplastic cells not only react with pan B-cell antibodies and show a single light chain, but also mark with CD38, an activation antigen often expressed on plasma cells and plasmacytoid lymphocytes. Immunohistochemistry on paraffin sections demonstrates cytoplasmic immunoglobulin and positive staining with plasma cell antibodies such as PCA-1 and PC-1.

Cytogenetic Analysis

Although cytogenetic abnormalities may be seen, they are nonspecific, so that cytogenetic studies are not usually indicated.

HEAVY CHAIN DISEASES

These are rare disorders producing an incomplete immunoglobulin composed solely of the heavy chain of IgG, IgA, or IgM and associated with proliferation of lymphocytes, plasma cells, or both. Heavy chain diseases produce paraproteins with defects in their hinge region, the site of conjugation of light chains, and consequently the heavy chain circulates without the light chain. These syndromes have clinical characteristics different from those of myeloma. Some have CLL or clinicopathologic features of Waldenström's macroglobulinemia. α-Heavy chain disease has a predilection for older children and young adults and presents either with enteric or respiratory forms of disease. Diagnosis of heavy chain diseases is based on finding a monoclonal protein in serum, urine, or both that reacts with antisera to γ, α, or μ heavy chains, but not with light chains. The distinction of these diseases from myeloma is important with regard to patient management and treatment decisions. Therapeutic decisions for heavy chain diseases should be based on the histologic features of the underlying lymphoproliferative disorder. Although some cases have been reported to respond to myeloma regimens, they are more effectively treated with a lymphoma protocol. In α-chain disease, antibiotics alone have induced long-lasting remission in some patients while others develop immunoblastic lymphoma.

PRIMARY AMYLOIDOSIS

Amyloidosis is the deposition of linear, nonbranching, hollow fibrils in tissues. The chemical composition of the fibrils may vary but their ultrastructure is similar. In primary amyloidosis, monoclonal plasma cells produce whole or partial immunoglobulin light chains which precipitate as amyloid in various tissues. Primary amyloidosis is associated with plasma cell myeloma in approximately 20% of cases. Secondary amyloidosis and familial amyloidosis are associated with deposition of nonimmunoglobulin proteins and have no relation to plasma cell dyscrasias; they will not be discussed here.

Incidence and Clinical Features

Primary amyloidosis is a rare disease of older adults. Common signs and symptoms include fatigue and weight loss. Carpal tunnel syndrome or pain related to peripheral neuropathy can be presenting manifestations. Other associated conditions include hemorrhage, congestive heart failure, nephrotic syndrome, or malabsorption. Factor X deficiency (due to binding of factor X by amyloid proteins) may produce hemorrhage. Physical findings include hepatomegaly and macroglossia. Splenomegaly and lymphadenopathy are uncommon.

Laboratory Evaluation

A monoclonal protein is found in most patients and is more common in urine than in serum. Laboratory evidence of factor X deficiency includes prolongation of PT and PTT. Diagnosis is made by demonstration of amyloid deposition in tissue, most commonly in the walls of blood vessels, as demonstrated by Congo red (which gives an apple green color to amyloid when viewed with polarized light) or Thioflavin T stains. Subcutaneous abdominal fat and rectal biopsies are diagnostic in a majority of cases. Skin and bone marrow can also be used and are positive in about 50% of cases. Renal biopsy is diagnostic in 90%, but is associated with a greater procedural risk.

Blood and Bone Marrow Findings

Although blood counts are usually normal at the time of diagnosis, anemia develops in many cases. The peripheral smear may show rouleaux or circulating plasma cells. The bone marrow is usually diagnostic in cases associated with myeloma but less than half of the nonmyeloma cases are diagnosed by marrow findings. Despite the lower yield, bone marrow examination should be performed in all cases to evaluate for multiple myeloma and rule out other disease processes. Most cases demonstrate less than 10% plasma cells, either monoclonal or polyclonal with immunohistochemical staining with light chain antibodies. Deposits of amyloid may be identified in some cases by Congo red or Thioflavin T staining. In some cases, use of electron microscopy will confirm the diagnosis by demonstrating rigid, linear, nonbranching aggregated 7–10 nm fibrils.

Treatment

Recent randomized clinical trials have indicated a survival advantage in amyloidosis patients treated with myeloma type therapy with melphalan and prednisone.

CHAPTER 27

Laboratory Evaluation of Hemostasis

LINDA G. BAUM

Hemostasis is a delicate balance between a need to respond to physical injury and prevent hemorrhage by initiating thrombosis, and the need to promote circulation. Three components are necessary for hemostasis. These are: (1) the vessel wall, (2) platelets, and (3) the coagulation system. This chapter will focus on the role of platelets and the coagulation system in hemostasis.

COMPONENTS OF THE HEMOSTATIC SYSTEM

Platelets

Primary hemostasis is carried out by platelets. Platelet functions include the following activities (Table 27.1).

Adhesion to Collagen at the Site of Vascular Injury

The adhesion of platelets to collagen exposed by disruption of the endothelium is mediated by an interaction between glycoprotein Ib on the platelet surface and von Willebrand factor which is released by endothelial cells. Von Willebrand factor is stored in Weibel-Palade bodies and released upon endothelial cell activation or physical disruption. The von Willebrand factor is believed to form a bridge between platelet glycoprotein Ib and collagen molecules in the subendothelial matrix.

Aggregation of Additional Platelets to "Plug" the Leak in the Blood Vessel

Platelet aggregation is distinct from platelet adhesion. Platelet aggregation is mediated by the glycoprotein IIb/IIIa–integrin protein complex on the platelet cell surface. Integrin molecules on the platelets increase their binding capacity when platelets are activated via adhesion. These integrin molecules can then bind soluble molecules such as fibrinogen or fibronectin which bridges the interacting platelets, resulting in the deposition of an aggregate of activated platelets at the site of injury.

Release of Platelet Contents to Promote Hemostasis

Platelet granules are rich in substances such as ADP and ATP, calcium, degradative enzymes, and a number of clotting factors. Release of many of these factors, as well as synthesis of the prostaglandin thromboxane A_2, promote platelet aggregation. In addition, thromboxane A_2 is the most potent vasoconstrictor known, assisting platelets in controlling bleeding by reducing blood flow.

Provision of a Phospholipid Surface to Assemble Proteins of the Coagulation Cascade

The phospholipid membrane of platelets is crucial for organizing and promoting interactions of clotting factors. Many of these factors require assembly into a complex for

Table 27.1.
Specific Platelet Functions and Their Molecular Mediators

Platelet Function	Mediators
Adhesion to Collagen	Glycoprotein Ib von Willebrand Factor (vWF)
Aggregation	Glycoprotein IIb/IIIa Fibrinogen
Secretion	Dense granules—ADP, Ca⁺⁺, Serotonin α-Granules—platelet factor IV; factor V, vWF, fibrinogen, platelet derived growth factor
Scaffold for coagulant protein assembly	Factor IX, VIII, X complex Factor X, V, II (thrombin) complex

full activity, such as factors VIIIa, IXa, and Xa, and factors Xa and Va. The assembly of these enzymes and cofactors in a complex on a phospholipid surface greatly enhances hemostatic activity.

The Coagulation Cascade

Secondary hemostasis is carried out by the coagulation system (Fig. 27.1). This consists of a number of proenzymes (zymogens) which circulate until activated. Historically,

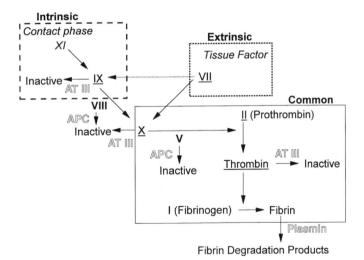

Figure 27.1. Simplified Essentials of the Coagulation Cascade. The intrinsic (dashed line) and extrinsic (dotted line) pathways are indicated, and are useful for laboratory diagnosis of coagulation defects. However, it is clear that factor VII activates factor IX, indicating that, in vivo, the pathways occur simultaneously. The components of the cascade include the activators (italics: contact phase, tissue factor and factor XI), the vitamin K–dependent serine proteases (underlined: factors IX, VII, X, II, and thrombin), the cofactors (bold: factors VIII and V), and fibrinogen. Coagulation is kept in check by the activity of clotting inhibitors (outline font). Protein C, in the presence of thrombin and protein S, is converted to active protein C (APC), which inactivates factors V and VIII, inhibiting coagulation. Antithrombin III (AT III), in the presence of heparin, inactivates thrombin. Plasmin, released from inactive plasminogen by a variety of factors, breaks down fibrin to degradation products, which inhibit further fibrin formation. Not shown in the diagram are calcium and platelet phospholipid; calcium is needed as a cofactor by the vitamin K–dependent factors VII, IX, X, and II, while phospholipid serves as a structural support for the common and intrinsic pathways.

the coagulation system has been divided into three systems, termed the **extrinsic, intrinsic,** and **common** pathways. While these terms are helpful for understanding in vitro laboratory tests and for recognizing specific factor deficiencies, these pathways are not separated in vivo, but feed each other. Disruption of endothelium exposes the protein **tissue factor** (thromboplastin) in subendothelial tissue, triggering the coagulation cascade by converting inactive factor VII into VIIa (activated), starting the extrinsic pathway. In addition to factor VII activation, endothelial disruption exposes collagen molecules in the vascular wall, activating the zymogens in the intrinsic pathway. In addition, factor VIIa can directly produce factor IXa, a key component of the intrinsic pathway. There are four major groups of factors in the coagulation cascade.

The Activators

As discussed above, tissue factor in subendothelial tissue activates factor VII, converting it to factor VIIa. Extracellular matrix components, such as collagen, will activate the **contact phase** proteins, composed of high molecular weight kininogen (HMWK), prekallikrein, and factor XII. The contact phase components then activate factor XI to factor XIa. It is easy to see that triggering of the extrinsic pathway by tissue factor and triggering of the intrinsic pathway via the contact phase activators must happen simultaneously in the body since disruption of the endothelial lining of a blood vessel would expose both tissue factor and collagen.

The Vitamin K–Dependent Factors

These are factors VII, IX, X, and II (prothrombin). During synthesis in the liver, these factors are enzymatically modified by a γ-carboxylase. The γ-carboxylation of glutamic acid residues on these factors allows them to bind calcium (necessary for optimal enzyme activity). Hepatocyte γ-carboxylase requires vitamin K as a co-factor. In the absence of vitamin K, γ-carboxylase activity is markedly reduced, and factors without the γ-carboxylation modification are released into the circulation. These unmodified factors have markedly reduced enzymatic activity, reducing activity of the clotting cascade. Vitamin K is synthesized by flora in the gastrointestinal tract and can also be obtained from leafy green vegetables. Thus, patients who are severely malnourished or who are receiving broad spectrum antibiotics that alter gastrointestinal flora can become vitamin K deficient. The drug coumadin (warfarin) inhibits vitamin K–dependent γ-carboxylation.

Cofactors

Two of the activated enzymes in the coagulation cascade, factor IXa and factor Xa, require cofactors for optimal activity. The factor IXa cofactor is factor VIIIa, while factor Xa cofactor is factor Va. Without these cofactors, these enzymes have reduced activity and clotting is impaired. It is important to note that both the vitamin K–dependent factors, factors VII, IX, X, and II, and the cofactors, factors VIII and V, are not consumed during coagulation. Thus, diminution of enzyme or cofactor does not significantly impair clotting until the plasma level is very low.

Fibrinogen

The conversion of fibrinogen to fibrin allows polymerization of fibrin monomers to produce a gel-phase or soft clot. The fibrin monomers polymerize via interactions at the termini of the molecules, resulting in interwoven strands of fibrin molecules. The soft clot is subsequently cross-linked and stabilized by the action of factor XIII.

Inhibitors of Coagulation

As with other body functions, there is a negative feedback on the process of coagulation, needed to prevent clotting from continuing unabated once begun. The activity of the coagulation cascade is regulated by a number of additional protein factors, illustrated in Figure 27.1. Deficiencies in any of these regulatory molecules will create a hypercoagulable state, resulting in an increased incidence of thrombotic events.

Plasminogen

The activation of the coagulation cascade simultaneously initiates the eventual destruction of the resulting thrombus. Both tissue plasminogen activator (in the presence of fibrin) and components of the contact phase convert circulating plasminogen into the active enzyme plasmin. Plasmin degrades fibrin, cleaving the cross-linked fibrin into small fragments termed fibrin degradation products (FDPs). Lipoprotein (a) (Chapter 8) competes for binding sites on fibrin and inhibits fibrin breakdown.

Antithrombin III

Antithrombin III (AT III) is a naturally occurring anticoagulant; in the presence of tissue heparin (from the vascular wall) or exogenous heparin, AT III is a serine protease inhibitor. Since the vitamin K–dependent factors are serine proteases, the AT III-heparin complex inhibits the enzymatic activity of factor IIa (thrombin) as well as the activity of factors Xa and IXa; however, for steric reasons, the AT III-heparin complex does not inhibit factor VIIa activity.

Protein C and Protein S

Activated protein C is an enzyme which cleaves and destroys cofactors VIIIa and Va (although not the common inherited variant, factor V Leiden). Protein S is a cofactor for protein C. Protein C is a vitamin K-dependent enzyme, just like factors VII, IX, X and II. Thus, protein C activity is also affected by vitamin K deficiency or coumadin therapy.

LABORATORY ASSAYS FOR PLATELET DISORDERS (TABLE 27.2)

Platelet Count

The reference interval for platelet count is typically $150–400 \times 10^3/\mu L$ ($150–400 \times 10^9/L$); hemorrhage is not usually apparent until platelet levels fall far below the lower reference limit. Below platelet levels of $50 \times 10^3/\mu L$ ($50 \times 10^9/L$), patients will bleed when challenged with trauma or surgery. Below platelet levels of $20 \times 10^3/\mu L$ ($20 \times 10^9/L$), patients may present with spontaneous bleeding. The likelihood of bleeding is also dependent on the age of the platelets; young platelets (as predominate in disorders associated with increased platelet destruction or after recovery from chemotherapy or other marrow suppression) function better than older platelets (as predominate in disorders associated with decreased platelet formation). In platelet destructive disor-

Table 27.2.
Laboratory Assays for Evaluating Platelet Function

Test	Reference Range	Utility
Platelet count	150–400 × 10³/μL (150–400 × 10⁹/L)	Detects quantitative abnormality
Bleeding time	<8 min	In vivo assay of platelet function, detects qualitative platelet defects with normal platelet count
Platelet aggregation	Response to each agonist compared to control	In vitro assay of response to specific platelet agonists; can be used to separate qualitative platelet dysfunctions
Bone marrow biopsy	Undefined	Differentiates decreased production from increased destruction

ders, spontaneous bleeding is not likely unless the platelet count is below $10 \times 10^3/\mu L$ ($10 \times 10^9/L$).

The Bleeding Time

This fairly primitive and nonspecific assay is the most commonly used test of in vivo platelet function (qualitative defects). Because the bleeding time is known to be prolonged in patients with thrombocytopenia, it is only useful for assessing platelet function in patients with platelet counts above $100 \times 10^3/\mu L$ ($100 \times 10^9/L$). In adults, the upper reference limit for bleeding time is typically 8–10 min, but varies with technique used. A number of studies suggest that bleeding times in normal pediatric patients may be longer than those of adults.

Platelet Aggregation Assays

Platelet aggregation assays can be used for evaluation of a number of platelet abnormalities. Platelet aggregation induced by the antibiotic ristocetin is impaired in von Willebrand's disease (discussed below). In patients who have intrinsic abnormalities in the contents of the platelet granules, termed storage pool deficiency, abnormal aggregation is seen in response to ADP and collagen. Patients who have defects in synthesis of thromboxane A_2, whether resulting from a congenital decrease in cyclooxygenase or the ingestion of aspirin, will have decreased aggregation in response to arachidonic acid. In addition, aggregation studies are useful to identify rare patients with congenital absence of glycoprotein Ib (**Bernard Soulier Syndrome,** failure to aggregate with ristocetin), or congenital absence of glycoprotein IIb/IIIa (**Glanzmann's Thrombasthenia,** failure to aggregate with ADP, collagen, or arachidonic acid). Platelet aggregation studies are also useful to identify heparin-induced thrombocytopenia. In these patients, autoantibodies to neoepitopes created by the interaction of heparin and platelet molecules cause immune mediated clearance of platelets. The serum of these patients causes aggregation of normal platelets in the presence of heparin.

Bone Marrow Examination

Examination of bone marrow aspirate and biopsy samples is useful to determine if thrombocytopenia results from increased destruction or decreased production of platelets; in the latter case, a decreased number of megakaryocytes is present. An increased number of megakaryocytes suggests that platelets are being destroyed peripherally, and that the marrow is responding with megakaryocytic hyperplasia. In addition, in myelodysplastic and myeloproliferative disorders (Chapter 25), megakaryocytes are often morphologically atypical.

LABORATORY TESTS OF THE COAGULATION SYSTEM (TABLE 27.3)

Causes of Artifactually Abnormal Coagulation System Results

Clotting time tests are among the most commonly affected by problems with specimen collection. Practitioners need to be aware of the common conditions interfering with clotting tests in order to recognize their presence and avoid unnecessary treatment of patients.

Abnormal Chelator Concentration

Blood for clotting tests is collected in tubes containing a calcium chelator, usually sodium citrate. Because addition of calcium in the reagents initiates clotting, a normal ratio of plasma to citrate is critical to prevent artifactual abnormalities in clotting assays. The most common cause of artifactual abnormalities in clotting times is the failure to completely fill tubes, causing higher than normal citrate concentration that allows chelation of calcium in the reagents and falsely prolonged clotting times. A similar phenomenon occurs in patients with polycythemia, who have less plasma in a volume of blood. Severe anemia causes inadequate chelation of calcium and falsely shortened clotting times.

Heparin Contamination

Another common cause of abnormal clotting times is contamination of the specimen with heparin. In critical care areas, blood is often drawn from catheters which may be coated with heparin, or from lines with access maintained patent by small doses of heparin. While normally collection of blood after discarding a volume of blood equal to the volume of the catheter prevents contamination, heparin concentration is so high

Table 27.3.
Laboratory Assays for Evaluating Coagulant Proteins

Test	Reference Range	Utility
Prothrombin time (PT)	11–12 s	Evaluates the extrinsic (factor VII) and common (factor X, V, II) pathways Coumadin monitoring
Partial thromboplastin time (aPTT)	22–33 s	Evaluates the intrinsic (factor XI, IX, VIII) and common (factor X, V, II) pathways Heparin monitoring Screen for lupus anticoagulant
Thrombin time	9–15 s	Evaluates conversion of fibrinogen to fibrin Screen for dysfibrinogenemia
Fibrinogen	200–400 mg/dL	Quantitative and qualitative fibrinogen abnormalities
Factor protein assays	50–80% of control	Detects specific factor or protein abnormalities, both qualitative and quantitative
D-Dimer	<100 ng/mL (μg/L)	Detects fragments of cross-linked fibrin, mainly in DIC
Activated protein C resistance	negative	Detects factor V Leiden mutation, predisposing to hyper-coagulable state

in such catheters that it may be necessary to discard 5–10 mL of blood to prevent contamination. Drawing blood above a line infusing heparin is also a common cause of heparin contamination.

Other Coagulation System Artifacts

Tissue factor is released during the process of venipuncture; specimens for coagulation testing should never be performed on the first tube collected through a needle. Collection above or through an intravenous line will dilute coagulation factors and cause falsely low results. Inadequate mixing of blood for platelet counts will often produce platelet aggregates, causing falsely low platelet counts (most laboratories examine a peripheral smear to detect aggregates and avoid reporting such erroneous counts; practitioners performing their own platelet counts should look at the edges of a smear to detect aggregates). Rarely, fragments of cells are counted as platelets by machines and may cause falsely increased platelet counts.

Prothrombin Time

The prothrombin time (PT) measures coagulation initiated by Factor VIIa. In this assay, tissue factor and calcium are added to patient plasma, and the time to form a fibrin clot is measured. Results are reported in seconds with a reference interval typically 11–12 s. Tissue factor preparations commonly in use are derived from biological materials, causing great variability in reagents used to measure PT. To reduce variability, the **International Normalized Ratio** (INR) has been adopted by most clinical laboratories. The INR is calculated from the patient's and control PTs and a factor describing the relative activity of tissue factor in the reagents, termed the **International Sensitivity Index** (ISI), calculated using Equation 27.1.

$$INR = \left(\frac{Patient\ PT}{Control\ PT}\right)^{ISI} \tag{1}$$

Although the INR allows comparison from one laboratory to another, high ISI numbers produce large changes in INR with small changes in PT, while low ISI numbers increase sensitivity to even minor deficiencies of clotting factors. It is now possible to purchase pure recombinant tissue factor, which has an ISI of 1.0. Use of recombinant tissue factor could eventually greatly reduce the variability currently seen with PT, although few laboratories are currently using it. Because factor VII has the shortest half-life of the vitamin K–dependent factors, the prothrombin time is typically used to assess the effects of coumadin on patients. When coumadin is started, the rapid change in Factor VII quickly causes the PT to increase; however, since other vitamin K–dependent factors have longer half-lives, PT does not accurately reflect the degree of anticoagulation for several days after starting or adjusting the dose of coumadin.

Activated Partial Thromboplastin Time

In the activated partial thromboplastin time (aPTT) assay, calcium and a contact phase activator such as kaolin are added to patient plasma; the tube or cup wall acts as a surface to assemble the members of the intrinsic pathway. As with PT, results are reported as the time to form a fibrin clot. The typical reference range for the aPTT is 22–33 s. Because AT III inhibits factors IX, X, and II, but not factor VII, the aPTT (rather than PT) is commonly used to assess the effect of heparin on patients.

Fibrinogen

Fibrinogen levels are determined by adding an excess of bovine thrombin (factor IIa) to patient plasma; time to form a fibrin clot is measured and compared to a standard curve to obtain fibrinogen level. Fibrinogen can also be estimated from the density of a clot formed during the PT test; this is sometimes termed semiquantitative fibrinogen or SQF. While SQF agrees well with quantitative measurements in most circumstances, it may be falsely high in the presence of dysfibrinogenemia. The typical reference interval for fibrinogen is 200–400 mg/dL.

Thrombin Time

The thrombin time (TT) uses exogenous thrombin to measure conversion of fibrinogen to fibrin; reference ranges are typically 9–15 s. In addition to low levels of fibrinogen, prolonged TT also occurs in the presence of heparin (heparin plus ATIII inactivates thrombin), fibrin degradation products, and abnormal forms of fibrinogen (**dysfibrino-genemia**), which can occur on a congenital basis or with liver disease.

Specific Factor and Protein Assays

Both immunologic and activity assays are commonly available for all hemostatic factors, including plasminogen, AT III, protein C, and protein S. In general, the activity assays are preferable to the immunologic assays, since many patients have qualitative rather than quantitative abnormalities of coagulation factors. Most of these assays use chromogenic substrates so that activity is related to the release of the specific chromogen product.

Fibrin Degradation Products

When fibrin is cleaved by plasmin, a number of small breakdown products are released; these are typically found in blood in a number of diseases in which thrombosis occurs, such as inflammation, myocardial infarction, sickle cell anemia, and venous thrombosis, but in highest concentrations in disseminated intravascular coagulation (DIC), discussed below. There are two different types of assays to measure these products. The D-dimer assay specifically measures one of these breakdown products by an immunoassay. The fibrin degradation (split) products (FDP or FSP) assay uses an antibody to breakdown products which cross-reacts with fibrinogen and its breakdown products; excess thrombin is present in special collection tubes to clot all fibrinogen in normal specimens. Levels of FDP (but not D-dimer) may be falsely elevated with inhibitors of thrombin (such as heparin), and is also high in primary fibrinolysis or dysfibrinogenemia. For this reason, many laboratories offer D-dimer measurement instead of FDP; D-dimer can also be measured in the same tubes used for normal coagulation testing, simplifying collection. It is important for practitioners to be aware which test is performed in the laboratories they use. The presence of the D-dimer fragment of fibrin in levels exceeding 500 ng/mL is strongly suggestive of DIC.

DISORDERS OF HEMOSTASIS

Disorders of hemostasis can be divided into disorders of platelets and disorders of the factors in the coagulation cascade.

When Not to Do Tests of the Coagulation System

Coagulation tests have not been found useful in screening patients before surgery or invasive procedures for a likelihood of bleeding. If the patient has no history of increased bleeding, no risk factors for bleeding (such as use of aspirin or nonsteroidal agents), and no history or laboratory evidence of liver disease, coagulation tests should not be performed. Tests for factor levels or lupus anticoagulants should not be done in patients with normal PT and aPTT. In addition, levels of many factors are increased by acute inflammation, and may be falsely high (or normal) in this situation; factor testing should be deferred in patients with acute inflammation. Coagulation inhibitors are also affected by acute illness; AT III increases, while proteins C and S decrease. Antithrombin III is decreased by heparin and proteins C and S are decreased by coumadin; testing should be deferred during acute illness and during anticoagulant therapy.

Disorders of Platelets

Platelet disorders typically result in generalized spontaneous bleeding. Since the primary function of platelets is to plug small holes, patients with platelet disorders typically present with small, oozing bleeds. These commonly present as petechiae, nosebleeds (epistaxis), and heavy menstrual periods (menorrhagia). These types of small bleeds, while not terribly alarming when present in skin or mucous membranes, can be devastating in other tissues such as the brain. Intracranial hemorrhage is a major cause of morbidity in patients with platelet disorders. Platelet disorders can be divided into two categories: (1) decreased numbers of circulating platelets (thrombocytopenia), and (2) abnormal platelet function.

Decreased Numbers of Platelets

Both acquired and congenital forms of thrombocytopenia have been described. Congenital thrombocytopenia is quite rare and is typically seen as a finding in syndromes such as TAR (thrombocytopenia with absent radii) or the Wiskott Aldrich Syndrome (thrombocytopenia, eczema, and T-cell dysfunction). Acquired thrombocytopenia, by far the more common form, can result from either decreased bone marrow production or increased peripheral destruction. Decreased production of platelets typically results from marrow failure, damage to the bone marrow, or replacement of the bone marrow with tumor or fibrosis. Increased destruction of platelets is seen in patients with a number of conditions. Joint prosthesis and heart valves can cause degranulation and destruction of platelets as they circulate. Autoimmune disorders can result in thrombocytopenia. Patients with **immune thrombocytopenic purpura** (ITP) have autoantibodies against their own platelets; antibody coated platelets are cleared by the reticuloendothelial system (particularly the spleen) resulting in thrombocytopenia. As mentioned earlier, heparin may induce an antibody mediated platelet destruction; occasionally, other drugs may produce a similar immune mediated thrombocytopenia. Platelet survival is decreased in patients with fever and in splenomegaly.

Thrombocytopenia is also an important component of **disseminated intravascular coagulation** (DIC). In DIC, systemic activation of coagulation with widespread thrombosis consumes platelets and fibrinogen, resulting in bleeding. This condition is seen in a number of disorders including traumatic tissue damage (especially head injury, since

Table 27.4.
Laboratory Abnormalities in DIC

Test	Result
D-Dimer	Positive, usually >500 ng/mL (μg/L)
PT	Prolonged (rising from baseline)
aPTT	Prolonged (rising from baseline)
Fibrinogen	Decreased (falling from baseline)
Platelet count	Decreased (falling from baseline)
Peripheral smear exam	Decreased platelets, most large (young) Schistocytes

Early in DIC, D-dimer may be below the detection limit. Repeat determinations are suggested if DIC is considered likely on a clinical basis.

the brain is rich in tissue factor), sepsis, tumor lysis, shock, and amniotic fluid embolization. Laboratory tests useful in making the diagnosis of DIC are listed in Table 27.4.

Decreased Platelet Function

Both acquired and congenital forms of platelet dysfunction have been described. The rare congenital disorders include cyclooxygenase deficiency, in which platelets cannot produce thromboxane A_2 and fail to aggregate. The most common congenital form of platelet dysfunction is von Willebrand's disease, discussed in detail below. Acquired functional abnormalities of platelets are quite common. Some are due to pharmacological agents; aspirin and nonsteroidal anti-inflammatory drugs inhibit platelet cyclooxygenase, inhibiting production of thromboxane A_2. Any evaluation of platelet function should always be performed when patients have been off aspirin for at least one week. Patients with uremia and liver failure often have impaired platelet function. In liver failure, decreased clearance allows accumulation of FDPs that adhere to platelets and interrupt normal platelet adhesion. Patients with myeloproliferative disorders, especially essential thrombocythemia, can produce abundant numbers of platelets; however, these are often defective and do not provide adequate hemostasis. Similar types of platelet functional defects have also been described in myelodysplastic syndromes.

Disorders of the Coagulation System

Coagulation system abnormalities can be divided into two categories: (1) decreased amount or activity of procoagulant factors which results in bleeding, and (2) decreased amount or activity of anticoagulant factors which results in hypercoagulability.

Disorders That Result in Bleeding

In contrast to the small bleeds seen in patients with platelet disorders, patients with defects in the coagulation system typically present with large bleeds, often in joints. Decreases or defects in coagulation factors can be acquired or congenital. Since the vitamin K–dependent enzymes and the cofactors are not consumed during coagulation, the levels of these proteins must be markedly decreased to see a clinical effect. More commonly, mild deficiencies are detected by prolongation of the PT or aPTT.

Acquired Coagulation Factor Deficiency

Since almost all coagulation factors are synthesized by the liver (factor VIII is made in endothelial cells), severe hepatocellular damage or portal hypertension (Chapter 11) results in decreased plasma coagulation factor levels. In addition, patients with vitamin K deficiency resulting from severe malnutrition or long term broad spectrum antibiotic treatment will have selective deficiency in factors VII, IX, X, and II activities.

Congenital Coagulation Factor Deficiency

Congenital abnormalities of all factors of the coagulation cascade have been described. Severe bleeding can occur with deficiencies in factors XI, VIII, VII, X, V, II, or fibrinogen; severity of bleeding depends on the level of functioning factor present. The most common congenital deficiency is **von Willebrand's disease,** due to one of several defects in production or function (usually inherited in an autosomal dominant fashion) of von Willebrand factor, a cofactor necessary for Factor VIII activity and platelet adhesion. In many cases, von Willebrand's disease is mild; symptomatic patients often have bleeding after surgical procedures, nosebleeds, and may bruise easily. While the aPTT may be abnormal, in many cases it is not prolonged. Specific tests include measurement of von Willebrand factor and impaired platelet aggregation in response to ristocetin.

The most common severe congenital coagulation deficiencies are the two forms of **hemophilia.** Patients with hemophilia often have bleeding into soft tissues or joints after only mild trauma, and also may have severe external bleeding after trauma or surgery. Bleeding in hemophilia is typically not present until the activity level of a factor falls below 30% of normal, and severe bleeding is not seen until the activity level of a factor is less than 1% of normal. Deficiencies in factor VIII (hemophilia A) and factor IX (hemophilia B) are the most common and are typically seen in males, since the genes for these two factors are on the X-chromosome. The other factors are on autosomes and thus the patients must have a defect in both genes to present with hemophilia.

Disorders That Result in Thrombosis

It is becoming increasingly clear that patients who present with a first thrombotic event relatively early in life or recurrent thrombotic events in later adult years often have deficiencies in specific plasma proteins leading to a hypercoagulable state.

Acquired Hypercoagulable States

The most common acquired condition resulting in hypercoagulability is the antiphospholipid syndrome (lupus anticoagulant). Patients with lupus and other autoimmune diseases often make antiphospholipid antibodies, discussed in more detail in Chapter 37. In the test tube, these antibodies bind to the phospholipids used to activate the intrinsic pathway in the aPTT assay, causing prolongation of the aPTT. However, in vivo, these patients are prone to thrombosis, although the mechanism of the hypercoagulability is not clearly understood. In patients with a prolonged aPTT, "lupus anticoagulants" can be recognized by performing mixing studies; when a prolonged aPTT is due to factor deficiencies, mixing with normal plasma will correct the result to normal, while antiphospholipid antibodies will inhibit normal coagulation as well and the aPTT will fail to correct to normal.

Congenital Hypercoagulable States

Congenital deficiencies in AT III, protein C, and protein S have all been described. Deficiencies in protein C appear to be the most common of the three. Patients with these deficiencies are typically heterozygotes who do not present with thrombosis until the second or third decade of life. When infants are born with a homozygous deficiency in protein C, these babies rapidly develop purpura fulminans, which is often fatal. In addition, approximately 5% of the population is heterzygous for a mutation in factor V (factor V Leiden), which makes factor V resistant to the enzymatic activity of protein C. The presence of this mutation appears to be a risk factor for the development of early thrombotic disease.

Abnormal Fibrinolysis

Disorders in the fibrinolytic system have also been described, including quantitative and qualitative abnormalities of plasminogen, as well as dysfibrogenemia in which the fibrin polymer is resistant to the proteolytic effect of plasmin. Interestingly, while factor XII is part of the contact factor complex which initiates coagulation in the test tube, factor XII deficiency clinically results in hypercoagulability. This may reflect the fact that factor XIIa participates in the conversion of plasminogen to plasmin.

MONITORING ANTICOAGULANT THERAPY

Anticoagulants are commonly used to manage patients with a number of medical problems. While levels of the two major anticoagulants, heparin and coumadin, can be measured, patients receiving these medications are better monitored by the effects of the drugs on coagulation.

Monitoring Coumadin Therapy

Coumadin is usually used for long term anticoagulation. As discussed earlier, coumadin impairs γ-carboxylation of factors VII, IX, X, and II, reducing their activity and mainly prolonging the PT. The short half-life of factor VII means that PT rapidly becomes abnormal after starting coumadin or increasing the dosage; PT should not be checked for at least three days after a change in coumadin therapy. The target for treatment should be based on INR; a value between 2 and 3 generally assures adequate anticoagulation with a low risk of increased bleeding.

Monitoring Heparin Therapy

Heparin is usually used when rapid anticoagulation is needed. While heparin may affect both the aPTT and PT, its effects on aPTT are usually used for monitoring therapy. The target for treatment is to increase the aPTT to 1.5–2.5 times the baseline value. In patients receiving low dose heparin, aPTT is not as reliable for monitoring treatment, and measurement of heparin levels is often required.

DIAGNOSIS AND MONITORING OF INFECTIONS

CHAPTER 28

Evaluation of Urinary Tract Infection

JOSEPH M. CAMPOS

Urinary tract infections, after respiratory tract infections, are the second most common type of infections reported in the U.S. They are responsible for more than 7 million visits to physician offices and more than 1 million hospitalizations in the U.S. each year. The majority are acute infections localized to the bladder or urethra. Others, however, may occur in or extend to the upper urinary tract or the prostate gland. They can become complicated by leading to invasive infection or by establishing a chronically infected state.

Under normal circumstances, microorganisms do not inhabit the urinary tract, except perhaps when bacteria colonize the distal urethra. Urine in the bladder should be sterile. Entry of microorganisms into the lower or upper tract, either by mechanical or invasive means, can result in microbial proliferation and infection. Uncomplicatea infections are relatively minor and respond promptly to antimicrobial therapy. However, urinary tract infections are a frequent cause of secondary bacteremia, and even uncomplicated infections are deserving of prompt medical attention.

TYPES OF URINARY TRACT INFECTION

The infections discussed in this chapter include asymptomatic bacteriuria, cystitis, urethritis, prostatitis, and pyelonephritis. The risk factors for these infections varies by age of the patient (Table 28.1).

Asymptomatic bacteriuria refers to the presence of bacteria in the urine of patients who are manifesting no obvious symptoms. This condition occurs in a high percentage of elderly patients (as many as 40%), pregnant women, patients who have experienced invasive urologic interventions, patients who have had recent removal of a chronic indwelling catheter, and young children. Routine detection and antimicrobial treatment of patients with asymptomatic bacteriuria who do not fall into one of the previously mentioned categories is not recommended because of the unnecessary risks of antimicrobial side effects and selection of antimicrobial resistance.

Cystitis is a term describing inflammation of the bladder and occurs mainly in young, sexually active women (Fig. 28.1). Cystitis presents typically with symptoms of dysuria, frequency, and urgency. Symptomatic patients should have urinalysis or other rapid screening tests performed and if findings are consistent with infection, should be treated empirically with an antimicrobial agent effective against the usual causes of infection. Single dose or short course therapy with an appropriate antimicrobial agent is generally all that is required. A urine culture should be performed if symptoms persist for more than 72 hours after the initiation of therapy.

Urethritis is most often found in patients suffering from one of several sexually transmitted diseases (see Chapter 30). However, urethritis can also be present in patients presenting with the symptoms of an ordinary urinary tract infection (acute urethral syndrome). Laboratory testing of these patients typically reveals an abundance

351

Table 28.1.
Age-specific Conditions or Activities Leading to Urinary
Tract Infection

<1 year	Abnormalities of the urinary tract
1–5 years	Abnormalities of the urinary tract, vesicoureteral reflux
6–15 years	Vesicoureteral reflux
16–35 years	Sexual activity
36–65 years	Sexual activity, catheterization, prostatic hypertrophy
>65 years	Catheterization, prostatic hypertrophy, incontinence

of inflammatory cells accompanied by low numbers of microorganisms. Management of these patients is the same as for patients with cystitis.

Prostatitis is an infection of male adults, but may occasionally affect male children as well (Fig. 28.2). There are two forms of prostatitis, acute and chronic, with the symptoms of acute disease being more severe. Acutely infected patients usually experience chills and fever accompanied by perineal discomfort. Symptoms of cystitis and urethritis are also commonly present.

Symptoms in chronically infected patients are variable and may include dysuria, urgency, frequency, hematuria, hematospermia, and discomfort in the lower back, perineum, penis, groin, testes, or thighs. Laboratory confirmation of infectious prostatitis entails collection of sequential specimens for colony count culture: the first 10 mL of voided urine (VB$_1$), a midstream urine specimen (VB$_2$), prostatic fluid collected after prostatic massage (EPS), and the first 10 mL of voided urine after the prostatic massage (VB$_3$). VB$_1$ results indicate the presence of urethral flora, VB$_2$ corresponds to the bladder, and EPS/VB$_3$ results delineate organisms present in the prostate. If the EPS/VB$_3$ colony counts are more than 10-fold higher than the other colony counts, a diagnosis

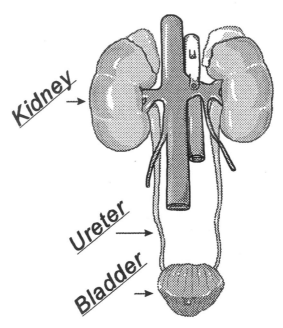

Figure 28.1. Human urinary tract.

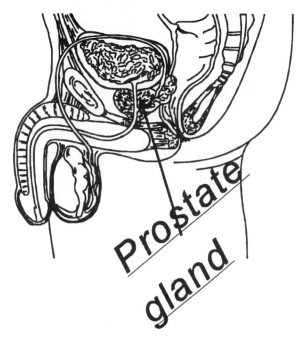

Figure 28.2. Male genitourinary tract.

of prostatitis is confirmed. Absence of a 10-fold difference in colony counts, however, does not rule out prostatitis unless the EPS/VB$_3$ cultures yield negative or very low colony counts.

Pyelonephritis refers to infection of the upper urinary tract (usually the kidneys) and is characterized by systemic symptoms (e.g. headache, nausea, vomiting, fever with chills) and unilateral or bilateral flank pain, lower back pain, or abdominal pain. Urinalysis, pretreatment and posttreatment cultures, and monitoring tests of renal function are indicated. Two weeks of outpatient treatment with an antimicrobial agent to which culture isolates are susceptible should be initiated.

Etiologic Agents of Urinary Tract Infections

The most frequent causes of urinary tract infection are bacteria, which routinely colonize the gastrointestinal tract or the perineal skin (Table 28.2). These organisms enter the host either from exogenous sources via the distal urinary tract, or from endogenous sources via the bloodstream and kidneys. Most commonly, urinary tract pathogens

Table 28.2.
Frequent Causes of Urinary Tract Infection

Infection	Microorganisms
Asymptomatic bacteriuria, cystitis, urethritis	*Escherichia coli, Staphylococcus saprophyticus, Proteus mirabilis, Klebsiella pneumoniae, Enterococcus* spp.
Prostatitis	*Escherichia coli, Proteus mirabilis, Klebsiella pneumoniae, Enterococcus* spp.
Pyelonephritis	*Escherichia coli, Proteus mirabilis, Klebsiella pneumoniae, Staphylococcus aureus*

originate from the gastrointestinal tract or from colonized periurethral sites and gain entry to the bladder through the urethra. The urethra in adult females is approximately 11 cm shorter than in adult males and is a major reason that these infections occur more commonly in women. Once in the urinary tract, infectious agents must avoid eradication by the host's humoral and cellular immune system if infection is to ensue.

Laboratory Diagnosis of Urinary Tract Infection

The laboratory is frequently called upon to assist in making the diagnosis of urinary tract infection. Tests commonly employed include macroscopic/microscopic urinalysis, manual/automated screens for markers of infection, and culture.

The success of laboratory testing is dependent upon the care with which specimens are collected and transported. Most important are (1) avoidance of specimen contamination with periurethral flora during collection, and (2) prevention of microbial growth during transport of specimens to the laboratory. Occurrence of either problem can ruin the diagnostic value of specimens.

The optimum time to sample urine for pathogens is in the morning, prior to or simultaneous with the day's first voiding. At this time infecting organisms are at their highest numbers, and discrimination between clinically significant and insignificant findings is easiest. Clean catch, catheterized or suprapubically aspirated specimens may be collected and should be placed in sterile, leak-proof containers.

Clean catch specimens from females and uncircumcised males require disinfection of the periurethral area prior to collection (Table 28.3). The instructions for uncircumcised males are similar to those in Table 28.3 except that the head of the penis is cleansed, rinsed, and the specimen collected while the foreskin is retracted with one hand. The specimen should be midstream urine to avoid gross contamination with residual intraurethral flora. A suitable midstream specimen is one in which the first 10 mL of voided urine is not collected. Despite these precautions, clean catch specimens inevitably are contaminated with small numbers of microorganisms, and care must be taken during specimen transport to the laboratory to prevent multiplication of contaminants. Maintenance of specimens at 4 C after collection and during transport is effective. Commercially available urine preservative tubes containing boric acid stabilize colony counts of pathogens and contaminants alike and are useful when long delays in specimen delivery are likely. Agar dipslide culturing devices that are inoculated immediately after specimen collection by medical care personnel can also be helpful in minimizing the problems associated with delayed specimen transport.

Table 28.3.
Collection of Clean Catch Urine Specimens from Women

Instructions
1. Wash hands with soap and water, rinse, and dry.
2. Separate the labia majora with one hand during cleansing and collection of the urine sample.
3. Soak four cotton gauze sponges with disinfectant soap and use each successively to cleanse the urethral area from front to back.
4. Soak four more cotton gauze sponges with warm water and use each successively to rinse the urethral area.
5. Void a small quantity of urine into the toilet, and then collect a sample of urine into the collection container without touching the container to the legs, genitalia, or clothing.
6. Apply the container lid in a manner that will prevent leakage and submit the specimen for testing.

Catheterized specimens are collected by introducing a sterile, narrow gauge tube (e.g. #12 French catheter) through the urethra and into the bladder. The initial flow of urine is discarded and a mid-flow specimen is collected, theoretically free of contamination from microorganisms colonizing the distal urethral mucosa. In reality, catheterized specimens are usually contaminated with small numbers of microorganisms carried into the bladder during the catheter insertion process. Such specimens should be handled and transported to the laboratory in the same manner as clean catch specimens.

For patients with indwelling urinary catheters, the catheter collection port should be disinfected and punctured directly with a needle and syringe. The specimen is aspirated, transferred to a sterile, leak-proof container, and delivered promptly to the laboratory.

Suprapubically aspirated urine is collected via aseptic needlestick puncture of the abdominal and bladder walls. Patients should have had high fluid intake and refrained from voiding for 1–2 hours prior to the procedure. The puncture site should be in the midline, approximately 5 cm above the pubic symphysis in adults, and thoroughly disinfected with povidone-iodine and cleansed with 70% ethanol. If performed properly, suprapubically aspirated urine is similar to other closed cavity body fluids and should be processed by the laboratory in the same manner as cerebrospinal fluid, synovial fluid, peritoneal fluid, etc. Care must be taken during needle insertion not to enter the large intestine and carry fecal material into the bladder.

Microscopic Urinalysis

Microscopic examination of unstained urine sediments during urinalysis is often the first direct laboratory evidence of infection. Leukocytosis, erythrocytosis, or bacteriuria, when present, are strong indicators of urinary tract infection. For laboratories which use a hemacytometer counting chamber for examining urine, significant leukocytosis has been defined as at least 8–10 leukocytes per mm^3 (excretion rate of more than 400,000 leukocytes per hour). Such findings are sufficient to prompt antimicrobial therapy in symptomatic patients with uncomplicated presentations and warrant follow-up cultures in other patients.

Gram Stain Microscopy

Examination of Gram-stained smears can also offer rapid laboratory evidence of infection. Observation of at least one organism per oil immersion field (1,000 ×) of stained, uncentrifuged urine is indicative of greater than 100,000 colony forming units per mL (cfu/mL). The Gram stain cannot be relied upon to accurately estimate colony counts less than 100,000 cfu/mL.

Gram-stained smears should be examined for the presence of leukocytes as well as microorganisms. The finding of many microorganisms in the absence of leukocytes in an immunologically normal host suggests specimen contamination. On the other hand, the presence of leukocytes without seeing microorganisms may indicate a sexually transmitted disease (e.g. *Chlamydia trachomatis* urethritis) or may be suggestive of acute urethral syndrome. Specimens from patients with unclear microscopic findings should be cultured.

Rapid Screening Tests

Several rapid urine screening tests are available today as aids for diagnosis of infection. They are potentially useful to practitioners to help decide whether patients require empirical antimicrobial therapy or whether specimens should be transported to the laboratory for culture. They are potentially useful to the laboratory to help decide which specimens warrant the time, effort, and expense of culture. The principal shortcoming of the rapid screens described below is their inability to reliably identify specimens with colony counts less than 100,000 cfu/mL.

Leukocyte Esterase

The leukocyte esterase (LE) test, now part of the standard urine dipstick, is a two minute screen for the presence of neutrophil granulocytes. The LE test thus screens for pyuria rather than bacteriuria. A positive test, evidenced by pinkish purple color development, indicates greater than 10 leukocytes per mm^3. The sensitivity and specificity of the leukocyte esterase test in identifying patients with more than 100,000 cfu/mL in urine has ranged from 70–90% in published studies. Obviously the test is of little to no value in screening specimens collected from neutropenic patients.

Urinary Nitrite

The nitrite test (NO_2) is also part of the standard urine dipstick and is a one minute screen for the presence of nitrite, an anion not normally present in human urine, but produced by many bacteria. Best results are obtained when testing first morning specimens, a time at which microbial colony counts are at their highest and sufficient time for microbial reduction of nitrate to nitrite has elapsed. The sensitivity of the test for identifying patients with greater than 100,000 cfu/mL in urine has ranged from 30–70% and the specificity has been more than 90%. The test is falsely negative in specimens harboring (1) microorganisms lacking the nitrate reductase system (e.g. *Enterococcus*), (2) bacteria which further reduce nitrite to ammonia or nitrogen gas (some *Pseudomonas* species), (3) nitrite concentrations below the detection capability of the test, (4) abnormal amounts of urobilinogen in urine, or (5) a urine pH below 6. A positive test result is denoted by pinkish red color development.

Colorimetric Filtration

Both bacteriuria and pyuria may be detected by colorimetric methods in less than two minutes. Specimens are passed through a filter, which traps both microorganisms and white blood cells. Safranin dye is then passed through the filter to stain captured material. Any degree of pinkness against the white background of the filter signifies a positive result. Specimens that contain precipitates or urinary pigments can interfere with test performance and interpretation by clogging the filter or imparting color to the filter. The sensitivity of these tests for identifying specimens with greater than 100,000 cfu/mL has been impressive, with results above 95% in most studies. As many as 15% of specimens have resulted in clogged filters and uninterpretable results, however.

Bioluminescence

Bioluminescence assays specific for bacterial adenosine triphosphate (ATP) are a relatively new approach toward rapid detection of bacteriuria. Specimens are first treated with somatic cell releasing agent, which ruptures the cell membranes of leukocytes and erythrocytes, releasing their ATP into solution. The ATP is destroyed by ATPase or removed by filtration. Intact microorganisms remaining in the specimen are lysed with a second reagent, and their ATP is used to supply energy for light production by the firefly luciferin–luciferase system. Light emission is measured with a luminometer, which provides data for a rough estimate of the colony count. Commercially available systems are capable of providing results in less than 30 minutes. The sensitivity of these assays has ranged between 85% and 97%, but false positive rates have been as high as 25%.

Culture

Culture remains the gold standard for laboratory diagnosis of urinary tract infection. The microorganisms most likely to cause infection, i.e., enteric Gram negative rods, enterococci, and staphylococci, dictate media selection. Searches for unusual infectious etiologies (e.g. *Neisseria gonorrhoea, Hemophilus* spp., fungi, and *Mycobacterium* spp.) necessitate alerting the laboratory so that special media can be inoculated and incubation temperature and duration adjusted.

Routine cultures are incubated overnight at 35 C under aerobic conditions. Since the most commonly encountered pathogens grow rapidly, there is no need to incubate cultures for longer periods of time, unless slowly growing organisms are being sought (e.g. fungi or mycobacteria), or specimens yielding positive Gram stains show no evidence of growth after one day of incubation.

INTERPRETATION OF LABORATORY TEST RESULTS

The rule of thumb used by most clinicians when evaluating laboratory results for the possibility of urinary tract infection in patients is (1) higher than normal erythrocyte or leukocyte counts in urine, (2) the presence of leukocyte esterase or nitrite in urine, or (3) culture colony counts of a single organism greater than 100,000 cfu/mL are all indicative of infection. Colony counts between 10,000 and 100,000 cfu/mL may be indicative of infection, and colony counts less than 10,000 cfu/mL are usually not indicative of infection in patients with cystitis. Specimens yielding growth of more than one organism generally suggest that contamination of urine with periurethral flora may be fully or partly responsible for the culture results. One must remember, however, that the above colony count guidelines were developed during studies of first morning voided urine from asymptomatic adult females. Specimens collected later in the day from symptomatically infected patients or infected patients who have been partially treated with antimicrobial agents may exhibit colony counts as low as 100 cfu/mL. Clinically significant colony counts from adult males and children also can be lower than 100,000 cfu/mL. Detection of any microorganisms in properly collected suprapubic aspirates is abnormal and should be considered evidence of infection. In sum, the clinician and the microbiologist must have an understanding, sometimes requiring communication on a case by case basis, concerning which laboratory results in which patients require further testing (e.g. antimicrobial susceptibility determination) be undertaken.

ANTIMICROBIAL SUSCEPTIBILITY TESTING

It has become clear that routine culture and antimicrobial susceptibility testing of all patients with evidence of urinary tract infection is unnecessary. Otherwise healthy adult ambulatory patients who present with classical symptoms of a nonrecurrent infection and who yield positive results on one of the rapid screening tests described earlier can be successfully managed with empirical, single dose antimicrobial therapy (e.g.

trimethoprim/sulfamethoxazole). In these cases, neither culture nor antimicrobial susceptibility testing is a cost-efficient practice. Should symptoms persist following single
dose therapy, then culture and antimicrobial susceptibility testing are indicated.

Standardized antimicrobial susceptibility test methods described in Chapter 34
can be used on clinically significant urinary tract isolates when testing is medically
indicated. Test batteries of antimicrobial agents should be selected to include agents
relevant to the treatment of urinary tract infections (e.g. ampicillin, first generation
cephalosporin, gentamicin, trimethoprim, sulfisoxazole, trimethoprim/sulfamethoxa-
zole, nitrofurantoin, and ciprofloxacin).

CHAPTER 29.

Respiratory Tract Infection

JOSEPH M. CAMPOS and D. ROBERT DUFOUR

CLINICAL PATTERNS OF RESPIRATORY TRACT INFECTION

The most frequent human infections are those of the upper respiratory tract. Respiratory infections range from the common minor, self-limiting disorders (rhinitis, pharyngitis) to severe, life-threatening infections (pneumonia, tuberculosis). Most respiratory tract infections are acquired following inhalation of organisms within microscopic droplets of respiratory secretions produced by coughing or sneezing, or less commonly droplets of water from aerosolizing machinery (cooling towers and *Legionella*). In some cases, organisms reach the respiratory tract following hand contact with contaminated surfaces or objects, subsequently allowing entry via the mouth, nose or eyes (e.g. respiratory syncytial virus). Respiratory infections can affect individuals of all ages, although otitis, epiglottitis, and bronchiolitis are much more common in children under age 5 years than older persons. The most common causes of differing respiratory tract infections are given in Table 29.1.

Infections of the Upper Respiratory Tract

Upper respiratory tract infections are the leading reason patients seek medical attention. While the majority are viral in nature and require only palliative therapy, a significant percentage are caused by other microorganisms and require antimicrobial therapy. Normally, the upper tract contains large numbers of aerobic (streptococci, *Lactobacillus*) and anaerobic (*Actinomyces, Peptostreptococcus*) organisms.

Pharyngitis

Inflammation of the throat may be infectious (viral or bacterial) or noninfectious (mucosal irritants, allergies, reflux of acidic stomach contents, etc.). Symptoms of pharyngitis range from mild but persistent scratchiness of the throat to severe throat discomfort associated with fever and cervical lymphadenitis. The latter are more common with bacterial pharyngitis (usually due to Group A streptococci). While viral and noninfectious pharyngitis require only symptomatic treatment, bacterial pharyngitis requires antimicrobial therapy. In streptococcal pharyngitis, treatment also prevents immunologic complications such as rheumatic fever or glomerulonephritis. Less commonly, pharyngitis may be due to *Neisseria gonorrheae* following oral sex with an infected individual, *Corynebacterium diptheriae* (which produces a tenacious "pseudomembrane" in the pharynx) in nonimmunized individuals, or *Arcanobacterium hemolyticum* (producing pharyngitis and rash, usually in adolescents and young adults). Most microbiology laboratories assume that pharyngeal swabs submitted for testing are to rule out infection with beta-hemolytic streptococci only, and will not culture for these other organisms unless informed of suspicion of atypical bacterial infection. It is critical for the practitioner to communicate with the laboratory when clinical features suggest infection with one of these organisms.

Table 29.1.
Frequent Causes of Respiratory Tract Infection

Infection	Microorganisms
Pharyngitis	*Streptococcus pyogenes* (Group A streptococci), *Streptococcus* Group C, *Arcanobacterium hemolyticum, Neisseria gonorrhoeae*, coronaviruses, rhinoviruses, adenoviruses
Sinusitis	*Streptococcus pneumoniae, Haemophilus influenzae* (nontypeable), *Staphylococcus aureus, Moraxella catarrhalis*, rhinoviruses
Otitis media	*Streptococcus pneumoniae, Haemophilus influenzae* (nontypeable), *Moraxella catarrhalis*
Otitis externa	*Pseudomonas aeruginosa, Aspergillus niger*
Epiglottitis	*Haemophilus influenzae* type b, *Streptococcus pyogenes* (Group A streptococci)
Laryngotracheobronchitis	Parainfluenza viruses, respiratory syncytial virus
Bronchiolitis	Respiratory syncytial virus, parainfluenza viruses, adenoviruses, influenza viruses
Acute bronchitis	Influenza viruses, adenoviruses, rhinoviruses, coronaviruses, *Mycoplasma pneumoniae, Chlamydia pneumoniae, Bordetella pertussis*
Community acquired pneumonia	*Streptococcus pneumoniae, Mycoplasma pneumoniae, Staphylococcus aureus, Klebsiella pneumoniae, Haemophilus influenzae, Legionella pneumophilia*, mixed anaerobic bacteria
Hospital acquired pneumonia	*Enterobacteriaceae, Pseudomonas aeruginosa, Legionella pneumophilia*
Interstitial pneumonia	Respiratory syncytial virus, influenza viruses, parainfluenza viruses, adenoviruses, *Pneumocystis carinii, Mycobacterium avium, Chlamydia pneumoniae*
Granulomas	*Mycobacterium tuberculosis, Histoplasma capsulatum, Blastomyces dermatitidis, Cryptococcus neoformans, Coccidioides immitis*

Sinusitis

Inflammation of the paranasal sinuses is usually acute, caused by bacteria in most cases; however, viruses, fungi, and even allergies may be causative. As many as 30% of adults suffer chronic sinusitis (inflammation lasting more than six weeks). Most cases of acute sinusitis follow a cold; features indicating progression include purulent nasal discharge and persistence of discharge for more than a week. Bacterial agents responsible for both acute and chronic sinusitis are usually normal upper respiratory tract flora (*Streptococcus pneumoniae, Haemophilus influenzae*). Since cefaclor or amoxicillin/clavulanic acid are generally effective against these organisms, many practitioners elect to treat infections empirically and do not perform culture. Patients not responding to empirical therapy require sinus aspirates for culture and susceptibility testing.

Otitis Media

Middle ear inflammation is one of the most common inflammatory disorders of infants and children below the age of 5, but it may also occur in older children and adults. In infants, the eustachian tube (connecting the middle ear with the nasopharynx) is nearly horizontal, allowing easier obstruction in young children than in older children and adults. Serous otitis describes accumulation of fluid in the middle ear, due to eustachian tube obstruction. It is usually separated from infectious otitis media (often simply termed acute otitis media) by the presence of fever, erythema, and bulging or fixation of the ear drum. Infection by upper respiratory bacteria (*S. pneumoniae*, nontypeable *H. influenzae, Moraxella catarrhalis*) often follows a viral infection which impairs drainage, and further swelling from acute inflammation worsens the obstruction and prevents bacterial clearance. While culture of middle ear fluid obtained by tympanocentesis allows identification of the causative organism, most cases are treated empirically and cultures are performed only with recurrent infection or primary infection refractory to antimicrobial therapy.

Otitis Externa

Inflammation of the outer ear canal (often called "swimmer's ear") is caused by bacteria (*Pseudomonas aeruginosa*), fungi (*Aspergillus niger*), or allergies. Symptoms include ear canal itching (often the first symptom), redness, extreme pain and swelling, sometimes associated with a foul smelling discharge; rarely, the swelling or exudate impairs hearing. Diagnosis is usually based on history and physical findings, while presumptive etiology can be determined by Gram stain of scrapings from inflamed areas of the ear canal. In cases that do not respond to empirical treatment, culture can be performed. Interpretation of smear or culture results should consider inevitable contamination by cutaneous flora (staphylococci, micrococci, diphtheroids).

Epiglottitis

Inflammation of the epiglottis and supraglottic structures is a childhood disease almost exclusively caused by *H. influenzae* type B, although the incidence has markedly declined since the introduction of *H. influenzae* vaccine. The organism invades the epiglottis or supraglottic tissues and, in most cases, the bloodstream. Epiglottitis has an abrupt onset of high fever, sore throat and dysphagia, moderate to severe respiratory distress, stridor, and lethargy. Visualization of the tip of the inflamed epiglottis (maraschino cherry sign) behind the tongue is the most obvious physical sign of infection. Documentation of the causative organism is usually based on positive blood culture, as attempts to visualize the epiglottis for culture can cause acute respiratory obstruction. Isolates should be tested for penicillin resistance to guide treatment.

Infections of the Lower Respiratory Tract

In contrast to the upper respiratory tract, the trachea, bronchi, and lungs typically have little bacterial flora present. Protective mechanisms in the lower respiratory tract include ciliary action by tracheal and bronchial cells, producing a physical "current" which washes out particulate matter, and the gag and cough reflexes which prevent upper respiratory material from reaching the lungs. The few bacteria which reach the lungs are usually handled by neutrophils and macrophages. Bacterial infection of the lungs is much more common in patients with damage to any of these protective barriers. Viruses are able to avoid these protective mechanisms; antibodies are the major protection against viral infection.

Laryngotracheobronchitis

Often termed croup, laryngotracheobronchitis is an acute viral infection of both upper and lower airways, generally affecting only infants and young children. Patients present with a barking cough, difficulty on inspiration (stridor), and occasionally with lung findings such as wheezing or ronchi. The major clinical findings are due to edema just below the larynx. Most cases are due to viruses, usually parainfluenza and, occasionally, respiratory syncitial virus (RSV). Culture is seldom indicated and treatment is usually nonspecific, using humidified air.

Bronchiolitis

Also a disease of young children, bronchiolitis typically presents with wheezing, cough, and respiratory distress. It is almost always caused by viruses, particularly RSV which is responsible for over half of cases. The virus initially infects upper airways and spreads to bronchioles, causing epithelial necrosis. The resultant edema and exudate cause partial or complete bronchiolar obstruction. Most cases occur as part of seasonal epidemics and are treated with humidified air. Severe cases or cases caused by RSV in children with complicating features (e.g. cardiac problems) are treated with aerosolized ribavirin. Recognition of RSV infection can be accomplished by culture, which takes several days to become positive. In most laboratories, detection of RSV antigen is usually employed instead of culture.

Bronchitis

Inflammation of large lung airways is usually caused by a virus, but may also be caused by bacteria or irritants in the air, such as allergens or air pollution. Acute bronchitis presents initially with cough, often productive of thick yellowish-gray sputum, often associated with fever, pleuritic chest pain, and wheezing. Common etiologies include *Mycoplasma pneumoniae* and *Chlamydia pneumoniae* which are usually treated empirically with oral clarithromycin or azithromycin; *S. pneumoniae* and *H. influenzae* can often be cultured from sputum in patients with chronic bronchitis and do not indicate acute infection or a need for antimicrobial therapy. Often, acute bronchitis develops in a patient with chronic bronchitis (clinically defined as productive cough on most days for more than three months during two years). A change in the amount or character of sputum production usually indicates acute infection. In contrast, chronic bronchitis is usually due to chronic airway irritation by tobacco smoke or air pollutants, and rarely is due to infection.

Airspace (Broncho-, Lobar) Pneumonia

Inflammation of alveolar spaces is the most common life-threatening infectious disease; approximately two million cases are recognized annually in the U.S. with an estimated 40,000 to 70,000 deaths. Pneumonia ranks sixth as a cause of death and is the most common fatal hospital-acquired infection. Clinically, it presents with fever, productive cough, and often with shortness of breath. Chest radiographs and clinical examination demonstrate the loss of airspaces. Airspace infection occurs when bacteria escape defense mechanisms; risk factors include agents damaging cilia (smoking), decreased immune response (old age, immunosuppression), decreased granulocytes, and impaired cough and gag mechanism (intoxication, debilitation). Rarely, aspiration of oral and gastric contents allows upper respiratory bacteria to directly reach the lung, often along with gastric acid which chemically damages cilia. Clinically, it is important to distinguish pneumonia that develops in ambulatory individuals ("community acquired pneumonia"), most commonly due to *S. pneumoniae* or *M. pneumoniae*, from hospital acquired pneumonia, often caused by other bacteria (e.g. *Escherichia coli, Serratia marcescens, Pseudomonas aeruginosa*). Because cultures are often nondiagnostic, especially in community acquired pneumonia, treatment is usually empirical unless cultures or lack of clinical response indicate a need to change therapy.

Interstitial Pneumonia

Inflammation affecting primarily the septa of alveoli is termed interstitial pneumonia. In addition to infection, interstitial damage may also be caused by early congestive heart failure, by idiopathic inflammatory disorders, and granulomatous disease. Clinically, interstitial pneumonia typically presents as shortness of breath, often with nonproductive or minimally productive cough. Affected patients often have low oxygen saturation on pulse oximetry, and respiratory alkalosis. A variety of organisms may cause interstitial pneumonia; viruses are most common, but *Pneumocystis carinii*, mycobacterial infections, and chlamydial species may also be responsible. Traditional bacterial cultures are not helpful in interstitial pneumonitis.

Granulomatous Inflammation

Infection of the lung by organisms that cannot be destroyed by neutrophils or macrophages (usually *Mycobacterium tuberculosis* and fungi such as *Histoplasma capsulatum*, *Blastomyces dermatitidis*, *Cryptococcus neoformans*, and *Coccidioides immitis*) typically leads to production of masses of modified macrophages (termed granulomas) which contain but do not destroy the organism. Granulomas typically present as one or more nodular lesions on a chest radiograph, often with enlargement of hilar lymph nodes. Calcification is common with some infectious agents, particularly *H. capsulatum*. With progression of infection, lesions often develop central necrosis and cavities develop when the inflammation erodes into an air space, allowing drainage of the necrotic material.

GENERAL TESTS OF USE IN IDENTIFYING RESPIRATORY TRACT INFECTION

Diagnosis of infection anywhere in the respiratory tract is complicated by the wide variety of microorganisms colonizing the upper respiratory tract. When infection occurs in the upper respiratory tract, the etiologic agent or agents sometimes must be identified among numerous saprophytic (i.e. currently harmless), but potentially pathogenic, microorganisms. When infection occurs in the lower respiratory tract, collection of specimens not contaminated with upper respiratory flora is virtually impossible, unless an invasive procedure bypassing the mouth, pharynx, and trachea is used. Interpretation of culture/smear results from respiratory tract specimens is difficult at best.

Pharyngeal (Throat) Cultures

Pharyngeal specimens should be collected by having patients open their mouths widely, depressing the tongue to improve visibility, and inserting the swab so that the tip makes contact with any exudative, inflamed regions on the posterior pharynx and tonsils. Carelessly collected specimens are likely to yield falsely negative results, especially when tested for Group A streptococcal antigen (discussed below). Cotton, rayon, or dacron swabs are all acceptable for culture, but swabs for antigen detection testing should be rayon or dacron only. Transport of pharyngeal swabs in modified Stuart's or Amie's medium is recommended for survival of pathogens other than Group A streptococci, which retain viability quite well on dry swabs. In fact, the yield of positive antigen and culture results for Group A streptococci is somewhat higher with dry swabs than with swabs moistened in transport medium.

Nasopharyngeal Cultures

Testing of nasopharyngeal specimens is recommended for diagnosis of pertussis and neonatal *Chlamydia trachomatis* pneumonia, even though the site of these infections is in the lower respiratory tract. The nasopharynx is also frequently colonized by pathogenic microorganisms; cultures for *Staphylococcus aureus, N. meningitidis* and *H. influenzae* type B can be performed to identify asymptomatic carriers during outbreaks. Nasopharyngeal specimens should be collected with a flexible, wire-shafted swab comprised of calcium alginate fibers, introduced through the nose and gently inserted until the tip reaches the posterior nasopharynx. The swab is then carefully rotated to collect mucus and mechanically dislodge ciliated epithelial cells containing chlamydial inclusions.

Other Upper Respiratory Cultures

Suspected Pharyngeal Abscess

Recognition of the cause of an abscess can be thwarted if specimens are contaminated by normal upper respiratory flora. Careful disinfection of the abscess aspiration site with a nonirritating, topical agent should precede specimen collection using a needle and syringe. Once obtained, specimens should be delivered promptly to the laboratory with a request for aerobic and anaerobic cultures.

Sinus Culture

Sinus aspirates should be collected aseptically with a needle and syringe following puncture of the cartilage encompassing the sinus cavity. The sinus cavity may be rinsed with sterile, nonbacteriostatic saline to facilitate aspiration. Specimens should be brought to the laboratory promptly for Gram stain, aerobic, anaerobic, and fungal cultures.

External Ear Culture

Ear canal culture specimens must be collected to minimize contamination by normal skin flora. Dried flakes and chunks of cerumen should be removed from the ear and discarded. Exudate should be absorbed onto a sterile minitip swab, carefully avoiding the unaffected ear wall while inserting, loading, and removing the swab. If Gram stain and culture are both needed, separate swabs should be submitted.

Middle Ear Culture

Collection of specimens from the middle ear, when needed, is best accomplished by tympanocentesis using a needle and syringe, avoiding contamination by normal external ear flora. The external ear canal and the tympanic membrane itself should be gently disinfected with 70% alcohol prior to tympanocentesis. If spontaneous tympanic membrane rupture has already occurred, residual fluid in the ear canal may be absorbed on a swab and submitted to the laboratory for testing. Test results, however, should be interpreted with caution since it is inevitable that such specimens are contaminated with external ear flora.

Lower Respiratory Tract Culture

Collection of specimens from the lower respiratory tract can be hampered by contamination with bacteria and fungi colonizing the upper respiratory tract. One solution is to bypass the upper respiratory tract and collect specimens directly from the lower respiratory tract; this would necessitate routine patient exposure to invasive procedures. More commonly, practitioners tolerate contamination of lower respiratory tract specimens with upper respiratory tract flora and rely upon the expertise of laboratory personnel and their own interpretive skills to derive useful information.

Sputum Culture

Expectorated or saline-induced sputum is usually used for diagnosis of pulmonary infection. Most "sputum specimens" contain little, if any, material from the lower tract, being either heavily contaminated by upper respiratory tract bacteria or consisting primarily of saliva. Gross examination of "sputum" revealing a thin, watery liquid without flecks of mucous suggests the specimen is predominantly saliva, and careful patient instruction on how to produce sputum may be needed. Laboratories examine Gram-stained smears before performing culture on sputum specimens; a predominance of epithelial cells over inflammatory cells indicates a poor specimen and culture is not performed. Sputum culture may be negative in patients with pneumococcal pneumonia, since the organisms do not survive well after specimens are collected. These cultures are positive for a single pathogen in less than half of cases of pneumonia.

Direct Culture

Specimens collected directly from the lung or pleural space via protected bronchoalveolar lavage, fine needle aspiration, thoracentesis, or open lung biopsy are superior to sputum for laboratory examination, particularly for diagnosis of opportunistic infections.

Gastric Aspirate

In children too young to produce sputum on demand, examination of gastric aspirates is an acceptable substitute. Gastric aspirates are especially useful for diagnosis of pulmonary tuberculosis since they can be expected to contain swallowed lower respiratory tract secretions. These specimens, like sputum, unavoidably become contaminated with upper respiratory flora, which can seriously mislead practitioners as to the etiology of infection. Specimens must be transported to the laboratory promptly, or refrigerated until transport is possible.

Microscopy

Microscopy is of minimal value for diagnosis of upper respiratory tract infection. Gram stained aspirates from patients with sinusitis and otitis media may be useful, if smears reveal predominance of a single, recognizable organism morphology. Microscopic examination of lower respiratory tract specimens can be extremely helpful. As mentioned earlier, sputum is assessed by Gram stain to determine specimen quality prior to further processing. Specimens containing more than 25 squamous epithelial cells per low power field are heavily contaminated with saliva and are not cultured. Gram stained smears of sputum specimens that contain neutrophils and large numbers of bacteria

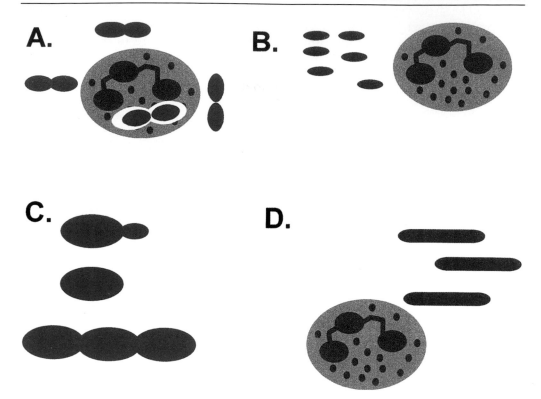

Figure 29.1. Common Lower Respiratory Pathogens. Gram stains are able to recognize most bacteria and fungi. The most common organism in bronchitis and pneumonia is *S. pneumoniae* (**A**), gram positive cocci in pairs. *H. influenzae* (**B**) produces small, gram negative cocci that resemble short bacilli. While *Candida albicans* (**C**) is part of normal flora and more commonly causes oral infections, it often causes pneumonia in immunocompromised patients. Gram negative bacilli such as *K. pneumoniae* (**D**) may cause community acquired pneumonia, but are more commonly seen in hospital acquired pneumonia, especially in antibiotic treated patients.

or fungi of a single type are suggestive of infection by that organism (Fig. 29.1). Specimens from patients with suspected tuberculosis should be acid-fast stained to obtain a rapid indication of infection (see below for more details). Microscopic examination of bronchoalveolar lavage, lung aspirate, and lung biopsy specimens generally furnish valuable results. Specimens may be Gram stained, acid-fast stained, calcofluor white stained, or toluidine blue stained to recognize bacterial, mycobacterial, fungal, or pneumocystis infections, respectively.

Antigen Detection

Detection of microbial antigens has become a popular means of diagnosing respiratory tract infections. Kits to detect Group A streptococcal antigen are available for use in practitioners' offices. The results can be read in fewer than ten minutes for most products. Antigen tests produce few false positive results, but are less sensitive than culture or DNA probe: practitioners should feel confident acting upon antigen positive results, but should wait for negative DNA probe or culture results before considering antigen negative patients free of infection. This requires collection of duplicate pharyngeal specimens from each patient and having to test both specimens in the majority of instances. Other respiratory tract pathogens for which antigen detection assays are available for laboratory use include *Bordetella pertussis, Legionella pneumophila, C. trachomatis,* influenza virus, parainfluenza virus, adenovirus, RSV, and *P. carinii.* The specimens of choice are nasopharyngeal swabs (*B. pertussis*), nasopharyngeal secretions (*C. trachomatis,* influenza A and B virus, parainfluenza virus, and RSV), bronchoalveolar lavage (*P. carinii*), and tissue impression smears or lung aspirates (*L. pneumophila*). Antigen detection assays for *B. pertussis* and *L. pneumophila* are significantly less sensitive than culture, and negative results should be confirmed by culture or amplification methods.

Nucleic Acid Probes

A DNA probe for detection of Group A streptococcal ribosomal RNA in pharyngeal swabs is commercially available. It is more sensitive than antigen detection, comparable in sensitivity to culture, but only requires approximately 60 minutes to complete. Probes for *M. tuberculosis* are discussed below.

METHODS TO DETECT SPECIFIC RESPIRATORY TRACT INFECTIONS

The techniques discussed in the previous section are adequate to identify the most common respiratory tract pathogens. In unusual situations, additional testing is needed to identify other pathogens, which are discussed in the section below. Because *M. pneumoniae* infection is typically diagnosed by serologic means, it is discussed in Chapter 35.

Anaerobic Bacteria

Anaerobic bacteria constitute a major portion of the upper respiratory flora, and are often involved in infection when aspiration of oral contents occurs (alcohol abuse, aspiration pneumonia). Documentation that anaerobes are causing lower respiratory infection demands that specimens avoid contamination with microorganisms from the upper respiratory tract. Accomplishing this requires direct lower respiratory culture by one of the techniques described above. Respiratory tract cultures from patients with anaerobic infections frequently yield growth of obligate anaerobes mixed with facultative anaerobes and aerotolerant anaerobes. As a result, a great deal of care must be taken by laboratory technologists to isolate each organism in pure culture and then determine its oxygen requirement. Since most anaerobes grow at slower rates than aerobes, a significant amount of time may pass before final culture results are available. Practitioners must learn to be patient with the laboratory during this process. Once isolated in pure culture, most anaerobes can be identified in less than 24 hours. Anaerobes frequently implicated in respiratory tract infection include the *Prevotella/Porphyromonas* group, *Fusobacterium, Peptostreptococcus, Actinomyces,* and *Veillonella.* These organisms are usually susceptible to standard antimicrobial agents, and rarely require susceptibility testing; however, the *Prevotella/Porphyromonas* group has been displaying increasing penicillin resistance.

Fungi

Fungal respiratory tract infections are often recognized by microscopic examination, but identification of specific etiologic agents usually requires culture. Many fungi can be temporary or permanent members of the upper respiratory tract flora. Thus, interpretation of culture results from specimens contaminated with upper respiratory secretions can be just as difficult with fungal cultures as for aerobic or anaerobic bacterial cultures. Pulmonary fungal infections are typically acquired by inhalation, and produce disseminated infections only in immunocompromised patients (Chapter 33). *H. capsulatum, B. dermatitidis,* and *C. immitis* are dimorphic fungi which grow as yeasts at 37 C and molds at lower temperatures. Colonies may be visible after as little as three days, but generally require several weeks for definitive identification (requiring demonstration of both phases of growth). The zygomycetes (*Mucor, Rhizopus, Rhizomucor,* and *Absidia*) can cause opportunistic pulmonary infections and often colonize the nose and paranasal sinuses in diabetic patients, often secondarily infecting the brain (rhinocerebral mucormycosis). These infections can often be suspected by finding black, necrotic material in the nose or sinuses in association with diabetes. These fungi grow extremely rapidly on bacteriologic and fungal media, so are not difficult to identify by culture.

Mycobacteria

The most important member of this group is *M. tuberculosis,* the cause of tuberculosis. Methods in use include nonspecific tests which detect the entire group of mycobacteria, and methods that allow differentiation of *M. tuberculosis* from other mycobacteria. The most important nontuberculosis pathogen, *M. avium,* is discussed in Chapter 33.

Screening Tests

Skin testing, which detects an immune response to *M. tuberculosis,* does not indicate active infection. In patients with suggestive clinical findings (fever, night sweats) and cavitary lesions, the current best screening test involves use of acid-fast staining techniques. To optimize detection, sputum should be collected early in the morning (when the number of organisms tends to be highest). Negative results should be confirmed with specimens on at least three consecutive days, while positive results indicate likely mycobacterial infection (but do not clearly indicate which member of the group is present). Laboratories use different techniques to perform acid-fast smears, which can affect the likelihood of positive results. Best results occur in laboratories which perform concentration and use fluorescent stains, which simplify screening. Because smears are much less sensitive than culture, negative screening tests should not be used to remove patients from isolation if clinical findings suggest tuberculosis.

Culture and Identification

Using traditional culture techniques, mycobacteria are notoriously slow growing; it may take 3–4 weeks or longer for an initial culture to become positive. Some laboratories use more rapid growth detection techniques, which may become positive in as little as 10–14 days. It is important for practitioners to be aware which technique is used in their laboratory to know how long to expect to wait for positive culture results. Once a positive culture occurs, the organism can be identified by either biochemical tests or DNA probes (which tend to be faster but more expensive). After the organism is identified, additional time is required to perform susceptibility studies (essential in areas with multidrug resistant tuberculosis), which will generally take the same amount of time to report as did the initial culture.

Amplification Techniques

Amplification-enhanced assays for detection of *M. tuberculosis* nucleic acid sequences are available for use on acid-fast smear positive lower respiratory tract specimens, allowing rapid identification of tuberculosis. They are not yet FDA-licensed for use on acid-fast smear negative specimens. Because there are false positive results, results should always be confirmed, but can be used to begin treatment for presumed tuberculosis.

Pneumocystis

One of the most common opportunistic pathogens, *P. carinii* most characteristically causes interstitial pneumonia. Standard sputum specimens are virtually worthless for diagnosis, although induced sputum specimens are helpful if positive; in patients with AIDS, induced sputum is positive in over 50% of cases. In patients with a high likelihood of *Pneumocystis* and negative induced sputum, bronchoalveolar lavage is considered the method of choice to establish the diagnosis. Laboratories use different types of stains to recognize the organism, which affect yield (particularly of induced sputum). Direct immunofluorescence is the most sensitive technique to identify *Pneumocystis*, however, many laboratories rely on histochemical stains, which have significantly lower sensitivity in induced sputum. It is important for practitioners to know which technique is used in their laboratory.

Viruses

Antigens of RSV, the most common cause of viral bronchitis, bronchiolitis, and pneumonia in young children, are readily detected by immunofluorescence and enzyme immunoassay. Antigens of influenza A virus, parainfluenza viruses 1–3, and adenovirus can also be detected by immunofluorescence. While herpes simplex virus and cytomegalovirus antigens can be detected by direct immunofluorescence, yield of DFA on sputum specimens is low. Viral culture is the most common approach toward etiologic diagnosis for agents not detectable by antigen assays. Details on proper collection and transport are given in Chapter 30.

Sexually Transmitted Diseases

JOSEPH M. CAMPOS and D. ROBERT DUFOUR

CLINICAL PATTERNS OF SEXUALLY TRANSMITTED DISEASES

Sexually transmitted diseases (STD, sometimes also called venereal diseases) are among the most common of human infections. Symptoms of these ailments can overlap so considerably that for centuries knowledge concerning the etiologic agents, routes of transmission, and numbers of distinct venereal diseases was scarce. Syphilis and gonorrhea, for example, were thought to be different manifestations of the same disease. Because of the many types of laboratory tests needed to identify all sexually transmitted infectious agents, it is essential for the practitioner to use clinical findings to select appropriate laboratory tests to diagnose the precise cause of infection. A summary of the most common infectious agents causing various STD is given in Table 30.1. While the title of this chapter implies that all diseases are spread only by sexual activity, the chapter will also cover genital infections that may be spread by other means.

Urethritis

While inflammation of the urethra may occur with urinary tract infection (Chapter 28), most cases are caused by STD. Clinically, these are often separated into gonococcal urethritis (caused by *Neisseria gonorrhoeae*) or nonspecific urethritis (usually caused by *Chlamydia trachomatis*). Urethritis typically presents as burning upon urination and a urethral discharge. with a heavier, thicker discharge usually suggestive of gonococcal urethritis. In some patients there may be no noticeable discharge and the main complaint may be a urethral itch.

Vulvovaginitis

While inflammation may affect exclusively the vulva or vagina, it often involves both. Vulvovaginitis can occur in females of all ages, and includes both infectious and noninfectious causes. Noninfectious causes include chemicals present in bubble baths, soaps, and perfumes, or environmental factors such as poor hygiene and allergens. Symptoms include irritation or itching of the genital area; inflammation of the labia majora, labia minora, or perineal area; vaginal discharge; foul vaginal odor; and discomfort or burning while urinating.

Candida Vulvovaginitis

Infection by yeast (usually *Candida albicans*) is not felt to be a sexually transmitted disease. It is most common in women of childbearing age, but also occurs in infants and in women with diabetes. Oral contraceptives may increase incidence as well. It can usually be recognized clinically as a thick, cottage cheese-like vaginal discharge or diffuse vulvar erythema (often with yellow-white papules) involving the vaginal opening and thighs.

Table 30.1.
Frequent Causes of Sexually Transmitted Diseases

Infection	Microorganisms
Urethritis	*Neisseria gonorrhoeae, Chlamydia trachomatis*
Vulvovaginitis	*Candida albicans, Trichomonas vaginalis*
Cervicitis	*Chlamydia trachomatis, Neisseria gonorrhoeae,* herpes simplex virus
Bacterial vaginosis	Combination of *Gardnerella vaginalis,* genital mycoplasmas, black-pigmented *Bacteroides* species, and *Mobiluncus* species
Pelvic inflammatory disease	*Neisseria gonorrhoeae, Chlamydia trachomatis,* genital mycoplasmas, along with anaerobic organisms
Genital ulcers	*Treponema pallidum, Haemophilus ducreyi,* herpes simplex type II

Trichomonal Vulvovaginitis

Because reporting of trichomonas is not required, the true incidence is not known but has been estimated at several million cases per year. Even this number is probably an underestimate since infection in males is usually asymptomatic. The organism is transmitted from person to person almost exclusively by sexual contact and adheres to epithelial cells of the genitourinary tract (preferentially in the vagina and urethra). *Trichomonas vaginalis* often causes a more foamy vaginal discharge, often associated with intense vulvar itching. On pelvic examination, there is often intense cervical inflammation with alternating red and white patches ("strawberry cervix").

Bacterial Vaginosis

While not technically an inflammatory disorder (although it was formerly called non-specific vaginitis), it is often in the differential diagnosis of vulvovaginitis. Bacterial vaginosis is an alteration in vaginal bacterial flora: disappearance of organic acid producing lactobacilli results in an elevation of vaginal pH and overgrowth by organisms associated with the syndrome. It produces no symptoms in nearly half of all affected women. When symptoms are present, they may include heavy, malodorous (often described as a "fish-like" smell) vaginal discharge, vaginal burning or itching, abdominal pain, and pain during sexual intercourse. The discharge is usually white and paste-like but can be thin and watery, frothy, or yellow. A few women also suffer from vulvar soreness. A number of bacteria are associated with bacterial vaginosis, as discussed below. While bacterial vaginosis is more common in sexually active women, it is not considered a sexually transmitted disease. There is also evidence that asymptomatic males may transmit the state to their sexual partners.

Condyloma Acuminata and Related Disorders

Genital infection with strains of human papilloma virus (HPV) is one of the most common sexually transmitted diseases. In the vulva, it most commonly presents as "genital warts" or condyloma acuminata, usually caused by HPV strains 6 and 11 (they are similar to warts on other parts of the body, caused by the other HPV strains 1 and 2). Infection by other HPV strains (notably HPV 16, 18, and 31) may cause intraepithelial neoplasia, a precursor to squamous cell carcinoma.

Cervicitis

Inflammation of the cervix is usually due to infection, particularly by *C. trachomatis.* Acute cervicitis, usually due to bacterial or viral infection, typically presents as a thick, yellow vaginal discharge. Chronic cervicitis, often the result of recurrent episodes of acute cervicitis, may present with slight vaginal discharge, backache, discomfort with urination, and painful sexual intercourse. More extensive chronic cervicitis often presents with profuse vaginal discharge, bleeding between menstrual periods, and spotting or bleeding after intercourse.

Genital Ulcers

While ulcers on the external genitals may be due to cancer, most genital ulcers are due to infection. While ulcerative diseases are among the most well known sexually transmitted disease, most are rare (except for herpes simplex) and are decreasing in incidence in much of North America.

Herpes Simplex

The most common ulcerating STD, genital herpes is typically due to infection with herpes simplex type II infection. Because the virus survives in ganglion cells, reactivation of infection can occur repeatedly. Primary infection typically begins as painful blisters which progress to shallow ulcers, often symmetrically placed. The recurrent lesions are similar but tend to have shorter duration.

Syphilis

The complete spectrum of syphilis (due to infection with the spirochete *Treponema pallidum*) is discussed more fully in Chapter 35. In primary syphilis, a painless ulcer (chancre) occurs at the site of bacterial entry through the skin several weeks after initial exposure. If untreated, it will eventually resolve after several weeks. In the secondary stage, genital lesions may again appear in the form of flat, broad elevated lesions termed condyloma lata.

Chancroid

Common in tropical regions and sometimes occurring as small outbreaks in more temperate climates, chancroid (due to infection by *Haemophilus ducreyii*) is most commonly found in uncircumcised males. Bacteria enter through a pre-existing injury, such as a small cut or scratch, initially presenting as one or more raised genital lesions 4–7 days after exposure. Initially, they form pustules surrounded by a narrow red border. The pustules eventually rupture to produce painful ulcers. Untreated cases may cause painful lymph node enlargement within 5–10 days, and the lymph nodes may ultimately rupture.

Pelvic Inflammatory Disease

Peritoneal inflammation is due to spread of an STD initially involving the lower female genital tract (such as gonorrhea or chlamydia) to pelvic organs, particularly the fallopian tubes (salpingitis) or ovaries (oophoritis, tuboovarian abscess). Superinfection with anaerobic organisms from the lower genital tract occurs in most cases. In the acute stage, it typically presents as fever and lower abdominal pain, and may mimic other inflammatory disorders of the abdomen, particularly appendicitis. Scarring of the pelvic organs may lead to sterility, ectopic pregnancy, and chronic pain.

GENERAL TESTS OF USE IN RECOGNIZING GENITAL TRACT INFECTIONS

Initial approach to suspected genital infection should be guided by the clinical features discussed above and aimed at detection of those organisms usually responsible for this clinical picture. In some cases, general tests will not be of use in identifying the causative agent; details on specific tests needed in such cases are discussed in the next section.

Microscopy

Examination of fluid obtained from patients with suspected infections is of most use in inflammation of the male genital tract and the lower female genital tract.

Gram Stain

Gram stain is the method of choice for diagnosis of symptomatic gonococcal urethritis in males, with identification of intracellular and extracellular Gram negative diplococci in a thin smear of urethral discharge as sensitive and specific as culture. Gram stain of cervical or vaginal discharge for diagnosis of gonorrhea in females yields only presumptive evidence of infection if intracellular Gram negative diplococci are found; other organisms found in normal vaginal flora may be indistinguishable from *N. gonorrhoeae*. Gram stains of vaginal discharge specimens from patients with nonspecific vaginosis may be examined for "clue cells" (epithelial cells coated with large numbers of bacteria). Smear results are as sensitive and more specific than cultures for *Gardnerella vaginalis*, a bacterium previously considered a cause of this infection. Gram stains of vaginal discharge specimens may also reveal fungi, usually considered diagnostic of *C. albicans*.

Vaginal Wet Preparation

The saline wet preparation is the most commonly performed test for diagnosis of vaginal and urethral trichomoniasis. A small drop of discharge is suspended in sterile normal saline and examined under low power for the presence of motile trophozoites. Wet preparation fails to detect 25% or more of culture proven cases, however, culture for *Trichomonas* is seldom performed.

Giemsa and Iodine Stain

Cervical and urethral scrapings can be used to demonstrate intracytoplasmic inclusion bodies of *C. trachomatis*. However, the sensitivity of these staining procedures is less than optimal, and most laboratories today use antigen detection, DNA probe, or culture.

Culture

"Bacterial" cultures of urethral and vaginal discharges may be of some benefit; *N. gonorrhoeae* and *C. albicans* will be cultured in all laboratories, although gram stain typically allows quicker recognition of presence of both organisms. Cultures for chlamydia and HSV can also be performed when necessary, but other tests to identify presence of the organism (discussed below) usually provide faster results.

Table 30.2.
Sites of Involvement of Genital Tract Infections

Agent	Annual Cases (per 100,000)	Organ(s) Involved	Clinical Presentation(s)
Gardnerella vaginalis Mobiluncus species	3,000	Vagina	Vaginal discharge (watery, foul smelling). Bacterial coated cells (clue cells) on Gram stain of discharge
Chlamydia trachomatis	270 (women) 43 (men)	Urethra, cervix, fallopian tubes	Pelvic inflammatory disease (PID), cervicitis, urethritis, infertility. Requires culture or direct laboratory identification
Trichomonas vaginalis	200	Vagina	Vaginal discharge (bubbly)—Motile organisms on wet preparation of discharge; often asymptomatic in men
Candida albicans	Unknown	Vulva, vagina	Vulva: Diffuse erythematous rash; Vagina: Thick white exudate. Organisms on KOH prep or Gram stain. More common with alteration in local defenses (diabetes, obesity, pregnancy)
Neisseria gonorrhoeae	200	Fallopian tubes, Bartholin's gland	Pelvic inflammatory disease (PID), Bartholin's abscess, urethritis
Human papilloma virus (HPV)	200	Vulva, cervix, penis	Condyloma acuminata (vulva, penis), flat condyloma/abnormal pap smear (cervix, vagina) with strains 6/11. Associated with increased risk of intraepithelial neoplasia and invasive carcinoma (strains 16, 18, 31)
Herpes simplex II	120 (new) 400 (recurrent)	Vulva, cervix, penis	Blisters which progress to ulcers. May be spread to infant with cervical infection causing severe infection
Treponema pallidum	13.7	Vulva, cervix, penis	Painless, hard ulcer (chancre) with primary, flat plaques (condyloma lata) with secondary

METHODS TO DETECT SPECIFIC GENITAL TRACT INFECTIONS

In contrast to infections in many other sites, where infection is caused primarily by easily cultured bacteria, routine culture and smear techniques have a low yield in determining the cause of some sexually transmitted diseases. Since tests of the most use to determine the cause of infection differ for each causative organism, they are grouped by organism rather than by type of test. A summary of the frequency, sites, and features of various sexually (and nonsexually) transmitted genital infections is given in Table 30.2.

Bacterial Vaginosis

Bacterial vaginosis is likely to have more than one microbial cause. Increased numbers of colonies of *Mobiluncus* species, black-pigmented *Bacteroides* species, *G. vaginalis,* and *Mycoplasma hominis* from vaginal discharge cultures are more commonly found in women with bacterial vaginosis than in asymptomatic controls. Concurrent with increased numbers of these bacteria are decreased numbers of normally present *Lactobacillus* species. The value of cultures for *G. vaginalis* is dubious; clinical symptoms correlate better with Gram stain findings of curved poorly staining rods (*Mobiluncus* species) and "clue cells" than with positive cultures for *G. vaginalis*.

Chlamydia

C. trachomatis, the most common sexually transmitted organism in the United States, is an intracellular bacterial form which cannot be cultured on routine bacteriology media. Laboratory diagnosis of *C. trachomatis* infection can be accomplished by several means which vary in sensitivity. Direct smears were discussed earlier.

Culture

Chlamydia can be cultured using cell culture techniques. Specimens should be placed in special chlamydial transport medium before culture (e.g. sucrose phosphate medium). Cell cultures are examined for chlamydial growth after 48–72 hours. Some laboratories blindly repeat negative cultures after 72 hours and recheck after another 48–72 hours to increase yield. A requirement for swabs limits the ability to screen large numbers of persons possibly exposed, as only symptomatic individuals are likely to seek medical care and have swabs made.

Antigen Tests

Tests to detect *C. trachomatis* antigens have become widely used. Accurate results from the antigen detection assays are highly dependent upon the quality of specimens. *C. trachomatis* is an intracellular pathogen of columnar epithelial cells, and unless these cells are scraped during specimen collection, the yield of positive results will be low. Most comparative evaluations demonstrate that soluble immunoassays are marginally more sensitive than direct fluorescent antibody (DFA), although DFA has the advantage that specimen adequacy may be judged at the same time as test results are read. While antigen assays are more rapid (several hours) than culture, culture is clearly more sensitive, especially when asymptomatic individuals are tested, and also more specific. Antigen tests should be used only when testing symptomatic populations with a high incidence of infection. Because of false positive results, antigen tests should not be used in screening or in asymptomatic sexual contacts of infected individuals.

Amplification Methods

Recently, amplification methods to detect chlamydial DNA have become available, and some of these assays can be performed on urine, markedly simplifying sample collection. Amplification assays also appear to be as sensitive and as specific as culture. At present, amplification assays are not in widespread use by most laboratories.

Gonorrhoea

N. gonorrhoeae is a gram negative diplococcus with fastidious growth requirements. Laboratory diagnosis of gonorrhoea is based upon microscopic examination of stained smears in most cases.

Culture

Swabs for culture of *N. gonorrhoeae* should be transported to the laboratory promptly and handled carefully to prevent drying of the swab; if not handled appropriately, false negative culture results may occur. *Neisseria* species propagate slowly by bacterial standards, and selective media (e.g. modified Thayer-Martin) facilitate detection of this organism by preventing overgrowth of other organisms. Occasional strains of vancomycin sensitive *N. gonorrhoeae* fail to grow on selective media, so some laboratories inoculate a nonselective chocolate agar plate to detect these strains. Cultures must be incubated for 72 hours to achieve maximal isolation rates. In areas where penicillin resistance is common, susceptibility testing should also be performed along with culture.

Antigen Tests

Detection of gonococcal antigens is possible and provides rapid results (2 hours). It is satisfactory for diagnosis in males, but is no more effective than Gram stain which yields results more rapidly and much less expensively. The assay lacks sensitivity in specimens from females, and negative results must be confirmed by culture. Perhaps the biggest drawback to gonococcal antigen detection is the inability to identify penicillin resistant strains.

Nucleic Acid Probes

Rapid in situ hybridization assays for *N. gonorrhoeae* are available, in some cases as a dual probe with *C. trachomatis*.

Herpes Simplex Virus (HSV)

Two different types of this double-stranded DNA virus produce human disease; HSV-1 generally causes oral and cutaneous infections while HSV-2 is the leading cause of genital ulceration. However, both types are capable of causing infection at any site. Diagnosis of HSV infection is usually based on clinical findings, with laboratory testing most often done only when the diagnosis is uncertain. In pregnant women with known herpes, asymptomatic shedding of virus from the cervix may infect the infant at birth. In these cases methods to recognize active virus replication can assist in management. Direct detection of HSV in lesion material, either via cytology examination (e.g. Tzanck preparation, smears made from the floor of a blister) or by various antigen detection assays, allows rapid diagnosis in symptomatic patients. Culture is the most sensitive test for herpes infection. Fluid from new blisters yields the most positives, while the positivity rate falls rapidly as lesions age and become crusted. Specimens in transport medium should be stored in refrigerators rather than frozen, since freezing and thawing destroys most HSV. HSV cultures may be positive in as little as 24 hours, with most positive results within 3 days. Amplification methods to detect viral DNA are also available, and provide more rapid results than culture.

Human Papilloma Virus (HPV)

In patients with condyloma acuminata, clinical diagnosis is usually sufficient and methods to identify the virus are not needed. In suspicious clinical lesions, the most commonly used test to determine HPV serotype is in situ hybridization of viral DNA in cervical or vulvar biopsies.

Pelvic Inflammatory Disease

By the time of presentation with pelvic inflammatory disease, the predominant organisms in fallopian tube or ovarian abscess fluid are typically anaerobic organisms from the lower female genital tract, while in only a minority of cases can more classic STD organisms be cultured. Cultures of the cervix are much more commonly positive for sexually transmitted organisms; Gram and Giemsa stain of a cervical swab will often reveal *N. gonorrhoeae* or *C. trachomatis*.

Syphilis

T. pallidum is longer (6–15 μm) and considerably thinner (0.15 μm) than most bacteria, making it virtually impossible to recognize the organism by conventional light microscopy. The organism is unable to grow on standard microbiologic media or in cell culture. In primary syphilis, the most sensitive test is demonstration of the causative organism by darkfield microscopy of exudate from the chancre. The lesion should be gently abraded with dry gauze, and a drop of exudate placed on a microscope slide; if necessary, a drop of saline may be mixed with the specimen. The prep should be coverslipped and examined promptly with a microscope equipped with a dark-field condenser. Positive specimens contain motile, tightly coiled spirochetes that flex and rotate around their longitudinal axes. In secondary syphilis, serologic tests (Chapter 35) are highly sensitive and can be used to establish the diagnosis in patients who have not recently received antibiotics for syphilis. In such treated patients, demonstration of organisms in lesions is the only way to prove residual active infection, although yield is not as great as in primary syphilis.

CHAPTER 31

Evaluation of Suspected Infectious Diarrhea

JOHN F. KEISER, SALOME MENDOZA, and D. ROBERT DUFOUR

PATHOGENESIS OF DIARRHEA

While the term diarrhea can mean different things to different patients, it generally is defined as a change in consistency and frequency of bowel movements, although some define it more specifically as three or more loose or watery bowel movements in a 24 hour period. Diarrhea is one of the most common infectious diseases, second only to upper respiratory infections (and more common in some settings). While in North America most cases are self-limiting and have limited long term consequences, worldwide diarrhea is a major cause of morbidity and mortality. Chronic diarrhea is a common finding in immunosuppressed patients and severe diarrhea is a major cause of morbidity in hospitalized patients. Many microbial agents may cause infectious diarrhea (Table 31.1), including bacteria, parasites, and viruses.

Normal Intestinal Fluid Handling

To be able to characterize the likely pathogenesis of diarrhea, it is helpful to understand the normal physiology of intestinal fluid handling. In the upper gastrointestinal tract (salivary glands, stomach, pancreas), fluid is added to the water in ingested food, producing a total volume of fluid of 7–8 L reaching the first part of the small intestine. Within the small bowel, additional fluid can be added through the action of adenyl cyclase; however, by the end of the small bowel, only about 1 L remains. The colon also absorbs water and electrolytes, although its maximum absorptive capacity is only about 2 L. With normal colonic function, stool is typically fairly solid with total water content of less than 0.2 L.

Protection Against Infectious Diarrhea

A number of host factors are important in protection against infectious diarrhea. Most bacteria are inactivated at normal gastric pH; bacterial caused diarrhea is thus more common in patients with an inability to produce acid, either due to disease (Chapter 21) or medications (antacids, H_2-antagonists). Intestinal bacteria, particularly anaerobic organisms, inhibit the growth of many potentially toxic bacteria. Normal immune response seems to inhibit the growth of certain bacteria and parasites. Damage to any of these normal protective barriers increases the likelihood of developing diarrhea.

Patterns of Diarrhea

Two major patterns of diarrhea occur, differing in their pathogenesis and location of damage; different organisms typically produce each of these types of diarrhea. A summary of these differences is given in Table 31.2.

Table 31.1.
Agents of Infectious Diarrhea

Bacteria—*Clostridium difficile, E. coli* (diarrheagenic strains), *Salmonella, Shigella, Vibrio, Campylobacter, Yersinia enterocolitica*
Viruses—Adenovirus, Rotavirus, Astrovirus, Calicivirus, Norwalk-like agents, Coronavirus
Parasites—*Giardia lamblia, Entamoeba histolytica, Cryptosporidium parvum, Cyclospora, Microsporidium* species

Small Bowel Diarrhea

The most severe forms of diarrhea are due to small bowel injury, usually due to production of a toxin which activates adenyl cyclase. The diarrhea is typically watery, and often the patient loses several liters of fluid each day. There is minimal inflammation in this type of diarrhea, and neutrophils are usually absent in stool.

Colonic Diarrhea

Diarrhea from colonic injury typically is less in volume than small bowel diarrhea, and often contains mucus and inflammatory cells. In some cases, it is associated with hemorrhage, suggesting an invasive organism such as enterohemorrhagic *E. coli* O157: H7, *Campylobacter,* or *Yersinia enterocolitica.*

CLINICAL FEATURES SUGGESTING CAUSES OF INFECTIOUS DIARRHEA

As mentioned earlier, in most cases diarrhea is self-limiting, and does not require laboratory testing to determine the etiology. Workup should be considered if diarrhea persists for more than 1–2 days, or is associated with severe clinical symptoms such as volume depletion, fever, or bloody diarrhea. A number of clinical features should suggest the possibility of specific etiologic agents, and should prompt a search for these organisms. Agents causing diarrhea in immunocompromised patients are discussed in Chapter 33.

Hospital Acquired Diarrhea

In patients with diarrhea developing in the hospital, almost all are due to pseudomembranous colitis caused by *Clostridium difficile* toxin. In most cases, the predisposing factor

Table 31.2.
Differential Features of Types of Diarrhea

Site of Injury	Small Bowel	Colon
Stool Consistency	Watery	Mucoid
Bloody Stools	Infrequent	Occur with certain types (see below)
Neutrophils	Uncommon	Seen with most agents
Pathogens	Bacteria: *Salmonella,*[a] *Vibrio, Yersinia enterocolitica,*[a] *E. Coli* (enterotoxigenic strains), Parasites: *Cryptosporidium parvum, Giardia lamblia, Microsporidium* Viruses: Rotavirus, Caliciviruses	Bacteria: *Campylobacter, Salmonella, Shigella, Yersinia enterocolitica, E. coli* (enteroinvasive, enterohemorrhagic strains), *C. difficile* Parasites: *Entamoeba histolytica*

[a] Indicates most common site for involvement

is treatment with antibiotics; however, *C. difficile* may also colonize the intestine in patients on chemotherapy, after surgery, and rarely after endoscopic procedures. Laboratory tests to recognize the presence of *C. difficile* or its toxin should be done early in the course of diarrhea, as repeated tests may be needed.

Recent Travel

Patients who develop diarrhea after traveling often have an infection with organisms not usually associated with diarrhea in the home area. With travel to tropical areas, infection with parasites such as *Entamoeba* and *Strongyloides* should be considered. After travel to areas with poor water sanitation, infection is often from parasites such as *Giardia* and *Cryptosporidium*. Infection with viruses such as Norwalk-like agents and rotavirus are also more common in patients who have traveled recently, as are some bacterial organisms.

Ingestion of Food

When diarrhea develops within 24 hours after food ingestion, toxins of organisms are usually at fault; the organisms are usually not identified in culture. In patients who develop diarrhea one to two days after ingestion of seafood, *Vibrio parahemolyticus* or *cholera*, and Norwalk-like agents are commonly at fault. When outbreaks of diarrhea develop after eating at a common site (restaurant, picnic, or party), unusual bacterial pathogens are often at fault. The laboratory should be notified, since certain strains of *E. coli* are often pathogenic in causing diarrhea. Because nontoxic strains are part of the normal flora, the laboratory may not do further testing unless it is aware of a possible epidemic of diarrhea following a common exposure.

Bloody Diarrhea

Most forms of diarrhea do not produce bleeding, although patients with persistent diarrhea may develop perianal skin erosions which may bleed after use of toilet paper following a diarrheal stool. It is important to get a careful history or to examine the stool directly to determine whether the blood is part of the stool or not. When bloody diarrhea is present, infection with invasive organisms such as *E. coli* O157:H7, *Shigella*, *Entamoeba*, or *Strongyloides* should be considered.

Neonatal Necrotizing Enterocolitis (NEC)

In premature infants, a combination of relatively increased susceptibility to colonization with unusual bacteria and sensitivity of intestinal mucosa to ischemia or toxins (from bacteria or catheters) often leads to damage to intestinal mucosa. This often sets up a vicious cycle, where bacterial toxins accumulate in a segment of bowel damaged by ischemia and cause further damage. Any intestinal symptoms in a premature infant (such as change in feeding, diarrhea, abdominal distention, or positive occult blood in the stool) should be followed by an abdominal radiograph to detect air in the bowel wall, peritoneal cavity, or portal venous system.

Enteric Fever

Organisms invading through intestinal mucosa often allows these organisms to spread to regional lymph nodes, allowing bacterial toxins to enter the circulation and producing fever. Common organisms producing this syndrome are *Salmonella* (especially *S. typhi*), *Y. enterocolitica* (often causing abdominal pain resembling appendicitis), or *Campylobacter fetus*. The latter two organisms often occur in patients with chronic liver disease.

LABORATORY TESTS OF USE IN SUSPECTED INFECTIOUS DIARRHEA

For the clinical microbiology laboratory to assist practitioners in making the correct diagnosis, it is essential for there to be close communication between the laboratory and the practitioner. While most bacteria causing diarrhea can be detected in a standard stool culture, some require special handling or media. In most settings, laboratories do not routinely test for viruses or leukocytes as part of stool culture, and specimens for ova and parasites require special processing rather than culture. Any special circumstances, such as outlined above, should be communicated to the laboratory by the practitioner.

When Not to do Tests for Infectious Diarrhea

In patients with community acquired diarrhea of less than 1–2 days duration, laboratory tests should not be requested unless the patient has any of the special clinical features discussed above. In community acquired diarrhea, *C. difficile* colitis is unusual unless the patient has been treated with antibiotics in the past month, and tests for *C. difficile* should not be requested. In patients with hospital acquired diarrhea, the vast majority of cases are due to *C. difficile*. In these circumstances routine stool cultures and tests for ova and parasites are seldom of use unless the patient is immunosuppressed, and should not be requested. Watery diarrhea is almost never associated with invasion of the mucosa, therefore tests for fecal leukocytes should not be requested in this situation. Tests for ova and parasites are not usually positive in patients living in urban areas unless the patient has recently traveled, is immunosuppressed, or is part of an epidemic related to problems with water contamination.

Collection and Transportation of Stool Specimens

Proper collection and transportation of stool specimens to the microbiology laboratory are critical. Certain pathogenic bacteria and parasites may become nonviable or unrecognizable if specimens are not rapidly transported to the laboratory. Diarrhea specimens should be delivered to the laboratory within 1–2 hours of passage to prevent overgrowth of nonpathogenic bacteria and death of fragile pathogens. If longer time delays are expected, use of a suitable transport medium (i.e. Carey-Blair) is recommended; specimens in transport media should be stored at 4–6 C until ready for plating. For *C. difficile*, specimens should reach the laboratory within 30 minutes of passage or be frozen to −20 C to prevent degeneration of toxin; the organism itself is not preserved well in most transport media. Specimens should be placed in a suitable transport container (screw top jar or cardboard container) except for a rectal biopsy, which should be submitted on a sterile moistened gauze pad inside of a tightly closed container. Rectal swabs are not routinely recommended for adults, however, newborns or young children may necessitate the use of swabs.

Tests on Stool

Further testing on diarrheal stools should be directed by the appearance of the stool specimen. Watery stools do not usually require examination for leukocytes. Bloody stool requires examination for agents commonly causing bloody diarrhea.

Fecal Leukocytes

The presence of leukocytes in a fresh stool smear suggests that the diarrhea has an inflammatory etiology and affects the colon (Table 31.2). Leukocytes can be identified by either Gram or methylene blue stains under 1000 × magnification. Both techniques are largely dependent on the skill, experience, and bias of the microscopist, and considerable variation may occur between different laboratory personnel. Additionally, some infectious agents (notably *C. difficile* and *Entamoeba histolytica*) cause degeneration of neutrophils and prevent their identification. The lactoferrin latex agglutination assay, an immunoassay for a neutrophil enzyme, is highly sensitive to the presence of polymorphonuclear neutrophils. This test requires minimal training and there is less subjectivity in reading agglutination reactions. Practitioners should be aware of which technique is being used by their laboratory before interpreting a negative test for leukocytes.

Gram Stain

Because bacteria are normally present in stool, Gram stains of stool are not as helpful as they are in normally sterile fluids such as urine, middle ear fluid, or sputum. There are situations where Gram stain can provide useful information. It can be used to screen for overgrowth by *Candida* species or large Gram-positive bacilli (*C. difficile*). *Campylobacter* species can be detected by using 1% basic fuchsin in a modified Gram stain.

Stool Culture

Most microbiology laboratories routinely culture for *Salmonella, Shigella, Campylobacter, Yersinia,* and *Vibrio.* Other enteric pathogens such as *Plesiomonas* species, *Aeromonas* species, *C. difficile,* and pathogenic strains of *E. coli* may also be cultured, depending on the information provided to the laboratory. The practitioner's input to the laboratory will influence the laboratory's decision to culture for certain additional organisms.

C. Difficile

Because of its importance in hospital-acquired diarrhea, tests for *C. difficile* are widely requested. The most sensitive routine test is culture; specimens are inoculated to a highly selective medium that prevents growth of most other organisms. Cultures may also be positive in asymptomatic individuals (particularly in neonates), so that a positive culture does not prove *C. difficile* as the cause of diarrhea, since some strains do not produce toxin. Tests for *C. difficile* toxin are most widely used to recognize colitis, however the usually employed immunoassays are not as sensitive as culture. Moreover, the toxin is labile at room temperature, so that specimens for toxin should be examined within 30 minutes of passage of the stool (or specimens should be frozen). Negative toxin tests should be repeated, particularly if there may have been a delay in transport. Amplification tests for the toxin producing gene have been developed, but are more expensive and not widely available.

Tests for Parasites

The most commonly employed method to detect parasitic disease is examination of stool for ova and parasites. Specimens should reach the laboratory within 30–60 minutes to prevent degeneration of parasites. If an extended delay is anticipated, 5–10% formalin and polyvinyl alcohol can be used as preservatives. Traditionally, three stool specimens are collected on an every other day basis; although some parasites shed continuously, this technique allows identification of those passed intermittently. Recent studies have shown that greater than 90% of pathogens can be detected with one stool specimen. Contamination of specimens with water from toilet bowls or bed pans will likely produce false positive results. Such specimens should not be submitted, as they will produce misleading results. Bismuth and mineral oil can prevent the detection of certain parasites, therefore specimen collection should be delayed at least 7–10 days after exposure to these chemicals. If GI imaging studies using barium have been performed, falsely negative results may persist for over one week. Again, collection should be delayed.

The ability of laboratory personnel to identify parasites varies not only from one laboratory to another, but also from one person to the next within a laboratory. Because of reorganization in laboratories, many are moving towards "cross-trained" technologists, rather than specialists; this may compromise the ability to identify rarely seen parasites. It is important for the practitioner to be aware of the ability of the laboratory to identify parasitic pathogens.

Direct Examination

Examination of stool specimens for motile trophozooites is usually performed on specimens obtained on endoscopy. Specimens should be examined immediately after their procurement. If this will be performed by the practitioner, examination with reduced light or phase microscopy allows easier recognition of motile amoebae. Certain protozoan cysts, along with helminth eggs and larvae, can also be observed in direct saline preparations.

Concentration Techniques

To detect low numbers of organisms, laboratories use a variety of methods to concentrate parasites from a stool specimen. Iodine is often used to stain sediment to increase yield, and acid-fast and trichrome stains are used in various laboratories to recognize certain pathogens. For example, in patients with AIDS, an "acid-fast screen" may be offered to detect common pathogens including *Cryptosporidium, Cyclospora, Isospora,* and *Mycobacteria* species.

Immunoassays

A number of laboratories are using immunologic techniques (Chapter 35) to identify parasites such as *Giardia lamblia, E. histolytica, Cryptosporidium parvum, Microsporidium,* and *Cyclospora*. Immunoassays are usually performed singly or in panels. Laboratories that use panels of immunoassays may not perform direct examination or concentration techniques, and thus may not identify less frequently observed parasites. It is important that practitioners be aware if immunoassay panels are used to screen for parasites, and to request microscopic examination when the clinical picture strongly suggests parasitic disease (recent travel to endemic area, lack of pathogens identified in stool culture) and immunoassay screens are negative.

Tests for Viruses

While viruses are the most common cause of infectious diarrhea worldwide, most are associated with self-limiting infections and an often expensive workup for viral pathogens may not be indicated.

Viral Identification Techniques

If viral identification procedures are needed, they should be obtained as soon as possible after onset of symptoms, when viral load in stool is highest; delayed culturing reduces the likelihood of obtaining a positive culture. As with cultures for bacteria, fresh stool specimens are preferred to rectal swabs (2–4 g or 1 tablespoon of semisolid stool, 10–30 mL sample of watery diarrhea). If transport to the laboratory will take more than 15–30 minutes, addition of 5–10 mL of viral transport medium will minimize false negative results. Because most laboratories do not perform viral identification in house, coordination with the laboratory to identify special culture requirements is essential to prevent false negative results. In addition to culture, electron microscopy (often with the use of antibodies to viruses to enhance sensitivity) is used in some laboratories to identify viral pathogens such as coronaviruses, astroviruses, caliciviruses, and Norwalk-like agents.

Serologic Tests

Because most viruses causing diarrhea are difficult to culture, detection of an acute increase in antibody titer against a virus or presence of IgM antibodies against a virus is often used to prove infection (Chapter 35). Because antibody tests are not positive for several days to weeks after onset of illness, such tests are often of more help from a public health point of view than for clinical diagnosis.

CHAPTER 32.

Wound And Body Fluid Infections

D. ROBERT DUFOUR

WOUND INFECTIONS

As discussed in Chapter 33, skin serves as one of the important barriers against infection. Wounds of various sorts break this barrier and allow organisms normally present on the skin surface, or on the surface of the object causing the injury, to gain access to underlying tissues. Any wound breaking the skin surface allows bacteria such as *Staphylococcus aureus* and a number of anaerobic organisms access to subcutaneous tissue; *S. aureus* is the single most common isolate from any wound infection. Some types of wound infections, particularly superficial and septic complications of burns and surgery, are discussed in more detail in Chapter 33. Some special aspects of particular types of wound infections are discussed here.

Determination of the Cause of Wound Infections

Obtaining appropriate specimens for stain and culture from wound infections depends on an understanding of where bacteria are normally encountered and how to avoid contamination from these locations.

Wound Cultures

In open wounds, a natural tendency is to obtain a swab from the surface of the injured site. Such cultures are worthless because surface bacteria (including *S. aureus* and *S. epidermidis*) will always be present, along with other normal surface flora, precluding identification of the etiologic agent. In addition, anaerobic organisms are frequently involved in pathogenesis of wound infections, and anaerobes will not survive in the transport media used for normal swab cultures. To reduce the possibility of contamination, specimens from wounds should be obtained by syringe after using topical antiseptics. Ideally, any air bubbles are expelled from the syringe, and the syringe is sealed by inserting the needle into a solid rubber stopper. This technique allows performance of both culture and Gram stain. If there will be a significant delay in transporting the specimen to the laboratory, some fluid from the aspirate should be injected into an anaerobic transport medium and the remainder left in the syringe or injected into an aerobic transport medium.

Gram Stain

Gram stains of wound specimens are often difficult to interpret, since most wound infections are due to infection by multiple organisms. In certain circumstances, however, a single organism may predominate and the Gram stain can allow rapid, presump-

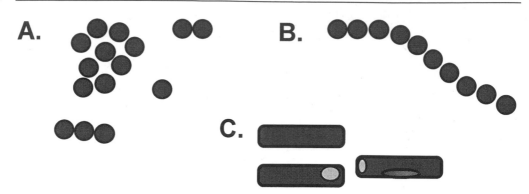

Figure 32.1. Important Organisms in Wound Infections. The three most important organisms in wound infections are illustrated in this representation of a Gram stain. *S. aureus* (**A**) is a gram positive coccus usually found in clusters, short chains, and single cells. *Streptococci* and *Enterococci* (**B**) are typically found as single cells or in long chains. *Clostridium* species (**C**), particularly *C. perfringens*, produces large Gram positive bacilli (often termed "box car" bacilli) which often form spores.

tive identification of that organism and facilitate selection of antibiotics. The most important organisms identified by gram stain are indicated in Figure 32.1.

Antibiotic Susceptibility

Testing for resistance to various antibiotics is essential for wound infections, especially for hospital acquired infections. Resistance to antibiotics is becoming increasingly common in hospitals, especially methicillin resistance in *S. aureus* (MRSA) and multiple antibiotic resistance (especially vancomycin) in *Enterococcus* (VRE).

Specific Patterns of Wound Infections

Differing patterns of wound infection suggest specific etiologic agents or groups of agents, which can be of help in interpreting Gram stains and selecting antibiotic therapy.

Superficial Skin Infections

Infection of skin often follows minor injury to the epidermis from factors such as increased skin moisture. Disorders such as impetigo (crusted skin infections), folliculitis (pustules within hair follicles), furuncles (deeper seated abscesses usually following folliculitis), and cellulitis (spreading erythematous infection of the dermal tissues) are usually caused by *S. aureus*, although a minority of cases of impetigo are due to Group A streptococci. In cellulitis following injury occurring in salt water or on exposure to salt water seafood, *Vibrio vulnificus* is often the etiologic agent. If culture is needed in impetigo, the exudate beneath a crust (after superficial disinfection) should be carefully collected with a swab, avoiding contact with the adjacent skin. Culture from areas of cellulitis, if indicated by unusual clinical history (such as salt water injury) or lack of response to therapy with antibiotics effective against staphylococci and streptococci, should be by needle aspirate of the advancing edge of cellulitis, although they will be positive in only about 30% of cases.

Gangrene

Infection associated with death of skin and soft tissue is termed gangrene. A number of clinical factors may indicate likely etiologic agents. Gangrene following minimal injury associated with rapid spread of injury in muscle is often caused by Group A streptococci (so-called "flesh eating bacteria"). Gangrene following local injury and associated with gas formation in tissue ("gas gangrene") is almost always caused by *Clostridium perfringens*. Gangrene occurring in the legs and feet of diabetic patients is usually caused by *S. aureus,* often MRSA. Common with prolonged infection is superinfection with other organisms, including *Enterococcus,* Gram negative bacteria, and anaerobic organisms. As discussed earlier, aspirate of areas of gangrene can be examined by Gram stain to look for a predominant organism and cultured for both aerobic and anaerobic organisms.

Bites

The large number of bacteria in the oral cavity often leads to infection following a bite, particularly if immediate treatment with antiseptic agents is not used. Because of the mixed flora present in the oral cavity (Chapter 29), infection with more than one organism is common. Following dog or cat bites, *Pasteurella multocida* is often involved in the infection, but *S. aureus* and anaerobic organisms are often isolated as well. After human bites, infection is more common than with animal bites because of the higher number of bacteria present in the human mouth. Streptococci and *S. aureus* are the most commonly isolated organisms, although anaerobic bacteria are also commonly found.

IDENTIFICATION OF INFECTION IN BLOOD AND BODY FLUID

Normally, the blood stream and internal body fluids (CSF, pleural, peritoneal, and joint) are considered sterile, with the presence of any bacteria in these sites abnormal and indicating infection. Because infection of these sites is usually serious and sometimes life threatening, rapid identification of the likelihood of infection is used to begin treatment, often before receiving the results of culture. While treatment is typically begun based on clinical suspicion of infection, documentation of infection is considered critical to continuing therapy and in determining if changes in antibiotic therapy are indicated. In the case of CSF infection, serologic tests are often used to rapidly determine the cause of infection. Specific organisms commonly seen with most body fluid infections are discussed in more detail in Chapter 20.

Gram Stain and Other Staining Techniques

In body fluid infection, the number of organisms present is often small, resulting in negative Gram stains in many infected individuals. Gram stains of blood have a low yield in most patients with sepsis, although Gram stain of a buffy coat (obtained by centrifugation of a sample of blood and making a smear of the white cell layer, which separates between plasma and red cells) increases yield in patients with meningococcal infection and some overwhelming infections with other organisms. In body fluids, Gram stain has a sensitivity of less than 70% in detecting bacteria present on culture, and in joint fluid and peritoneal fluid less than half of culture positive cases have bacteria detected by Gram stain. In effusions caused by tuberculosis, acid-fast stains are positive in less than 10% of cases (although the yield is higher on pleural biopsy specimens). Negative results of Gram and acid-fast stains are thus not useful in ruling out infection, while positive results are helpful findings.

Body Fluid Culture

Since body cavity fluids are normally sterile, a positive culture is strong evidence of infection. The major problem in interpreting positive culture results is the possibility of contamination. For collection of blood and body fluid specimens for culture, careful disinfection of the surface overlying the site of puncture used to obtain fluid is essential to prevent contamination. Cultures positive for weakly pathogenic organisms normally found on skin surfaces (diptheroids, coagulase negative staphylococci) often represent contamination rather than infection. Cultures positive for other normal skin flora (*S. aureus*, streptococci) may also represent contamination. Practitioners should carefully interpret positive cultures in light of the care taken in preparing the site for culture.

CSF Culture

The major considerations in CSF culture are possible contamination and relatively low numbers of organisms. While most bacteria can be reliably identified in CSF specimens of 1 mL or greater, fungi and mycobacteria are usually present in smaller numbers, and at least 3–5 mL of fluid should be obtained to maximize the likelihood of positive cultures. Most viruses causing meningitis or encephalitis cannot be cultured from CSF specimens. For these diagnosis is usually based on detection of antibodies to the virus. Direct fluorescent antibody tests for herpes simplex and cytomegalovirus are also available, and amplification methods to detect these viruses are available from many laboratories. Tests to detect Lyme disease and syphilis are discussed in Chapter 35.

Body Fluid Culture

As with CSF, bacterial cultures usually are successful if 1–2 mL of fluid is collected. Particularly with pleural and peritoneal fluid, specimens should also be handled to allow culture of anaerobic organisms (discussed above under wound infections). If tuberculosis is suspected, at least 10–15 mL of fluid should be submitted; this is centrifuged and the sediment used for culture.

Blood Culture

As with body fluid cultures, careful decontamination of skin is essential in preventing falsely positive cultures. Generally, blood is collected with a syringe, and a minimum of 5 mL of blood should be obtained for each culture performed. Most authorities recommend collecting a minimum of two venipunctures, ideally at different sites, using 10 mL of blood from each venipuncture and inoculating 5 mL into each of two different culture containers. The use of two sets of culture tubes results in over 98% sensitivity for detecting bacteremia. Use of two sets of tubes also increases the ability to distinguish contaminants from significant positive results: a positive culture of normal skin flora organisms in only one out of four tubes identifies false positive results. Laboratories typically use commercial collection sets that use a variety of techniques to recognize bacterial metabolic products to identify growth of microorganisms. In patients receiving antibiotics at the time of collection of blood cultures, use of antibiotic binding resins will reduce the likelihood of false negative results.

Serologic and Nonspecific Tests

Tests to identify bacterial antigens are widely used on CSF specimens to allow rapid recognition of the causative organism, with antigen tests available for *Cryptococcus neoformans, Neisseria meningitidis, Streptococcus pneumoniae,* and *Haemophilus influenzae,* responsible for most cases of meningitis. Nonspecific tests such as cell count, protein, lactic acid, and pH are often helpful in making a presumptive diagnosis of body fluid infection. These tests are discussed in more detail in Chapter 20.

CHAPTER 33

Opportunistic Infections

D. ROBERT DUFOUR

NORMAL DEFENSES AGAINST INFECTION

The likelihood of infection is based upon the balance between virulence of an organism and body defenses against it. While many infectious agents discussed earlier can cause disease even in persons with normal defenses, in many cases the failure of protective systems allows relatively harmless organisms to cause infection. A number of factors (Table 33.1) are important in protecting against damage to tissues by microorganisms. Damage to one of these defense components increases the risk of infection, while the types of organisms gaining access to tissue vary with each component injured. Awareness of these factors will allow for appropriate laboratory testing to detect unusual infectious agents and selection of appropriate antimicrobial therapy while awaiting results.

Intact Epithelial Surfaces

The most important barrier to infection is the layer of epithelial cells which physically separates tissues from the external environment. Most obviously, the skin forms a protective layer from the omnipresent bacteria distributed through the air, water, and on solid surfaces (including the skin). Internally, the mucosa lining the upper and lower respiratory tract, intestinal tract, urinary tract, and female genital tract prevent bacteria normally present in these sites from invading tissue. Mechanical injuries (surgery, burns, abrasions on skin, foreign bodies and stool in internal organs) or chemicals (including chemotherapeutic agents) may damage these surfaces and allow bacteria to invade tissues and produce infection. Insertion of catheters also damages these barriers and predisposes to infection.

Normal Drainage of Hollow Organs

In organs such as the lungs, middle ear, urinary tract, and gall bladder, free flow of fluid helps to wash out bacteria which normally gain entrance to these cavities. In addition, in the case of the respiratory tract, cilia (finger-like projections) produce waves within the fluid to assist in removing organisms. Obstruction of drainage or damage to cilia (such as by smoking) allows bacteria to proliferate and produce infection.

Presence of Normal Bacterial Flora

In the mouth, lower female genital tract, and lower intestine, bacteria coexist with tissues without producing harm. The use of antibiotics which reduce the numbers of these bacteria may allow proliferation of resistant bacteria or more dangerous organisms.

Table 33.1.
Host Factors Protecting Against Infection

- Epithelial surfaces
- Normal drainage of organs
- Normal bacterial flora
- Neutrophilic white blood cells
- Liver and spleen phagocytic cells
- Antibody production (B lymphocytes)
- Cell mediated immunity (T lymphocytes)

Granulocytes

White blood cells (WBCs) of the granulocytic series form a line of defense primarily directed against large organisms such as bacteria and fungi. Unlike the immune response, WBCs do not require prior exposure to be able to attack and destroy most organisms. Many bacteria gain access to the circulation daily, often through the mouth during food ingestion or from the intestinal tract, and these are usually promptly destroyed by WBCs. Granulocytes can ingest (phagocytize) organisms and then destroy most of them by enzymatic and chemical reactions; this process is enhanced when an antibody or complement "marks" organisms as foreign (a process termed **opsonization**). A decrease in the number of granulocytes (from replacement of the bone marrow, toxic chemicals such as chemotherapeutic agents, or other causes discussed in Chapter 25) or impairment of WBC function (diabetes, chronic myelogenous leukemia, rare inherited defects such as chronic granulomatous disease) typically leads to infection.

Phagocytic Cells

The spleen and liver have large numbers of phagocytic cells which can ingest foreign particles, particularly microorganisms, once they have been marked by the immune system. Removal of the spleen or presence of portal hypertension allows bacteria which cannot be digested by granulocytes to produce infection.

Damage to the Immune System

The final line of defense against infection remains the immune system, which allows protection against foreign substances (such as microorganisms) once the body recognizes the presence of an intruding antigen. Patients with immunodeficiencies (Chapter 36) are also prone to develop infections. Decreased B-cell function occurs in patients with congenital immune deficiency, with defective T-helper function (as occurs in AIDS), with many lymphomas, plasma cell dyscrasias, and chronic lymphocytic leukemia, and with high dose corticosteroid treatment. Deficiency of immunoglobulin producing B lymphocytes typically causes infection by organisms that cannot be destroyed by granulocytes due to lack of antibody production. Deficiency of T-cell function typically occurs with congenital deficiency states, with lymphomas, AIDS, and with immunosuppressive therapy following transplantation or in the treatment of serious autoimmune diseases. Deficiency of T lymphocytes typically causes infections by organisms resistant to granulocytes and phagocytic cells, particularly by otherwise relatively innocuous organisms.

COMMON PATTERNS OF INFECTIONS WITH SPECIFIC DAMAGE TO HOST DEFENSES

As mentioned above, the types of defense offered by specific components dictates the classes of organisms which may thrive when that component is injured. Opportunistic infections are particularly common in the elderly, in patients receiving antibiotics and cancer chemotherapeutic agents, and in patients with immunodeficiencies. While the normal culture media used by most laboratories will allow identification of most of these organisms, some may be ignored as contaminants unless the laboratory is aware the patient has impaired defense mechanisms. This is particularly likely to be a problem with urine cultures in patients with catheters, as discussed in Chapter 28; while low colony counts and growth of organisms such as coagulase negative *staphylococci* are usually considered negative results, these often indicate urinary tract infection in catheterized patients. Practitioners should routinely notify the laboratory of the patient's clinical condition when performing cultures on patients with impaired host defenses.

Damage to Mucosal Surfaces

Mucosal injury allows normal bacterial flora in a particular site to gain access to tissue. With skin injury by burns or surgery, the most common infective organisms are *staphylococcus aureus* (often methicillin resistant (MRSA), reflecting the use of antibiotics and the prevalence of antibiotic resistance in hospitals), *enterobacter cloacae, pseudomonas aeruginosa,* and *enterococci.* After "clean" surgery, a similar pattern of infective organisms is seen, although coagulase negative *staphylococci* and *escherichia coli* are also commonly involved. With injury to intestinal epithelium by ischemia or chemotherapy, enteric organisms such as *E. coli, Klebsiella pneumoniae,* enterococci, and *Pseudomonas* are commonly encountered infections. Insertion of catheters allows normal surface flora access to tissues. For example, with intravenous or intra-arterial catheters, staphylococci and streptococci are often involved, while with bladder catheters the same organisms responsible for urinary tract infections (Chapter 28) are typically involved.

Obstruction of Drainage

Failure of drainage of a hollow organ allows bacteria normally found in that area to proliferate. In the respiratory tract, obstruction is often associated with infection by staphylococci or streptococci. Obstruction of the intestinal tract (such as the appendix) or bile duct often causes infection with *E. coli, K. pneumoniae,* and enterococci. Urinary tract obstruction often is associated with infection with the same organisms, *S. aureus, P. aeruginosa,* proteus species, and candida.

Alteration of Normal Bacterial Flora

Use of broad spectrum antibiotics allows colonization of body cavities by a different type of bacteria and overgrowth of resistant organisms, altering the pattern of infection seen in various organs. In the oral cavity, gram negative organisms often become prevalent, particularly *P. aeruginosa.* In the intestinal tract, use of antibiotics without significant activity against anaerobes (such as cephalosporins and sulfonamides) does not typically allow resistant organisms to emerge, whereas use of broad spectrum antibiotics often allows emergence of *Clostridium difficile* (Chapter 33) and multiply resistant (vancomycin-resistant) enterococci (VRE) and MRSA. Fungi such as *Candida albicans* also increase in number. While diarrhea in patients receiving antibiotics almost always is due to *C. difficile,* urinary tract infections and septicemia are often due to one of these other resistant organisms.

Granulocytopenia

A number of organisms are capable of entering the blood stream from sources such as the oral cavity and the intestine in small numbers; they are normally destroyed by granulocytes. When total granulocyte count falls below $0.5 \times 10^3/\mu L$ ($0.5 \times 10^9/L$), and particularly with granulocyte counts below $0.1 \times 10^3/\mu L$ ($0.1 \times 10^9/L$), normal defenses cannot prevent proliferation of organisms and infection frequently develops. The vast majority of infections in granulocytopenic patients are caused by relatively few organisms: bacteria include staphylococci (both *S. aureus* and coagulase-negative staph), α-hemolytic streptococci, *P. aeruginosa, E. coli,* and *K. pneumoniae.* In addition, the fungi *C. albicans* and aspergillus species are also common causes of infection. Because fungi may grow more slowly than bacteria, practitioners should notify the laboratory to incubate cultures for additional time to allow detection of fungal infections in granulocytopenic patients.

Defects in Phagocytic Function

The liver and spleen are important in the defense against bacteria. In patients with liver failure, particularly in portal hypertension in cirrhosis, intestinal bacteria can gain entry to normally sterile fluids such as ascitic fluid, producing spontaneous bacterial peritonitis. In addition, septicemia and bacterial endocarditis due to gram negative organisms and enterococcus are much more common in patients with portal hypertension. After splenectomy, encapsulated organisms such as *S. pneumoniae, Hemophilus influenzae,* and *Neisseria meningitidis* are not removed readily from the circulation and are more likely to produce serious infections, including septicemia.

Immune System Compromise

The most classic forms of opportunistic infection occur in patients with defective immune function. The pattern of infection differs between patients with deficient B-cell and T-cell function.

Deficient B-Cell Function

With deficient B-cell function, antibody levels fall (or remain low in infants with congenital immune deficiency). In children, this causes failure of vaccination against common childhood ailments. In both children and adults, lack of immunoglobulins allows bacteria which require an antibody attachment in order to be ingested by granulocytes or monocytes ("opsonization") to escape host defenses. The major organisms producing infection are similar to those in splenectomized patients, mainly encapsulated organisms such as *S. pneumoniae, N. meningitidis,* and *H. influenzae,* along with *E. coli.*

Deficient T-Cell Function

In patients with deficient cellular immunity, a number of unusual pathogens often produce infection. In addition to the unusual opportunistic infections discussed below, a number of other infectious agents are more commonly found in patients with deficient cell mediated immunity, including *Listeria monocytogenes,* salmonella, *Legionella pneumophila,* and *Mycobacterium tuberculosis.*

Pneumocystis

The protozoan *Pneumocystis carinii* is a common cause of pneumonia in patients with defective cell mediated immunity. Most normal individuals have evidence of previous exposure to this organism and have little risk of infection. With immunosuppression, pneumocystis typically causes mild fever, shortness of breath, and a nonproductive cough. Chest radiographs often reveal a patchy pattern of infiltrates and interstitial pneumonia; blood gases reveal a respiratory alkalosis and hypoxemia with an increased A-a gradient. Examination of regular sputum specimens has a low yield and is not recommended. Use of induced sputum has a better yield, while bronchoalveolar lavage has a sensitivity of nearly 100% for pneumocystis. The organism can be demonstrated using special stains, such as toluidine blue or silver stains, but many laboratories use fluorescent-labeled antibodies to detect pneumocystis.

Atypical Mycobacteria

While tuberculosis is more commonly encountered in patients with T-cell deficiency, other mycobacteria are often isolated in patients with immunosuppression. Because skin tests rely on normal cell mediated immunity, practitioners should remember that a negative PPD is not helpful in ruling out tuberculosis in immunocompromised patients. *Mycobacterium avium-intracellulare* (MAI) rarely causes severe infections in patients with normal immune status. With defective T-cell function, especially in AIDS, MAI is a common infection, and ultimately affects over one-third of AIDS patients. Although often starting as a pulmonary infection, dissemination to other parts of the body is common; bacteremia occurs frequently in patients with CD4 counts less than $0.1 \times 10^3/\mu L$ ($0.1 \times 10^9/L$). Once dissemination occurs, infection may develop in many organs, including the liver, spleen, the gastrointestinal tract, and bone marrow. Cultures are usually obtained from sputum and blood; like other mycobacteria, slow growth can delay diagnosis. Identification of an acid-fast organism in a patient with immunosuppression should lead to coverage for both tuberculosis and MAI. In other forms of deficient T-cell function, other atypical mycobacteria may predominate; in hairy cell leukemia, *Mycobacterium kansasii* is commonly found.

Fungal Infections

In patients with T-cell deficiency, fungal infections often cause severe or chronic infections. The most common fungal infection is due to *C. albicans,* which often produces severe topical infections in the mouth and esophagus (thrush), frequently recognizable as a whitish exudate on an erythematous surface. Demonstration of fungal pseudohyphae on a KOH preparation is usually all that is required for diagnosis. Candida can also cause urinary tract infections and septicemia in immunosuppressed patients. *Cryptococcus neoformans* is much more frequently encountered in patients with T-cell dysfunction, most commonly as meningitis. While culture is possible, methods to quickly identify cryptococcus are needed to begin treatment rapidly. India ink preparations can identify cryptococcus in many cases. When the smear is negative, detection of cryptococcal antigen is diagnostic in most cases. Both serum and CSF should be tested to achieve maximal sensitivity. *Histoplasma capsulatum* typically produces chronic pulmonary infection in patients with normal immune function. In patients with T-cell deficiency, histoplasma may produce disseminated infection. As with cryptococcus, detection of the fungal antigen can produce a rapid diagnosis. Urinary tests for histoplasma antigen will detect over 90% of cases of disseminated infection. The reference laboratory at Wishard Memorial Hospital in Indianapolis provides rapid availability of urine histoplasma antigen tests.

Viral Infections

Initial infection with viruses is not more common in patients with T-cell dysfunction. A number of viruses that remain dormant after initial infection often produce recurrent disease in patients with defective cell mediated immunity; these include herpes simplex and herpes zoster. Cytomegalovirus (CMV) often produces disseminated infection in patients with severe T-cell dysfunction. When necessary, CMV can be isolated by culture or amplification methods; IgM antibodies can also document recent infection. Direct examination of tissue can identify CMV antigen in tissue, and in severe cases viral inclusions can often be detected using cytology from fluids in infected organisms (urine, sputum, esophageal brushings). Herpes simplex can also produce encephalitis in patients with immunosuppression; herpes viral DNA can be detected by culture or amplification methods.

Parasites

Toxoplasma gondii is a common infection in adults, particularly those who are exposed to cats. When T-cell function is suppressed, infections may reactivate, commonly producing infections in the retina and the brain, and less commonly causing pneumonia. In the retina, it usually occurs following infection of the brain, causing pain and necrotizing lesions. In the brain, toxoplasma usually produces abscesses with ring enhancement on contrast imaging studies. The organism can be detected in biopsies when needed to establish the diagnosis. Negative serologic studies can be helpful in ruling out infection. If the titer is positive, a rise in titer may indicate reactivation, but takes 1–2 weeks for documentation. *Cryptosporidium* commonly causes diarrhea in immunodeficient patients, responsible for 10–20% of cases; the parasite can be demonstrated in stool using Giemsa stain or modified acid-fast stains. Fluorescent antibody tests are also used in some laboratories and have increased sensitivity. Less commonly, *Cryptosporidium* may colonize the biliary tract and cause cholecystitis or cholangitis and obstructive jaundice. *Microsporidia* are much smaller pathogens than *Cryptosporidium*, most commonly causing chronic diarrhea and less frequently cholangitis, similar to *Cryptosporidium*. Although historically tissue biopsies using either light or electron microscopy have been used to establish the diagnosis, recently a fluorochrome stain has become available to detect *Microsporidia* in stool specimens.

CHAPTER 34

Selecting and Monitoring Antibiotic Therapy

D. ROBERT DUFOUR

SELECTION OF ANTIBIOTICS TO TREAT BACTERIAL INFECTIONS

In most instances, bacteria identified by culture are tested to determine which antibiotics are able to inhibit bacterial growth; this is termed antibiotic susceptibility testing. To determine susceptibility, organisms must be isolated in pure culture, which takes at least 1–2 days after the culture specimen is submitted to the laboratory, and often longer in the presence of mixed infections. Unfortunately, this means that a significant delay occurs between the time the specimen is submitted to the laboratory and when the results of susceptibility testing become available. Knowledge of bacterial susceptibility is most likely to be helpful when patients are responding poorly to antibiotics selected before culture results were known. Studies have also shown that practitioners seldom use susceptibility results to change treatment when patients are responding clinically to therapy. If the practitioner understands and uses susceptibility testing, it may be possible to improve cost effective treatment of patients with bacterial infections.

Methods Used to Determine Susceptibility

Regardless of method used, bacteria are typically classified as susceptible, moderately susceptible (or intermediate), or resistant to a particular antibiotic agent.

Limitations of Susceptibility Testing

Susceptibility determinations are based upon the average concentrations of an antibiotic achievable *in vivo*, and may not indicate the actual ability of an antibiotic to control infection. For example, in patients with urinary tract infection, extremely high concentrations of antibiotics in urine allow virtually any antibiotic to control infection with most organisms (even those which seem "resistant" in vitro). However, in renal failure, the lack of urinary excretion of most antibiotics (other than penicillins) may cause failure of an antibiotic even though laboratory testing indicates that the organism is susceptible to the antibiotic. Organisms which penetrate poorly into body fluids, or are inactivated at certain pH levels, will be ineffective even if testing indicates susceptibility. With intermediate susceptibility, it may be possible to use larger doses of the antibiotic to produce higher concentrations that may inhibit bacterial growth.

Types of Susceptibility Testing

Laboratories employ two major types of methods to determine susceptibility, outlined in Figure 34.1. In both, a relatively standardized concentration of a pure culture of the organism is tested against a number of different antibiotics. Because laboratory measurements of antibiotic concentration in the patient are not available for most drugs, there is little advantage to one type of test or reporting system over another,

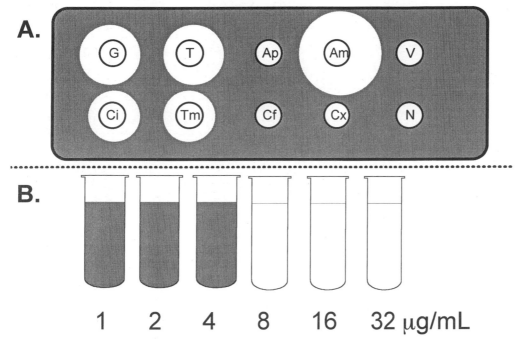

Figure 34.1. Antibiotic Susceptibility Methods. In disc diffusion methods (**A**), circular discs containing a known concentration of antibiotic are placed on a culture plate. After incubation, the diameter of the zone in which bacterial growth is inhibited is measured for each antibiotic and compared to results from organisms known to be susceptible, intermediately susceptible, and resistant. In the illustration, the organism is susceptible to gentamicin (G), tobramycin (T), and ampicillin (Am), intermediately susceptible to ciprofloxacin (Ci) and trimethoprim (Tm), and resistant to other antibiotics. With serial dilution methods (**B**), varying concentrations of multiple antibiotics are used, and the minimum concentration of antibiotic inhibiting bacterial growth (minimum inhibitory concentration, MIC) is determined. This may either be reported (in concentration units, such as μg/mL) or the organism classified by comparison to other strains as with disc testing. In the illustration, testing with gentamicin, the MIC is 8 μg/mL which would make the organism intermediately susceptible (In both A and B, dark areas indicate bacterial growth).

and results of the two techniques are generally equivalent; however, dilution methods are often available more rapidly than disc diffusion methods.

Hospital Antibiograms

On a periodic basis, hospital microbiology laboratories analyze results of susceptibility tests from all patients seen over a specific period of time (usually a year). The percentage of organisms susceptible to each antibiotic is reported for each of the most common bacteria cultured by that laboratory. This can be helpful once culture results are available in evaluating whether current antibiotics are likely to be effective in treating the infection.

MONITORING ANTIBIOTIC THERAPY

Once antibiotic therapy has been started, clinical response is the most widely used method to evaluate therapy. When antibiotics are toxic (aminoglycosides, vancomycin), measurement of antibiotic levels can prevent toxicity. Failure of response to antibiotics

Table 34.1.
Therapeutic Ranges for Aminoglycosides Antibiotics and Vancomycin

Drug	Half-life (hrs)	Therapeutic Peak (μg/mL)	Therapeutic Trough (μg/mL)
Amikacin	2–3	20–25	5–10
Gentamicin	2–3	4–10	1–2
Tobramycin	2–3	4–10	1–2
Vancomycin	3–5	30–40	5–10

may be due to a subtherapeutic concentration of antibiotics; measurement of antibiotic level may be helpful in changing dosage to improve response. With serious infections (such as bacterial endocarditis), assuring adequate antibiotic concentrations can prevent treatment failure and improve response.

Antibiotic Levels

The aminoglycoside antibiotics and vancomycin have a low therapeutic index, and are often associated with renal tubular damage and hearing loss. Use of antibiotic levels to adjust therapy lowers the risk of complications and assures adequate therapeutic doses. In general, toxic complications are likely when trough concentrations exceed therapeutic limits, and poor antibiotic response is associated with low peak drug concentration. Antibiotic levels should not be drawn for 4–5 half-lives after starting therapy if no loading dose is given; this generally occurs after 2 doses of drug. Because these drugs are excreted by the kidney, initial intervals should be adjusted using the formula in Equation 18.5. Levels can be used to adjust therapy so that both peak and trough levels are within therapeutic ranges, using the approach in Chapter 18. Therapeutic ranges for aminoglycosides and vancomycin are shown in Table 34.1.

Concentration of Other Antibiotics

When patients show poor response during treatment with antibiotics to which the organism is susceptible, low blood levels may be the cause. This may be due to underdosing or to poor drug absorption. Unfortunately, most hospital laboratories do not have the capability to measure the concentration of antibiotics other than those listed above. A few reference laboratories can indirectly determine drug concentration by comparing the ability of patient serum to inhibit growth of a particular organism when compared to standard responses to known antibiotic concentrations. Such indirect methods work only when patients are given a single antibiotic; they cannot be used in patients on multiple antibiotic agents. Results often take several days to return, so are only likely to be useful in patients who require long term antibiotic therapy. Specimens are usually drawn as trough specimens, just before the next dose of antibiotic.

Serum Bactericidal Concentration

In patients with bacterial endocarditis, the likelihood of bacteriologic cure is related to the ability of an antibiotic to not simply inhibit growth, but to kill the organism. Some authorities have advocated use of serum bactericidal titers to determine the relative ability of drug in a patient's blood to destroy the organism responsible for endocarditis. Samples for bactericidal titers should be drawn using the same aseptic technique used for obtaining blood cultures, requiring the use of special bacteria free tubes for blood collection. Failure to follow appropriate precautions in specimen collection will cause falsely low results and may lead to unnecessary changes in antibiotic treatment. Usually, both peak and trough specimens are obtained. The patient's serum is incubated overnight with a standard concentration of the organism (obtained from previous cultures). If no gross bacterial growth is seen, the serum specimen (containing bacteria) is then cultured to see if any viable organisms remain. The highest titer in which no organisms can be cultured is termed the bactericidal titer. About one-third of patients with titers less than 1:16 on peak specimens or less than 1:8 on trough specimens failed therapy, while almost all patients with peak titers greater than 1:64 and trough titers greater than 1:32 were cured; intermediate results are difficult to interpret. Since a significant percentage of patients with low titers will be cured, it is controversial whether to increase dosages in patients with low titers, although this is recommended by most authorities if the drug therapy used does not have significant toxicity.

CHAPTER 35

Use of Serologic Procedures to Diagnose Infections

D. ROBERT DUFOUR

ADVANTAGES AND DISADVANTAGES OF SEROLOGIC PROCEDURES

The term "serologic" procedure was initially used to describe serum tests to identify antibodies to infectious agents; such procedures have been available for many years. Currently, the term is often used for tests to identify infections without culturing the causative agent. The types of procedures used have increased over the past 10 years, allowing increasing numbers of infections to be recognized and changing the testing used for diagnosis of many infectious diseases.

Advantages of Serologic Procedures

In some infections, the organism is difficult to culture, either because of the growth requirements of the organism (many viruses, agents causing sexually transmitted diseases) or prior antibiotic treatment. In some cases, a culture is not attempted because of significant risk to laboratory workers. In other infections, a culture requires a significant amount of time to become positive (fungi, mycobacteria). In such circumstances, serologic procedures often allow diagnosis to be made in a timely fashion. In yet other infections, serologic methods can provide prognostic information and can be used to monitor therapy (viral load testing in HIV and chronic hepatitis). Nucleic acid probes can often detect infectious agents earlier than culture or other serologic tests.

Disadvantages of Serologic Procedures

Serologic tests which measure host immune response to an organism are not positive for 10–14 days after an infection, and with some viral infections (HIV, hepatitis B and C) may not be present for weeks to months. While IgM antibodies are only present transiently, IgG antibodies often persist for years, and in many instances are present for life. In patients with immunodeficiency, antibody response may be blunted or nonexistent, impairing the ability to use serologic procedures to establish a diagnosis. Finally, the antibody detected may have been made against another organism, and represents a falsely positive test for the suspected organism. Serologic procedures to detect antigens produced by an organism are typically positive earlier than antibody tests, but are not be available for as many infectious agents as are antibody tests. Nucleic acid probes tend to be expensive, subject to problems with contamination if not performed under extremely careful isolation techniques, and are still not widely available.

TYPES OF SEROLOGIC PROCEDURES

An understanding of the methods used in serologic procedures will make it easier for the practitioner to interpret the test results obtained in their patients and to understand the likelihood of an erroneous result in a patient.

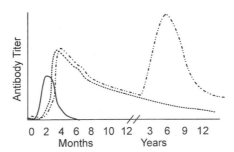

Figure 35.1. Patterns of Antibody Response. Within about 7–10 days after most infections, IgM antibodies (solid line) against an agent appear. They reach peak levels before 2 months and typically resolve by 4–6 months. IgG antibodies (dotted line) follow within 2–4 weeks after an IgM response, reach a peak by about 2–3 months, and generally remain positive for life. On re-exposure to an agent, an anamnestic response (dotted-dashed line) causes antibody to transiently rise to even higher levels before rapidly returning to near baseline levels. While presence of IgM antibodies to an agent indicate acute infection, a rise in antibody amount is also reliable evidence of recent infection.

Tests to Detect Antibody Production

The most common serologic tests are those that detect antibodies to a particular organism. A prototypical antibody response to an infectious agent is illustrated in Figure 35.1. IgM antibodies to an organism are the earliest response to infection. Testing for IgM antibodies to an agent is particularly important in neonates, since IgG antibodies can cross the placenta and may represent previous exposure of the mother to an organism, rather than infection of the baby. IgM antibodies against an organism are also important when there is a high frequency of asymptomatic infection. In these instances, IgG antibodies could represent either current infection or remote exposure to the organism. If it is not possible to measure IgM antibodies separately, then detection of a rise in titer between specimens taken 1–2 weeks apart ("acute" and "convalescent" serum) indicates recent infection. Three basic types of tests to detect antibodies are used; the significance of positive results and the way of expressing positive results varies for each.

Serial Dilution Methods

In this earliest type of serologic test, serum from a patient is progressively diluted 1:2, producing progressively lower amounts of antibody in each tube. A constant amount of antigen from an infectious agent is then added to each tube, often attached to an indicator such as latex beads or red cells. The greatest dilution of serum that produces a positive response is reported (e.g., 1:16, 1:128, etc.). Serial dilution methods are not very precise; a difference of one tube in dilution is not considered to be a significant difference in determining the presence of recent infection (e.g., 1:4 and 1:8 are not significantly different, while 1:4 and 1:16 would be).

Enzyme-Linked Immunosorbent Assay (ELISA) and Related Techniques

For most antibody tests, laboratories are using a variant of ELISA testing, illustrated in Figure 35.2. In ELISA, results are not reported as a titer; instead, they are reported in one of several ways, related to the relative amount of signal generated by the patient's serum when compared to that of a known, usually weakly positive, serum. Results are

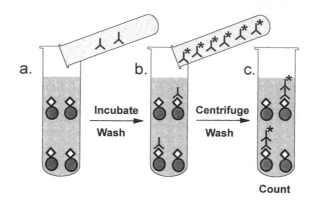

Figure 35.2. Principle of ELISA and Similar Tests. A solid support, such as a bead (circle) is coated with an antigen (diamond). A sample of serum is added, and after incubation and washing, any antibody to the antigen will be attached to the bead. An antibody from another animal that recognizes human immunoglobulin (either all immunoglobulin or specific for either IgG or IgM) is labeled with an enzyme to detect presence of antibody from the patient's serum. If this is incubated with the beads after the initial washing, an amount of enzyme-labeled antibody will attach to the bead in proportion to the amount of antibody present in the patient's serum. By measuring the activity of the enzyme, it is possible to quantify the amount of antibody in the patient. This procedure can be modified to detect antigen in serum by attaching antibody to an antigen to the beads instead of antigen.

reported either as relative units with a numerical reference range (e.g., 10–30 U/mL), or as a ratio of results in the sample to those in the low positive control (e.g., patient 12 U/mL, control 10 U/mL, ratio 1.2). The exact relationship between ELISA results and serial dilution methods varies with each test, making it impossible to directly compare the results of the two types of tests. There is a roughly linear relationship in each assay between the result and the amount of antibody present, so that a doubling in the result means a two-fold rise in the amount of antibody.

Purified Antigen Tests (Western and Other Blots)

As mentioned earlier, antibody tests are often subject to false positive results due to cross-reactivity. Because most infectious agents produce multiple antigens, it is unlikely that a cross-reactive antibody would react with more than one antigen. By separating the antigens of an organism in some fashion and testing for antibodies to multiple antigens (Figure 35.3), it is usually possible to conclusively demonstrate that antibodies are being produced in response to infection with a specific organism. Such tests are considered virtually 100% specific.

Tests for Antigens Produced by an Organism

Because antibody response takes some time to become positive, tests for antibody to an organism are best used when there is no specific therapy available. When treatment is based upon documentation of the presence of a specific organism, tests that directly detect antigens produced by that organism are more likely to establish the diagnosis in a timely fashion. There are a number of antigen tests available to detect infectious agents.

Tests on Body Fluids

Many infectious organisms produce proteins that can be identified in serum, urine, sputum, cerebrospinal fluid, or exudates on body surfaces such as the throat. Tests to

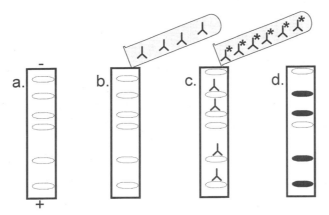

Figure 35.3. Principle of Western Blot and Related Tests. In Western blot (illustrated), antigens are obtained by fractionating organisms, and the antigens are separated by electrophoresis. To facilitate testing, the separated antigens are "blotted" onto a membrane. The membrane is then incubated with serum from a patient and, after washing, the membrane is incubated with labeled antibody to human immunoglobulin. After washing, the label can be detected wherever antibody from serum attaches to antigens. In the related immunoblot testing, antigens from an organism are obtained in pure form, often by recombinant techniques and applied to the membrane in discrete "dots." The incubation and detection steps are otherwise similar to western blot. By showing presence of antibody to multiple antigens of an organism, it is usually possible to eliminate false positive results due to cross-reacting antibodies and prove infection by a specific organism.

detect these antigens are similar in principle to those outlined above for antibody tests. In variants of the tube tests, an antibody to an antigen is attached to a solid support such as a latex bead or red cells; the antigen allows agglutination of the particles by formation of antigen-antibody complexes. In variants of the ELISA technique, antibody to the antigen is attached to the solid support; when a second, labeled antibody is added, only the presence of the antigen allows formation of an antibody-antigen-antibody "sandwich." Such direct antigen tests are widely available for many infectious agents, often in forms that can be used in a practitioner's office. Because reagents may deteriorate over time, it is important to always test known positive and negative samples along with the patient's sample to assure that the test is working as intended. Antigen tests are generally somewhat less sensitive than culture, but provide a diagnosis earlier.

Tests on Tissue

Some infectious agents do not produce significant amounts of antigen that can be detected in body fluids, but remain predominantly within cells. With such agents, examination of cells with antibody to infectious agents may allow detection of infection. Typically, this is accomplished by direct immunofluorescence or related techniques (Figure 35.4). Careful attention to technique and inclusion of positive and negative controls are essential for correct interpretation of results.

Tests for Nucleic Acids of an Organism

The fastest growing area of serologic testing involves tests to detect the nucleic acids (DNA or RNA) of an infectious agent (Figure 35.5). Sequences of nucleic acids form the genetic material of an organism, and are relatively specific for a given infectious ᵊnt. Nucleic acids usually exist as matching pairs of strands, in which the nucleic

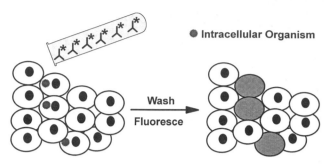

Figure 35.4. Principle of Direct Immunofluorescence. Some organisms, mostly viruses but sometimes other organisms such as pneumocystis, chlamydia, and legionella, are found within samples of tissue or body fluids. The sample is incubated with antibody against an antigen from the organism that is labeled in some way, most typically with a fluorescent compound. After washing the sample, any fluorescence indicates the presence of antigen from the organism. Direct fluorescent techniques are typically the most rapidly available means to demonstrate an organism.

acids are exact mirror images of each other. By incubating a labeled string of nucleic acids derived from the organism (or synthesized to match the nucleic acids of the organism) with material thought to contain an organism (after separating the two strands of DNA or RNA), it is possible to determine whether the organism is present. In general, these tests are much more expensive than antibody or antigen tests. They are typically used to document infection in cases where culture is difficult or impossible, or takes too long to allow timely treatment of a patient. Amplification tests can also be used to quantify the amount of an organism present, and as such are useful for prognosis and monitoring of treatment, particularly with HIV and hepatitis B and C infections.

In Situ Hybridization

Once material containing an infectious agent is available (either by obtaining tissue by biopsy or cytology, or following culture), use of a labeled nucleic acid probe can identify the presence of an organism. In situ hybridization tests are less sensitive than amplification methods, and are generally reserved for those situations where there is likely to be a large quantity of the infectious agent (tissue biopsies, culture preparations). Controls must be run to assure that there is no nonspecific binding of the probe to other genes.

Amplification Methods

The natural function of nucleic acids is to replicate; amplification allows detection of replication of a specific sequence found only in the probe and the organism. Amplification methods allow detection of "growth" of an organism, much as does culture; however, amplification methods often provide results much earlier than do cultures. In addition, amplification methods can provide an estimate of the number of copies of a particular gene and, by extension, the number of organisms present. There are a number of limitations to amplification methods which must be kept in mind when interpreting results. As with culture, amplification methods are prone to produce falsely positive results when contamination occurs. Because amplification methods are typically performed in laboratories that repeatedly attempt to detect specific infectious

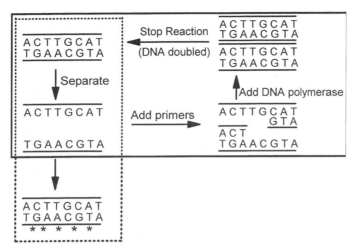

Figure 35.5. Principle of Nucleic Acid Detection Methods. The two major types of methods to detect genetic material (DNA or RNA) from an organism are in situ hybridization (dotted box) and amplification methods (solid box). In in situ hybridization, strands of nucleic acid are separated and a probe, consisting of a length of nucleic acid labeled in some way, is added; it will bind to tissue only when the complementary strand is present. By detecting the label, it is possible to prove the presence of nucleic acids of the organism. In amplification methods (polymerase chain reaction, PCR, is illustrated here), copies of specific genes are made by incubating separated strands of nucleic acids with two short sequences of DNA in the presence of the enzyme DNA polymerase. The genes will replicate only if a complementary strand to the probes is present. By repeating the process several times before incubating with a labeled probe, it is possible to make multiple copies of specific DNA. This procedure can be used not only to detect the presence of nucleic acids of an organism, but also to quantify how many copies have been made (which will be directly proportional to the number of copies originally present.)

agents, contamination is a constant possibility. When used for quantitation, amplification methods are not highly reproducible; it is not unusual for results on the same specimen to differ by 20–25% when tested repeatedly in the same laboratory. For this reason, as with tumor markers, either a trend over three consecutive specimens or a marked change in results is needed to confirm a change in the amount of virus present. Finally, a specific minimum amount of nucleic acid must be present for the assay to detect a positive result; this may vary from one assay to another. While laboratories may report results below this level as "negative" or "undetectable," this does not rule out the presence of small numbers of the organism.

SPECIFIC INFECTIOUS AGENTS AND THEIR SEROLOGIC TESTS

For a number of infectious agents, serologic tests are widely used to diagnose and monitor infection. Some of these agents are discussed in other chapters; for example, antigen tests for streptococci are discussed in Chapter 29, tests for *Clostridium difficile* are found in Chapter 31, hepatitis B and C virus are discussed in Chapter 11, and tests for *Helicobacter pylori* are found in Chapter 21. Although serologic tests can be used to screen for almost any infectious disease, they form the major means to diagnose and monitor patients with the relatively few infections discussed below.

Human Immunodeficiency Virus

Human immunodeficiency virus (HIV), the cause of acquired immunodeficiency syndrome (AIDS), has become one of the most common infections in many parts of the world. While it is possible to culture HIV, in almost all cases diagnosis of HIV infection is based on serologic tests. Recently, amplification methods have been developed and are widely used to monitor treatment with protease inhibitors.

Detection of Antibody to HIV Infection

After infection, HIV specific antibodies appear after an average of 2 months; however, in some patients, antibody may not appear until as long as 6 months following infection. Human immunodeficiency virus antibody assays use either proteins derived from viral infected cells or, in some cases, proteins produced by recombinant techniques (HIV nucleic genes added to bacterial cells). Antibody tests ultimately detect close to 100% of patients infected by HIV. These assays have a relatively high rate of false positive results, so that no more than 15–25% of positive results indicate actual antibody to HIV; the remainder are false positive results. For this reason, positive results are confirmed by first repeating the test; specimens positive in both tests are usually confirmed as positive by Western blot (although some other procedures have been used for this purpose). A Western blot which has positive staining for at least two of the three HIV specific bands (p24, gp41, gp120/160) confirms antibody to HIV-1. If less than two of these specific bands is present, usually along with other less specific bands, the Western blot is termed indeterminate and repeat testing should be performed after 3–6 months.

HIV Antigen Detection

Within about 2–3 weeks of infection, most patients develop a phase in which HIV is present in the circulation; this viremia can be detected by demonstrating the presence of the p24 antigen of HIV, the earliest routine marker. In blood donor testing, this is now mandatory; p24 antigen is felt to detect infection an average of 2–3 weeks earlier than antibody tests. After development of antibody, p24 antigen is seldom detectable in blood until the late stages of infection when symptoms of AIDS develop.

Viral Load Testing

Measurement of the amount of circulating viral RNA has been found to correlate well with risk of progression of HIV infection to AIDS, and also to reflect response of HIV infection to treatment. In general, patients with fewer than 5,000 copies of RNA per mL of plasma have a low rate of progression, while those with greater than 50,000 copies/mL have a high rate of progression. A recent report from an international panel recommends treating asymptomatic patients with normal CD4 lymphocyte counts but viral load of greater than 30,000–50,000 copies/mL, or patients with a CD4 count of $350–500 \times 10^3/\mu L$ ($0.35–0.50 \times 10^9/L$) and greater than 5,000–10,000 copies/mL. Once treatment has started, repeat testing should be done at about 1 month to see if there has been a significant fall in viral load; if so, repeat testing should be done every 3–6 months. Because viral load measurements are not highly reproducible, successful treatment should lower the number of copies by $0.5 \times \log_{10}$. Lack of response or rising viral load suggests the need to add or change therapy.

Infectious Mononucleosis and Epstein-Barr Virus

One of the most common viral infections of adolescents, Epstein-Barr virus (EBV) commonly causes the clinical picture of infectious mononucleosis; however, a significant number of individuals infected are totally asymptomatic. Infectious mononucleosis

Table 35.1.
EBV Antibodies in Infectious Mononucleosis

Time Since Exposure	IgM anti-VCA	IgG anti-VCA	Anti-early Ags	Anti-EBV Nuclear Ag
Recent	Positive	Negative	Negative	Negative
Recovery (1–2 months)	Wk. Positive-Negative	Positive	Positive	Negative-Positive
Remote	Negative	Positive	Negative	Positive

typically presents with fever, enlarged lymph nodes, sore throat, and splenomegaly, and most cases resolve spontaneously over several weeks. An increase in lymphocyte count is found in the majority of patients, and the lymphocytes are often "atypical" (Chapter 25). In over 90% of cases, antibodies react with red blood cells of horse and sheep (termed "heterophile" antibodies). If heterophile antibodies are negative, there are more specific antibodies to EBV antigens that can be used to establish the diagnosis. The earliest antibody to appear is the IgM antibody to EBV viral capsid antigen (VCA), which remains positive for about 1–2 months; the IgM antibody must be measured specifically, since IgG antibodies appear to persist for life. Following this, antibodies to "early antigens" appear and remain positive for only 3–6 months. Antibodies to nuclear antigens develop late after infection and persist for life. The pattern of antibodies (Table 35.1) can help to clarify the time course of an EBV infection.

Syphilis

Caused by the spirochete *Treponema pallidum,* syphilis has become progressively less common in North America. There are three recognized clinical phases. In primary syphilis, infection is typically limited to the site of entry of the organism through the skin or mucous membranes, producing a painless chancre an average of 3 weeks after exposure. During this stage, infection is usually based on demonstration of the organism by darkfield examination. In secondary syphilis, the infection becomes disseminated, often involving skin and CNS, although other organs can be infected. In tertiary syphilis, chronic organ damage occurs, usually affecting the CNS or aorta. There are often long periods when the disease is asymptomatic (termed latent syphilis). During all stages except the chancre, diagnosis is best established by serologic tests.

Nonspecific Antiphospholipid (Reagin) Tests

The most common tests used to screen for syphilis are those detecting antibody to phospholipids (termed "cardiolipins"); such antibodies have been termed reagin. Although historically the most common reagin test was the Venereal Disease Research Laboratory (VDRL) test, most laboratories now use modifications, most commonly the Rapid Plasma Reagin (RPR) test; the tests are roughly equivalent. Reagin antibodies are not specific for syphilis; false positive results are especially common with autoimmune disease (see discussion on antiphospholipid antibodies in Chapter 27), with a variety of other infections, and in older individuals. Positive results on a reagin test should always be confirmed with antibodies specific for syphilis. Reagin antibodies are found in about 70–80% of patients with primary syphilis, but in almost 100% of patients with secondary and early latent syphilis. In late tertiary and latent syphilis, about 25% of patients will have negative results. With successful treatment of syphilis, antibodies often disappear, although the length of time to become negative depends on the duration of infection before treatment. Reagin tests are also preferred for use in CSF to diagnose neurosyphilis, but here confirmatory testing is not done.

Antitreponemal Antibodies

Although a number of tests to detect antibody to *treponema pallidum* have been used, the only tests still widely used are the Fluorescent Treponemal Antibody–Absorbed (FTA-ABS) and the Microhemagglutination–*Treponema Pallidum* (MHA-TP). Both tests have slightly higher sensitivity than reagin tests in primary syphilis, but are still less sensitive than darkfield examination. In addition to their specificity, these tests seldom become negative in latent syphilis or in patients treated for syphilis (only about 10% of those treated in early syphilis become negative). While this is an advantage in detection of late disease, antitreponemal tests cannot be used to judge success of treatment. Once an antitreponemal test is positive, it should not be repeated.

Lyme Disease

Caused by the spirochete *Borrelia burgdorferi*, Lyme disease is acquired by bites from ticks transmitting the organism from other infected individuals. In the initial stage, Lyme disease typically presents as a centrally clearing area of redness (erythema chronicum migrans) before disseminating. In early systemic disease, it often presents with neurologic manifestations, joint swelling, or generalized skin rash. The disease may then become asymptomatic, similar to latent syphilis, before again becoming symptomatic months to years later.

Antibody Tests

The major tests for Lyme disease measure antibodies to borrelia in blood or, with neurologic involvement, in CSF. IgM antibodies are present at the time of initial presentation with skin involvement in only about 40% of patients. By 6 weeks after infection, almost 90% of patients have IgG antibodies to *B. burgdorferi*. Antibody may disappear after treatment, but usually remains positive for life. Although theoretically the protein antigens are specific for Lyme disease, false positive tests are common with standard ELISA-type tests. For this reason, positive results are usually confirmed with Western blot, which can be performed using antibodies to either IgM or IgG. If the clinical symptoms and history suggest infection has occurred in the past 4 weeks, both IgM and IgG Western blot should be performed; if symptoms are present for over 1 month, only IgG Western blot should be requested.

Amplification Methods

In patients with equivocal results, or in whom symptoms persist after therapy, demonstration of nucleic acids of *B. burgdorferi* provides evidence of infection. In patients with Lyme arthritis, amplification methods detect borrelia DNA in synovial fluid in almost 100% of patients; DNA becomes negative with successful treatment. In CSF, borrelia DNA is detected in less than half of patients with suspected CNS Lyme disease, so that positive results are helpful but negative results do not rule out infection.

Mycoplasma Pneumonia

Primary atypical pneumonia, a clinical disorder in which pneumonia is not caused by usual bacteria, is most often caused by infection with *Mycoplasma pneumoniae*.

Mycoplasma are small, bacteria-like organisms that are difficult to culture on normal bacterial culture media, although *M. pneumoniae* will grow slowly on certain media, often taking several weeks to become positive. Mycoplasma pneumonia is a relatively common infection, particularly in children and young adults, and often occurs in epidemics. Because diagnosis is difficult by other means, serologic tests are usually used to recognize *M. pneumoniae* infections.

Cold Agglutinins

In about 50–70% of patients with *M. pneumoniae* infection, high titer IgM antibodies that react with the I blood group antigen present on virtually all adult red blood cells (but not on fetal red cells) develop early in infection. Because IgM antibodies react best at cold temperatures, a quick bedside test is to collect 1 mL of blood into a tube containing an anticoagulant (usually blue top tubes containing sodium citrate) and place the tube into iced water for 3–4 minutes. When the tube is tilted, red cell agglutination can be detected as "clumps" that cling to the sides of the tube. Laboratories can perform titers using a similar technique; titers greater than 1:32 are relatively specific for *M. pneumoniae* infection. Both false positive and false negative results are relatively common, so that diagnosis usually requires detection of anti-mycoplasma antibodies.

Anti-mycoplasma Antibodies

An ELISA-like test is available to detect IgM antibodies to *M. pneumoniae;* it will generally not become positive for 7–10 days after infection, ultimately detecting almost all infected patients. The specificity of the assay is much higher than cold agglutinin assays, usually around 99%. IgM antibody typically persists for approximately 3–4 months. Because *M. pneumoniae* is a relatively common asymptomatic infection, detection of IgG antibodies is usually of no benefit in diagnosis.

SECTION V.
IMMUNOLOGY

CHAPTER 36

Laboratory Assessment of Immunologic Function

RICHARD A. McPHERSON

Clinical evaluation of immune function is usually prompted by the findings of repeated infections in a patient. Such an immunodeficient state may be hereditary and evident from early life, or may be acquired later in life. This chapter details the various tests that are useful in assessing immune function. Generally they fall into three broad categories: 1) humoral immunity (antibodies), 2) cellular immunity, and 3) complement.

HUMORAL IMMUNITY

Antibody Structure and Clonality

The immunoglobulin molecule consists of two heavy chains (H) and two light chains (L) that are linked to one another through disulfide bonds (Fig. 36.1). The region of the immunoglobulin molecule that binds to antigens is designated F_{ab}; the region that binds complement is F_c. The F_c region is also relatively constant in composition between different antibodies, whereas the F_{ab} region is highly variable allowing individual antibodies to bind to vastly different antigens. Both the heavy chain and the light chain have constant and variable regions. Any particular immunoglobulin synthesizing cell produces only a single type of molecule with a fixed heavy chain and a fixed light chain. This property is called *clonality,* and a population of cells that make a single type of immunoglobulin is termed *monoclonal.* Immune responses to immunogenic challenge such as infection generally stimulate the formation of multiple different antibodies; this response is termed *polyclonal.* Many laboratory assays are designed to determine whether elevations of antibodies in a patient's sample are monoclonal (implying unregulated synthesis due to malignancy) or polyclonal (implying normal response to infection or other stimulus).

The class of an antibody is determined by its heavy chain type. IgG has γ heavy chains, IgM has μ heavy chains, IgA has α heavy chains, IgD has δ heavy chains, and IgE has ϵ heavy chains. The heavy chains are encoded on chromosome 14. Each immunoglobulin has either κ or λ light chains. κ Light chains are encoded on chromosome 2; λ light chains are encoded on chromosome 22. Examination of a patient's immunoglobulins for clonality usually focuses on the light chain type; monoclonal populations are *restricted* to a single light chain type, whereas polyclonal ones have a mixture of both types.

An IgG molecule has two γ chains and two light chains (either κ or λ) as depicted in Figure 36.1. An IgM molecule is a pentamer of five basic antibody units that are linked by a peptide segment called the *joining fragment.* Thus an IgM molecule contains ten μ chains and ten light chains, and it has ten F_{ab} regions through which it can theoretically bind to ten individual antigens. IgA circulating in the blood has a structure similar to IgG; IgA secreted at mucosal surfaces consists of a dimer of two antibody units that are linked by a peptide called a *secretory piece.* The overall structures of IgD and IgE are similar to that of IgG; IgD and IgE are present at far lower concentrations in serum than IgG, IgM, or IgA. IgG is further divided into four subclasses and IgA into two subclasses according to heavy chain uniqueness. Most individuals make all subclasses, but selected deficiencies of subclasses are noted clinically.

413

Immunoglobulin Structure

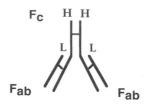

Figure 36.1. Basic structure of immunoglobulin with two heavy (H) and two light (L) chains linked into a configuration with two regions that bind to antigens (F$_{ab}$) and a region that can bind complement (F$_c$).

Immunoglobulin Gene Coding and Rearrangement

The immunoglobulin heavy chain gene structure is outlined in Figure 36.2. It contains separate coding regions for *variable, diversity, joining,* and *constant* segments of the final protein product. Each immunoglobulin class expresses a single constant region. The other segments are chosen from many possible ones by gene rearrangement in which one of about 100 variable gene segments, one diversity segment (from 15 to 20), and a particular joining segment (out of 6) are linked together with excision of the extra DNA segments. This rearranged gene is then transcribed into mRNA that is further processed by splicing out extra joining segments and linking the translatable region to the constant segment. The rearranged gene is passed on to all its daughter cells; they are a clone and all make the same immunoglobulin molecule. A similar process occurs with rearrangement of the κ light chain genes and then the λ light chain genes resulting in expression of only a single light chain. The normal process of immunoglobulin gene rearrangement can also lead to nontranslatable forms. If the heavy chain gene on one chromosome rearranges nonfunctionally, the allele on the other chromosome then attempts rearrangement. Similarly the light chains rearrange in the order of each κ chain and then each λ chain gene until the first successful rearrangement. If none of the genes rearranges successfully, the cell dies.

An immune response usually begins with antibody formation of the IgM type. Later response is switched to IgG synthesis against the same antigens. Subsequent stimulation with the same immunogen results in synthesis of IgG as the *anamnestic response*. This process entails retaining the same variable, diversity, and joining sites on the heavy chains but changing the heavy chain constant region from μ to γ by a secondary rearrangement that removes the μ gene and places one of the γ genes next to the joining segment. Similarly the choice of one of the other constant region genes such as δ, one of the two α, or ε results in immunoglobulin D, A, or E. This process of gene rearrangement accounts for the enormous repertoire of immunoglobulins that can be made by the human immune system.

LABORATORY METHODS FOR ASSESSING HUMORAL IMMUNITY

Quantitative Immunoglobulins

Quantitation of serum immunoglobulins is frequently performed to indicate the overall capacity of the immune system to synthesize antibodies. Methods for measuring concentrations of immunoglobulins are based on precipitation reactions with antihuman immunoglobulin antibodies that are generally produced in animals such as goats or rabbits. The first general kind of these assays is *radial immunodiffusion* (*RID*), in which

Synthesis of Immunoglobulin Heavy Chain Gene

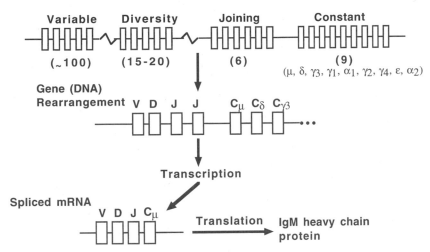

Figure 36.2. Mechanism by which the immunoglobulin heavy chain gene rearranges to form a specific combination of DNA segments that encode the mRNA for a particular antibody.

the antihuman immunoglobulin is dissolved in a layer of agarose. Wells a few millimeters in diameter are cut in the agarose; serum samples are loaded into the wells and allowed to diffuse into the agarose layer where the human immunoglobulins form precipitin rings around each well. The area within each ring is proportional to the concentration of immunoglobulin in the sample. Ring diameters are measured at 24 and 48 hours for samples and standards, allowing the concentration in each sample to be calculated from a calibration curve based on measurements with the standards. Radial immunodiffusion is still used in many laboratories; however, due to the prolonged time for completion (one to two days), very laborious technique, and relative lack of precision, RID has largely been replaced with automated instrumentation for *nephelometry*. This second general method is based on the turbidity and light scattering in solution that results from precipitation of antigen (human immunoglobulin) with antibody. This turbidity occurs quite rapidly and can be detected with automated instruments within minutes of beginning an assay. Nephelometry has enormous advantages over RID in speed, labor savings, and relatively high precision.

Standard measurements of immunoglobulins include quantitation of IgG, IgA, and IgM. IgE is present in much lower concentrations; it is also conveniently measured by nephelometry, but typically separately for evaluation of allergies (Chapter 9).

Another method commonly used for quantitation of proteins is enzyme linked immunosorbent assay (ELISA) (Fig. 36.3). ELISA is conveniently performed in 96-well plates for simultaneous analysis of multiple specimens and standards. In ELISAs, an antibody directed against the target of interest is coated onto the bottom of the wells. In the first step, samples are placed into wells and allowed to bind to this solid phase antibody. After washing, a second antibody is added. This antibody also binds to the antigen and has an enzyme linked to it so that for every molecule of antigen bound, enzyme activity is also bound. After another wash, the substrate for the marker enzyme is added in a solution to each well. This substrate is colorless but is converted to a colored product by the enzyme. Thus the final detection step is one of measuring the

Format of ELISA

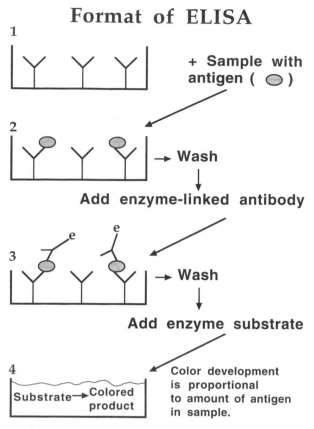

Figure 36.3. Outline of the steps in performance of enzyme linked immunosorbent assay (ELISA).

amount of color change in each well, which is proportional to the amount of antigen applied. ELISAs have been adapted to an extremely wide range of analytes including both antigens and antibodies. Despite the apparent complexity of multiple pipetting, washing, and final spectrophotometric steps, ELISAs have been highly automated and can deliver very good performance.

Specific Antibody Measurements

Specific antibody titers are also used to assess B-cell function. These assays include the *ABO blood group isoagglutinins,* as well as serum antibodies against *diphtheria* and *tetanus toxins* (protein antigens; T-cell dependent B-cell response), and against *pneumococcus* and *Hemophilus influenzae* (carbohydrate antigens; T-cell independent B-cell response). Most persons have had immunizations with these antigens or exposure during natural infections, so that the rate of positive antibodies is generally high. If the titer is negative, patients can be given immunization, and the assay is repeated weeks later to document the ability of the immune system to respond.

Qualitative Assessment of Immunoglobulin Proteins

The primary question to be answered about the qualitative nature of serum immuno-globulins is whether only a monoclonal spike of immunoglobulin is present, or if the distribution is polyclonal. This description is based on the appearance of the γ-globulin fraction in serum protein electrophoresis (discussed in Chapter 9). Protein electrophoresis can also be done on urine for evidence of monoclonal protein. A disorder such as multiple myeloma, in which a monoclonal protein is synthesized, may also show excess synthesis of the immunoglobulin light chain. Such free light chains are easily filtered by the kidney due to their low molecular size (ca. 25,000 daltons). Renal tubule cells can resorb some of the light chains, but their capacity to do so is ultimately overwhelmed in part due to toxicity from large intracellular loads of the light chain (clinically manifested as myeloma kidney). The free light chains then accumulate in the urine where they can be detected as a spike on protein electrophoresis of a concentrated specimen. Parallel electrophoreses of serum and urine from a patient with multiple myeloma can show monoclonal peaks in each with quite different positions because the protein in serum is usually the whole immunoglobulin molecule (two heavy chains plus two light chains; molecular weight 150,000 daltons) whereas the urine can contain some of the intact immunoglobulin but a larger amount of the free light chain. Identification of monoclonal bands is usually accomplished by immunofixation electrophoresis (IFE) or immunoelectrophoresis (IEP) (Chapter 9).

Monoclonal protein peaks are presumptively diagnosed from serum protein electrophoresis, and confirmed by IEP and IFE based on the single associated heavy chain but more importantly on the single type of light chain. This phenomenon is termed "light chain restriction" because only one type is expressed by a monoclonal population, whereas both are expressed in a polyclonal one. Tissue biopsies of lymph nodes or tumor can also be stained by immunoperoxidase methods using similarly specific antibodies that recognize T-lymphocyte markers, B-lymphocyte markers, and immunoglobulin heavy and light chains. Light chain restriction enables the diagnosis of clonal B-cell proliferation by establishing the single light chain expressed. Without a comparable marker for T cells, clonality of T-cell proliferations can only be inferred from protein markers and not conclusively proven.

Cryoglobulins

Some immunoglobulins have the tendency to crystallize and precipitate from plasma at temperatures lower than normal body core temperature. They are called *cryoglobulins* in recognition of this characteristic. Patients who have cryoglobulins frequently have symptoms relating to clogging of small blood vessels in exposed areas of the body (e.g., skin on the ears, nose, digits), especially during cold weather. Laboratory detection and quantitation of cryoglobulins begins with collection and handling of a blood specimen in warm conditions (e.g., the tube of blood is transported in a cup of warm water to the laboratory) to prevent loss of the cryoglobulin by precipitation before analysis. Properly processed serum is then refrigerated in a specially graduated tube for one to two days to permit any cryoglobulins to precipitate and sink to the bottom of the tube, where they are read as a percentage of *cryocrit* (analogous to hematocrit) to indicate the relative amount. Repeat measurements can be done to assess treatments intended to reduce circulating levels of cryoglobulins.

There are three general categories of cryoglobulins. Type I is a monoclonal immunoglobulin that crystallizes by itself; it typically occurs in a plasma cell dyscrasia such as multiple myeloma. Type II is a monoclonal rheumatoid factor; it is characterized by a precipitate of monoclonal IgM (the rheumatoid factor) and polyclonal IgG (the antigen in immune complexes). Type III is a rheumatoid factor consisting of polyclonal IgM that reacts with polyclonal IgG. These three types can be readily distinguished by performing immunofixation on the precipitate. The second and third types are designated *mixed cryoglobulins* due to the presence of IgG and IgM. Cryoglobulins are common in chronic hepatitis B and C.

Serum Viscosity

Elevated concentrations of monoclonal immunoglobulins (paraproteins) can cause symptoms in patients by increasing plasma viscosity, leading to impaired blood circulation in small vessels. In those patients, circulatory symptoms are generally related to the concentration of the paraprotein; however, not all paraproteins have the same effect on viscosity (although in general, IgM has a significant effect). Therefore it is necessary to assess individual patients with such symptoms by direct measurement of *serum viscosity.* It is quantitated by measuring the time required for serum to flow through a glass device with narrow tubing, with reference to the time required for water (viscosity = 1.0) to follow the same path.

Circulating Immune Complexes

Simultaneous presence of high concentrations of antigen and its specific antibody in blood can lead to the formation of *circulating immune complexes (CIC)* that are then filtered from the blood by small vessels such as renal glomeruli. Circulating immune complexes also bind and activate complement leading to tissue damage wherever the CIC deposit. Circulating immune complexes may occur in autoimmune diseases and also in infectious diseases where there is chronic production of microbial antigen in the face of an antibody response (e.g., hepatitis B surface antigen and antibody). Typical clinical findings include glomerulonephritis, arthritis, and neuropathy.

Although CIC are the immediate cause of the disease effects, measurements of CIC are not often useful clinically, in part because the amount deposited in tissues is much more significant than what is circulating. Perhaps more important is that laboratory measurement and quantitation of CIC are difficult to perform and are susceptible to many false positive and false negative results. A more satisfactory strategy is to measure the effects of CIC such as end organ damage (e.g., serum creatinine, urinalysis) or C3 and C4 concentrations which are depressed due to consumption during CIC-induced activation of complement.

Rheumatoid Factor

One of the special forms of circulating immune complexes is *rheumatoid factor,* which is actually an IgM molecule that acts as an antibody to bind other immunoglobulins as antigens. Rheumatoid factor is typically measured in the laboratory by virtue of its ability to cause various agglutination reactions that can be observed visually or detected by nephelometric methods. Rheumatoid factor is used as a marker for diagnosis of rheumatoid arthritis, and its titer is useful for monitoring and predicting clinical status.

Immunoglobulin Gene Rearrangement Studies

Because all of the cells of a B-cell clone have the same rearrangement of immunoglobulin heavy and light chain genes, examination of their DNA can be used to establish clonality and cell lineage. The process of *gene rearrangement* produces a combination of gene segments unique to a particular clone that allows it to be distinguished from

DNA ANALYSIS BY SOUTHERN BLOT

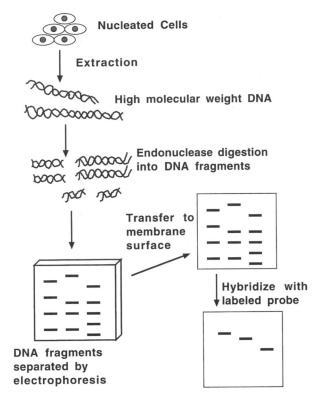

Figure 36.4. Outline of the steps of DNA analysis by Southern blot.

unrearranged (germ line) DNA. To perform analysis by *Southern blot* (Fig. 36.4), DNA is extracted from tissue biopsy or nucleated cells of peripheral blood. This high molecular weight DNA is cut into shorter, characteristic pieces with enzymes called *restriction endonucleases* so that they can be separated electrophoretically in agarose gels. After electrophoresis, the DNA fragments are transferred to the surface of a *membrane* (blotting); the membrane is then incubated with a labeled *nucleic acid probe* that *hybridizes* to specific sequences of target DNA. The final result demonstrates bands of DNA that contain the sequences being investigated, separated by molecular weight.

In the case of immunoglobulin gene rearrangements, a clonal population has the same rearranged genes in all cells, resulting in DNA bands that are readily distinguished from germ line DNA by Southern blot. In contrast, a polyclonal population has hundreds or more different gene rearrangements throughout all its individual subclones; this multitude of different rearrangements does not allow any one clone to be predominant on the Southern blot which therefore shows the germ line pattern.

For most patients with B-cell abnormalities, protein markers are generally sufficient to make a diagnosis of clonality and cell lineage. Examinations include serum protein electrophoresis and cell surface marker analysis by flow cytometry on circulating cells, or immunoperoxidase on biopsies. Gene rearrangement studies are generally reserved for cases in which the diagnosis may be equivocal based on protein markers. DNA studies may also be very useful to detect very small amounts of tumor following

Table 36.1.
Leukocyte Surface Markers

Antigen	Function/Role
CD2	T cells, NK cells
CD3	Pan T-cell marker; part of antigen receptor complex
CD4	Helper/inducer T cells
CD5	Pan T-cell marker; present on some B cells
CD8	Suppressor/cytotoxic T cells
CD10	Common acute lymphatic leukemia antigen (CALLA)
CD14	Monocytes, granulocytes
CD16	NK cells
CD19	Pan B-cell marker
CD20	Pan B-cell marker
CD25	IL-2 receptor; activated T cells, B cells
CD34	Hematopoietic stem cell marker
CD56	NK cells
CD71	Transferrin receptor

ablative therapy; thus they can have a role to play in detecting minimal residual disease. Southern blot analysis can detect a clonal band when the clone consists of approximately 5% or more of all the cells. Consequently it may not be sensitive enough for minimal residual disease detection; however, nucleic acid amplification techniques such as polymerase chain reaction (PCR) are well suited for this purpose.

CELLULAR IMMUNE FUNCTION

The cellular immune response is effected by lymphocytes that have on their surfaces antigen receptors that are homologous to immunoglobulins. The *T-cell antigen receptor* consists of two subunits: either α and β, or γ and δ. These proteins have variable and constant regions that derive from genes that undergo rearrangements, just as the immunoglobulin genes do in B lymphocytes. Once the T-cell antigen receptor gene has successfully rearranged in a lymphocyte, that receptor then binds to the external surface of the cell. Protein antigens are processed by monocytes (also termed macrophages) and presented in association with *MHC* (*major histocompatibility complex*) antigens to the antigen receptor on T lymphocytes. Specific T lymphocytes are stimulated to proliferate in response to such antigens. This antigen-directed T-lymphocyte activation is a critical portion of the immune response, especially against viruses and fungal organisms. It also is a major component of many autoimmune diseases, and similarly it is largely responsible for rejection of allogeneic (from a genetically different individual) organ transplant.

Lymphocytes are also categorized into subsets defined by other protein markers that are found on their surfaces (Table 36.1). These markers are referred to according to their *CD* (for *cluster designation*) numbers. B lymphocytes are marked with CD19 and CD20, T lymphocytes are marked with CD2 and CD3 (pan T-cell markers present on all T cells), helper inducer T cells with CD4, and suppressor cytotoxic T cells with CD8. Another group of lymphocytes is called natural killer (NK) cells because they do not respond to specific antigens but rather display cytotoxicity wherever they infiltrate. The NK cells are marked by CD16 and CD56.

The process of lymphocyte proliferation is also regulated by cytokines which are stimulatory factors such as interleukin-1 (IL-1, lymphocyte activating factor; endogenous pyrogen), interleukin-2 (IL-2, T-cell growth factor), interleukin-3 (IL-3, multicolony stimulating factor), interleukin-4 (IL-4, T-cell derived B-cell growth factor), interleukin-5 (IL-5, B-cell growth factor), interleukin-6 (IL-6, B-cell stimulatory factor 2), interleukin-8 (IL-8, neutrophil chemotactic factor), monocyte chemoattractant protein, and tumor necrosis factor (cachectin). Measurement of the cytokines is not generally necessary for clinical diagnosis as the end results of cell counts and activities can be directly examined.

LABORATORY METHODS FOR ASSESSING CELLULAR IMMUNITY

A complete blood count with differential count of leukocytes establishes whether a patient has adequate numbers of granulocytes and lymphocytes, and if there are indications of qualitative abnormalities such as abnormal granules, thrombocytopenia, or other aberrant cells. The next step is to perform more specific tests of cell type or function.

Lymphocyte Subset Enumeration

Subsets of lymphocytes are conveniently analyzed by *flow cytometry* in which *fluorescent-labeled monoclonal antibodies* against individual lymphocyte surface markers are mixed with blood samples. The cells are then examined automatically by the flow cytometer which quantitates the amount of fluorescence bound to each cell. By using two or more different fluorescent dyes on different monoclonal antibody reagents, it is possible to search for multiple markers simultaneously. For evaluation of cellular immune function, assessment is made of B cells (usually CD20), total T cells (using a pan T-cell marker such as CD3), helper (CD4) T cells, suppressor (CD8) T cells, monocytes (CD14), and NK cells (CD16 and CD56). Results are expressed as a percentage of mononuclear cells and also as absolute cell counts. The ratio of CD4 cells/CD8 cells is also calculated from these results.

Skin Tests

Lymphocyte function may be assessed directly in the patient (in vivo) by *delayed hypersensitivity skin tests* that use antigens from commonly encountered microorganisms. Skin tests evaluate the entire cellular immune response (including presentation of antigen by monocytes, mobilization of T cells, and the resulting inflammatory response of T cells sensitized to the antigen) with typical wheel and flare of induration and erythema. A major disadvantage of skin tests is that they may be negative in infants who have not yet been exposed to many naturally occurring microorganisms. Lack of a positive response to standard skin tests is termed *anergy*. It suggests paralysis of the cellular immune response such as occurs with primary immunodeficiency, but it may also be found with viral infections, malnutrition, granulomatous diseases, cancer, and chemotherapy. In the course of acquired immunodeficiency syndrome (AIDS), the progressive loss of CD4 cells over a period of years corresponds to sequential diminution and loss of previously positive skin tests.

Lymphocyte Function Tests

Lymphocyte function may be tested in vitro as a *proliferative response* when presented with certain antigens. These include mitogens such as *phytohemagglutinin (PHA)* and *poke weed mitogen (PWM)* which nonspecifically activate both CD4 and CD8 lymphocytes. Alloantigens such as those on cells from another individual (*mixed lymphocyte culture, MLC*) are also used to determine the likelihood of allogeneic organ transplant rejection, or to measure lymphocyte responsiveness. Tests more specific for the ability to resist infections use antigens from common microorganisms or those to which most persons have been immunized (e.g., tetanus, polio, candida, streptococcal proteins).

The proliferative response is typically measured as incorporation of radiolabeled thymidine into the DNA of dividing lymphocytes a few days after stimulation with the antigen. The entire assay takes several days due to the prolonged nature of the cellular response. Assays based on proliferative responses are therefore very labor intensive and can only be performed in laboratories with a high degree of technical expertise. They also show a great deal of variability between replicate analyses of the same patient's cells. Consequently they are more appropriately used as qualitative assessments of immune function rather than as quantitative ones.

Natural killer cells do not have immunoglobulin or T-cell antigen receptors on their surfaces. Natural killer cells have the innate ability to kill bacteria, virus-infected cells, or tumor cells without priming by antigen; however, they can be made to react more specifically by antibody. The usual method for testing the function of NK cells is through their cytotoxicity for radioactively labeled K-562 cells.

Neutrophil Function

Neutrophils normally act by phagocytizing particles such as bacteria coated with immunoglobulins and complement. Ingestion occurs into a *phagocytic vacuole* that then merges with *azurophilic granules* (*degranulation*). The ingested bacteria are killed by a combination of enzymatic actions plus *hydrogen peroxide* and *halides*. Defects in the killing process allow bacteria to live and the patient may have repeated bouts of bacterial infections, as in the X-linked *chronic granulomatous disease* (*CGD*) due to defective generation of superoxide by the enzyme NADPH-oxidase with the catalyzing action of neutrophil cytochrome b.

Laboratory assessment of neutrophil function includes examination of a peripheral blood smear to identify any qualitative cellular abnormalities. The *nitroblue tetrazolium* (*NBT*) test is performed by incubating the cells with NBT, which is converted to an insoluble blue pigment within normal granulocytes but not in those without adequate hydrogen peroxide-generating capacity. A further refinement on this assay is direct measurement of *superoxide production*. Bacterial killing assays have also been employed as *colony counts following phagocytosis*. In CGD phagocytosis may be normal, but the bacteria persist or multiply leading to high colony counts. Further tests of granulocyte function include *phagocytosis* and *chemotaxis*. Assays of granulocyte function are quite esoteric and require special technical expertise as well as considerable experience in their interpretation.

Allergies

Allergies are usually mediated by release of vasoactive substances such as *histamine* from *mast cells* and *basophils* that have IgE on their surfaces. Contact with a *specific allergen* causes the surface IgE to transmit a signal into the cell, which then releases histamine extracellularly from its granules. Chemotactic factors for eosinophils are also released leading to *eosinophilia*. Serial peripheral eosinophil counts can be used to gauge the degree of allergic activation. In addition, examination of smears for eosinophils in body fluids such as *nasal discharge* may be used to distinguish allergic from other etiologies.

Laboratory evaluation of allergies includes skin testing with specific candidate allergens, quantitation of total *serum IgE* (which tends to be elevated in patients with allergic reactivities), and tests for allergen-specific IgE antibodies. These latter assays have been termed *radioallergosorbent tests (RAST)*, in which the patient's serum is reacted with individual specific allergens bound to a solid phase in a format similar to the ELISA. Many different allergens can be tested by this means without directly exposing the patient to them. This testing does not completely predict a patient's response to allergens as it examines only a portion of the immune system in vitro. Nevertheless allergen-specific testing can provide extremely valuable information about possibly severe reactions with specific foods, drugs, bee venom, etc.

COMPLEMENT

The complement system can be considered the means by which immunoglobulins cause damage and mediate inflammation (Fig. 36.5). Complement activation also results in the formation of small peptide cleavage products such as C3a, C4a, and C5a which are designated *anaphylatoxins*. They have biological activities on smooth muscle, small blood vessels, mast cells, and circulating leukocytes. They are the direct mediators of increased vascular permeability, degranulation of mast cells and basophils, granulocyte aggregation, and smooth muscle contraction, all of which lead to increased blood flow to an inflamed region and can cause substantial tissue damage if left unchecked.

Down regulation of complement activation is accomplished by various inhibitor proteins. Activated C1 is destroyed by *C1 inhibitor (C1-Inh)*; congenital deficiency of this protein leads to the chronic inflammatory state called *hereditary angio(neurotic)edema*. In this disorder, trauma or stress induces acute formation of edema in skin and mucosa frequently involving the face and extremities, and also laryngeal and intestinal mucosa that can be life-threatening. Other specific inhibitor proteins similarly block the action of later components.

Autoimmune disorders such as systemic lupus erythematosus are sometimes associated with congenital deficiencies of the early components such as C1q, C1r, C1s, C4, C2, C3, and C5. Repeated bacterial infections are associated with hereditary deficiencies of some of the later components such as C3, C5, C6, C7, C8, and C9.

LABORATORY METHODS FOR ASSESSING COMPLEMENT

The most abundant components in normal serum are C3 and C4; consequently, these two assays are widely available by automated nephelometric methods and are frequently used to monitor clinical progress in patients with systemic autoimmune diseases. Active systemic rheumatic diseases typically consume complement, lowering serum concentrations of C3 and C4.

For cases in which a congenital deficiency of some component of complement is suspected, the *CH50 (hemolytic complement)* can be employed. In the CH50, a patient's serum is used as a source of complement for the hemolysis of sheep erythrocytes that are sensitized with bound antibodies. Minor reductions of the CH50 are consistent with partial reductions of any or all of the components as might occur during activation and consumption of complement. The CH50 is a difficult assay to standardize, so it is not appropriate to use for monitoring patients (use C3 and C4 instead). Major reductions of the CH50 suggest possible complete (congenital) deficiency of a single component. Once it is determined that the CH50 is markedly abnormal, each of the individual components should be quantitated by immunoassay. The C1-Inh measure-

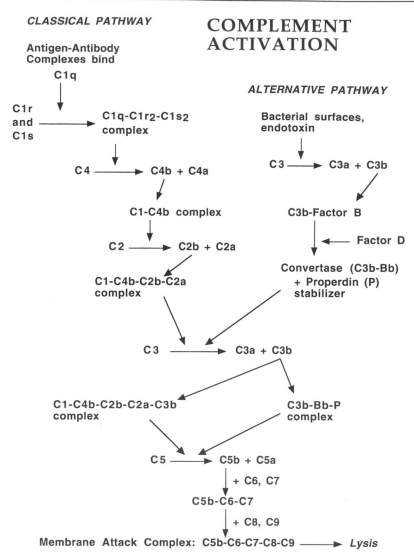

CLASSICAL PATHWAY

COMPLEMENT ACTIVATION

Figure 36.5. Complement activation cascade. The *classical pathway* of complement activation entails binding of complement component C1 to the F_c region of antibodies combined with their specific antigens, forming immune complexes. IgM antibodies are more efficient at this step of binding C1 than are IgG ones due to the presence of more F_c regions per immunoglobulin molecule. The sequence of events includes binding and cleavage of C4, C2, C3, C5, C6, C7, C8, and C9; the complete complement complex creates enzymes capable of creating holes in membranes (e.g., the *membrane attack complex, MAC*). The target of these activities is specified by the location of the immune complexes, whether on the surface of a bacterial cell (an appropriate immune response) or on the basement membrane of renal glomeruli (an undesirable autoimmune response). Complement can also be activated by the *alternative pathway* in which C3 is the first component activated and proceeds to activate the later components.

ment is also useful for the evaluation of patients with symptoms suggestive of angi-oedema; secondary cases of this disorder can also be acquired.

CONGENITAL IMMUNODEFICIENCIES

These disorders are generally apparent early in life (i.e., in the first year) when mater-nally transferred immunity wanes and the infant is exposed to a variety of naturally occurring infectious agents. In general, humoral (antibody, B-cell) immune deficiencies leave an individual susceptible to bacterial infections, whereas cellular (T-cell) immune deficiencies lead to infections with viruses, fungi, intracellular bacteria, and protozoa. Immunodeficient patients may also have a higher incidence of cancers, especially those caused by oncogenic viruses (e.g., Epstein-Barr virus).

B-Cell Immunodeficiencies

X-linked (Bruton's) agammaglobulinemia is marked by an absence of IgG. Inheritance is through the X chromosome so the disorder generally affects males; heterozygous fe-males are asymptomatic carriers. The responsible gene does not encode immunoglobu-lins, but rather has some action on the maturation of pre-B cells. To avoid fatal infec-tions, these patients must be treated regularly with injections of exogenous γ-globulins pooled from normal individuals who have antibodies against common microorganisms. Roughly one-fifth of these patients develop autoimmune disorders.

Selective IgA deficiency is the most common primary immunodeficiency, affecting 1 in 700 persons of Caucasian ancestry. IgG and IgM tend to be normal or even elevated, perhaps because of response to infections. The resulting clinical state varies, ranging from no apparent abnormality, to occasional mild infections, up to more severe infec-tions of the respiratory and gastrointestinal tracts along with autoimmune disease for-mation. Persons with IgA deficiency are at risk of anaphylactic response to IgA con-tained in transfused blood products following some initial sensitization by transfusion; they should be transfused with products collected from other IgA-deficient persons.

Selective IgM deficiency is a rare disorder resulting in severe bacterial infections, especially pneumococcal and meningococcal meningitis. *Selective deficiencies of IgG subclasses* are usually normal clinically. *Decreased IgG and IgA with increased IgM* is an X-linked disorder that results in susceptibility to bacterial infections; the IgM anti-bodies formed include autoantibodies against erythrocytes, leukocytes, and platelets, thereby exacerbating infections.

Common variable immunodeficiency may appear in children at various ages or in early adulthood with development of bacterial infections as those individuals develop hypo-gammaglobulinemia. The etiology is failure of B-cell maturation that may be due to different causes. The disorder is also called *acquired agammaglobulinemia*.

T-Cell Immunodeficiencies

Selective T-cell deficiency (DiGeorge syndrome) results from a congenital malformation of the third and fourth pharyngeal pouches that normally develop into the thymus and the parathyroids plus aortic arch and parts of the lips and ears. Therefore this immuno-deficiency may also present with absence of the parathyroids (abnormal regulation of calcium metabolism), abnormal vasculature, and facial malformation. Immunologically the defect affects maturation of T cells with very few or no T cells in peripheral blood; most blood lymphocytes in these persons are B cells as opposed to only 10–20% B cells in normals. Antibody levels are generally normal, but may be depressed in some cases. Diagnosis is made by lymphocyte subset enumeration (using flow cytometry) and lymphocyte stimulation test which are markedly depressed. These patients are susceptible to infections with viruses, fungi, and mycobacteria. Treatment has been done with fetal thymic transplant; however, after several years of life, T-cell function recovers (as does parathyroid function) apparently due to ectopic sites of thymic tissue expansion.

Other rare defects in T-cell responses have been associated with clinical immunodeficiencies probably due to abnormalities in cytokine production or cytokine receptors.

Combined Immunodeficiencies

Mixed defects affecting both B cells and T cells are heterogeneous disorders that demonstrate lymphopenia, defective cell-mediated immunity, and agammaglobulinemia (originally termed Swiss type agammaglobulinemia). They are also called *severe combined immunodeficiency* (*SCID*). All immune functions are deficient in these individuals who usually have serious infections leading to death in the first year of life. About one-fifth of SCID cases are due to deficiency of the enzyme *adenosine deaminase* (*ADA*); these cases may be treated with transfer of the ADA gene into bone marrow cells and transplantation. Another enzyme responsible for some cases of SCID is *purine nucleoside phosphorylase*.

Other examples of mixed B-cell and T-cell immunodeficiency occur in *Wiskott-Aldrich syndrome* (an X-linked disorder with eczema, thrombocytopenia, small lymphocytes, and an inability to synthesize antibodies against polysaccharide antigens such as those from encapsulated bacteria) and *ataxia telangiectasia* (an autosomal recessive disorder with abnormal gait, microvascular abnormalities, neurologic defects, frequent cancers, and respiratory tract infections).

Other Leukocyte Disorders

Chronic granulomatous disease (*CGD*) affects about 1 in 1,000,000 persons, of which two-thirds are X-linked recessive cases (mostly males) and one-third are autosomal recessive (males and females). These individuals suffer frequent bacterial infections, and in response form granulomas consisting of activated macrophages. Death results early in life.

The abnormality in CGD is a defect in production of the superoxide anion which neutrophils use to kill phagocytized bacteria. X-linked CGD has an abnormality of neutrophil cytochrome b which participates in generation of superoxide. The autosomal recessive cases are apparently due to defects in NADPH-oxidase which mediates superoxide generation. Diagnosis can be made by testing the patient's neutrophils for phagocytosis and bactericidal functions and for superoxide generation; DNA tests are also done for the specific gene mutations. Treatment with interferon-gamma stimulates superoxide production in normal and CGD neutrophils and is used clinically.

Chediak-Higashi syndrome shows partial oculocutaneous albinism, lymphocytic infiltration of tissues, and giant cytoplasmic granules in neutrophils, lymphocytes, and monocytes. The cellular defect is one in which cytoplasmic granules tend to fuse thereby causing loss of function. Phagocytic cells are less able to combat infections, platelets do not function well (causing bleeding problems), and melanocytes and nerve cells are affected.

Leukocyte adhesion defects result in impaired wound healing and recurrent infections with bacteria and fungi. Functions of adherence, aggregation, chemotaxis, phagocytosis, and cytotoxicity of neutrophils, T lymphocytes, and NK cells are affected. Effective therapy for this very rare disorder will likely arise from gene transfer in bone marrow transplantation.

ACQUIRED IMMUNODEFICIENCY SYNDROME (AIDS)

Because of its high prevalence, AIDS must be considered as a likely cause of any case of immunodeficiency. Laboratory testing can contribute a great deal to the diagnosis and monitoring of human immunodeficiency virus-1 (HIV-1) infection and AIDS. Following the initial clinical suspicion of AIDS due to opportunistic infections, *HIV-1 antibody screening* is done on serum by ELISA. Present day assays usually can detect antibodies against both HIV-1 and HIV-2. A positive result is followed by repeat ELISA. If both are positive, *Western blot analysis* is performed as *confirmatory testing* by which antibodies against specific viral proteins are detected. HIV testing is also widely done on blood donors and upon physical examinations for life insurance policies leading to detection of unsuspected cases. It is also used to evaluate patients who have had exposure to other sexually transmitted diseases and thus are at higher risk for HIV infection as well.

Viral antigen has also been used to monitor HIV infection or to make a diagnosis when the serological measurements may be indeterminate due to presence of only one antibody (i.e., not yet characteristic of a typical immune response to the virus). The *viral antigen* most commonly measured in serum is *p24*. Because p24 may be complexed with antibody in the circulation, these immune complexes can be dissociated chemically in the laboratory to facilitate detection of p24.

After initial exposure to HIV-1, the p24 antigen rises briefly for a few weeks in serum coincident with high level viremia during primary infection. At this time the patient may have an acute viral syndrome with fever, rash, lymphadenopathy, and pharyngitis. HIV-1 antibody tests are negative at this early stage. After about six weeks, antibodies against HIV-1 appear in the serum, an the infection enters an asymptomatic phase that can last for years. The specific antibodies that arise and are tested for by Western blot confirmation are directed against the viral proteins GAG (group-specific antigens: p55, p24, and p18), POL (polymerase: p65, p51, and p32), and ENV (envelope: gp160, gp120, and gp41–gp43).

Western blots are interpreted by scoring the presence and intensity of antibody bands from the patient's serum onto locations on the strips where each of these proteins is located. Absence of any reactive bands on a strip indicates a negative result. Reactivity of 1+ or greater to any two of the major products of the structural genes GAG (p24) and ENV (gp120/gp160, gp41) constitutes a positive result. A pattern with one or more reactive bands that do not meet the positive criteria is deemed indeterminate. Patients who have indeterminate results should be followed with repeat testing over succeeding weeks or months to establish diagnosis and progression. Infants with maternally transferred HIV-1 antibodies can convert from positive to indeterminate to negative patterns as the antibody clears over a period of months if they are not infected. Nonspecific binding to some HIV-1 antigens (e.g., p18, p24, and p55) may persist in some persons without evolution over time to the more diagnostic patterns. As the disease progresses, AIDS patients may lose the antibody to p24 due to impaired synthesis of antibody and to extensive production of the p24 antigen as the virus replicates.

Direct evaluation of a patient's immune function in AIDS is usually done by lymphocyte enumeration using flow cytometry to count the numbers of CD4 and CD8 T cells. CD4 cells are infected by HIV, and their numbers decrease during the progression of AIDS; the CD4/CD8 ratio also falls progressively. A CD4 count below 400 cells/ NL^3 is an indicator for AIDS along with positive serologies for HIV-1, presence of opportunistic infections, and other diseases (such as some lymphomas) according to surveillance definition from the Centers for Disease Control. Patients with CD4 counts less than 250 cells/NL^3 are at great risk for opportunistic infection. Critical levels of CD4 counts are also used to recommend specific treatments. As long as the CD4 count remains above 500 cells/NL^3, repeat counts are done every 3–6 months. Below 500 cells/mL^3, zidovudine may be started to treat the HIV-1 infection. When the CD4 counts fall below 200 cells/NL^3, the patient is at high risk of developing *Pneumocystis carinii* pneumonia and should begin prophylactic therapy for that agent.

With the success of new antiviral agents such as protease inhibitors, the natural course of HIV-1 infection can be markedly altered with improvement in lymphocyte function, increased CD4 counts, recovery from opportunistic infections, cessation of HIV-1 replication, and possibly clearance of the virus from the body. Current standard of practice for monitoring active HIV replication in infected patients is quantitation of the viral genomic RNA using reverse transcriptase (RT, to make DNA from RNA) polymerase chain reaction (PCR, to amplify the DNA to easily detected concentrations). Circulating concentrations of HIV RNA are now considered the most sensitive indicator of active infection for use in monitoring treatment with antiviral agents. In a recent multicenter study of HIV-1 positive hemophiliacs, levels of HIV-1 RNA in serum ranged from 200 to more than 1,000,000 viral genome copies per milliliter. The level of HIV-1 RNA predicted time to develop AIDS: 72% of those with 100,000 copies/mL or more developed AIDS in 10 years, 52% of those with 10,000 to 99,999 copies/mL, 22% of those with 1,000 to 9,999 copies/mL, and of those with below 1,000 copies/mL, none developed AIDS in 10 years.

LABORATORY APPROACH TO THE IMMUNODEFICIENT PATIENT

Patients with suspected primary immunodeficiency should be tested in a sequence that places first the easiest tests with greatest potential for identifying the most common abnormalities. If those tests are normal, further more esoteric procedures can be done to diagnose rarer disorders.

The primary tests to be performed begin with a complete blood count and differential to quantitate total lymphocytes and to detect any qualitative morphologic abnormalities of neutrophils, lymphocytes, or platelets. Next is examination of serum immunoglobulins including quantitation of IgG, IgA, and IgM (may also do subclass measurements of IgG or IgA) and specific titers such as isohemagglutinins against ABO blood group antigens and antibodies against diphtheria, tetanus, pneumococcus, and *Hemophilus influenzae*. Quantitative IgE measurement may also be performed. Complement function is assessed by CH50 to screen for congenital deficiency of a component followed by individual component measurements (most commonly available ones are C3 and C4). Lymphocyte function is assessed with delayed hypersensitivity skin testing and by surface marker analysis for enumeration of B cells, T cells, T-cell subsets (CD4, CD8), and NK cells. Lymphocyte proliferation and cytotoxicity assays would then be used.

The final level of most specialized tests includes measurement of enzymes (e.g., adenosine deaminase) and cytokines associated with lymphocyte function. Chronic bacterial infections should prompt further evaluation of neutrophil function including the NBT test and assays of phagocytosis, superoxide generation, and chemotaxis.

CHAPTER 37

Laboratory Evaluation of Autoimmunity

RICHARD A. McPHERSON

Autoimmune disorders and their etiologies have become well understood through the study of many components of the immune system. These biochemical factors are well known to medical personnel who have been introduced to the principles of pathogenesis; however, only a restricted number of these factors are actually useful in diagnosing and monitoring autoimmune diseases. This chapter emphasizes the most useful laboratory procedures for assessing autoimmunity.

SYSTEMIC RHEUMATIC DISEASE

The biochemical basis of autoimmune disease is deposition of human immunoglobulins and complement in tissues of affected organs, and frequently lymphocytic infiltrations as well. Renal and skin biopsies are used to diagnose diseases affecting these organs. Such biopsy material is examined by *direct immunofluorescence assay (DFA)* to demonstrate deposits of immunoglobulins in the patient's own tissue. A DFA (Fig. 37.1) is performed by mounting a section of the biopsy on a slide and incubating with fluorescent antihuman immunoglobulin (from an animal such as goat or rabbit that has been immunized with human immunoglobulins). After washing off excess fluorescent reagent, the biopsy section is examined microscopically under ultraviolet illumination. If the patient's biopsy has deposits of immunoglobulins, they will be detected as yellow-green fluorescence. By using fluorescent antihuman C3, complement binding in the tissues can similarly be demonstrated.

Indirect immunofluorescence assays (IFAs) (Fig. 37.2) are used to demonstrate presence of an antibody in a patient's serum. In this procedure, a dilution (usually starting at 1:40, to minimize background staining) of the patient's serum is layered over the cells fixed to a glass slide. If the patient's serum contains an antibody that reacts with any of the cellular antigens, it will bind to the cells. The patient's serum is then washed off the cells and antihuman immunoglobulin that is labeled with the fluorescent dye fluorescein is placed over them to detect the human antibodies. This second antibody is then washed off, and the slide is viewed under a microscope with illumination from an ultraviolet light source. Sites of fluorescence indicate binding by the patient's antibody to a cellular antigen. The intracellular distribution of the fluorescence is interpreted as a pattern (e.g., homogeneous, speckled, nucleolar, centromere, etc.). Indirect immunofluorescence assays require both special equipment and additional expertise that may not be available directly through smaller laboratories; requests for such studies may therefore be sent to a reference laboratory. More recent technologies have made it possible to perform screening ANA with enzyme linked immunosorbent assay (ELISA) that is automated and done in large numbers using purified autoantigens.

Antinuclear Antibody

The most common screening procedure for systemic rheumatic disease is the *antinuclear antibody (ANA)* which detects autoantibodies that react with protein or nucleic acids in the nuclei of cells. Typically these antigens are preserved between different species (e.g., the chemical nature of DNA is the same across species), and so testing

Direct Immunofluorescence Assay

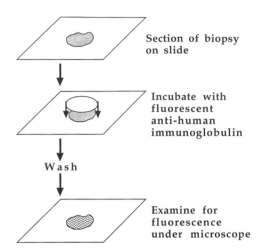

Section of biopsy
on slide

Incubate with
fluorescent
anti-human
immunoglobulin

Wash

Examine for
fluorescence
under microscope

Figure 37.1. Scheme for performing direct fluorescence assay (DFA) which is used to demonstrate presence of human immunoglobulins or complement in patient tissue biopsies.

can be done with human or animal cells to detect these autoantibodies; most laboratories today use a human epithelial cell line called HEp2 cells. It should be remembered that patients may have antibodies to more than one cellular antigen; only the antibody present in highest titer may be identified by IFA studies if its pattern obscures other patterns.

Antinuclear antibodies of low titer occur as nonspecific findings in about 1% of normal individuals; this percentage rises to as much as a 50% incidence in persons 80 years and over. High titer ANAs are strongly associated with active systemic lupus erythematosus, although they can also arise in other rheumatic diseases. Following are general guidelines for interpreting positive ANA results.

Homogeneous Pattern

The homogeneous (or diffuse) pattern is one with solid staining of the nucleus; mitotic cells show clear staining of the metaphase chromosomes (Fig. 37.3). The autoantibodies producing the homogeneous pattern are directed against double stranded DNA (dsDNA) or histones. Additional testing usually entails measuring specific dsDNA antibody by such means as immunofluorescence using *Crithidia* (a protozoan which has a kinetoplast of pure dsDNA without histone), or ELISA. The dsDNA antibody is frequently found in systemic lupus erythematosus (SLE) and has an association with nephritis (especially at the higher titers), but it may be present in other connective tissue diseases such as rheumatoid arthritis, mixed connective tissue disease (MCTD), Sjögren's syndrome, scleroderma, and also chronic active hepatitis and primary biliary cirrhosis. If the dsDNA antibody is negative, additional testing would involve measuring antibodies against histones (especially if the clinical situation suggests drug-induced SLE). Anti-dsDNA antibody titers are generally related to severity of disease as higher titers correlate well with low levels of C3 and C4 presumably due to activation and consumption of complement.

IgA and IgM anti-dsDNA antibodies are usually not clinically significant, but they

Indirect Immunofluorescence Assay

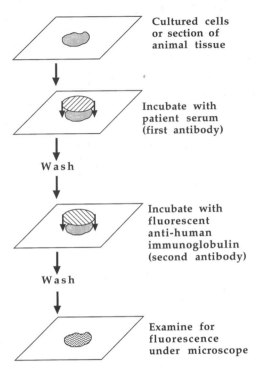

Figure 37.2. Scheme for performing indirect fluorescence assay (IFA) which is used to detect circulating autoantibodies in patient serum.

can give positive results with *Crithidia* and DNA binding. Some laboratories also measure anti-single stranded DNA (ssDNA) antibodies. Titers of this antibody do not correlate well with diagnosis or clinical course, and consequently anti-ssDNA antibody is thought by many not to be very useful clinically.

Peripheral Pattern

The peripheral (or rim) pattern is a variant in which dsDNA antibody stains more intensely in the outer region of the nucleus and more weakly at its center; metaphase chromosomes stain strongly positive. The peripheral pattern is highly suggestive of active SLE. Autoantibodies against the nuclear membrane should be distinguished from a true peripheral pattern as the antinuclear membrane carries no known clinical significance.

Speckled Pattern

The most common ANAs are speckled patterns in which the nuclei show fine to coarse staining, but the chromosomes in mitotic cells and nucleoli show no staining (Fig. 37.4). Many different autoantibodies can give rise to speckled nuclear patterns, especially those directed against the extractable nuclear antigens (ENA): Sm, RNP (ribonucleoprotein), SS A (or Ro), SS B (or La), and Scl-70. Consequently the finding of a speckled pattern should be confirmed with a panel of these specific autoantibodies.

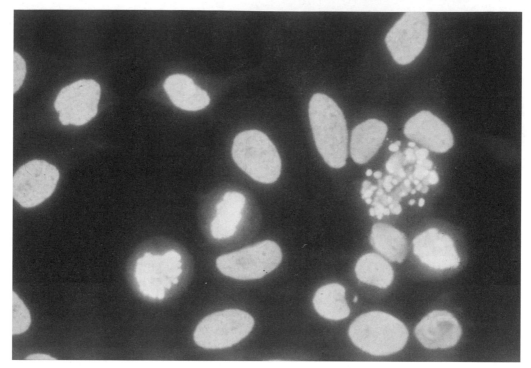

Figure 37.3. Homogeneous pattern of antinuclear antibody by IFA on HEp2 cells. Note uniform staining in interphase nuclei and intense staining of metaphase chromosomes with individual chromosomes visible in one cell.

Low titers of autoantibodies against the ENAs are generally considered to be nonspecific indicators of connective tissue disease, although they may actually signify no clinical abnormality (biological false positives). High titer antibodies to Sm are strongly associated with SLE. High titer anti-RNP autoantibodies are found in mixed connective tissue disease (MCTD) but may also appear with SLE; they indicate a low risk of nephritis in anti-DNA negative SLE. In MCTD with high titers of anti-RNP, changes in titer may be used to follow the disease course and response to therapy. Anti-SS A (Ro) and anti-SS B (La) antibodies are both demonstrated in Sjögren's syndrome, although either may be present in SLE where they imply a particular subset of clinical findings. Anti-SS A antibody, when present in lupus, generally portends prominent cutaneous involvement and photosensitivity. It may be present in ANA-negative lupus as well as neonatal lupus. Anti-SS B antibody alternatively may signify a low risk of renal disease when detected in SLE.

The Scl-70 antibody is generally associated with scleroderma. This antibody may be found together with the nucleolar antibody.

Nucleolar Pattern

The nucleolar pattern consists of six or fewer large coarse speckles or granules (the nucleoli) in the nucleus (Fig. 37.5). The nucleoli can stain in a variety of ways (homogeneous, clumpy, speckled, etc.), but the usual nomenclature simply calls them "nucleolar" without further subclassification. The target antigens are nuclear proteins in association with small RNA molecules. Antinucleolar antibodies are associated with

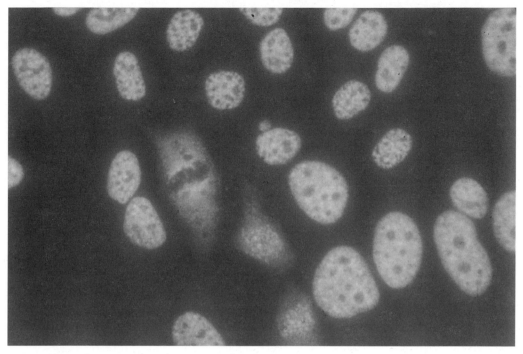

Figure 37.4. Speckled pattern of antinuclear antibody by IFA on HEp2 cells. The nuclei contain many brightly staining speckles, but metaphase chromosomes and nucleoli are negative.

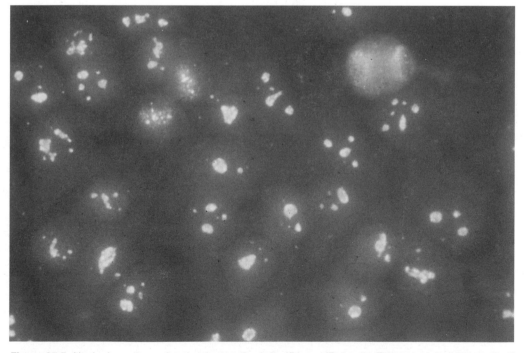

Figure 37.5. Nucleolar pattern of antinuclear antibody by IFA on HEp2 cells. There are only a few nucleoli in each nucleus.

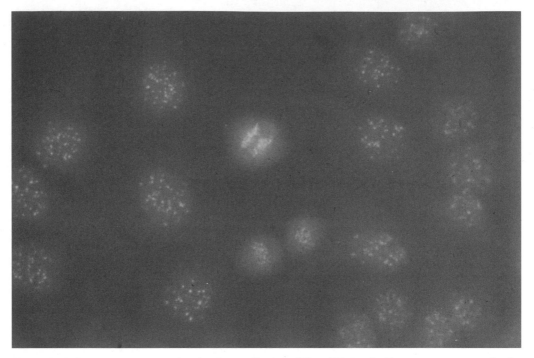

Figure 37.6. Centromere pattern of antinuclear antibody by IFA on HEp2 cells. The centromeres are distributed throughout the nuclei in interphase cells but line up in metaphase nuclei.

scleroderma (progressive systemic sclerosis) and Sjögren's syndrome. They may also be present as nonspecific findings in other autoimmune diseases.

Centromere Pattern

The centromere pattern (ACA) shows discrete speckled staining numerically related to the 46 chromosomes in human cells (Fig. 37.6). Interphase cells demonstrate centromeric staining distributed throughout the nucleus, whereas mitotic cells show the centromeres to be lined up along the metaphase plate (by chromosomal attachment to the mitotic spindle apparatus). Clinically the *anticentromere antibody (ACA)* is associated with the CREST (calcinosis, Raynaud's phenomenon, esophageal dysmotility, sclerodactyly, and telangiectasia) syndrome variant of scleroderma. Because of this strong diagnostic association with a complex disorder that may be confused with other entities, the ACA is sometimes requested by practitioners as a separately named test. The ACA is in fact tested for each time an ANA is performed on HEp2 cells. Part of the confusion about this test may have arisen from earlier ANA assays that used tissue sections (such as liver) that did not contain many mitotic cells and in which centromeres were hardly detectable. Present day ANA tests using HEp2 cells guarantee excellent detection of ACA.

True ACAs should be distinguished from pseudo-centromere antibodies which have no known disease association. The pseudo-centromere pattern shows bright discrete speckles in interphase cells, but the chromosomes do not stain in metaphase cells.

Proliferating Cell Nuclear Antigen Pattern

The anti-proliferating cell nuclear antigen (PCNA) pattern contains nuclear speckling that varies markedly in intensity from cell to cell. Nuclei of quiescent cells are negative; positive cells reflect cellular proliferation due to DNA synthesis prior to mitosis (mitotic cells are negative). The antigen is actually a polymeric form of the cofactor for DNA polymerase δ. The variable speckling of PCNA must be distinguished from a true speckled pattern that shows uniform staining over all cells. Proliferating cell nuclear antigen is considered to be a very significant finding in a patient as it essentially always indicates a diagnosis of SLE; however, fewer than 5% of patients with SLE have positive PCNA antibody making it not a very sensitive disease marker.

Cytoplasmic Antibodies

HEp2 cells present a variety of cytoplasmic antigens in addition to nuclear ones. Occasionally the cytoplasm will stain intensely positive in patterns that suggest specific autoantibodies. These patterns include antimitochondrial antibody (AMA), antiactin antibody which is equivalent to antismooth muscle antibody (ASMA), antiribosomal antibody, anti-Golgi antibody, and various other antifilament antibodies such as vimentin. Of these antibodies, the most significant ones are AMA and ASMA. Unfortunately it is not possible to rely on immunofluorescent staining of HEp2 cells to identify them. Such positive cytoplasmic patterns should be further analyzed using mouse stomach and kidney sections to confirm autoantibody identity by specific staining on differentiated tissues that contain the antigens in different cells.

Rheumatoid Factor

This IgM autoantibody reacts with the F_c region of IgG and is typically detected by agglutination or nephelometric methods. Rheumatoid factor (RF) is commonly present in the serum of adult patients with rheumatoid arthritis. Rheumatoid factor may also occur as a nonspecific finding in elderly persons with no clinical illness. Children with juvenile rheumatoid arthritis often are negative for RF. Other rheumatic or chronic inflammatory conditions may demonstrate RF including syphilis, tuberculosis, subacute bacterial endocarditis, hepatitis, malaria, sarcoidosis, and infectious mononucleosis. Low titer RF generally has little diagnostic significance; patients with high titer RF tend to have severe disease that is systemic. Titers of RF are frequently used to monitor progression of rheumatoid arthritis.

Phospholipid Antibody Syndrome

Patients with antiphospholipid antibodies (APL) (Chapter 27) often demonstrate prolongation of the activated partial thromboplastin time (APTT). Despite the presence of this circulating anticoagulant (lupus anticoagulant), these patients paradoxically have an increased tendency for both arterial and venous thrombosis. Pregnant women with APL are at greater risk for spontaneous abortions. A small number of patients may also have neurologic symptoms such as chorea. Antiphospholipid antibodies occur in over half of patients with SLE, but also in a wide variety of other disorders including cancer and infections.

Antiphospholipid antibodies can be detected by various modifications of the APTT using mixtures with normal plasma. They can also be detected by ELISA using cardiolipin and other phospholipid antigens. Antiphospholipid antibodies frequently give rise to biological false positive results of the VDRL.

Assessing Systemic Disease Activity

Most autoantibodies in systemic rheumatic diseases carry more significance for diagnosis than for serial monitoring of disease activity. A major exception is anti-dsDNA antibody where the titer quite accurately reflects and predicts disease activity. Thus, patients who have this antibody should have periodic measurements of the titer as well as quantitation of serum concentrations of the complement components C3 and C4 which are consumed during active disease. Although the pathogenetic mechanism of complement consumption involves circulating immune complexes (CIC), measuring their concentration is rarely, if ever, useful clinically. (CIC can be quantitated by methods that involve binding of C1q or by Raji cells that have receptors for the F_c portion of immunoglobulins. CIC assays are generally only available from reference laboratories and so should not be relied on for acute medical management decisions.) The presence of CIC can be inferred from the end effects of low C3 and C4 levels as well as target organ damage such as to the kidneys. Thus serum creatinine and urine sedimentary analysis for erythrocytes and erythrocyte casts can be useful in diagnosing and monitoring SLE.

A very general marker for inflammation is the erythrocyte sedimentation rate (ESR) which becomes elevated as a response to disease activity. C-reactive protein (CRP) (Chapter 9) also rises generally in response to inflammation and tends to be very high in exacerbations of rheumatoid arthritis. Paradoxically, CRP remains low (generally within the reference range) in active SLE.

ORGAN SPECIFIC AUTOIMMUNE DISEASES

Tissue Antibodies

Many autoantibodies can be detected using IFA with sections of tissues containing differentiated cells that express particular antigens such as mitochondria or smooth muscle. The most useful screening test for a wide spectrum of these antibodies uses sections of mouse stomach and kidney as the substrate, which can detect antibodies to mitochondria, smooth muscle (actin), liver-kidney microsomes (in renal tubules), and gastric parietal cells. Autoimmune thyroiditis (e.g., Hashimoto's thyroiditis) and Graves' disease are usually associated with thyroid autoantibodies detected by IFA using thyroid tissue sections or agglutination reactions (Chapter 13).

Autoimmune Liver Disease

Homogeneous and speckled patterns of ANA are frequently found in autoimmune hepatitis (up to 80% of cases), in 60% of patients with primary biliary cirrhosis, in 50% of patients with alcoholic liver disease, and in 40% of patients with chronic viral hepatitis. Thus the ANA may be useful for suggesting autoimmune etiology of liver disease, but must be followed with other assays to differentiate the disease.

Antimitochondrial antibodies (*AMAs*) are commonly detected by IFA on sections of mouse stomach (by staining gastric mucosal cells) and kidney (by staining renal tubule cells). Western blot analysis has shown that AMAs can be further divided on the basis of autoantigen reactivity into nine types designated M1 through M9; the M2 and M9 types in high titer are associated with primary biliary cirrhosis. The M2 autoantigen has been identified as a mixture of subunits of pyruvate dehydrogenase and branched-chain oxo-ketoacid dehydrogenase. Most clinical laboratories still use IFA to detect AMAs, but they cannot discriminate between the various types on the basis of the immunofluorescent pattern. Consequently, we should expect to find new ELISAs in the near future for specific measurement of the M2 type of AMA.

Smooth muscle antibodies (*SMAs*) are detected by IFA on mouse stomach and kidney (gastric wall muscle, arteriole smooth muscle). The autoantigen for SMA is F-actin, a component of the cytoskeleton. Smooth muscle antibodies occur in about half of patients with autoimmune hepatitis in relatively high titers. Low titers of AMA are also seen in other autoimmune diseases and even in apparently healthy individuals.

Liver-kidney microsomal autoantibodies (*LKMAs*) are detected by a characteristic pattern of staining proximal but not distal renal tubule cells. Three subtypes of LKMA have been identified in different patient groups, including some who have chronic infection with hepatitis C virus.

Several markers of autoimmune liver disease have been developed to assist in the diagnosis of various subgroups of patients. These include antibodies against soluble liver antigens (SLA), asialoglycoprotein receptor (ASGP; apparently the receptor molecule by which hepatitis B virus enters hepatocytes), liver membrane, cytoskeletal antigens, etc. In coming years, some of these assays will probably come into prominence, particularly if medical treatments will require them for monitoring.

Kidney Disease

Glomerulonephritis is mediated by activation of complement in the renal glomeruli in response to immune complexes depositing there and binding complement from circulating blood. *Circulating immune complexes* (*CICs*) may form when both antigen and antibody are present in substantial amounts, such as in hepatitis B when infected hepatocytes are releasing large amounts of HB surface antigen and the immune system is simultaneously making large amounts of anti-HBs antibody. Heavy burdens of CIC are filtered out into renal glomeruli and may also cause arthritis and peripheral neuropathies. Diagnosis of glomerulonephritis must be guided by microscopic urinalysis for evidence of erythrocytes, by serum creatinine and urea measurements, and by examination for antibodies that are known to be etiologic. Foremost of these is the *anti-DNA antibody* which is frequently found in SLE. It may be that anti-DNA antibodies can bind directly to the glomerular basement membrane on a charge basis without previously forming CIC with DNA.

Renal biopsy is used to establish the nature of glomerulonephritis. Needle biopsies are directly stained with fluorescent antihuman immunoglobulins and antihuman complement to demonstrate where in the glomeruli there are deposits of IgG, IgA, IgM, and C3. The pattern of antibody deposition is generally granular for CIC, whereas for *antiglomerular basement membrane* (*GBM*) antibody, the pattern is linear. Frequently the diagnosis cannot be made from direct staining of renal biopsy due to rapidly progressive disease that has destroyed most of the glomeruli available for examination. Further testing in that situation would entail looking for anti-GBM antibody in serum (Fig. 37.7); this antibody is the etiologic factor in Goodpasture's syndrome: hemorrhagic alveolitis associated with rapid progression to glomerulonephritis. Success of immunosuppression in this disorder can be predicted by serial titers of serum anti-GBM antibody.

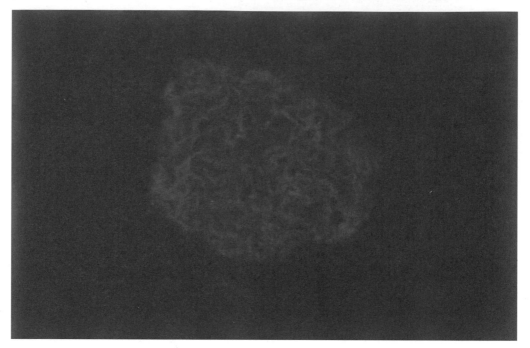

Figure 37.7. Antineutrophil cytoplasmic antibody pattern by IFA on human neutrophils.

Wegener's Granulomatosis

This disorder is a necrotizing vasculitis that affects the upper and lower respiratory tract. The kidneys are also affected, causing glomerulonephritis and frequently leading to death from renal and pulmonary failure. Because Wegener's granulomatosis is fatal if untreated and long-term remissions can be achieved in most cases with immunosuppression (cyclophosphamide and steroids), the diagnosis is critical. Biopsies of lung and kidney may not be specific; however, circulating antineutrophil cytoplasmic antibodies (ANCAs) are strongly indicative of Wegener's granulomatosis.

The presence of ANCAs may be demonstrated with IFA using human neutrophils (Fig. 37.8). Cytoplasmic staining (c-ANCA pattern) is due to autoantibody against proteinase 3. Perinuclear staining (p-ANCA) is due to autoantibody against myeloperoxidase. Antiproteinase 3 and antimyeloperoxidase are quantitated by ELISA. They are both found clinically with Wegener's granulomatosis (a small vessel vasculitis that typically presents with pneumonia, sinusitis, and hematuria). They may be seen with other forms of vasculitis such as periarteritis nodosa, Churg-Strauss syndrome (medium vessel vasculitis), and pauci-immune necrotizing and crescentic glomerulonephritis. The c-ANCA pattern is more strongly associated with Wegener's granulomatosis, whereas p-ANCA may be found in Wegener's and in the other vasculitides. Some studies have found a p-ANCA pattern associated with inflammatory bowel and biliary diseases, although the target neutrophil antigen in those cases is different from myeloperoxidase.

Gastrointestinal

Pernicious anemia is associated with *antigastric parietal cell autoantibody* in the majority of cases (at least 90%) and *autoantibody against intrinsic factor* in up to 75% percent of

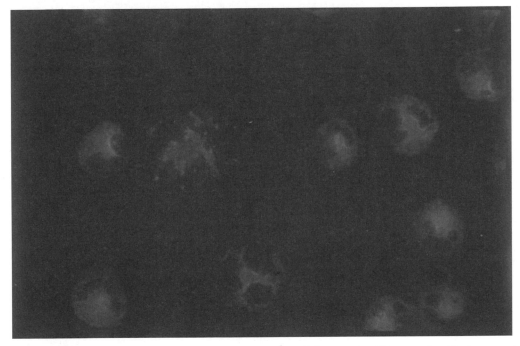

Figure 37.8. Antiglomerular basement membrane antibody by IFA on monkey kidney section. The basement membrane shows linear staining in the glomerulus; the surrounding renal tubules are not stained.

cases. Parietal cell antibodies are identified by IFA with the same mouse stomach and kidney slides that are used for detecting AMA and SMA. The finding of a macrocytic anemia with low vitamin B_{12} levels may prompt a search for parietal cell antibodies; however, parietal cell antibodies are not completely specific for pernicious anemia and may occur with other autoimmune disorders and in asymptomatic elderly persons at low titer. Autoantibodies against intrinsic factor are usually measured by radioimmunoassay. They can either block the binding of vitamin B_{12} to intrinsic factor (type 1) or bind to vitamin B_{12} and thereby block the action of intrinsic factor (type 2). Diagnosis of pernicious anemia usually does not require the measurement of autoantibodies. However, pernicious anemia may be associated with other autoimmune disorders of the endocrine system including thyroiditis and Addison's disease (autoimmune primary adrenocortical insufficiency), in which case autoantibody detection can elucidate the full scope of the disorder.

Gluten sensitive enteropathy or celiac disease is an inflammatory disorder of the small intestine that is initiated by an immunologic response to the wheat protein gluten (also termed gliadin). Avoidance of gluten is usually sufficient to reverse the inflammation. This disorder results in flattening of the intestinal mucosa, loss of absorptive surface, and diarrhea leading to malabsorption and failure to thrive in children. Because the treatment of avoiding dietary gluten can be so effective (but very difficult to maintain long term), definitive diagnosis is essential. The gold standard of diagnosis has been intestinal mucosal biopsies on full diet, again after institution of gluten-free diet to demonstrate return of normal mucosal surfaces, and a third time after reinstitution of full diet to demonstrate that gluten exposure can stimulate the disorder. Patients with celiac disease also demonstrate some unique serum antibodies that can be used for diagnosis. These include antibodies against gluten (gliadin) and *autoantibodies against reticulin and endomysium.* Antireticulin antibodies are relatively nonspecific as they are seen in other disorders as well. IgA antigliadin and antiendomysial antibodies can be used in monitoring for compliance with a gluten-free diet as titers fall when exposure ceases. Antiendomysial antibodies appear to be completely specific for celiac disease and have been used for screening or for diagnosis in questionable cases.

Pancreas

Type 1 diabetes mellitus (insulin dependent diabetes mellitus, IDDM; discussed in Chapter 7) is an autoimmune disease in which genetically susceptible persons undergo selective destruction of the β cells of the islets of Langerhans in the pancreas. Prior to onset, IDDM patients demonstrate autoantibodies that may be significant for initiating the destructive process. *Islet-cell autoantibodies (ICAs)* can be detected by IFA using frozen sections of human pancreas. Islet-cell autoantibodies are titered against reference serum calibrated in Juvenile Diabetes Foundation units. Islet-cell autoantibodies are usually detected in patients with newly diagnosed IDDM but also in a small number of their nondiabetic relatives. *Insulin-associated autoantibodies (IAA)* can be found in about half of IDDM patients at time of diagnosis. They also arise later in response to insulin therapy. *Antiglutamic acid decarboxylase (GAD) autoantibodies* are found in most IDDM patients at diagnosis and also in a large proportion of their relatives who later develop IDDM themselves. There are two forms of GAD occurring in islet cells (GAD65) and nerves (GAD67). Anti-GAD autoantibodies are associated with the stiff-man syndrome due to interference with the neurotransmitter γ-aminobutyric acid.

None of these autoantibodies is useful or necessary for diagnosing IDDM, but they do have promise for predicting the onset of IDDM in patients at high risk (i.e., first-degree relatives of already affected patients). Presumably immunotherapy may someday be successful in preventing progression with destruction of islet cells. The best predictive value appears to be afforded by anti-GAD along with ICA or IAA. After onset of IDDM, the titers of these autoantibodies fall, perhaps because no autoantigen remains to stimulate the immune system.

Skin

Autoimmune cutaneous disease may be diagnosed with a combination of DFA on skin biopsies and IFA using the patient's serum to react with tissue sections such as esophagus of guinea pig or monkey. Direct immunofluorescence assays demonstrate deposition of human immunoglobulins (autoantibodies) in the patient's own tissues. Indirect immunofluorescence assays demonstrate antigen specificity of the autoantibodies. The particular autoantibodies associated with skin diseases are directed primarily against basement membrane zone (BMZ) and epidermal intercellular substance (ICS). These tests can be used for differential diagnosis of skin lesions.

In *pemphigus,* autoantibodies react with a glycoprotein of keratinocytes that shows up on fluorescence assays as binding to ICS; IFA shows binding to desmosomes. Disease activity corresponds roughly to titer in serum; however, lesions can occur without circulating titers (such as on oral mucosa) and so must be diagnosed by DFA. *Bullous pemphigoid* shows circulating autoantibody to BMZ by IFA and deposition of IgG and C3 in a linear pattern by DFA in biopsy of skin or oral mucosa. *Paraneoplastic pemphigus* has occurred in malignancies such as lymphomas, squamous cell carcinoma, and poorly differentiated sarcoma. It is characterized by autoantibodies against ICS and BMZ. *Dermatitis herpetiformis* shows granular deposits of IgA in dermal papillae that lead to subepidermal bullous formation. This skin disorder is associated with gluten-sensitive enteropathy (celiac disease); those cases demonstrate reticulin and endomysial autoantibodies.

Muscle

Skeletal muscle is affected in polymyositis and dermatomyositis. Serologic markers of these diseases include autoantibodies against PM-1 and Jo-1 antigens. Skeletal muscle autoantibodies can be detected with IFA on frozen sections of monkey muscle; unfortunately skeletal muscle autoantibodies are not very specific as they are frequently seen at low titers in healthy individuals. Skeletal muscle inflammation can be monitored by measuring creatine kinase enzymatic activity in serum. *Anti-Jo-1 antibodies* may indicate an increased risk for developing pulmonary disease in polymyositis patients.

Autoantibodies against myocardial muscle may develop after damage to the heart as from myocardial infarction, cardiac surgery, or cardiomyopathy. Myocardial antibodies may be detected by IFA using sections of monkey heart.

Neurologic

Myasthenia gravis is marked by antiacetylcholine receptor (anti-AChR) autoantibodies that block acetylcholine from interacting with its receptor at postsynaptic sites on skeletal muscle. The clinical result is failure of muscle to contract in response to motor nerve impulses; interference with neuromuscular transmission causes muscle weakness. Measurement of anti-AChR in serum is useful for diagnosing myasthenia gravis; serial titers of this autoantibody are also useful for monitoring therapy such as plasmapheresis, as clinical status is directly related to titer. The assay is almost always sent to a reference laboratory due to its complexity. It entails immunoprecipitation of the autoantibody with the receptor and radiolabeled bungarotoxin that in turn is bound to the receptor. There are at least three forms of anti-AChR based on their abilities to bind, block, or modulate the receptor.

The Lambert-Eaton syndrome presents a similar clinical picture of muscle weakness that is usually due to paraneoplastic autoimmunity. It is caused by autoantibodies against presynaptic voltage-dependent calcium channels on nerve terminals. This autoantibody frequently is associated with small-cell lung carcinoma. Finding a myasthenic syndrome without anti-AChR should prompt a search for this autoantibody, and if positive, should lead to further evaluation for occult malignancy.

Multiple sclerosis (MS) causes demyelination of the central nervous system and is generally diagnosed on clinical findings. Objective laboratory data supportive of immunologic activation (suggesting MS) in the central nervous system include oligoclonal bands of immunoglobulin in cerebrospinal fluid that do not appear in serum; however, such clonal bands may also be seen in a wide variety of infections and other disease (Chapter 20). Current understanding of MS indicates that a unique subset of T lymphocytes is responsible for disease progression. Definitive laboratory testing for MS and for monitoring its progression in the future will probably focus on identifying that unique group of lymphocytes.

Neuronal

Autoantibodies against several different neuronal antigens have recently been discovered to cause neuropathies and other neurologic syndromes. Some patients have IgM paraproteins that cause peripheral neuropathies due to interactions with glycosphin-golipid components of the nerve. Other patients have autoantibodies that exhibit the same reactivities and result in the same sensory and motor neuropathies. These antigens include ganglioside GM1, sulfatides, and myelin associated glycoprotein. Measurements of these autoantibodies use ELISAs that are usually grouped in a panel of different antigens, as the syndromes they cause are overlapping and cannot be distinguished on clinical grounds. Of all patients with neuropathies, those with an autoimmune etiology are a small fraction, but they are important to diagnose accurately as therapy is based on immunosuppression and can be quite successful.

Paraneoplastic neurologic syndromes result from an immune response against a tumor that cross-reacts with a neuronal antigen. Notable among these antibodies are *anti-Yo* that affects Purkinje cells causing cerebellar degeneration. The autoantibodies *anti-Ri* and *anti-Hu* can cause abnormalities such as opsoclonus, encephalomyelitis, and sensory-motor disorders. Associated malignancies include breast and small-cell lung carcinoma. The major significance in discovering a paraneoplastic neuronal antibody is then to initiate a search for the primary malignancy which may be occult in part due to the intensity of the immune response. Therapy is directed at the malignancy; the neurologic syndrome may improve as the immune response wanes after removal of neoplastic immunogen.

A final caution about autoimmune testing is that laboratory procedures are in general not useful to screen for autoimmune diseases in asymptomatic individuals. Many healthy persons can have circulating autoantibodies that either have no clinical significance or do not initiate disease processes (i.e., they are merely markers of disease but can also be present without the disease). Thus screening an entire population would give rise to many false positive results. A better approach to the use of autoantibody testing is to apply those assays to patients who demonstrate clinical evidence of disease and may have other supporting laboratory data (such as abnormal serum creatinine, urinalysis, erythrocyte sedimentation rate, etc.) that suggest the presence of an inflammatory disorder.

FACTORS AFFECTING LABORATORY TESTS

CHAPTER 38

Factors Affecting Laboratory Tests

D. ROBERT DUFOUR

As has been discussed in Chapters 1 and 2, laboratory test results must be interpreted in light of the population to which the individual belongs, and of physiologic and other factors which can alter test results from those in the individual's baseline state. This chapter attempts to outline the major factors which affect results for the most common laboratory tests.

Table 38.1 is arranged alphabetically by test name, with extensive cross-references provided for alternate test names. Reference ranges are given both for units commonly used in the United States and for the SI system, as well as the factor for converting between the two. The conversion is straightforward: to convert from U.S. units to SI units, multiply by the factor; to convert from SI to U.S. units, divide by the factor. An exception is for enzymes, where the SI unit, the katal, is not appreciably different in meaning from the longer accepted International Unit. Moreover, for enzymes, selection of the method for performing the measurement is a more important variable. Practitioners should always check with the laboratory they are using for reference values for enzymes.

The next three columns list major factors affecting results for each test. The column titled "Nondisease Causes of Changes" first lists changes expected in healthy individuals, giving random (intraday), day to day (interday) variation and any cyclic variation observed. Next are listed physiologic factors which either increase or decrease the test result. Finally, differences in reference values based on age, pregnancy, sex, or ethnic group are given; these represent the general types of changes seen. Complete information on different reference ranges in children, older individuals, and during pregnancy can be found in the references at the end of the introduction. The column titled "Disease Related Changes" includes the most common disorders which increase or decrease the test result; uncommon or rare diseases are not given, but may be found in the references provided. "Drug Related Changes" also includes the most commonly used drugs which increase or decrease test results; again, uncommon drugs which affect tests can be found in the references.

The final column, "Common Conditions for Use of Test," lists the most common indications for performing the test and a summary of interpretive information found in the individual chapters. This is meant to provide a ready reference for test users who have simple questions about use of tests. For more complete information, the reader should refer to the appropriate chapter or use the index to find more information on the test of interest.

REFERENCES

Faulkner WR, Meites S, eds. Geriatric clinical chemistry, reference values. Washington, D.C.: American Association for Clinical Chemistry, 1993.

Lokitch G. Handbook of diagnostic biochemistry and hematology in normal pregnancy. Cleveland: CRC Press, 1993.

Soldin SJ, Hicks JM, eds. Pediatric reference ranges. Washington, D.C.: American Association for Clinical Chemistry, 1995.

Young DS. Effects of disease on clinical laboratory tests, 3rd edition. Washington, D.C.: American Association for Clinical Chemistry, 1996.

Young, DS. Effects of drugs on clinical laboratory tests, 4th edition. Washington, D.C.: American Association for Clinical Chemistry, 1996.

Table 38.1.
Factors Affecting Laboratory Tests

Test Name	Reference Range			Nondisease Causes of Changes	Disease Related Changes	Drug Related Changes	Common Conditions for Use of Test
	Standard	Factor	SI Units				
ACE (see Angiotensin converting enzyme)							
Acetone (see Ketones)							
Acetylcholinesterase	7,816–11,666 IU/L	1	7,816–11,666 IU/L	DEC: Ethanol.	INC: Hemolytic anemia (activity higher in young erythrocytes). DEC: Organophosphate poisoning (best test for chronic exposure), megaloblastic anemia.	DEC: Pyridostigmine, organophosphates.	Used for monitoring chronic organophosphate exposure; use plasma cholinesterase to monitor response to therapy for acute exposure, or in presence of hemolytic anemia.
Acid phosphatase	0–0.5 U/L	1	0–0.5 U/L	Interday variation 50–100%; intraday variation 25–50%; highest in PM with nadir in AM. Higher in males than in females. In males, increases after prostatic examination or biopsy. Increases 50% in males by age 60. INC: Hemolysis. DEC: Specimen storage.	INC: Prostatic carcinoma, rarely with benign prostatic hyperplasia, Gaucher's disease, increased bone turnover, bone metastases, diabetes, amyloidosis, myocardial infarction.	INC: Androgens (in females).	Total acid phosphatase is seldom used currently. Prostatic acid phosphatase can be helpful in patients with prostatic cancer treated with antiandrogens, when PSA may be falsely low. Tartrate-resistant acid phosphatase mainly measures bone isoenzyme, and can be used to monitor metabolic bone disease.

(continued)

Table 38.1 *(continued)*

ACTH (see Adrenocorticotropic hormone)

ADH (see Vasopressin)

Test Name	Reference Range			Nondisease Causes of Changes	Disease Related Changes	Drug Related Changes	Common Conditions for Use of Test
	Standard	Factor	SI Units				
Adrenocorticotropic hormone	7–51 ng/L	1	7–51 ng/L	Highest shortly before waking, 50% lower in early sleep; released in episodic spikes. INC: Stress, exercise, hypoglycemia. DEC: Hyperglycemia.	INC: Cushing's disease, Addison's disease, congenital adrenal hyperplasia, ectopic ACTH production. DEC: Hypopituitarism, adrenal Cushing's syndrome.	INC: Insulin, desipramine, ketoconazole, L-dopa, RU 486, vasopressin. DEC: Glucocorticoids, clonidine.	Used in diagnosis of adrenal hyperfunction and hypofunction. Basal levels are of limited value unless cortisol is markedly abnormal. Response of ACTH to known stimuli is of more use in determining state of pituitary. Normally, dexamethasone will suppress ACTH production (see *Dexamethasone suppression tests*). Insulin hypoglycemia is a potent stimulus to ACTH production; glucose must fall below 40 mg/dL to be able to interpret results. Other stimuli, such as CRH, metyrapone, and naloxone are used less frequently.

Test		Reference range	Physiologic factors	Drugs/Other	Comments
Alanine aminotransferase (ALT, SGPT)	1	M: 8–45 U/L F: 6–38 U/L	Interday variation 5–30%. Slightly higher in males than females. INC: Obesity. DEC: Physical fitness, renal failure (falsely low in most assays). About 10% lower during first two trimesters of pregnancy, returns to normal by delivery. Lower in children by 5–10 U/L until adolescence.	INC: Hepatocellular injury, large myocardial infarction, severe skeletal muscle disease, severe hemolysis, gall stone disease, renal infarct. DEC: Vitamin B$_6$ deficiency.	ALT is relatively specific for hepatocyte injury. Mild elevations (often <5× normal) in chronic hepatitis, elevated 10–40× normal in most acute hepatitis, and >40× normal in toxic or ischemic hepatitis. Generally, AST:ALT ratio is >3:1 with muscle injury, between 2:1 and 4:1 with alcoholic hepatitis or very acute liver injury, and <1:1 in most liver diseases.
				INC: Drugs injuring liver or muscle.	
Albumin	10	3.7–5.0 g/dL 37–50 g/L	Interday variation 2–4%. INC: Hemoconcentration, exercise. DEC: Smoking. Gradually decreases in pregnancy by an average 20% by 20 weeks, remains low during lactation. In children, higher by age 6, remains higher in young adults; typical reference range 4.5–5.4 g/dL.	DEC: Chronic liver disease, nephrotic syndrome, malnutrition, acute inflammation, burns, malignancies.	Used as a marker of nutritional status. With poor nutrition, albumin is usually decreased to a similar degree as is total protein. With chronic infections, myeloma, and chronic liver disease, albumin is decreased more than is total protein. Has been used to classify severity of illness and malnutrition; levels <2.1 g/dL indicate severe malnutrition and high mortality.
				DEC: Drugs damaging liver, amiodarone, estrogens, oral contraceptives, high dose steroids.	

(continued)

Table 38.1 *(continued)*

Albuminuria (see Microalbuminuria)

Alcohol, ethyl (see Ethanol)

AFP (see α-Fetoprotein)

Test Name	Reference Range			Nondisease Causes of Changes	Disease Related Changes	Drug Related Changes	Common Conditions for Use of Test
	Standard	Factor	SI Units				
Aldosterone	Serum: <16 ng/dL Urine: 6–25 μg/day	0.0277 2.77	<0.44 nmol/L 17–69 nmol/day	Interday variation 30%. While supine, decreases during day; when upright, increases progressively and remains elevated for 6 hours. INC: Obesity, high temperatures, prolonged fast, upright posture, low salt diet, exercise, smoking, ethanol. DEC: High altitude, ethanol, severe acute illness, high salt diet. In females, higher in late luteal phase. Increases in early pregnancy, remains elevated until term. In children highest in neonates, reaches adult levels by 3 months. In adults, decreases with age. Lower in blacks than whites.	INC: Primary hyperaldosteronism, secondary hyperaldosteronism, dehydration, accelerated hypertension, hyperkalemia, chronic obstructive lung disease, congestive heart failure, nephrotic syndrome, hyperkalemia, cirrhosis. DEC: Diabetes, Addison's disease, hyporeninemic hypoaldosteronism, hypokalemia.	INC: Volume depleting agents, lithium, spironolactone, verapamil. DEC: Licorice, heparin, propranolol, angiotensin converting enzyme inhibitors, nonsteroidal anti-inflammatory agents, ranitidine. Nifedipine decreases the response to the upright position.	Used in evaluation of patients with hypertension and hypokalemia or in evaluation of hyperkalemia, especially when associated with hyponatremia and volume depletion. Should always be combined with renin measurement. Patient must be properly prepared, off drugs affecting aldosterone, and with normal plasma potassium. Salt intake should be known.
Alkaline phosphatase	30–130 U/L	1	30–130 U/L	Interday variation 5–10%. No diurnal variation. INC: After meals in some persons. DEC: Following blood transfusion, specimens collected with EDTA, citrate.	INC: Biliary tract obstruction, intrahepatic mass lesions (metastatic cancer, granulomatous diseases), drug-related hepatitis, primary biliary cirrhosis, increased	INC: Drugs causing cholestasis, estrogens, cyclosporin, lithium, anticonvulsants (especially phenytoin). DEC: Oral contraceptives, clofibrate, tamoxifen, glucocorticoids.	Mainly used to detect and monitor liver or bone diseases; often the only liver abnormality present with mass lesions. Degree of elevation related to extent

Test	Factor	Reference range		Physiologic/collection factors	Disease (INC/DEC)	Drugs (INC/DEC)	Comments
				In pregnancy, increases gradually; 100% higher by 20 weeks, 3–4 times higher at term. In children, approximately 2× adult values in infants, gradually increases to 4× adult values by age 10, falls in late adolescence, reaches adult values by age 20. In older adults, increases with age >50, typically up to 160 U/L. Higher in blacks than whites. Higher in males than females until menopause.	bone turnover (osteomalacia, Paget's disease, renal osteodystrophy), osteosarcoma, metastatic cancer to bone, following fractures, hyperthyroidism. DEC: Congenital hypothyroidism, zinc or magnesium deficiency, vitamin B_{12} deficiency, hypoparathyroidism, malnutrition.		and duration of liver pathology. Seldom increased >2× in most forms of hepatitis. With bone disease, may also be only routine laboratory abnormality. Useful marker of success of treatment in Paget's disease, renal osteodystrophy. Asymptomatic elevations best evaluated with alkaline phosphatase isoenzymes.
Alkaline phosphatase isoenzymes	0.01	Bone: 25–91% Liver: 13–67% Other: Trace or less	Bone: 0.25–0.91 Liver: 0.13–0.67	See above. In adolescence, bone isoenzyme increases. In pregnancy, placental isoenzyme increases.	INC (bone): High bone turnover. INC (liver): Hepatobiliary diseases. Often, a second liver isoenzyme band is present. INC (intestine): Inflammatory bowel disease, bowel ischemia, renal failure. INC (placental): Pregnancy, malignancy (especially germ cell tumors).	INC (bone): Lithium. DEC (bone): Clofibrate. INC (liver): Anticonvulsants (especially phenytoin), drugs causing cholestasis. DEC (liver): Oral contraceptives.	Used to evaluate unexplained elevation of alkaline phosphatase. A separate immunoassay for bone isoenzyme can be used to monitor treatment of metabolic bone diseases. Heat fractionation, still offered by some laboratories, is unreliable.
Aluminum	0.371	0–6 µg/L	0–2.2 µmol/L	Highest at 9 AM, lowest at 6 PM. INC: Pregnancy, contamination of specimen; must use special collection sets.	INC: Hemoconcentration, renal failure, Hodgkin's disease, cystic fibrosis, liver disease, leukemia. DEC: Gastric ulcers, pernicious anemia, diabetes.	INC: Aluminum containing antacids, sucralfate (in renal failure).	Used primarily to monitor exposure in patients with chronic renal failure on dialysis. Sources of aluminum are oral antacids and water.

(continued)

Table 38.1 *(continued)*

Test Name	Reference Range			Nondisease Causes of Changes	Disease Related Changes	Drug Related Changes	Common Conditions for Use of Test
	Standard	Factor	SI Units				
Alpha-1 antitrypsin (see α_1-Antitrypsin)							
Alpha-fetoprotein (see α-Fetoprotein)							
Ammonia (NH$_3$)	15–45 µg/dL	0.71	11–32 µmol/L	INC: Delay in specimen analysis, storage at room temperature, parenteral nutrition, high protein diet, exercise, blood transfusion, shock (if venous ammonia measured). DEC: Smoking. In children, values 4–6× adult values in neonates, remain 2–3× adult values through first two years of life, reach adult levels by adolescence.	INC: Liver failure, Reye's syndrome, inborn errors of urea cycle enzymes, congestive heart failure, chronic obstructive lung disease. DEC: Renal failure.	INC: Ammonium salts, barbiturates, diuretics, valproic acid. DEC: Nonabsorbable antibiotics given orally.	Most commonly used in severe liver disease. While often used to "diagnose" hepatic encephalopathy, degree of ammonia elevation correlates poorly with degree of encephalopathy. High levels generally indicate severe liver injury.
Amylase	44–128 U/L	1	44–128 U/L	Interday variation 5–10%. INC: Smoking, postsurgery (thought to be due to absorption of salivary amylase during ventilation). In AIDS and in older individuals, macroamylase can cause increased values. DEC: Hypertriglyceridemia (interference). In children, very low before age 1 (<30% of adult), reaches adult values by age 1. In pregnancy, increases by 70%. After age 65, amylase averages about 20% lower than in younger	INC: Acute pancreatitis, pancreatic pseydocyst, salivary gland inflammation, intestinal ischemia, diabetic ketoacidosis, renal failure, ovarian carcinoma, ectopic pregnancy, acute illness. DEC: Pancreatic insufficiency, hyperthyroidism, malnutrition, severe liver disease.	INC: Drugs causing pancreatic damage (ethanol, pentamidine most commonly), drugs causing constriction of pancreatic duct outlet (narcotic analgesics).	Used to diagnose pancreatitis, but less specific than lipase. May remain elevated as little as 36–48 hours after onset of pancreatitis. When amylase elevated but lipase normal, amylase isoenzymes can be helpful in determining the type of enzyme increased. Low urine amylase in the presence of elevated plasma

amylase identifies the presence of macroamylase.

adults. Higher in females than males. Higher (2×) in blacks than whites.

ANA (see Antinuclear antibodies)

ANCA (see Antineutrophil cytoplasmic antibodies)

Test			Factors affecting	Associated diseases	Drugs affecting	Comments
Angiotensin coverting enzyme	8–52 U/L	8–52 U/L [1]	Interday variation 8–12%. INC: Ethanol. DEC: Collection with EDTA, following heavy meals, in hemolyzed specimens, smoking, acute illness. In pregnancy, falls by approximately 20%. In children, highest in neonates, falls to adult levels by 6 months before rising again after age 4. Returns to adult levels by late adolescence.	INC: Granulomatous diseases (especially sarcoidosis), HIV infection, ethanol abuse, autoimmune diseases, hyperthyroidism, renal failure, diabetes. DEC: Hypothyroidism, advanced lung neoplasms, chronic lymphocytic leukemia, multiple myeloma, Crohn's disease.	INC: Thyroid hormone replacement. DEC: Angiotensin converting enzyme inhibitors, propranolol.	Used to monitor patients with granulomatous disease, especially sarcoidosis. Level correlates with the extent of disease, especially the degree of pulmonary disease.
Anion gap	7–16 mEq/L	7–16 mmol/L [1]	Interday variation 10%. "Normal" values differ depending on method used to measure electrolytes; check with laboratory. During pregnancy, increases 1–2 mmol/L.	INC: Lactic acidosis, ketoacidosis, oliguric renal failure, rare congenital metabolic errors, toxin ingestion. DEC: Decreased albumin (cirrhosis, malnutrition, nephrotic syndrome), increased globulins (multiple myeloma, Waldenstrom's, HIV, autoimmune diseases).	INC: Ethylene glycol, methanol, paraldehyde, aspirin.	Used in evaluation of acid-base disorders. Indicates the presence of increased organic acids. Calculated by using the formula $Na - (Cl + HCO_3^-)$.
Anticardiolipin antibodies (phospholipid antibodies)	Negative	Negative		INC: Systemic lupus erythematosus, hypercoagulable states.		Most commonly used in the evaluation of patients with hypercoagulable states, particularly arterial thromboses, and in recurrent miscarriages. Also used to evaluate prolonged PTT.

(continued)

Table 38.1 *(continued)*

Test Name	Reference Range			Nondisease Causes of Changes	Disease Related Changes	Drug Related Changes	Common Conditions for Use of Test
	Standard	Factor	SI Units				
Antidiuretic hormone (see Vasopressin)							
Antidouble stranded DNA	Negative		Negative		INC: Systemic lupus erythematosus.		Found in about 70% of patients with SLE, particularly with renal involvement. Levels correlate somewhat with disease activity. Also found in 25% of patients with mixed connective tissue disease, diabetes mellitus.
Antiendomysial antibodies	Negative		Negative		INC: Celiac disease.		Used in diagnosis of celiac disease; thought to be 100% specific.
Antiextractable nuclear antigens (ENA)	Negative		Negative				Includes a panel of antibodies which typically includes anti-Sm, anti-RNP, anti-SS A, and anti-SS B. Used to further evaluate persons with a positive ANA, particularly if the pattern is speckled.
Antiglomerular basement membrane antibodies (anti-GBM)	Negative		Negative		INC: Goodpasture's syndrome, rapidly progressive glomerulonephritis.		Used to evaluate patients with nephritic syndrome and rapid onset of renal failure; found in 90% of patients

			with Goodpasture's, 25% of patients with RPGN without pulmonary involvement.
Antiglutamic acid decarboxylase	Negative	Negative	INC: Type I diabetes.	Used to screen first degree relatives of type I diabetes patients for risk of developing diabetes, often along with anti-islet cell antibodies. Present several years before diagnosis, and persists for a variable period after diagnosis before eventually disappearing. May also be used to differentiate type I from type II diabetes; will be absent in the latter.
Antihistone antibodies	Negative	Negative	INC: Drug induced systemic lupus erythematosus, systemic lupus erythematosus, rheumatoid arthritis.	Used to detect drug induced lupus (positive in 100% of cases); also positive in 50% of other cases of lupus and in 15% of cases of rheumatoid arthritis.

(continued)

Table 38.1 *(continued)*

Test Name	Reference Range			Nondisease Causes of Changes	Disease Related Changes	Drug Related Changes	Common Conditions for Use of Test
	Standard	Factor	SI Units				
Anti-insulin antibodies	Negative		Negative		INC: Type I diabetes (before insulin treatment), autoimmune disease, type I and type II diabetes (after insulin treatment), insulin resistance.	INC: Insulin.	Used most commonly to recognize insulin resistance states and in workup of hypoglycemia. Anti-insulin antibodies may occur spontaneously and cause both hyperglycemia and hypoglycemia, but may also occur after insulin injection. Less useful for detecting the risk of type I diabetes than anti-GAD or anti-islet cell antibodies.
Anti-islet cell antibodies	Negative		Negative		INC: Type I diabetes (before insulin treatment).		Used to screen first degree relatives of type I diabetes patients for risk of developing diabetes, often along with antiglutamic acid decarboxylase. Present several years before diagnosis, and persist for a variable period after diagnosis before eventually disappearing. May also be used to

Test		Causes of abnormal value	Comments
Anti-intrinsic factor antibodies	Negative	INC: Pernicious anemia, hyperthyroidism, type I diabetes.	differentiate type I from type II diabetes; will be absent in the latter. Positive in 50% of patients with pernicious anemia, rarely in association with hyperthyroidism or diabetes. INC: Vitamin B$_{12}$.
Anti-La (anti-SS B)	Negative	INC: Sjogren's syndrome, systemic lupus erythematosus.	Found in 50% of patients with Sjogren's syndrome and 10% with systemic lupus.
Antimicrosomal antibodies (see Antithyroid peroxidase)	Negative		
Antimitochondrial antibodies	Negative	INC: Primary biliary cirrhosis, chronic hepatitis, acute hepatitis.	Often used to investigate elevated alkaline phosphatase of liver origin. High titer of antibodies strongly suggests the presence of primary biliary cirrhosis.

(continued)

Table 38.1 *(continued)*

Test Name	Reference Range			Nondisease Causes of Changes	Disease Related Changes	Drug Related Changes	Common Conditions for Use of Test
	Standard	Factor	SI Units				
Antineutrophil cytoplasmic antibodies (ANCA)	Negative		Negative		INC: Wegener's granulomatosis, polyarteritis nodosa, other forms of vasculitis, sclerosing cholangitis, inflammatory bowel disease.		Antibodies to myeloperoxidase (perinuclear or P-ANCA) occur predominantly in Wegener's, occasionally in glomerulonephritis without other findings of Wegener's. Antibodies to proteinase 3 (cytoplasmic or C-ANCA) are found in other disorders mentioned. Commonly used in patients with pulmonary or renal diseases suggesting Wegener's or glomerulonephritis.
Antinuclear antibodies (ANA)	Negative		Negative	INC: Smoking. Increases in frequency with increasing age over 60.	INC: Autoimmune diseases, leprosy, viral hepatitis, mononucleosis, renal failure.	INC: Methyldopa, procainamide, tocainide, hydralazine, other drugs causing a lupus-like picture.	Used in screening for autoimmune disease; if the results are negative, other autoantibodies are almost always negative as well and are rarely indicated. Low titer of antibodies is commonly found with increasing age.

Antiphospholipid antibodies (see Anticardiolipin antibodies)

Antiribonucleoprotein (Anti-RNP)	Negative	Negative	INC: Mixed connective tissue disease, systemic lupus erythematosus.	Found in almost all patients with mixed connective tissue disease and 50% of patients with systemic lupus; rarely positive with other autoimmune diseases. Higher titer of antibodies suggest an autoimmune disease. Followed-up with more specific autoimmune markers to determine likely etiology.
Anti-Ro (Anti-SS A)	Negative	Negative	INC: Sjogren's syndrome, systemic and cutaneous lupus erythematosus, scleroderma, rheumatoid arthritis.	Found in 70% of patients with Sjogren's syndrome, 50% with systemic lupus, and may be found in cutaneous lupus, 33% of patients with scleroderma, rarely with rheumatoid arthritis.
Anti-Sm	Negative	Negative	INC: Systemic lupus erythematosus, mixed connective tissue disease, scleroderma.	Found in 30% of patients with systemic lupus, rarely with mixed connective tissue disease or scleroderma.

(continued)

Table 38.1 *(continued)*

Test Name	Reference Range			Nondisease Causes of Changes	Disease Related Changes	Drug Related Changes	Common Conditions for Use of Test
	Standard	Factor	SI Units				
Antismooth muscle antibodies	Negative		Negative	Occasionally found in some normal individuals.	INC: Autoimmune chronic hepatitis, primary biliary cirrhosis; rarely with obstructive jaundice, acute hepatitis.	INC: Methyldopa, nitrofurantoin.	Used in evaluation of patients with chronic hepatitis and negative viral serologies. Elevated in high titers in autoimmune chronic hepatitis (70% of cases).
Anti-SS A (see Anti-Ro)							
Anti-SS B (see Anti-La)							
Antithrombin III	85–115%	0.01	0.85–1.15	Interday variation 3%. INC: In females at time of menstruation, acute inflammation. In pregnancy, decreases in last trimester.	INC: Acute liver disease, renal transplant. DEC: Disseminated intravascular coagulation, congenital deficiency, cirrhosis, liver failure, nephrotic syndrome.	INC: Anabolic steroids, warfarin. DEC: Heparin, estrogens, oral contraceptives, tamoxifen.	Used to screen for congenital deficiency in patients with recurrent thrombosis. Also used as diagnostic test for DIC.
α_1-Antitrypsin	77–173 mg/dL	10	770–1,730 mg/L	Interday variation 5–10%. INC: Hemoconcentration, exercise, acute inflammation. In pregnancy, increases gradually up to 100% higher by term. About 2× adult levels at birth, similar in children, 50% higher during adolescence. Average 30 mg/dL higher in females than males.	INC: Malignancy, tissue damage, acute hepatitis. DEC: Congenital deficiency, malnutrition, cirrhosis, nephrotic syndrome, hypothyroidism, respiratory distress syndrome of the newborn.	INC: Estrogens, oral contraceptives, tamoxifen.	Used primarily to detect α_1-antitrypsin deficiency. Should not be done when the patient is acutely ill. In situations listed where results may be affected, can also perform α_1-antitrypsin phenotyping.
Antithyroglobulin	0–59 IU/L	1	0–59 IU/L	Increased in frequency with increasing age.	INC: Graves' disease, thyroiditis, thyroid carcinoma, cirrhosis.		Less sensitive or specific than antithyroid

peroxidase antibodies, not routinely useful in evaluation for thyroiditis. Useful in patients with differentiated thyroid carcinoma; if positive, thyroglobulin measurements will not be accurate. Persistence of antibody increases the likelihood of recurrent thyroid cancer.

| **Antithyroid peroxidase** | 0–0.3 U/mL | 1 | 0–0.3 U/mL | Increased in frequency during pregnancy. Increases in frequency with increasing age. | INC: Graves' disease, thyroiditis. | Used in evaluation for thyroiditis in patients with goiter. In subclinical hypothyroidism, high titers suggest likely progression to clinical hypothyroidism. |

(continued)

Table 38.1 *(continued)*

Test Name	Reference Range			Nondisease Causes of Changes	Disease Related Changes	Drug Related Changes	Common Conditions for Use of Test
	Standard	Factor	SI Units				
Apolipoprotein A1	119–240 mg/dL	0.01	1.2–2.4 g/L	Interday variation 5–10%. Highest at 8 PM, 7% lower at 6 AM. INC: Ethanol, hemoconcentration, exercise. DEC: Smoking, weight loss, acute stress. During pregnancy, increases by 30% by the third trimester. In children, about 33% of adult levels in neonates, reaches adult levels by 1–2 months; falls in males at puberty. Higher in females than males and in blacks than in whites.	INC: Familial hyperalphalipoprotein-emia. DEC: Tangier disease, uncontrolled diabetes, chronic liver disease, nephrotic syndrome, chronic renal failure, septicemia.	INC: Oral contraceptives, estrogens, clofibrate, HMG-CoA reductase inhibitors, gemfibrozil, niacin. DEC: Estrogen/progesterone cycling, probucol, Norplant, phenytoin, valproic acid.	Used to assess the risk of coronary artery disease; in general correlates with HDL-cholesterol.
Apolipoprotein B	52–163 mg/dL	0.01	0.5–1.6 g/L	Interday variation 5–10%. No diurnal variation. INC: Smoking, hemoconcentration. DEC: Weight loss. In pregnancy, increases by 100% by the third trimester. In children, about 50% of adult levels in neonates, reaches adult levels by 1–2 months. Increases with age till about age 55. Higher in males than in females, and in whites than in blacks.	INC: Hyperlipidemia, diabetes, hypothyroidism, nephrotic syndrome, renal failure, obstructive jaundice. DEC: Tangier disease, abetalipoproteinemia, malignancies, malnutrition, hyperthyroidism, acute illness (up to a 40% drop).	INC: Chlorthalidone, retinoids (>100%), progestational agents. DEC: HMG-CoA reductase inhibitors, phenytoin, phenobarbital, valproic acid.	Used to assess risk of coronary artery disease; in general, correlates with LDL-cholesterol.
Aspartate aminotransferase (AST, SGOT)	8–40 U/L	1	8–40 U/L	Interday variation 8–12%. INC: Exercise, hemolysis, IM injection.	INC: Liver injury (acute and chronic hepatitis, slightly in obstructive	INC: Drugs inducing liver or muscle injury.	Usually used as a test for liver injury. Mild increases are

typical of chronic hepatitis and alcoholic hepatitis; in the former, AST is typically greater than ALT. With acute hepatitis of most types, AST is elevated to a lesser degree than is ALT, and is usually increased 10–40×. Very high values occur with ischemic and toxic hepatitis, and AST is transiently higher than ALT. With muscle injury, AST is usually 3–5× higher than ALT.

jaundice), myocardial infarction, skeletal muscle disease, hemolytic anemias, gallstone pancreatitis, pulmonary infarction. DEC: Chronic renal failure.

In pregnancy, about 10–20% lower in the first two trimesters, near normal in the third trimester. Highest in young adults, decreases with increasing age.

Bence Jones protein (see Protein electrophoresis, urine)

Beta-2-microglobulin (see β₂-Microglobulin)

Bicarbonate 22–28 mEq/L 1 22–28 mmol/L

Interday variation 5%. Highest in AM, 30% lower in PM. INC: After meals. DEC: Exercise, prolonged fasting, delay in analyzing specimen, prolonged tourniquet use. In pregnancy, decreases by an average 15% throughout gestation. In neonates and infants, may be up to 5–8 mmol/L lower due to hyperventilation.

INC: Respiratory acidosis, metabolic alkalosis (vomiting, Cushing's syndrome, volume depletion, hyperaldosteronism). DEC: Respiratory alkalosis, metabolic acidosis (ketoacidosis, lactic acidosis, diarrhea, renal tubular acidosis, renal failure).

INC: Diuretics, mineralocorticoids, carbenicillin, glucocorticoids. DEC: Carbonic anhydrase inhibitors, spironolactone, ethylene glycol, methanol, aspirin, paraldehyde.

Used in evaluation of acid-base disorders, interpreted along with anion gap, electrolytes, and blood gases (see the algorithm in Chapter 4). Should agree closely with calculated bicarbonate from blood gases; a lack of agreement suggests erroneous results and blood gases should be repeated.

(continued)

Table 38.1 *(continued)*

Test Name	Reference Range			Nondisease Causes of Changes	Disease Related Changes	Drug Related Changes	Common Conditions for Use of Test
	Standard	Factor	SI Units				
Bilirubin, direct	0–0.2 mg/dL	17.1	0–3.4 μmol/L	Interday variation 40%. INC: Dubin-Johnson, Rotor syndromes. DEC: Specimen storage.	INC: Liver or biliary tract diseases.	INC: Drugs causing liver injury.	Measures predominantly biliprotein and conjugated bilirubin; only a small amount of unconjugated bilirubin reacts. Most sensitive test of liver function in acute and chronic hepatitis. Usually 50–80% of total bilirubin in patients with liver or biliary tract disease. Will remain elevated with recovery because biliprotein is also measured in the direct reaction. High total bilirubin with <20% direct suggests prehepatic causes (Gilbert's syndrome, hemolysis). When direct bilirubin is initially elevated but fails to rise with worsening jaundice, strongly suggestive of massive hepatic injury.

| **Bilirubin, total** | 0.3–1.7 mg/dL | 17.1 | 5–29 μmol/L | Interday variation 15–20%. INC: Fasting, Gilbert's syndrome. DEC: Specimen storage. In pregnancy, about 50% lower in first trimester, rises to 25% below baseline by term. In neonates, markedly elevated (up to 10× normal from 3–5 days), falls to adult levels by 1 month. In older persons, about 33% lower than in younger adults. Higher in males than in females and in whites than in blacks. | INC: Acute liver or biliary tract disease, hemolytic anemia, hypothyroidism, hematomas, congestive heart failure. | INC: Drugs causing liver injury or hemolysis. DEC: Oral contraceptives, estrogens. | Used along with direct bilirubin, predominantly in liver disease. When direct bilirubin <20% of total, suggestive of hemolysis or Gilbert's syndrome, a common benign inherited trait. With fasting, bilirubin rises faster in Gilbert's syndrome than in normal individuals. Usually normal until late in chronic liver disease. |
| **Bleeding time** | 2–8 min | 1 | 2–8 min | INC: Edema, ethanol. | INC: Thrombocytopenia, platelet dysfunction, chronic renal failure, liver disease, toxemia. | INC: Aspirin (for 7–10 days), nonsteroidal anti-inflammatory agents, penicillins, heparin, warfarin. DEC: Desmopressin, erythropoietin. | Used to assess platelet function. In immune thrombocytopenia, bleeding time is much better than expected from the platelet count. Reproducibility is poor. While other tests of platelet aggregation can be used in vitro, bleeding time assesses all phases of the formation of the initial hemostatic plug. |

(continued)

Table 38.1 *(continued)*

Test Name	Reference Range			Nondisease Causes of Changes	Disease Related Changes	Drug Related Changes	Common Conditions for Use of Test
	Standard	Factor	SI Units				

Blood urea nitrogen (see BUN)

Bone alkaline phosphatase (see Alkaline phosphatase, bone isoenzyme)

Bone Gla protein (see Osteocalcin)

Test Name	Standard	Factor	SI Units	Nondisease Causes of Changes	Disease Related Changes	Drug Related Changes	Common Conditions for Use of Test
BUN (blood urea nitrogen)	8–22 mg/dL	0.36	2.9–7.9 mmol/L	Interday variation 5–15%. Highest at midnight, lowest at 5 PM. INC: Dehydration, high protein intake, exercise, blood transfusions. DEC: Low protein intake, high water intake, after meals, smoking, specimens collected with fluoride, hemolysis. In pregnancy, decreases an average of 30% by 12 weeks, 40% by mid-pregnancy, 20% below baseline near term. In children, about 20% lower until puberty. In adults, increases with age after 40; about 50% higher by age 90. Slightly higher in males than females.	INC: Renal failure, dehydration, protein catabolic states, upper GI bleeding, congestive heart failure. DEC: Malnutrition, cirrhosis, overhydration, acromegaly.	INC: Androgens, glucocorticoids, tetracycline, drugs causing kidney damage.	Used along with creatinine to assess renal function. Normal BUN: creatinine ratio (when both are in mg/dL) is 10:1–20:1. Increased ratio with high BUN suggests protein catabolic states, prerenal azotemia (heart failure, volume depletion), upper GI bleeding or acute urinary obstruction. Normal ratio with increased BUN occurs with acute tubular necrosis and chronic renal disease. Low ratio with increased BUN may occur in renal diseases associated with malnutrition, cirrhosis, or dialysis.

C3 (see Complement component C3)
C4 (see Complement component C4)
Ca (see Calcium)

CA 125	1	0–35 U/mL 0–35 kU/L	Interday variation up to 40%. INC: Up to 2× during menses. During pregnancy, increases 25% in first trimester, higher with multiple gestations. In females, higher in secretory phase, acute rise with menses.	INC: Epithelial ovarian carcinoma (except mucinous), endometriosis, carcinomas of endometrium, pancreas, liver, and lung, cirrhosis, ascites, peritonitis, pelvic inflammatory disease.	Used primarily to follow patients with surface epithelial tumors of the ovary. Increased levels occur mainly with metastatic disease, making the test insensitive for early ovarian carcinoma. Not useful for identification of a tumor as being of ovarian origin.
CA 15-3	1	0–30 U/mL 0–30 kU/L	Interday variation 25%.	INC: Breast carcinoma, liver disease.	Used primarily to follow breast carcinoma, elevated in only about 60% of patients with metastatic disease.

(continued)

Table 38.1 (continued)

Test Name	Reference Range			Nondisease Causes of Changes	Disease Related Changes	Drug Related Changes	Common Conditions for Use of Test
	Standard	Factor	SI Units				
CA 19-9	0–37 U/mL	1	0–37 kU/L		INC: Pancreatic, gastric, colon, and lung carcinomas, chronic pancreatitis, cholangitis, liver disease, obstructive jaundice.		Used primarily to diagnose and monitor pancreatic carcinoma. Increased in about 90% of pancreatic carcinomas >4 cm in diameter. Not useful for identifying a carcinoma as being of pancreatic origin. Biliary obstruction also increases CA 19–9; testing should be deferred, if possible, until 1–2 weeks after stenting to relieve obstruction.
Calcitonin	<100 ng/L	0.29	<29 pmol/L	DEC: Exercise. Increases during pregnancy. In children, highest in neonates, decreases with age. Higher in males than females. In females, decreases after menopause.	INC: Medullary thyroid cancer, small cell lung cancer, carcinoid tumors, burns with lung injury, renal failure. DEC: Thyroidectomy.	INC: Epinephrine, oral contraceptives, calcium (IV), pentagastrin. DEC: Phenytoin.	Used primarily to diagnose medullary thyroid cancer and C-cell hyperplasia in families with multiple endocrine neoplasia syndromes. Basal levels not as sensitive as increase after calcium or pentagastrin. Normal persons will show peak values of <200 with either

Test	Reference range			Physiological factors	Conditions	Drugs	Comments
							stimulus, <350 after use of both; in females, the response is less than in males with peak values after combined stimulation <100.
Calcium, free (ionized)	4.7–5.2 mg/dL	0.25	1.17–1.30 mmol/L	Interday variation 2%. Highest at 8 AM. INC: Prolonged tourniquet use, prolonged immobilization, exercise, delayed processing of blood. DEC: Acute illness, following blood transfusions, after meals. About 10% higher in neonates, decreases through childhood to reach adult levels by adolescence. Declines slightly with increasing age in adults.	INC: Primary hyperparathyroidism, malignancies producing PTHrP, multiple myeloma, bone metastases, sarcoidosis, acidosis. DEC: Renal failure, hypoparathyroidism, vitamin D deficiency, magnesium deficiency, malnutrition, alkalosis.	INC: Androgens, diethylstilbestrol, thiazides, chlorthalidone, calcium carbonate, vitamin D, lithium. DEC: Carbamazepine, phenytoin, estrogens, fluorides, foscarnet, furosemide, glucocorticoids.	More accurately reflects calcium than total calcium levels, but requires handling of the specimen similar to blood gases. In ambulatory patients, provides little additional information to total calcium corrected for albumin. In acutely ill individuals, usually needed to assess calcium status.

(continued)

Table 38.1 (continued)

| Test Name | Reference Range | | | Nondisease Causes of Changes | Disease Related Changes | Drug Related Changes | Common Conditions for Use of Test |
	Standard	Factor	SI Units				
Calcium, total	8.9–10.5 mg/dL Urine <250 mg/day	0.25 0.025	2.23–2.63 mmol/L Urine <63 mmol/day	Interday variation 1–3% (serum), 20–30% (urine). Highest at 8 PM, lowest at 4 AM. INC: Hemoconcentration, upright posture, exercise, tourniquet use, prolonged immobilization. DEC: Low serum albumin. About 10% lower throughout pregnancy and lactation. In children, highest in neonates, decreases to adult levels by 1 year. Slightly higher in adolescents (up to 10.7 mg/dL) and young adults, decreases after age 50. Urine calcium higher in whites than in blacks, and in males than in females.	INC: Primary hyperparathyroidism, malignancies producing PTHrP, multiple myeloma, bone metastases, sarcoidosis, acidosis, dehydration. DEC: Renal failure, hypoparathyroidism, vitamin D deficiency, magnesium deficiency, alkalosis, cirrhosis, nephrotic syndrome, acute illness, malnutrition.	Same as for free (ionized) calcium.	Used to detect abnormalities of calcium metabolism. More accurate when corrected for abnormal albumin: Corrected calcium = total calcium + $0.8 \times (4.0 -$ serum albumin).
Carbon dioxide (see pCO$_2$)							
Carboxyhemoglobin (carbon monoxide)	0–2.5% of total hemoglobin	0.01	0–0.025 of total hemoglobin	INC: Smoking, decreased caloric intake, living in urban areas, heparin. DEC: Exercise.	INC: Carbon monoxide poisoning, hemolytic anemia, GI bleeding.		Used to detect carbon monoxide poisoning. Typically done along with blood gases when oxygen saturation is measured, not calculated or estimated using pulse oximeters.

Test	Reference range	Factor	SI units	Factors affecting	Increased/Decreased in disease	Comments
Carcinoembryonic antigen (CEA)	0–5 ng/mL	1	0–5 µg/L	Interday variation 35%. INC: Smoking, hemoconcentration. DEC: Heparin anticoagulants.	INC: Cancers of colon, pancreas, stomach, lung, breast, and cervix, inflammatory bowel disease, diverticulosis, cirrhosis, pulmonary infections, emphysema, renal failure.	Primarily used to follow patients with cancers of organs producing CEA. Some assays may give falsely low results with individual patient's samples due to differences in CEA from one person to another.
Carotene	10–85 µg/dL	0.0186	0.19–1.6 µmol/L	Interday variation 5–10%. INC: After meals, hyperlipidemia, hemoconcentration, vegetarian diet, vitamin supplements. DEC: Smoking, ethanol use, fever. Increases gradually in pregnancy, highest at term. Low in neonates, transient rise from 6–12 months, falls until age 2, slight rise to age 6 and fall to adult levels by age 14. Gradual decrease in persons over age 40. Higher in females than males.	INC: Hyperlipidemia, hepatitis, hypothyroidism, nephrotic syndrome, diabetes. DEC: Malabsorption, pancreatic insufficiency, malnutrition, hypolipidemia.	DEC: Cholestipol, estrogens. Used primarily to diagnose malabsorption; requires normal carotene intake for interpretation. Carotene is unstable in light, so specimens must be wrapped in foil after collection.

(continued)

Table 38.1 *(continued)*

Test Name	Reference Range			Nondisease Causes of Changes	Disease Related Changes	Drug Related Changes	Common Conditions for Use of Test
	Standard	Factor	SI Units				
Catecholamines	Norepinephrine Plasma: 65–400 ng/L	5.91	Norepinephrine 380–2365 pmol/L	Interday variation 10–20%, lowest for dopamine. In plasma, released in spikes with marked variation; lowest at night, highest at 6 PM. INC: Stress, acute illness, upright posture, exercise, smoking, ethanol, caffeine, bananas. DEC: After meals. In females, highest at mid-luteal phase. In children, total values increase with age, but ratio of catecholamines to creatinine decreases to reach adult levels by age 12.	INC: Pheochromocytoma, neuroblastoma, hypothyroidism, bipolar disorder, myocardial infarction. DEC: Peripheral neuropathy, Parkinson's disease, diabetes, hyperthyroidism, depression.	INC: Calcium channel blockers, monoamine oxidase inhibitors, theophylline, phenothiazines, nitroglycerin, propranolol (plasma), L-dopa (dopamine only), nifedipine, tricyclic antidepressants (norepinephrine only), nicotine patch, isoproterenol. DEC: Clonidine, bromcriptine, dexamethasone, radiographic contrast agents (urine).	Urine catecholamines used for diagnosis of pheochromocytoma. Generally better sensitivity than catecholamine metabolites (such as VMA or metanephrines) for diagnosis, but may be normal in malignant pheochromocytoma. Many substances may cross react, depending on the type of assay used; practitioners should check with their laboratory. Plasma catecholamines used if urine results normal and patient has widely separated episodes of hypertension. Less useful than metabolite assays in neuroblastoma. If stress related increase is suspected, values should fall to normal within 3 hours after 200 mg clonidine; test not useful if plasma catecholamines <2× normal.
	Urine: 10–80 mg/day	5.46	59–470 nmol/day				
	Epinephrine Plasma: 0–70 ng/L	6.53	Epinephrine 0–380 pmol/L				
	Urine: 0–20 µg/day		0–109 nmol/day				
	Dopamine Plasma: 0–35 ng/L		Dopamine 0–230 pmol/L				
	Urine: 65–400 µg/day		425–2610 nmol/day				

CEA *(see Carcinoembryonic antigen)*

Ceruloplasmin 21–51 mg/dL 10 210–510 mg/L

Interday variation 10–15%. INC: Acute illness, smoking, exercise, hemoconcentration. DEC: Specimen storage. In pregnancy, increases by about 100% by 20 weeks. In children, 50% lower in neonates, rises rapidly to adult female levels, falls in males after puberty. Higher in females than males after puberty until before menopause. After age 50, increases slightly (average 10% higher).

INC: Malignancies, acute inflammation, biliary cirrhosis, trauma. DEC: Wilson's disease, cirrhosis, malnutrition, ovarian failure, nephrotic syndrome.

INC: Androgens, oral contraceptives, estrogens, phenytoin, phenobarbital, tamoxifen.

Used in patients with signs or symptoms suggestive of Wilson's disease. Test should not be done to screen for Wilson's disease if the patient is on drugs increasing ceruloplasmin, during pregnancy, or in acutely ill patients. Test is of little value in patients with chronic liver disease and low serum albumin, as all liver produced proteins will be low.

CH_{50} *(see Complement, total)*

Chloride 100–109 mEq/L 1 100–109 mmol/L

Interday variation 1%. INC: Ethanol. DEC: After meals, blindness. In females, slight increase just prior to menses. Decreases slightly after age 60 (average 2–3 mmol/L lower).

INC: Hypernatremia, renal tubular acidosis, diarrhea, primary hyperparathyroidism, respiratory alkalosis. DEC: Hyponatremia, vomiting, respiratory acidosis, metabolic alkalosis.

INC: Androgens, carbonic anhydrase inhibitors, cholestyramine, estrogens, drugs causing metabolic acidosis. DEC: Antacids, glucocorticoids, florinef, theophylline, drugs causing metabolic alkalosis.

Of little use in routine laboratory testing, typically follows sodium changes in hyponatremia and hypernatremia. Of most use in evaluation of acid-base disorders (see Chapter 4).

(continued)

Table 38.1 (continued)

Test Name	Reference Range			Nondisease Causes of Changes	Disease Related Changes	Drug Related Changes	Common Conditions for Use of Test
	Standard	Factor	SI Units				
Cholecalciferol (see Vitamin D)							
Cholesterol	Borderline high: >200 mg/dL, High: >240 mg/dL	0.0259	Borderline high: >5.18 mmol/L High: >6.22 mmol/L	Interday variation 5–7%. Higher in winter by 3–5%. INC: Smoking, hemoconcentration, stress, ethanol, blindness. DEC: Acute illness (falls up to 40%), exercise. In females, 10–20% lower in luteal phase of cycle, lowest during menstruation. In pregnancy, increases by 75% by the third trimester. In children, falls after puberty in males; levels before puberty are poorly predictive of adult levels. In adults, increases gradually (5–10 mg/dL per decade) until age 60, declines slightly after age 65. In females, may rise sharply after menopause.	INC: Hyperlipidemias, obstructive jaundice, nephrotic syndrome, hypothyroidism, chronic renal failure, diabetes. DEC: Lipoprotein deficiency states, cirrhosis, malignancies, malabsorption, malnutrition, megaloblastic anemia.	INC: Amiodarone, cyclosporine, glucocorticoids, phenothiazines, phenytoin, chlorthalidone, thiazides, aspirin, retinoids, some oral contraceptives, β-adrenergic antagonists. DEC: Chlorpropamide, haloperidol, estrogens, neomycin, thyroid hormones, ketoconazole, calcium channel blockers, hypolipidemic agents.	Used mainly to screen for risk of coronary artery disease; decisions on treatment should be based on LDL-cholesterol levels. Results are about 5% lower if the laboratory uses EDTA plasma instead of serum. Tests should never be done during periods of acute illness; results remain low for an average of 1–3 months.

Cholesterol, HDL (see High density lipoprotein cholesterol)
Cholesterol, LDL (see Low density lipoprotein cholesterol)
Cholinesterase, red cell (see Acetylcholinesterase)

Test Name	Standard	Factor	SI Units	Nondisease Causes of Changes	Disease Related Changes	Drug Related Changes	Common Conditions for Use of Test
Cholinesterase, plasma (pseudocholinesterase)	4.9–11.9 U/mL	1	4.9–11.9 kU/L	Interday variation 6%. INC: Ethanol. DEC: Inflammatory disorders, use of serum separator tubes or	INC: Nephrotic syndrome, breast cancer, increased triglycerides. DEC: Organophosphate exposure, acute and	DEC: Androgens, estrogens, glucocorticoids, H$_2$-blockers, lithium, oral contraceptives,	Used to detect cholinesterase variants with susceptibility to prolonged paralysis

Test	Conventional	Factor	SI	Physiological Influences	Disease Influences	Drug Influences	Comments
				anticoagulants. In children, values markedly decreased for first 6 months of life, reach values 40% over adult levels by 5 years, gradually decrease to reach adult levels at puberty.	chronic liver disease, malnutrition, inherited cholinesterase deficiency, tetanus.	phenothiazines, drugs causing liver damage.	after use of succinylcholine. Those showing abnormal inhibition by dibucaine or fluoride have increased effect. Also used to follow organophosphate poisoning recovery, but is less sensitive than acetylcholinesterase for detection of toxicity.
Chorionic gonadotrophin, human	Nonpregnant: <5 mIU/mL Values during pregnancy are found in Table 17.1	1	<5 IU/L	INC (urine): Proteinuria, urinary tract infection, hematuria, multiple gestations. DEC: 20% lower in pregnant smokers, dilute urine. Released in episodic spikes during first trimester of pregnancy. Gradually rises during first trimester, falls to a plateau by 16–20 weeks.	INC: Trophoblastic neoplasia, toxemia, germ cell tumors, breast carcinoma, rarely with other malignancies. DEC: Ectopic pregnancy, spontaneous abortion.	INC: Menopausal urine gonadotropins may cross-react.	Serum HCG becomes positive about the same times as urine HCG and is not needed to diagnose pregnancy. In ectopic pregnancy, the rate of doubling is >2 days in most cases, but <2 days in normal pregnancy. In miscarriage, levels fall. With hydatidiform mole, values often higher than in normal pregnancy; after therapy, fall with half-life of about 2 days.

(continued)

Table 38.1 *(continued)*

Test Name	Reference Range			Nondisease Causes of Changes	Disease Related Changes	Drug Related Changes	Common Conditions for Use of Test
	Standard	Factor	SI Units				
CK (see Creatine kinase)							
Cl (see Chloride)							
Complement component C3	50–90 mg/dL	10	0.5–0.9 g/L	Interday variation 6%. INC: Acute inflammation. DEC: Specimen storage. In pregnancy, increases an average of 25–30%. In adults, increases slightly (5%) by age 65.	INC: Infections, malignancies, diabetes, amyloidosis. DEC: Congenital deficiency, autoimmune disease, immune complex diseases, membranoproliferative glomerulonephritis, bacterial endocarditis, septicemia, cirrhosis.	INC: Oral contraceptives. DEC: Danazol.	Used to detect activation of complement through classic or alternate pathway. May be normal in patients with complement consumption who also have factors increasing complement production.
Complement component C4	10–40 mg/dL	10	100–400 mg/L	Interday variation 12%. INC: Acute inflammation. In pregnancy, increases an average of 25%.	INC: Infections, malignancies, diabetes, amyloidosis. DEC: Congenital deficiency, autoimmune disease, immune complex diseases, mixed cryoglobulinemia, bacterial endocarditis, septicemia, cirrhosis.	INC: Oral contraceptives. DEC: Danazol.	Used to detect activation of complement through classic pathway. May be normal in patients with complement consumption who also have factors increasing complement production.
Complement, total (CH_{50})	55–160%	0.01	0.55–1.6	INC: Acute inflammation. DEC: Collection in tubes containing EDTA or citrate. In pregnancy, increases an average of 25%.	INC: Infections, malignancies, diabetes, amyloidosis. DEC: Congenital deficiency, autoimmune disease, immune complex diseases, cirrhosis, membranoproliferative	INC: Oral contraceptives. DEC: Danazol.	Used to detect congenital deficiency of complement components other than C3 or C4. Not as sensitive as C3 or C4 to complement

CO (see Carboxyhemoglobin)

CO₂, blood (see pCO₂)

CO₂ content (see Bicarbonate)

Test	Conventional	Factor	SI	Physiologic/Other Factors	Disease States	Drugs	Comments
					glomerulonephritis, bacterial endocarditis, septicemia, malnutrition.		consumption, not useful as routine test if C3 and C4 levels are available.
Copper	70–155 µg/dL Urine: <60 µg/day	0.157 0.0157	11–24 µmol/L <0.94 µmol/day	Interday variation 5%. Lowest in AM, highest in mid-afternoon. INC: Hemoconcentration, after meals, acute inflammation, anemia, ethanol, proteinuria (urine). DEC: Heavy exercise, vegetarian diet. In pregnancy, increases gradually up to 2 × basal by 20 weeks, remains elevated during lactation. In neonates, about 33% of adult values, reaches adult levels by 4–5 months. In adults, peaks about age 60 (averages 10–20% higher). Higher in females than males.	INC: Infections, leukemia, malignancies, thyroid disease, autoimmune disease. DEC: Wilson's disease, malabsorption, pancreatic insufficiency, malnutrition, ovarian failure, nephrotic syndrome, renal insufficiency (urine).	INC: Oral contraceptives, estrogens, carbamazepine, phenytoin, phenobarbital. DEC: Penicillamine.	Serum copper generally used to screen for Wilson's disease, adds little to measurement of ceruloplasmin; the same factors affecting ceruloplasmin also affect serum copper. Urine copper is less affected than serum copper or ceruloplasmin, but will be adversely affected by renal disease.

(continued)

Table 38.1 *(continued)*

Corticotropin (see Adrenocorticotropic hormone)

Test Name	Reference Range			Nondisease Causes of Changes	Disease Related Changes	Drug Related Changes	Common Conditions for Use of Test
	Standard	Factor	SI Units				
Cortisol	8 AM: 5–25 μg/dL 4 PM: <9 μg/dL 11 PM: <5 μg/dL Urine Free: 10–90 μg/day	27.6 2.76	140–690 μmol/L <260 μmol/L <140 μmol/L Urine Free: 28–250 nmol/day	Interday variation 15%. Highest near time of rising, lowest around 4 AM; in persons working nights, pattern changes. INC: Stress, exercise, fasting, ethanol (both urine and serum); obesity, smoking, upright posture, hemoconcentration (serum only). DEC: Blindness. In pregnancy, increases 2× by 20 weeks, 2× more by term. About 20% lower in neonates, reaches adult levels by 2 months.	INC: Cushing's syndrome, acute inflammation, malignancy, following surgery (up to 2–3× normal), critical illness (up to 10× normal); diurnal pattern lost or blunted in all of these states. DEC: Addison's disease, secondary adrenal insufficiency, congenital adrenal hyperplasia, respiratory distress syndrome of the newborn.	INC: Amphetamines, carbamazepine, estrogens, oral contraceptives, RU 486, vasopressin, tricyclic antidepressants; licorice, oral contraceptives increase urine free cortisol. DEC: Some glucocorticoids, lithium, L-dopa, megestrol acetate, clonidine, ketoconazole, danazol, ephedrine; diuretics, ketoconazole decrease urine free cortisol.	Serum and urine used to screen for adrenal disease. For Cushing's disease, urine free cortisol more sensitive than plasma cortisol. Lack of diurnal variation occurs in Cushing's syndrome, acute illness; cortisol at 11 PM is more sensitive for Cushing's syndrome. For adrenal insufficiency, plasma values >20 μg/dL rule out the diagnosis. Dynamic tests are usually needed to fully evaluate adrenal cortical function.
Cortrosyn stimulation test	Peak: >20 μg/dL Increment: >7 μg/dL	27.6	>550 μmol/L >190 μmol/L	Interday variation 10%. Lower in the afternoon and evening than in the morning. INC: Stress.	INC: Cushing's syndrome, acute inflammation, malignancy. DEC: Addison's disease, secondary adrenal insufficiency, congenital adrenal hyperplasia, iron deficiency.	DEC: Ketoconazole, long term synthetic glucocorticoids.	Used to recognize adrenal suppression or insufficiency. In the normal test, 250 ng of cortrosyn (synthetic ACTH) is given as a bolus; cortisol is drawn at baseline, 30, and 60 minutes. In a

normal response, both increment and peak will be above criteria. In secondary adrenal insufficiency or moderate dose glucocorticoid therapy, a normal response may occur. A lower dose of cortrosyn (1 ng) produces the same response in normal persons, but improves sensitivity for adrenal dysfunction.

Test					Comments
C-Peptide (Insulin)	Serum: 0.5–3.0 µg/L	33.3	17–100 nmol/L	Interday variation 10%. INC: After meals, obesity. Increases with age >60. Higher in Hispanics than in whites.	INC: Type II diabetes, insulinoma, renal failure. DEC: Pancreatic insufficiency, type I diabetes, insulin administration.	Same as for insulin. Used to assess insulin production. In type I diabetes, will be reduced, even in face of hyperglycemia, following meals, or after glucagon injection. In hypoglycemia, used to distinguish endogenous insulin production from insulin injection (will be low in the latter). Use of oral hypoglycemic agents also increases C-peptide. Should only be done in fasting state for insulinoma work-up.

(continued)

Table 38.1 *(continued)*

CPK (see Creatine kinase)

Test Name	Reference Range			Nondisease Causes of Changes	Disease Related Changes	Drug Related Changes	Common Conditions for Use of Test
	Standard	Factor	SI Units				
C-Reactive protein (CRP)	0–0.5 mg/dL	10	0–5 mg/L	INC: Smoking exercise. Increased in pregnancy, doubles during labor. Lower in neonates (only 0.05× adult levels)	INC: Acute inflammation, bacterial infections, malignancy, trauma, following surgery, renal failure. DEC: Liver disease, malnutrition.	INC: Estrogens, oral contraceptives.	Used to recognize the presence of inflammation in a variety of settings, particularly bacterial infections and autoimmune disease. Rises more rapidly than erythrocyte sedimentation rate, roughly correlates with severity of inflammation.
Creatine kinase (CK, CPK)	M: 50–300 U/L F: 30–200 U/L	1	M: 50–300 U/L F: 30–200 U/L	Interday variation 20–30%. INC: Exercise, IM injection, cardioversion, respiratory distress, coughing. DEC: Inactivity, EDTA or citrate containing tubes. In pregnancy, falls to a low at about 12 weeks. In children, upper normal limits increase in adolescence, remain higher in young adults (up to about 2–3× adult levels). Levels decrease with age, average about 20–30% lower after age 60. Higher (50–100%) in blacks than in whites.	INC: Muscle trauma, myopathies, rhabdomyolysis, muscular dystrophy, myocardial infarction, hypothyroidism, nephrotic syndrome, diabetic ketoacidosis, malignant hyperthermia, neuroleptic malignant syndrome, following surgery, psychoses. DEC: Malnutrition, hyperthyroidism.	INC: Drugs injuring skeletal muscle. DEC: Prednisone.	Most commonly used to recognize skeletal muscle injury or myocardial infarction, although CK MB is more specific for myocardial injury than total CK. Because of many non-disease states affecting CK, a rise in CK is more indicative of muscle injury than total CK; values up to 30× normal can occur after strenuous exercise, and up to 10× normal after IM injection.

Test						
Creatine kinase isoenzyme	96–100% CK MM 0–4% CK MB 0% CK BB	0.01	0.96–1.0 CK MM 0–0.04 CK MB 0 CK BB	INC: CK MB in respiratory distress, ethanol, strenuous exercise. In pregnancy, increased CK BB in the third trimester. In neonates, increased CK MB and CK BB in neonates (up to 5% CK MB, up to 12% CK BB). An abnormal isoenzyme (macro CK-1) occurs with increasing age (up to 1% of patients >60 years).	INC (CK MB): Myocardial infarction, chronic myopathies, renal failure, hypothyroidism. INC (CK BB): Intestinal ischemia, severe brain trauma, malignancy (usually prostate, GI tract, small cell carcinoma of lung). INC (macro CK-1): AIDS, autoimmune disease.	INC (CK MB): Drugs causing skeletal muscle injury.

All CK isoenzymes can only be quantified by electrophoresis. Used in patients with elevated CK of uncertain etiology. Less sensitive than measurement of CK MB by immunoassay to detect myocardial infarction.

Test						
Creatine kinase MB isoenzyme	0–5 ng/mL Relative Index <2.5	1	0–5 µg/L Relative Index <2.5	Interday variation 15–30%. INC: Respiratory distress, ethanol, strenuous exercise. Increased in neonates.	INC: Myocardial infarction, myocarditis, cardiac contusion, chronic myopathies, renal failure, hypothyroidism, skeletal muscle injury (total CK MB, not relative index).	INC: Drugs injuring skeletal muscle (total CK MB, not relative index).

Immunoassay specific for CK MB, used to diagnose myocardial infarction. Use of relative index improves specificity for myocardial injury. Some laboratories still measure CK MB by immunoinhibition assay, which gives frequent false positive results (hemolysis, liver disease, CK BB, macro CK-1); this can be recognized by CK MB reported in U/L. Remains elevated for 24–36 hours following myocardial infarction or injury.

(continued)

Table 38.1 *(continued)*

Test Name	Reference Range			Nondisease Causes of Changes	Disease Related Changes	Drug Related Changes	Common Conditions for Use of Test
	Standard	Factor	SI Units				
Creatinine	0.7–1.5 mg/dL Urine: 1–2 g/day	88.4 8.8	62–133 µmol/L 8.8–17.6 mmol/day	Interday variation 15–20%. Up to 30% higher in PM than in AM. INC: Strenuous exercise, following meat ingestion, fasting. DEC: Vegetarian diet. In pregnancy, 30% lower by 12 weeks, 20% lower by the third trimester. In children, near adult levels in neonates, falls to about 25–50% of adult levels by 2 months, gradually rises to adult levels during adolescence. Urine creatinine rises during childhood and decreases gradually after age 30. Higher in males than females and in blacks than whites.	INC: Renal insufficiency and failure, acromegaly, hyperthyroidism, rhabdomyolysis, dehydration. DEC: Malnutrition, water intoxication, inappropriate antidiuresis.	INC: Nephrotoxic agents; cimetidine, aspirin, trimethoprim-sulfamethoxazole (all inhibit tubular secretion of creatinine).	Used along with BUN to evaluate renal function (see comments under BUN). Because creatinine production decreases with age, similar creatinine values indicate worse renal function in older individuals; can estimate creatinine clearance from serum creatinine and patient age using formula in Chapter 6. In some assays, ketones and cephalosporine may cross-react, causing falsely increased creatinine in ketoacidosis or antibiotic therapy.
Creatinine clearance	M: 90–150 mL/min F: 70–120 mL/min	1	M: 90–150 mL/min F: 70–120 mL/min	Interday variation 10–15%. INC: High protein intake. DEC: Vegetarian diet, low protein intake, heavy exercise. Increases in pregnancy by up to 50% in the first trimester, remains elevated until term. In females, 20% higher in	INC: Early diabetes, anemia. DEC: Renal insufficiency and failure, dehydration, congestive heart failure, shock, hepatorenal syndrome.	INC: Furosemide, glucocorticoids. DEC: Nephrotoxic agents, cimetidine, aspirin, trimethoprim-sulfamethoxazole, diazoxide, thiazides.	Requires collection of 24 hour urine and measurement of plasma creatinine during collection. Calculated using the formulas in Chapter 6. Will overestimate true glomerular filtration

Test	Reference value	Factor	SI units	Physiological variation	In vivo effects	Drugs	Comments
				luteal phase than at menses. In children, about 1/2 adult levels in neonates, falls to about 1/3 of adult levels in first year, slowly increases to about 2/3 of adult levels by puberty. After age 30, falls by 5–10 mL/min per decade.			rate; degree of overestimation increases as renal insufficiency worsens.
Cu (see Copper)							
D-Dimer (see also Fibrin degradation products)	<100 ng/mL	1	<100 µg/L	INC: Thrombocytopenia. Increases during pregnancy.	INC: Disseminated intravascular coagulation, arterial or venous thrombi, inflammatory disorders (slightly increased), malignancy, postsurgery.	INC: Tissue plasminogen activator, streptokinase.	D-Dimer is a major breakdown product of fibrin; its presence indicates fibrin formation and lysis. Most commonly used to recognize DIC.
Dehydroepiandrosterone sulfate	M: 800–5,600 µg/L F: 350–4,300 µg/L	0.0026	M: 2.1–14.6 µmol/L F: 0.9–11.2 µmol/L	Interday variation 1% in males, 5% in females. Highest in AM, lowest in PM. INC: Exercise, fasting, smoking. DEC: Ethanol, weight loss. In pregnancy, decreases 50% by 20 weeks, then stable until term. In children, markedly decreased after 1 month, low until adolescence, reaches adult levels by 20 years. In adults, gradually decreases after age 40 to about 20% of adult levels by age 80 years. Higher in blacks than whites.	INC: Cushing's syndrome, congenital adrenal hyperplasia, polycystic ovary syndrome. DEC: Adrenal insufficiency, malnutrition, acute illness.	INC: Clomiphene, danazol. DEC: Glucocorticoids, carbamazepine, phenytoin, ketoconazole, oral contraceptives.	Used to evaluate patients with hirsutism, represents adrenal androgen production. Mildly elevated levels often seen with polycystic ovary syndrome. Marked elevations usually indicate adrenal sources (tumor, congenital hyperplasia).

(continued)

Table 38.1 *(continued)*

Test Name	Reference Range			Nondisease Causes of Changes	Disease Related Changes	Drug Related Changes	Common Conditions for Use of Test
	Standard	Factor	SI Units				
Deoxypyridinoline (see Pyridinoline cross-links)							
Dexamethasone suppression effect on urine free cortisol	2 mg/day: <20 mg/day; 8 mg/day: <20% of basal in Cushing's disease	2.8; 1	2 mg/day: <56 mmol/L; 8 mg/day: <20% of basal in Cushing's disease	Nonsuppressed (2 mg/day): Ethanol withdrawal.	Nonsuppressed: Ectopic ACTH production, adrenal tumors.		Used in differential diagnosis of patients with Cushing's syndrome; cortisol production rate falls with Cushing's disease (pituitary ACTH overproduction), but not in other causes. In Cushing's disease, may require larger doses to demonstrate a fall in cortisol production.
Dexamethasone suppression, overnight effect on AM cortisol	<5 μg/dL	27.6	<140 nmol/L	Nonsuppressed: Obesity, stress, pregnancy, ethanol.	Nonsuppressed: Cushing's syndrome, infections, malignancy, renal failure, malabsorption, depression, acute illness.	Nonsuppressed: Phenytoin.	Used as screening test for Cushing's syndrome; detects virtually all cases, but has many false positive results. Suppression effectively rules out Cushing's syndrome. May produce more false positive than urine free cortisol, but easier to perform.

DHEA-S (see Dehydroepiandrosterone sulfate)

1,25-Dihydroxycholecalciferol (see Vitamin D, 1,25-dihydroxyl)

Dopamine (see Catecholamines)

Epinephrine (see Catecholamines)

Test	Reference interval	Factor	Reference interval	Physiological variation	Disease/condition effects	Drug effects	Comments
Erythrocyte sedimentation rate	M: 0–15 mm/h F: 0–20 mm/h	1	M: 0–15 mm/h F: 0–20 mm/h	Interday variation 10 mm/h for males and 18 mm/h for females. Highest in afternoon. INC: Ethanol, high cholesterol or fibrinogen. In pregnancy, increases markedly after the second trimester. In males, increases with increasing age; in females, falls with increasing age.	INC: Inflammation, infection, malignancy, multiple myeloma. DEC: Abnormal red cell shapes, low fibrinogen, polycythemia vera, congestive heart failure.	INC: Dextran, oral contraceptives, vitamin A. DEC: Glucocorticoids, cyclophosphamide, tamoxifen.	Used to evaluate the activity of inflammatory response. Subject to more interferences than is C-reactive protein, which is more commonly used in Europe. Is usually available readily in most laboratories, however, where CRP measurements are less commonly available.
Erythropoietin	0–32.6 mIU/mL	1	0–32.6 IU/L	Lowest in early afternoon, increases to peak around midnight; 60% intraday variation. INC: Exercise, high altitude, smoking. Increases 100% during pregnancy. In children, highest in neonates, decreases to adult levels by age 4 years. Increases after age 60 years.	INC: Anemia due to red cell destruction or lack of production, chronic hypoxemia, erythropoietin producing tumors (renal, hepatic primarily), high oxygen affinity hemoglobin, renal transplant rejection, toxemia. DEC: Renal failure, malignancy, chronic inflammation, polycythemia vera.	INC: Androgens. DEC: Angiotensin converting enzyme inhibitors, amphotericin.	Most commonly used in evaluation of polycythemia; increased values seen in all secondary polycythemia, but low values occur in polycythemia vera. Also used in patients with chronic anemia and low reticulocyte count to determine if erythropoietin therapy will be effective; values <15–20× normal usually benefit from erythropoietin therapy.

(continued)

Table 38.1 *(continued)*

Test Name	Reference Range			Nondisease Causes of Changes	Disease Related Changes	Drug Related Changes	Common Conditions for Use of Test
	Standard	Factor	SI Units				
ESR (see Erythrocyte sedimentation rate)							
Estradiol	M, post-menopausal F: 10–60 ng/L Menstruating F: <400 ng/L	3.67 0.0037	37–220 pmol/L <1.45 nmol/L	Interday variation 25%. Highest in late afternoon, 50% greater than lowest values at night. INC: Smoking (in males). DEC: Heavy exercise, low fat diet, serum separator gels. In menstruating females, rises during follicular phase with sharp peak 2–3 days before ovulation, then a later rise in mid-luteal phase. In pregnancy, increases markedly during latter half. In children, very low until puberty, gradually rises to adult levels by late pubertal period. Increases with age over 55 in males. In females, begins to decline after about age 35.	INC: Estrogen producing tumors, cirrhosis, hyperthyroidism, gynecomastia. DEC: Hypogonadism, hypopituitarism, malnutrition, acute illness, toxemia.	INC: Clomiphene, tamoxifen. DEC: Oral contraceptives, ketoconazole, megestrol; cimetidine decreases mid-cycle peak.	Most commonly used in evaluation of infertility or during attempted assisted fertilization to assure adequate estrogen production. Also used in males with gynecomastia. Significantly lower results when collected in tubes containing separator gels.
Estriol	Nonpregnant: <2 ng/mL	3.47	<7 nmol/L	High random diurnal variation (50%), even for samples 5–15 min apart; highest about noon. INC: Hemoconcentration, multiple gestations. DEC: High altitude, smoking. In pregnancy, continuous slow rise in the first two trimesters, rapid increase during the third trimester (1 ng/mL per week).	DEC: (in pregnancy) intrauterine growth retardation, hemolytic disease of the newborn, fetal distress, anencephaly, toxemia, chromosomal abnormalities.	INC: Glucocorticoids (in pregnancy), spironolactone (in males). DEC: Ampicillin, penicillin, aspirin, probenecid, thyroxine, albuterol (most effects seen only in pregnancy).	RIA: Most commonly used to evaluate fetal well being during pregnancy, although less useful than clinical evaluation because of wide variation in values. Also used along with α-fetoprotein and β-HCG to detect fetuses with chromosome abnormalities.

Ethanol (alcohol, ethyl)	<10 mg/dL	0.22	<2 mmol/L	INC: Use of ethanol swabs to clean skin; may be falsely increased with delayed analysis and bacterial contamination, with ingestion of other alcohols. DEC: Delayed separation.	INC: Ethanol intoxication.	Used to detect ethanol intoxication; a rough correlation exists between levels and degree of impairment (see Table 19.2). In many states, reported as the relative concentration which equals result in mg/dL divided by 1,000.
Factor VIII antigen (see Von Willebrand factor)						
Factor VIII procoagulant	0.01		0.5–1.5 U/mL	INC: Strenuous exercise, stress, ethanol. In pregnancy, increases 100% during last trimester.	INC: Acute inflammation, cirrhosis, renal failure. DEC: Hemophilia A, Von Willebrand's disease, DIC.	INC: Desmopressin, epinephrine. DEC: Heparin, tissue plasminogen activator, streptokinase.	Used in patients with prolonged PTT, particularly if present in childhood, to evaluate for hemophilia A and Von Willebrand's disease.

(continued)

Table 38.1 *(continued)*

Test Name	Reference Range			Nondisease Causes of Changes	Disease Related Changes	Drug Related Changes	Common Conditions for Use of Test
	Standard	Factor	SI Units				
Fat, fecal	0–7 g/day	1	0–7 g/day	DEC: Low fat diet.	INC: Malabsorption, pancreatic insufficiency, cirrhosis, obstructive jaundice, hyperthyroidism, adrenal insufficiency, pernicious anemia.	INC: Aspirin (high doses), cholestipol, cholestyramine, nonabsorbable antibiotics.	Used to diagnose malabsorption; will be increased in intestinal, pancreatic, or biliary disorders. Requires a relatively standardized fat intake and collection of stool for 72 hours to adjust for marked interday variation in fat excretion. Semi-quantitative estimation of fat droplets after fat stains is slightly less sensitive but significantly easier to accomplish.
Fe (see Iron)							
Ferritin	M: 30–284 ng/mL F: 10–120 ng/mL	1	M: 30–284 µg/L F: 10–120 µg/L	Interday variation 10–20%. INC: Fasting, ethanol. DEC: Heavy exercise. In pregnancy, decreases gradually, 50% lower by 20 weeks, 70% lower by the third trimester. In children, increased 2–3× by first month of life, falls to near adult levels by 2 months, then similar to adult female	INC: Hemochromatosis, acute hepatitis, alcoholic liver disease, malignancy, acute inflammation, acute leukemia. DEC: Iron deficiency, celiac disease.	INC: Oral contraceptives.	Used to document iron deficiency. Test is quite useful in otherwise healthy individuals, but often increased by tissue injury from infection, inflammation, and malignancy, which can mask iron deficiency. While

Fetal hemoglobin (see Hemoglobin F)

Test	Conventional		SI		
				levels throughout childhood and adolescence. In adults, increases with age.	high levels occur with hemochromatosis, ferritin is not as sensitive as transferrin saturation for early detection.
α-Fetoprotein	0–8.9 ng/mL	1	0–8.9 µg/L	During pregnancy, increases gradually to reach values 6–8× normal by 20 weeks. In children, markedly elevated in neonates (20,000 ng/mL), falls to adult levels by 1–2 years.	INC: Acute or chronic hepatitis, hepatocellular carcinoma, hepatoblastoma, germ cell tumors; other malignancies (rarely). In pregnancy, increased levels occur with multiple gestations, incorrect dates, fetal neural tube defects, fetal abdominal wall defects, fetal death. DEC: In pregnancy, low levels are associated with trophoblastic neoplasia, trisomies.	Most commonly used to screen for fetal abnormalities during pregnancy; accurate information on duration of pregnancy, maternal weight, race, and diabetes must be provided to the laboratory (see Chapter 17). Also used to screen high risk individuals for hepatocellular carcinoma, and for monitoring patients with liver tumors or germ cell tumors.

(continued)

Table 38.1 *(continued)*

Test Name	Reference Range			Nondisease Causes of Changes	Disease Related Changes	Drug Related Changes	Common Conditions for Use of Test
	Standard	Factor	SI Units				
Fibrinogen	200–400 mg/dL	10	2–4 g/L	Highest at noon, lowest at midnight. INC: Acute illness, obesity. DEC: Exercise, ethanol, unsaturated fatty acids. In pregnancy, increases 25% by 12 weeks, 50% by third trimester. In females, highest during menstruation.	INC: Acute inflammation or infection, malignancy, nephrotic syndrome. DEC: Cirrhosis, liver failure, DIC, malnutrition.	INC: Aspirin, estrogens, oral contraceptives. DEC: Androgens, valproic acid.	Usually measured by clotting assays; immunoassays may produce false elevations in patients with abnormally functioning fibrinogen (dysfibrinogenemia). Often estimated with prothrombin time (semi-quantitative fibrinogen, SQF), which is accurate enough for most uses, but will not detect dysfibrinogenemia.
Fibrin split products (FSP) (see also D-Dimer)	<10 μg/mL	1	<10 mg/L	INC: Failure of specimens to clot completely, as often occurs in patients receiving heparin or thrombolytic agents; prolonged tourniquet use, excess shaking of tube. In pregnancy, increases gradually after 20 weeks.	INC: Disseminated intravascular coagulation, arterial or venous thrombosis, infection, inflammation, malignancy, cirrhosis, toxemia.	INC: Tissue plasminogen activator, streptokinase, heparin.	Used to recognize production and breakdown of fibrin, most commonly in DIC. Test is less specific than the D-dimer test, as failure of specimen to clot will give false increases in FSP but not in D-dimer.

Test	Reference	Conversion factor	SI units	Physiologic factors	Disease/condition factors	Drug factors	Comments
							Rheumatoid factor can agglutinate the latex beads used to detect the split products and can produce false elevations.
Foam stability test	Mature: >47	1	Mature: >47	INC: Blood, meconium contamination of amniotic fluid.	INC: Mature infants; hypoxemia, hypothermia, hypoglycemia produce high values in immature infants. DEC: Immature fetus (respiratory distress syndrome).		Used as bedside test for fetal lung maturity. Not as sensitive as phosphatidyl glycerol for presence of surfactant.
Folate	Serum: 3–13 ng/mL RBC: 150–600 ng/mL	2.27	6.8–29.5 nmol/L 340–1,560 nmol/L	Highest in winter, lower in summer. INC: Vegetarian diet, recent folate intake (serum folate). DEC: Smoking, ethanol, malnutrition. In pregnancy, decreases by 10%. In children, falls to 30–50% of adult levels by age 1 year, remains low throughout adolescence.	INC: Vitamin B_{12} deficiency (serum folate), viral hepatitis. DEC: Folate deficiency, malnutrition, malabsorption, hemolytic anemia, malignancy; vitamin B_{12} deficiency (RBC folate).	INC: Phenformin. DEC: Anticonvulsants, folic acid antagonists, colchicine, oral contraceptives, isoniazid, triamterene, aspirin, estrogens, pentamidine, antacids, trimethoprim.	Used to diagnose folate deficiency as a cause of anemia. RBC folate is generally more reliable than serum folate, except in vitamin B_{12} deficiency or early folate deficiency; however, serum folate is rapidly affected by normal intake. Because anemia and macrocytosis develop rapidly after RBC folate becomes low, folate is not a useful test in nonpregnant patients who are not anemic.

(continued)

Table 38.1 *(continued)*

Test Name	Reference Range			Nondisease Causes of Changes	Disease Related Changes	Drug Related Changes	Common Conditions for Use of Test
	Standard	Factor	SI Units				
Follicle stimulating hormone	1–14 mIU/mL Postmenopausal F: 34–96 mIU/mL	1	1–14 IU/L 34–96 IU/L	Interday variation 40%. Pulsatile release during day (50% variation). DEC: Obesity, malnutrition. In menstruating females, spikes at mid-cycle. In children, low during childhood, increases at adolescence. Suppressed during pregnancy and lactation. Increases markedly after menopause.	INC: Gonadal failure, Kleinfelter's syndrome, ethanol abuse. DEC: Hypopituitarism, hypogonadotrophic hypogonadism, acute illness, increased prolactin.	INC: Cimetidine, L-dopa, clomiphene, ketoconazole. DEC: Anticonvulsants, glucocorticoids, oral contraceptives, estrogens, gonadotropin-releasing hormone analogues, megestrol, phenothiazines.	Used in evaluation of hypogonadism; should be increased in primary gonadal failure, while should be decreased with pituitary or hypothalamic disease. Ratio of FSH:LH usually <1:2 in polycystic ovary syndrome, usually >1 in most other states. Should always be collected as multiple samples (combining serum) in males and premenopausal females.

Free erythrocyte protoporphyrin (see Protoporphyrin, zinc)
Free thyroxine (see Thyroxine, free)

| **Fructosamine** | 174–286 mmol/L | 1 | 174–286 mmol/L | Interday variation 8%. INC: High IgA. DEC: Low serum albumin, obesity, heparin Decreases by 20% during pregnancy. Lower in infants, increases to adult levels by 6 years. | INC: Diabetes mellitus, renal failure, hypothyroidism. DEC: Nephrotic syndrome, diabetic nephropathy, hyperthyroidism. | | Used to follow short term (1–2 week) diabetic control. Preferred test for monitoring diabetic treatment during pregnancy, or when short term changes in glucose control need to be assessed. Little data on values indicating good control and |

Gamma-glutamyl transferase (see γ-Glutamyl transferase)

G6PD (see Glucose-6-phosphate dehydrogenase)

				likelihood of diabetic complications. Not useful in patients with proteinuria.
Gastrin	<100 ng/L	1	Lowest in early AM, 3× higher by evening, 90% fall in values during night. INC: After meals, caffeine, *Helicobacter pylori* infection. In children, highest at birth, gradually decreases to adult levels. Increases after age 60 years.	INC: Zollinger-Ellison syndrome, atrophic gastritis, pernicious anemia, chronic renal failure, hyperthyroidism, hyperparathyroidism. DEC: Hypothyroidism.	INC: Calcium, catecholamines, cimetidine, insulin, omeprazole, ranitidine. DEC: Atropine, lithium, octreotide.	Used to diagnose Zollinger-Ellison syndrome. High gastrin in the face of acid production strongly suggests the diagnosis. Patients with high gastrin levels should always have gastric pH checked to rule out atrophic gastritis. Gastrin levels increase after calcium or secretin administration with pancreatic tumors producing gastrin, but will not increase significantly in most other states.

(continued)

Table 38.1 *(continued)*

Test Name	Reference Range			Nondisease Causes of Changes	Disease Related Changes	Drug Related Changes	Common Conditions for Use of Test
	Standard	Factor	SI Units				
GGT (see γ-Glutamyl transferase)							
GH (see Growth hormone)							
Glucose	65–115 mg/dL	0.055	3.6–6.4 mmol/L	Interday variation 5–10%, higher for postprandial glucose. INC: Stress, after meals, mild exercise, ethanol, smoking. DEC: Prolonged exercise, fever, prolonged fasting, delayed separation of serum from red cells. In pregnancy, fasting about 10% lower; postprandial glucose slightly higher. Postprandial (but not fasting) glucose increases with increasing age.	INC: Diabetes mellitus, hyperthyroidism, Cushing's disease, acromegaly, pheochromocytoma, acute illness. DEC: Insulin producing tumor, adrenal insufficiency, growth hormone deficiency, hypopituitarism, renal failure, sepsis, liver failure, rare tumors producing IGF-2.	INC: Thiazides, phenothiazines, caffeine, estrogens, epinephrine, glucocorticoids, lithium. DEC: Anabolic steroids, amphetamines, pentamidine, propranolol.	Plasma glucose used to screen for and monitor diabetes mellitus. Bedside glucose instruments often inaccurate in patients with decreased or increased pO_2 or hematocrit, and are affected by inadequate amount of blood or improper storage of reagents. CSF glucose used in evaluation for meningeal diseases; will be low in bacterial, sometimes with fungal meningitis, and also with metastatic carcinomas to the meninges. Values for CSF glucose are based on normal plasma glucose; CSF glucose will average 50–75% of plasma glucose up to plasma vales of 300 mg/dL; above
	CSF: 45–80 mg/dL		2.5–4.4 mmol/L				

this point, CSF glucose will not rise as rapidly as plasma. When plasma glucose is rapidly changing, as in diabetics, CSF glucose takes 6–8 hours to reflect new stable plasma glucose concentrations and will be difficult to interpret during the intervening time period.

| Glucose tolerance test | See Figure 7.3 | Increase in glucose lower in afternoon than morning. Improved tolerance: Smoking. Worsened tolerance: Ethanol, mental stress, inactivity, low carbohydrate intake. In normal pregnancy, glucose tolerance worsens in second trimester. | Improved tolerance: Malabsorption, adrenal insufficiency, hypothyroidism, hypopituitarism. Worsened tolerance: Diabetes mellitus, hyperthyroidism, pheochromocytoma, acromegaly, cirrhosis, infections, acute illness. | Improved tolerance: Phenytoin. Worsened tolerance: B blockers, calcium channel blockers, chlorthalidone, danazol, estrogens, glucocorticoids, lithium, oral contraceptives, thiazides. | Used to diagnose diabetes in children and during pregnancy; seldom needed to diagnose diabetes in adults. Patient must be properly prepared before performing test; results must be abnormal on two or more occasions (except during pregnancy). |

(continued)

Table 38.1 *(continued)*

Test Name	Reference Range			Nondisease Causes of Changes	Disease Related Changes	Drug Related Changes	Common Conditions for Use of Test
	Standard	Factor	SI Units				
Glucose-6-phosphate dehydrogenase	7.9–16.3 U/g Hgb	0.065	0.52–1.04 MU/mol Hgb	INC: Reticulocytosis. Higher in neonates by 50%.	INC: Hemolytic anemia. DEC: Congenital deficiency.	INC: Drugs causing hemolysis in G6PD deficient persons.	Used to detect deficiency of this enzyme as a cause of hemolytic anemia. Hemolysis in the African form usually follows exposure to oxidant drugs such as quinolines, quinidine. In the Mediterranean form, hemolysis may occur with lesser stresses. As enzyme activity is higher in younger cells (especially in the African form), levels will be higher and may be normal immediately after an episode of hemolysis; testing should be deferred.

Glutamic acid decarboxylase antibodies (see Antiglutamic acid decarboxylase)

Test Name	Reference Range			Nondisease Causes of Changes	Disease Related Changes	Drug Related Changes	Common Conditions for Use of Test
	Standard	Factor	SI Units				
γ-Glutamyl transferase	M: 11–49 U/L F: 7–32 U/L	1	M: 11–49 U/L F: 7–32 U/L	Interday variation 8–15%. INC: Ethanol, obesity, smoking. DEC: Exercise. In pregnancy, about 15–20% lower in first trimester, near normal in third trimester. In neonates, 2–3× higher, falls to levels 50% lower than adult during	INC: Obstructive jaundice, hepatitis, cirrhosis, metastatic cancer to liver, prostate cancer, pancreatitis, hyperthyroidism, diabetes. DEC: Hypothyroidism.	INC: Barbiturates, carbamazepine, estrogens, heparin, oral contraceptives, phenytoin, primidone, propoxyphene. DEC: Ascorbic acid, fibric acids.	Used to confirm source of elevated alkaline phosphatase; less expensive but not as accurate as alkaline phosphatase isoenzymes. Often used to detect ethanol abuse,

Test			Physiological factors	Disease states	Drug effects	Comments
			childhood, reaches adult levels in adolescence. Increases 20% with age up to 60 years.			although only 70% of ethanol abusers show increased GGT. Often used as a general screen for liver disease; highly sensitive, but many false positive results.

Glycated (glycosylated) hemoglobin (see Hemoglobin A$_1$c)

Test			Physiological factors	Disease states	Drug effects	Comments
Growth hormone	<6.5 µg/L	1 <6.5 µg/L	Highest just after sleep; released in episodic spikes during the day. Highest in fall, lowest in spring. INC: After protein meals, hypoglycemia, stress, exercise, starvation. DEC: Obesity, hyperglycemia. In pregnancy, decreases. In children, 2–3× higher during adolescence. In adults, decreases with increasing age. Responsiveness to stimuli decreases with increasing age.	INC: Acromegaly, gigantism, Laron dwarfism, renal failure, cirrhosis, anorexia nervosa, diabetes. DEC: Hypopituitarism, Cushing's syndrome, acute illness.	INC: Amphetamines, clonidine, desipramine, diazepam, estrogens, glucocorticoids (short term), indomethacin, L-dopa, propranolol, phenytoin, valproic acid. DEC: Bromcriptine, glucocorticoids (long term), octreotide, phenothiazines, probucol.	Used to recognize growth hormone excess or deficiency. Basal levels are usually not adequate to identify abnormalities. IGF-1 is more useful as a screening test and to follow therapy of excess growth hormone. To evaluate growth hormone deficiency, must show failure of GH to rise in response to two stimuli (sleep, L-dopa, insulin hypoglycemia, arginine, clonidine, or GHRH). For growth hormone excess, will fail to suppress with hyperglycemia.

(continued)

Table 38.1 *(continued)*

| Test Name | Reference Range | | | Nondisease Causes of Changes | Disease Related Changes | Drug Related Changes | Common Conditions for Use of Test |
	Standard	Factor	SI Units				
Haptoglobin	50–320 mg/dL	0.01	0.5–3.2 g/L	Interday variation 20%. INC: Exercise, ethanol. In children, low in neonates, rises to near adult levels by 6 months. Increases by average of 100% from young to old adults.	INC: Acute inflammation, infections, nephrotic syndrome, obstructive jaundice, malignancies. DEC: Hemolytic anemia, cirrhosis, malnutrition.	INC: Androgens, glucocorticoids. DEC: Estrogens, oral contraceptives, tamoxifen, drugs causing hemolysis.	Used to document hemolysis. Because genetic variants affect absolute levels, best used by demonstrating a change in concentration (either fall from previous or rise to normal after recovery from suspected hemolysis). About 5% of blacks congenitally lack haptoglobin.

HCG (see Chorionic gonadotropin, human)

HDL Cholesterol (see High density lipoprotein cholesterol)

Hematocrit	M: 39–49% F: 35–45%	0.01	M: 0.39–0.49 F: 0.35–0.45	Interday variation 3%. Highest in AM, lowest in PM. INC: Hemoconcentration, high altitude, exercise, upright posture. DEC: Supine posture. In pregnancy, decreases 10%. In children, up to 25% higher in neonates, decreases to 10% lower than adult levels by 6 months, increases to adult levels by adolescence.	INC: Polycythemia vera, chronic obstructive lung disease, erythropoietin producing tumors (mainly kidney, liver), high affinity hemoglobin variants. DEC: Bone marrow replacement or failure, hemolysis, bleeding, malignancies.	INC: Androgens, oral contraceptives. DEC: Interferon, drugs causing hemolysis or bone marrow depression.	Used along with hemoglobin to recognize anemia and polycythemia. May be falsely elevated when cold agglutinins are present and hematocrit is calculated (as in most automated cell counters).

| Hemoglobin | M: 13.2–17.3 g/dL F: 11.7–15.5 g/dL | 10 | M: 132–173 g/L F: 117–155 g/L | Same as for hematocrit. INC: Hyperbilirubinemia (interference). | Same as for hematocrit. | Same as for hematocrit. | Same as for hematocrit. |
| **Hemoglobin electrophoresis** | Hemoglobin A >95% No abnormal variants. | 0.01 | Hemoglobin A >0.95 No abnormal variants. | Abnormal variants identified in hemoglobinopathies. | | | Used to identify congenital hemoglobin variants. Initial screening usually performed at pH 8.6, which identifies most variants but may not separate each from other variants. Laboratories will perform additional tests as needed to separate variants, which may include acid electrophoresis and globin chain electrophoresis. In heterozygous states, hemoglobin A usually is about 60% and the variant about 40%. Coexistent β-thalassemia usually causes the variant to be 50% or higher. |

(continued)

Table 38.1 *(continued)*

Test Name	Reference Range			Nondisease Causes of Changes	Disease Related Changes	Drug Related Changes	Common Conditions for Use of Test
	Standard	Factor	SI Units				
Hemoglobin A₁c	<7.25% for good diabetic control	0.01	<0.0725 for good diabetic control	INC: Prolonged red cell survival (splenectomy, iron deficiency), stress; salicylates, renal failure, ethanol interfere with total A₁ methods but not true A₁c. DEC: Hemolytic anemias, bleeding, blood transfusion. In pregnancy, decreases by 8%. Lower in diabetic males than diabetic females. Increases with age after 60 years.	INC: Diabetes mellitus, other states of glucose intolerance, iron deficiency, splenectomy. DEC: Hypoglycemia, renal failure.	INC: Drugs increasing glucose, combination oral contraceptives.	Used to monitor glucose control over the past 1–2 months. ADA target values are based on true hemoglobin A₁c, and may differ with other methods. Other methods may cause false increases (see Chapter 7). Adversely affected by recent episodes of high glucose. Falsely low with decreased red cell survival, and falsely high with iron deficiency or following splenectomy; in such states, fructosamine should be used instead.
Hemoglobin A₂	1.5–3.5%	0.01	0.015–0.035	Lower in infants, reaches adult levels by 1 year.	INC: β-Thalassemia, megaloblastic anemia. DEC: Iron deficiency.		Used in differentiation of α-thalassemia and β-thalassemia; will be high in the latter and normal in the former.
Hemoglobin F	0–2.0% of Hgb	0.01	0–0.02 of Hgb	Increases during pregnancy, particularly with fetomaternal hemorrhage. In	INC: Hemoglobinopathies, hereditary persistence of hemoglobin F,		In adults, usually used in evaluation for thalassemia minor, not elevated in

α-thalassemia, only in β-thalassemia. In pregnancy, used to estimate amount of fetal-maternal hemorrhage, which can help to guide Rh immune globulin administration in Rh negative mothers with Rh positive infants; one vial neutralizes 15 mL of fetal red blood cells.

IgM antibody to virus used to diagnose acute hepatitis A. Some laboratories measure total antibody, which will be positive in a high percentage of children and adults due to previous infection or after hepatitis A vaccination (although may be negative after vaccine).

β-thalassemias, myelodysplastic syndromes, leukemia, chronic renal failure, hydatidiform mole.

INC: Acute hepatitis A, previous exposure to hepatitis A.

neonates, represents majority of hemoglobin; gradually falls to 5% by 6 months of age and reaches adult levels by 9–12 months.

INC: Hepatitis A vaccination.

Hemoglobin saturation (see Oxygen saturation)

Hepatitis A antibody Negative

Negative

(continued)

Table 38.1 *(continued)*

Test Name	Reference Range			Nondisease Causes of Changes	Disease Related Changes	Drug Related Changes	Common Conditions for Use of Test
	Standard	Factor	SI Units				
Hepatitis B core antibody (HB$_c$Ab)	Negative		Negative		INC: Acute or chronic hepatitis B, previous exposure to hepatitis B.		IgM antibody to core antigen used to diagnose acute hepatitis B; IgM antibody may persist at low levels in chronic hepatitis B. Some laboratories measure total antibody, which will be positive in any person exposed to virus; antibody remains detectable for life. Will be negative after receiving hepatitis B vaccine.
Hepatitis B surface antibody (HB$_s$AB)	Negative		Negative	INC: Hepatitis B vaccination.	INC: Hepatitis B infection.		Development of antibody in acute or chronic hepatitis B indicates resolution of infection. Antibody thought to persist for life, but may become undetectable while core antibody persists many years after infection. Also used to document success of immunization against hepatitis B.

Hepatitis B surface antigen (HBsAg)	Negative	Negative	INC: Acute or chronic hepatitis B.	Used to document active infection with hepatitis B virus. Will be positive before any other markers with acute infection, may have been cleared before clinical diagnosis in acute hepatitis B. In chronic hepatitis B or with carrier state (occurring with infection early in life), antigen persists. HBsAg is absent following vaccination.
Hepatitis C antibody	Negative	Negative	INC: Influenza vaccination.	INC: Hepatitis C.	Used to recognize hepatitis C infection. In addition to transient elevations of antibody following influenza vaccine, false positive results may occur. Test can be confirmed, if needed, by testing for antibodies to isolated hepatitis C antigens (RIBA test) or demonstrating HCV RNA in the circulation; the two tests have equivalent sensitivity and cost. Antibody may not be detectable for as long as 6 months after infection.

(continued)

Table 38.1 *(continued)*

Test Name	Reference Range			Nondisease Causes of Changes	Disease Related Changes	Drug Related Changes	Common Conditions for Use of Test
	Standard	Factor	SI Units				
5-HIAA (see 5-Hydroxyindoleacetic acid)							
High density lipoprotein cholesterol	NCEP Decision Level: High Risk: <35 mg/dL Low Risk: >60 mg/dL	0.026	<0.9 mmol/L >1.6 mmol/L	Interday variation 5–8%. INC: Exercise, ethanol, hemoconcentration. DEC: Obesity, prolonged fasting, smoking, stress. In pregnancy, increases by 25% by 12 weeks. In adolescence, decreases in males by 10–20%. Higher in blacks than whites and in females than males.	INC: Chronic hepatitis, primary biliary cirrhosis. DEC: Acute infections, diabetes, chronic liver disease, chronic renal failure, nephrotic syndrome.	INC: Estrogens, phenytoin, cimetidine, fibric acids, HMG-CoA reductase inhibitors, niacin. DEC: Androgens, thiazides, β-blockers, progesterone, Norplant, probucol, phenothiazines, isotretinoin, danazol, spironolactone.	Used to evaluate risk of coronary artery disease. High levels are associated with decreased risk, while low levels show increased risk.
Homocysteine	5.1–13.9 μmol/L	1	5.1–13.9 μmol/L	INC: Delayed separation. DEC: After meals, delayed storage. In pregnancy, decreases by 50%.	INC: Renal failure, inherited disorders of homocysteine metabolism, folate deficiency, vitamin B_{12} deficiency.		Used to evaluate risk of premature atherosclerosis and thrombotic disorders (associated with high homocysteine levels). In patients with low vitamin B_{12} levels, can also provide evidence of tissue B_{12} deficiency, although not as frequently elevated as methylmalonic acid.
Human chorionic gonadotropin (see Chorionic gonadotropin, human)							
25-Hydroxycholecalciferol (see Vitamin D, 25-hydroxy)							
5-Hydroxyindoleacetic acid	<6 mg/day	5.2	<31.2 μmol/day	Highest in winter, 50% lower in summer. INC: Smoking, foods containing serotonin (bananas, avocado,	INC: Carcinoid tumors, sprue, small cell carcinoma of lung, migraine headaches. DEC: Malabsorption,	INC: Atenolol, 5-FU, reserpine. DEC: Acetaminophen, methyldopa, L-dopa, isoniazid, ranitidine,	Used to diagnose and monitor carcinoid tumors. A number of drugs (including vitamin C) may

				plums, pineapple, kiwi fruit, most nuts, tomatoes, eggplant). DEC: Ethanol, alkaline urine. Increases moderately in pregnancy. In children, decreases with increasing age. Lower in persons > age 60 years.	depression, phenylpyruvic aciduria.	imipramine, guaiacol.	cause falsely low results with some assays; check with laboratory for interferences before performing test.
Hydroxyproline	0.0076	Urine: 25–80 mg/day	0.19–0.61 mmol/day	Interday variation 20%. Excretion higher at night. Highest in spring, fall; lower in winter. INC: Dietary protein, especially gelatin; prolonged bed rest. In pregnancy, increases in the third trimester, highest after delivery. Lower in children before puberty, increases to highest levels during adolescence. Decreases with age from 20–60 years, then increases up to 50% > age 60 years in males, in females increases further.	INC: Metabolic bone diseases with high turnover (hyperparathyroidism, hyperthyroidism, Paget's disease, osteomalacia), bone metastases, severe burns, fractures, orchiectomy, sarcoidosis. DEC: Malnutrition, hypothyroidism, hypopituitarism.	INC: Barbiturates, glucocorticoids, phenytoin, tolbutamide, thyroxine. DEC: Antineoplastic agents, aspirin, estrogens, mithramycin, omeprazole, bisphosphonates; propranolol (in hyperthyroidism).	Used to monitor turnover of collagen. Less sensitive marker of bone turnover than pyridinoline cross-links. Markedly affected by dietary collagen, especially gelatin found in many foods. If used, should always be done on 24 h urine with dietary restrictions.

(continued)

Table 38.1 *(continued)*

IFE (see Immunofixation electrophoresis)

Ig (see specific Immunoglobulin)

Test Name	Reference Range			Nondisease Causes of Changes	Disease Related Changes	Drug Related Changes	Common Conditions for Use of Test
	Standard	Factor	SI Units				
Immunofixation electrophoresis	No abnormal bands.		No abnormal bands.	Transient faint bands commonly are found after acute illness.	Monoclonal band present: Multiple myeloma, Waldenstrom's macroglobulinemia, monoclonal gammopathy of undetermined significance, mycosis fungoides, chronic lymphocytic leukemia.		Used to confirm the presence of a monoclonal band seen on protein electrophoresis and to identify the type of heavy and light chain present. Although slightly more sensitive than regular electrophoresis, not usually done if no abnormal band seen on standard electrophoresis. Not useful for serial monitoring after initial diagnosis.
Immunoglobulin A	100–490 mg/dL	0.01	1.0–4.9 g/L	Interday variation 5–10%. INC: Smoking exercise. DEC: Plasmapheresis. In pregnancy, decreases 20%. About 80% lower in neonates, rises to adult levels by adolescence.	INC (polyclonal): Cirrhosis, chronic GI or respiratory infections, inflammatory bowel disease, autoimmune disease. INC (monoclonal): IgA producing multiple myeloma. DEC: Congenital IgA deficiency, ataxia-telangiectasia, Bruton's agammaglobulinemia, multiple myeloma (non-IgA producing), chronic	DEC: Carbamazepine, estrogens, glucocorticoids, oral contraceptives, phenytoin, valproic acid.	Used in evaluation of suspected immunodeficiency disorders, usually ordered along with IgG and IgM. Selective deficiency of IgA occurs in about 1 in 600, associated with transfusion reactions, GI symptoms. Quantitative IgA is not recommended

Test	Reference Range		SI Range	Factors	Causes of Increase/Decrease	Drugs	Comments
					lymphocytic leukemia, nephrotic syndrome.		for following patients with IgA producing myeloma because it significantly underestimates actual IgA concentration; protein electrophoresis should be used instead.
Immunoglobulin E	0–180 U/mL	1	0–180 kU/L	INC: Smoking. DEC: Plasmapheresis. In childhood, virtually undetectable in neonates, increases to 50% of adult levels by 1 year, reaches 2× adult levels in adolescence. Higher in males than females.	INC (polyclonal): Allergies, parasitic infections, bronchopulmonary aspergillosis, IgA deficiency, nephrotic syndrome. INC (monoclonal): IgE producing multiple myeloma (rare). DEC: Bruton's agammaglobulinemia.	DEC: Phenytoin.	Used to recognize allergic disorders; total IgE roughly correlates with severity of allergic symptoms, particularly asthma. Levels over 5× normal are highly specific for allergic disorders.
Immunoglobulin G	500–1,700 mg/dL	0.01	5.0–17.0 g/L	Interday variation 5%. DEC: Plasmapheresis. In pregnancy, decreases by 25% by 12 weeks, 33% by third trimester. Low in neonates, reaches adult levels by 1 year. Decreases in older individuals.	INC (polyclonal): AIDS, autoimmune disease, sarcoidosis, cirrhosis, chronic infections, parasitic disease. INC (monoclonal): Multiple myeloma, monoclonal gammopathy of undetermined significance, mycosis fungoides. DEC: Bruton's agammaglobulinemia, multiple myeloma (non-IgG producing), chronic lymphocytic leukemia, nephrotic syndrome, burns, malnutrition.	INC: Methadone, propylthiouracil, drugs causing lupus. DEC: Diazoxide, gold, glucocorticoids, phenytoin.	Used in evaluation of suspected immunodeficiency disorders and in evaluation of increased globulins (total protein—albumin). Quantitative IgG is not recommended for following monoclonal IgG because of variation in results from patient to patient; protein electrophoresis should be used instead.

(continued)

Table 38.1 *(continued)*

Test Name	Reference Range			Nondisease Causes of Changes	Disease Related Changes	Drug Related Changes	Common Conditions for Use of Test
	Standard	Factor	SI Units				
Immunoglobulin G index, CSF	0.3–0.6	1	0.3–0.6		INC: Multiple sclerosis, AIDS, subacute sclerosing panencephalitis, Lyme disease, Guillain-Barre syndrome, CNS syphilis, CNS lupus erythematosus.		Similar to oligoclonal band demonstration with CSF electrophoresis in identifying disorders associated with synthesis of IgG in central nervous system; calculated using formula in Equation 20.1. Requires less CSF than does electrophoresis and often is less expensive. Is not useful for serial monitoring of patients with multiple sclerosis.
Immunoglobulin M	50–300 mg/dL	0.01	0.5–3.0 g/L	Interday variation 5–10%. In pregnancy, decreases by 20%. In children, very low levels in neonates, reaches adult levels by 1 year.	INC (polyclonal): Viral infections, autoimmune disease, primary biliary cirrhosis, sarcoidosis, nephrotic syndrome. INC (monoclonal): Waldenstrom's macroglobulinemia, chronic lymphocytic leukemia, malignant lymphomas. DEC: Multiple myeloma, burns, malnutrition, immunodeficiency disorders.	INC: Chlorpromazine. DEC: Carbamazepine, gold.	Used in evaluation of suspected immunodeficiency disorders or increased globulins, often measured along with IgA and IgG. Quantitative IgM is not recommended for following patients with monoclonal IgM because of significant overestimation of actual IgM

Insulin	0–20 mIU/L	7.18	0–144 pmol/L	Interday variation 15%. Intraday variation up to 70% with pulsatile secretion. INC: After meals, stress, obesity. DEC: Ethanol, fasting, exercise, physically fit individuals. Increases 15–20% during pregnancy. Higher in Hispanics than whites.	INC: Insulinoma, type II diabetes, renal failure, cirrhosis, acromegaly, Cushing's syndrome. DEC: Type I diabetes, hypopituitarism, pheochromocytoma, malnutrition, cystic fibrosis.	INC: Danazol, L-dopa, megestrol, oral antibiotics, oral contraceptives, spironolactone. DEC: Diuretics, cimetidine, propranolol, fibric acids, nifedipine, phenytoin.	concentration; protein electrophoresis should be used instead. Used most commonly in evaluation of hypoglycemia. High ratio of insulin to glucose (>0.3 with insulin in mU/mL and glucose in mg/dL) indicates excess insulin. Further evaluated with C-peptide; high levels of both indicate endogenous production, while high insulin but low C-peptide indicates insulin injection. Sometimes used to distinguish type I and type II diabetes; most useful when stimulated insulin (after glucagon or meals) is used.

(continued)

Table 38.1 *(continued)*

Test Name	Reference Range			Nondisease Causes of Changes	Disease Related Changes	Drug Related Changes	Common Conditions for Use of Test
	Standard	Factor	SI Units				
Insulin antibodies (see Anti-insulin antibodies)							
Insulin C-peptide (see C-Peptide)							
Insulin-like growth factor-1 (IGF-1, somatomedin C)	123–463 ng/mL	1	123–463 µg/L	Approximately 15% variation during day, 30% fall at onset of sleep with rise to highest values at 4 AM. INC: Hemoconcentration, exercise. DEC: fasting, obesity. In females, higher in luteal than follicular phase. In pregnancy, gradually increases; 100% higher by the third trimester. In children, may be undetectable until age 5 years, peaks about 10 years, elevated in adolescence. Declines gradually throughout adult life. Higher in females than males.	INC: Acromegaly, Cushing's syndrome, renal failure. DEC: Pituitary dwarfism, hypopituitarism, hypothyroidism, cirrhosis, malnutrition, acute illness.	INC: Androgens, clonidine, dexamethasone. DEC: Estrogens, tamoxifen.	Used in diagnosis of growth hormone excess or deficiency. Best test for screening, follow-up of patients with acromegaly or gigantism. For growth hormone deficiency, useful for screening in children over 5 years; however, growth hormone response to stimuli is considered more reliable, especially in younger children.
Intrinsic factor antibodies (see Anti-intrinsic factor)							
Iron	44–136 µg/dL	0.18	7.9–24.5 µmol/L	Interday variation 25%. Up to 40% diurnal variation, highest in AM, lowest at night. INC: Hemoconcentration, transfusions (for 24–36 hours), hemolysis, ethanol. DEC: Exercise, stress; EDTA, desferoxamine (interfere with assay). In females, highest in luteal	INC: Hemochromatosis, iron poisoning, chronic transfusion, bone marrow failure, pernicious anemia, lead poisoning, acute leukemia, acute hepatitis, chronic hepatitis C, porphyria. DEC: Iron deficiency, chronic inflammation, hypothyroidism,	INC: Cisplatin, estrogens, methotrexate, oral contraceptives. DEC: Allopurinol, androgens, aspirin, cholestyramine, glucocorticoids.	Used in evaluation of anemia or iron excess. In iron deficiency, will have low iron with high iron binding capacity (TIBC). In chronic disease, iron and TIBC both low. Becomes abnormal later than ferritin in

Test	Conventional range	Conversion factor	SI range	Physiological factors	Disease factors	Drug factors	Comments
				phase, lowest after menstruation. In pregnancy, decreases 5–10%. Decreases with age >70 years.	nephrotic syndrome, malabsorption, malnutrition, septicemia.		uncomplicated iron deficiency, but not affected as much as ferritin by tissue injury. In iron poisoning, iron high with saturation >100%; level used to determine need for treatment (see Chapter 19). In hemochromatosis, high iron and low TIBC with saturation (Fe/TIBC × 100) >62% in males or >50% in females; abnormal earlier than ferritin. Ferritin better test for monitoring therapy.
Iron binding capacity	229–365 µg/dL	0.18	41.2–65.7 µmol/L	Interday variation 2–3%. INC: Hemoconcentration, exercise. In pregnancy, increases gradually, up to 50% higher by term. Higher in females than males.	INC: Iron deficiency, thalassemia. DEC: Hemochromatosis, inflammation, malignancies, nephrotic syndrome, malnutrition, hypothyroidism.	INC: Estrogens, oral contraceptives. DEC: Androgens, glucocorticoids.	Used to estimate transferrin (the major iron transport protein); can be converted using the formula: transferrin = (0.8 × TIBC) − 43. Used along with serum iron to diagnose disorders of iron metabolism.

(continued)

Table 38.1 *(continued)*

Islet cell antibodies (see Anti-islet cell antibodies)

K (see Potassium)

Test Name	Reference Range			Nondisease Causes of Changes	Disease Related Changes	Drug Related Changes	Common Conditions for Use of Test
	Standard	Factor	SI Units				
Ketones	<10 mg/dL (negative)	0.1	<1 mmol/L (negative)	INC: Fasting, exercise, ethanol.	INC: Diabetic ketoacidosis, isopropanol intoxication, starvation ketoacidosis, hyperthyroidism.	INC: Aspirin, isopropanol toxicity, albuterol, nifedipine. DEC: Valproic acid.	Used to recognize ketoacidosis. Detects acetoacetate and, in some assays, acetone; hydroxybutyrate predominates early in ketoacidosis. With treatment, as hydroxybutyrate is converted to acetoacetate, ketones rise. Anion gap is preferred test to monitor ketoacidosis initially; ketones can be used once anion gap reaches normal.
Lactate	Venous: 3.6–18.9 mg/dL Arterial: 4.5–15.4 mg/dL	0.11	0.4–2.1 mmol/L 0.5–1.7 mmol/L	Interday variation 25%. INC: Exercise, hyperventilation, ethanol, fasting, prolonged tourniquet use, delayed separation of plasma. DEC: Weight loss. Slightly higher in females than males.	INC: Hypotension, hypoxemia, severe volume depletion, rapidly growing malignancies (primarily leukemias, lymphoma, small cell carcinoma, renal failure, seizures. DEC: Toxemia.	INC: Albuterol, carbamazepine, catecholamines, oral contraceptives, phenobarbital, valproic acid, propylene glycol. DEC: Morphine.	Used to recognize lactic acidosis. Specimens must be collected using tubes containing sodium fluoride. In CSF, high lactate most commonly seen with bacterial or fungal meningitis, but also occurs with cerebral ischemia,

| Lactate dehydrogenase (LDH) | 100–212 U/L | 1 | 100–212 U/L | Interday variation 5–10%. INC: Exercise, hemolyzed specimens, delayed separation. In children, 2–4× higher in neonates, remains 1–2× higher in children, reaches adult levels by late adolescence. Increases by 10% by age 60 years. Higher in males than females. | INC: Hemolytic anemias, megaloblastic anemia, malignancies, shock, acute hepatitis, myocardial infarction. | INC: Amiodarone, drugs causing hemolysis or hepatitis. | hemorrhage, and metastatic carcinomas. Nonspecific marker of cell injury, elevated with injury to most cell types. Generally of most use in seeking damage to cells without other enzymatic markers (red cells, malignancies), and of less use in detecting damage to solid organs (liver, heart, skeletal muscle) because of higher levels of other markers. Hemolyzed specimens are a major source of false elevations. |

(continued)

Table 38.1 *(continued)*

Test Name	Reference Range			Nondisease Causes of Changes	Disease Related Changes	Drug Related Changes	Common Conditions for Use of Test
	Standard	Factor	SI Units				
Lactate dehydrogenase isoenzymes	LDH 1: 18–33% LDH 2: 28–40% LDH 3: 18–30% LDH 4: 6–16% LDH 5: 2–18%	0.01	LDH 1: 0.18–0.33 LDH 2: 0.28–0.40 LDH 3: 0.18–0.30 LDH 4: 0.06–0.16 LDH 5: 0.02–0.18	INC (LDH 1): Hemolyzed specimens, delayed separation. INC (LDH 5): Strenuous exercise. DEC (LDH 5): Specimen storage.	INC (LDH 1): Hemolytic anemia, megaloblastic anemia, myocardial infarction, germ cell tumors, renal cell carcinoma. INC (LDH 2,3,4): Pulmonary infarction, leukemia, lymphoma, infectious mononucleosis. INC (LDH 4,5): Rhabdomyolysis, inflammatory myopathies, acute hepatitis (especially due to shock or toxins). INC (all isoenzymes): Shock, malignancies, multiple organ damage.	INC (LDH 1): Drugs causing hemolysis. INC (LDH 5): Drugs causing skeletal muscle or liver injury.	Used to identify source of elevated LDH. Of limited use if LDH <2× normal. Used previously to diagnose myocardial infarction in patients with late presentation, now replaced by troponin.

LAP (see Leukocyte alkaline phosphatase)

LDH (see Lactate dehydrogenase)

LDL-Cholesterol (see Low density lipoprotein cholesterol)

| **Lead** | Adult: <40 μg/dL Child: <25 μg/dL | 0.048 | <1.93 μmol/L <1.21 μmol/L | Interday levels fluctuate; magnitude of fluctuation not reported. INC: Smoking, ethanol; using regular collection tubes (interference). In children, decreases with age until 16 years, then continuously increases throughout adult life. Higher in males than females and in blacks than whites. | INC: Lead poisoning. | | Used to detect active lead poisoning. In children, lead levels >10 μg/dL are considered potentially dangerous. In patients with remote lead exposure, blood lead typically normal; increased urine lead after |

Test				Comments	Factors
				administration of 50 mg/kg EDTA (>1 μg/mg EDTA) indicates increased body lead. While zinc protoporphyrin has been used to screen for lead poisoning, it is insensitive at lead levels <25 μg/dL, where blood lead is the preferred test.	
Lecithin/sphingomyelin ratio	Mature: >2:1	1	Mature: >2:1	Used to identify fetal lung surfactant production. Ratios <2.0 may be associated with surfactant but have high false positive results. In infants of diabetic mothers, ratios as high as 3.5 may still be associated with immature lungs.	INC: Fetal blood, meconium, vaginal mucus.	INC: Glucocorticoids.	INC: Maternal diabetes. DEC: Immature infants.
Leukocyte alkaline phosphatase	40–130	1	40–130	In pregnancy, averages 2× higher.	INC: Polycythemia vera, infections, lymphoma, multiple myeloma, myeloproliferative diseases. DEC: Chronic myelogenous leukemia, sideroblastic anemia, sickle cell disease, paroxysmal nocturnal hemoglobinuria, cirrhosis, diabetes, sarcoidosis, pernicious anemia, many malignancies.	INC: Glucocorticoids.	Used in evaluation of patients with leukocytosis to determine likelihood of chronic myelogenous leukemia.

(continued)

Table 38.1 *(continued)*

| Test Name | Reference Range | | | Nondisease Causes of Changes | Disease Related Changes | Drug Related Changes | Common Conditions for Use of Test |
	Standard	Factor	SI Units				
Leukocyte esterase	Negative		Negative	DEC: Proteinuria, highly concentrated urine.	INC: Urinary tract infections, trichomoniasis, interstitial nephritis.	INC: Drugs discoloring urine. DEC: Vitamin C.	Used to detect inflammatory cells in urine, usually as a result of urinary tract infection. Reliably positive when >10 WBC/hpf of urine. May be positive when microscopic negative in dilute urine or with delay in analysis.
LH (see Luteinizing hormone)							
Lipase	50–240 U/L	1	50–240 U/L	Interday variation 10%. DEC: Hepatitis, obstructive jaundice (falsely low). In children, 2× higher in neonates, reaches adult levels by one month. Increases slightly after age 60 in females.	INC: Pancreatitis, pancreatic pseudocyst, intestinal injury, renal failure. DEC: Pancreatic insufficiency.	INC: Drugs causing pancreatic injury, heparin. DEC: Protamine.	Used to diagnose pancreatitis. Remains elevated longer than amylase, rises at approximately same time. Both are elevated with intestinal injury and renal failure.
Lipoprotein (a)	0–30 mg/dL	10	0–300 mg/L	Interday variation 8–10%; no diurnal variation. INC: Hemoconcentration, ethanol withdrawal. In pregnancy, increases by 100% by third trimester. Lowest in neonates, gradually rises over first 6 months of life. Slight increase with increasing age. Values highest in blacks, intermediate in whites and Asians, lowest in Hispanics.	INC: Diabetes, acute illness, renal failure, hypothyroidism. DEC: Hyperthyroidism.	INC: Cyclosporine, some oral contraceptives. DEC: Androgens, danazol, estrogens.	Used to identify increased levels of apo(a), which correlates with increased risk of atherosclerosis and thrombosis in whites. Correlation between apo(a) levels and risk is not clear in blacks.

Test	Conventional reference range	Conversion factor	SI reference range	Physiologic variation	Disease (INC/DEC)	Drugs (INC/DEC)	Comments
Low density lipoprotein cholesterol	NCEP Target: No risk: <160 mg/dL High risk: <130 mg/dL CAD: <100 mg/dL	0.026	NCEP Target: No risk: <4.1 mmol/L Hi risk: <3.4 mmol/L CAD: <2.6 mmol/L	Interday variation 10–15%. INC: High fat diet, obesity. DEC: Low fat diet, exercise. In pregnancy, decreases by 20% by 12 weeks, gradually rises to 50% above baseline by third trimester. In adults, gradually increases to age 65. Higher in females than in males and in whites than blacks.	INC: Congenital hyperlipidemias, hypothyroidism, nephrotic syndrome, obstructive jaundice, chronic renal failure, Cushing's syndrome. DEC: Acute illness (falls by up to 40%), abetalipoproteinemia, hyperthyroidism, malabsorption, malnutrition, cirrhosis, malignancies.	INC: Androgens, β-blockers, cyclosporine, danazol, glucocorticoids, isotretinoin, progestins, thiazides. DEC: Lipid lowering agents, estrogens, interferon, thyroxine.	Used to identify risk of coronary artery disease. Can either be measured directly or calculated from total cholesterol, HDL-cholesterol, and triglycerides; both types of assays require fasting specimens and triglycerides <400 mg/dL for accurate results.
Luteinizing hormone	M: 2.4–15.9 mIU/mL F: 0–27 mIU/mL Postmeno-pausal F: 40–104 mIU/mL	1	M: 2.4–15.9 IU/L F: 0–27 IU/L Postmeno-pausal F: 40–104 IU/L	Interday variation 30%. Within day, released in spikes, highest in early sleep, lowest in late afternoon. Highest in summer, lowest in winter. INC: Psychologic stress, ethanol. DEC: Obesity, starvation, high altitude, heavy exercise, blindness. In females, sharp spike prior to ovulation. Decreased during pregnancy. In children, undetectable until adolescence.	INC: Renal failure, menopause, gonadal failure, polycystic ovary syndrome, gonadotropin producing pituitary adenoma, hyperthyroidism. DEC: Acute illness, hypopituitarism, elevated prolactin, anorexia nervosa, malnutrition.	INC: Clomiphene, propranolol (in males), ketoconazole, naloxone, phenytoin, tamoxifen. DEC: Androgens, oral contraceptives, estrogens, phenothiazines, digoxin, progesterones; propranolol (in females).	Used in evaluation of hypogonadism. Also used to screen for polycystic ovary syndrome in patients with hirsutism and menstrual irregularities; ratio of 3 LH:FSH >3:1 is virtually diagnostic. False elevations can also occur with high HCG or very high TSH.

(continued)

Table 38.1 (continued)

Test Name	Reference Range			Nondisease Causes of Changes	Disease Related Changes	Drug Related Changes	Common Conditions for Use of Test
	Standard	Factor	SI Units				
Mean cell volume (MCV)	80–97 fL	1	80–97 fL	Interday variation 1%. INC: Cold agglutinins, ethanol, smoking. In children, markedly increased in neonates (up to 120), then gradually decreases (range 70–85) by 6 months, then gradually increases to adult levels by adolescence. Slightly higher in females than males. Increases slightly with age over 50 years.	INC: Megaloblastic anemia, hemolysis, liver disease, malignancies, hypothyroidism. DEC: Iron deficiency, thalassemias, chronic disease, hyperthyroidism, porphyrias.	INC: Zidovudine, drugs causing hemolysis or megaloblastic changes.	Used to estimate red blood cell size, as an aid to determining cause of anemia. Because it represents an average, may be normal with mixed types of anemia. Immature red blood cells, as occurs with hemolysis, will increase MCV. High MCV is seen with megaloblastic anemia, hemolytic anemia, myelodysplastic syndromes, and liver diseases. Low MCV indicates impaired hemoglobin synthesis in iron deficiency, thalassemia, lead poisoning, and in some anemia of chronic disease. Most other anemias are normocytic (normal MCV). Sometimes, large platelets will be measured as red cells and falsely lower MCV.

Magnesium	1.4–2.5 mg/dL	0.41	0.6–1.0 mmol/L	Interday variation 3–5%. Highest in winter, lowest in summer. INC: Dehydration, hemoconcentration, hypoglycemia, hemolyzed specimens, delayed separation. DEC: Malabsorption, ethanol, hyperglycemia. In pregnancy, about 10% lower.	INC: Renal failure, diabetic ketoacidosis, Addison's disease, hypothyroidism, cell lysis syndromes, hemolytic anemia. DEC: Malabsorption, malnutrition, renal tubular injury, hypoparathyroidism, diarrhea, SIADH.	Used most commonly to recognize magnesium deficiency. Serum does not reflect total body stores of magnesium, making magnesium levels a poor test to follow magnesium therapy.
	Urine: 14–290 mg/day	0.041	0.6–12 mmol/day			
Metanephrines	0.3–0.9 mg/day	5.07	1.5–4.6 μmol/day	INC: Stress, exercise, caffeine.	INC: Amphetamines, hydrazines, monoamine oxidase inhibitors, prochloperazine, theophylline. DEC: L-dopa.	Used to screen for pheochromocy-toma. May miss pheochromocy-tomas which produce only epinephrine; fractionated catecholamines are better for such cases. Of less use than VMA and HVA in children with neuroblastoma.
Methylmalonic acid	0.85–3.19 μg/dL	85	73–271 nmol/L	Interday variation 25%.	INC: Vitamin B$_{12}$ deficiency, renal insufficiency, methylmalonic aciduria.	Used to confirm vitamin B$_{12}$ deficiency in patients with low B$_{12}$ levels. Can be difficult to interpret in patients with renal insufficiency.

Table 38.1 *(continued)*

Test Name	Reference Range Standard	Factor	SI Units	Nondisease Causes of Changes	Disease Related Changes	Drug Related Changes	Common Conditions for Use of Test
β_2-**Microglobulin**	1.0–2.4 μg/mL	1	1.0–2.4 mg/L		INC: Acute inflammation, AIDS, autoimmune disease, lymphocytic malignancies, viral infection, renal failure, toxemia. DEC: Renal tubular disorders.	INC: Cefuroxime, cyclosporine, gentamicin, lithium. DEC: Drugs causing proximal renal tubular injury.	Used for initial staging in patients with B-cell lymphomas and multiple myeloma. Not commonly used to follow myeloma, where quantitation of immunoglobulin from protein electrophoresis is preferred.
Mg (see Magnesium)							
Microalbuminuria	0–40 mg/day 0–32 μg/mg creatinine	1 0.11	0–40 mg/day 0–3.6 μg/mmol creatinine	Interday variation 30–70%, lower for first morning urine. INC: Fever, exercise, upright posture, acute illness, ethanol, high fat diet, x-ray contrast agents. DEC: High fiber diet.	INC: Glomerular injury (diabetes, hypertension, glomerulopathies), renal tubular damage, urinary tract infection, toxemia.	INC: Drugs damaging renal tubules.	Urinary albumin is used to detect early renal injury, particularly in patients with diabetes. Treatment of early injury can prevent progression in diabetics.
Myelin basic protein	0–5 ng/mL	1	0–5 μg/L		INC: Multiple sclerosis, subacute sclerosing panencephalitis, viral encephalitis, cerebrovascular accident, metastatic carcinoma to brain, brain trauma.		Used to measure activity of disorders destroying myelin within the central nervous system. In multiple sclerosis, inferior to CSF electrophoresis in sensitivity, but is a better marker of disease activity.

Test	Conventional	Factor	SI Units	Factors Causing Variation	Disorders	Drugs	Comments
Myeglobin	M: 20–90 ng/mL F: 10–75 ng/mL	1	M: 20–90 µg/L F: 10–75 µg/L	INC: Exercise, IM injection. Increases with age over 50 years, up to 100% higher by age 75 years.	INC: Skeletal muscle injury (see CK), myocardial infarction, renal failure, seizures.	INC: Drugs damaging muscle, succinylcholine.	Used to recognize muscle injury. In some hospitals used as an early marker to recognize myocardial infarction; however, because of inability to distinguish skeletal and cardiac muscle injury, must be confirmed if coexisting muscle injury or renal failure is present or suspected. Remains elevated for shortest period of time of any myocardial marker.
Na (see Sodium)							
Nitrite	Negative		Negative	INC: Open storage of bottles containing reagent strips, prolonged storage of specimen, contamination with talc from gloves. DEC: Vitamin C.	INC: Urinary tract infection with most gram negative bacilli.	INC: Drugs discoloring urine. DEC: Vitamin C.	Used to screen for urinary tract infection along with leukocyte esterase. May be falsely negative with bacteria not producing nitrite (gram positive organisms, some pseudomonas), with low levels of infection, or with severe frequency of urination. Ideally should be performed on first morning specimen to minimize effects of low level infection and frequency.

(continued)

Table 38.1 *(continued)*

Test Name	Reference Range			Nondisease Causes of Changes	Disease Related Changes	Drug Related Changes	Common Conditions for Use of Test
	Standard	Factor	SI Units				
Norepinephrine (see Catecholamines)							
O₂ blood (see pO₂)							
O₂ saturation (see Oxygen saturation)							
Occult blood, stool	Negative		Negative	INC: Meat ingestion, betadine contamination, strenuous exercise. DEC: Constipation, excessively dry stools.	INC: Upper or lower gastrointestinal tract bleeding.	INC: Drugs causing intestinal bleeding, iron. DEC: Ascorbic acid.	Used to screen for intestinal bleeding, often an early sign of intestinal tumors (both benign and malignant). Results may be falsely positive with ingestion of red meat or vegetables containing peroxidases (radishes, horseradish, turnips). May be falsely negative with delayed intestinal transit, with high levels of ascorbic acid, with upper GI bleeding. Solid stool specimens should not be tested immediately, as they may be falsely negative if the heme has not penetrated the paper before the developer is added. Rehydration of strips improves sensitivity.

| **Osmolality** | 275–295 mOsm/kg | 1 | 275–295 mOsm/kg | Interday variation 1–2%. Highest in morning, 7.5% lower in evening. INC: Exercise, ethanol. DEC: High altitude. Decreases during pregnancy in parallel to sodium, urea. | INC: Dehydration, diabetes insipidus, diabetes mellitus, renal failure, overdose of ethylene glycol, isopropanol, or methanol. DEC: Hyponatremia, adrenal insufficiency, hypopituitarism, water intoxication, inappropriate ADH production. | INC: Steroids causing salt retention, lithium, glycine, hydroxyethyl starch, mannitol. DEC: Diuretics, vincristine, carbamazepine, cyclophosphamide, drugs causing hyponatremia. | Main use is to detect osmotic gap, the difference between measured and calculated osmolality (see Chapter 4), to detect toxin ingestion. Some laboratories use vapor pressure osmometers, which will not detect alcohols. Plasma osmolality often ordered to detect "pseudohyponatremia," but not usually needed for this purpose. Urine osmolality is best test of urine concentrating ability, and can help calculate free water clearance (Chapter 6) to evaluate tubular function. Urine osmolality also of use in evaluation of hyponatremia and hypernatremia as an indirect indicator of ADH related urine concentration (Chapter 5). |

(continued)

Table 38.1 *(continued)*

Test Name	Reference Range			Nondisease Causes of Changes	Disease Related Changes	Drug Related Changes	Common Conditions for Use of Test
	Standard	Factor	SI Units				
Osteocalcin (bone Gla protein)	2–12 ng/mL	1	2–12 µg/L	Interday variation > 50%. Highest at night, 50–100% lower in early afternoon. INC: Obesity. DEC: Ethanol. In females, higher in luteal than follicular phase. Decreases in first trimester of pregnancy, returns to normal by term, increased during lactation. In children, peaks during periods of bone growth, adult levels by age 20. In adults, increases about 50% after age 50 in females, about 10% higher in older males. Higher in whites than blacks.	INC: Increased bone formation (Paget's disease, osteomalacia, hyperparathyroidism, bone metastases), renal failure. DEC: Acute illness, primary biliary cirrhosis, growth hormone deficiency.	INC: Calcitriol, omeprazole, rarely with phenytoin-related vitamin D deficiency. DEC: Glucocorticoids, coumadin, estrogens, oral contraceptives, tamoxifen, thiazides.	Used as marker of bone formation, more sensitive than total alkaline phosphatase to changes in bone formation rate. Cannot be used in patients taking coumadin. Because of marked diurnal variation, should always be drawn at 8 AM to compare serial results.
Oxygen (see PO₂)							
Oxygen saturation	94–98%	0.01	0.94–0.98	INC: Hyperventilation; lipemia (interference). DEC: Hypotension, hypothermia, arrhythmias cause false decreases using pulse oximeters.	INC: Oxygen therapy. DEC: Pneumonia, interstitial lung disease, pulmonary emboli, chronic obstructive lung disease, CNS depression, congestive heart failure, right to left shunt, cirrhosis.	INC: Aspirin. DEC: Drugs inhibiting respiration.	Usually determined by pulse oximeters, which measure only oxyhemoglobin and deoxyhemoglobin. While this allows calculation of oxygen saturation, it may be inaccurate in patients with carboxyhemoglobin or methemoglobin. Cannot be used to

Test	Reference value	Factor	SI units	Physiological factors	Disease / Drug factors	Comments
						reliably estimate pO_2 in patients receiving high levels of oxygen where saturation is high. Usually inaccurate in neonates because of fetal hemoglobin.
P (see Phosphate)						
Parathyroid hormone, intact	10–65 pg/L	0.1	1.0–6.5 pmol/L	Within day variation 30%, highest at 4 PM, lowest at 8 AM. Higher in summer than winter. INC: After meals, obesity. DEC: Exercise, high protein diet, ethanol. In females, gradually increases to peak at mid-cycle. In pregnancy, increases in early pregnancy but falls to below normal by term, increases with lactation. In children, undetectable in neonates, reaches adult levels by 2–3 days. Increases with age >40 years. Higher in blacks than whites.	INC: Primary hyperparathyroidism, renal failure, hypocalcemia, malabsorption. DEC: Hypoparathyroidism, hypercalcemia, magnesium deficiency, acute illness, hyperthyroidism. INC: Estrogens, glucocorticoids, octreotide, omeprazole, phosphate, lithium, phenytoin. DEC: Pindolol, cimetidine (mid-molecule only), thiazides.	Used to detect primary and secondary diseases of parathyroid glands. PTH should always be interpreted in light of serum free calcium. In patients with hypercalcemia due to other disease, PTH should be suppressed below normal. With hypocalcemia of other causes, PTH should be increased. In renal failure, PTH much higher than expected for serum calcium due to lack of feedback inhibition from calcitriol.

(continued)

Table 38.1 *(continued)*

Test Name	Reference Range			Nondisease Causes of Changes	Disease Related Changes	Drug Related Changes	Common Conditions for Use of Test
	Standard	Factor	SI Units				
Parathyroid hormone-related peptide	0–1.5 pmol/L	1	0–1.5 pmol/L	INC: Lactation. Similar in neonates, children, and adults.	INC: PTHrP producing malignancies (squamous cell carcinoma, breast carcinoma, renal cell carcinoma most commonly).		Used to detect PTHrP production as a cause of hypercalcemia. Since this is usually due to malignancy, test needed in patients with hypercalcemia without obvious malignancy by clinical evaluation.
Partial thromboplastin time (PTT)	22–33 s	1	22–33 s	Interday variation 3–8%. INC: Incompletely filled tubes, high hematocrit, delayed storage. DEC: Hemolysis, exercise, anemia. In pregnancy, decreased 5–10%.	INC: Hemophilia, disseminated intravascular coagulation, Von Willebrand's disease, liver failure, antiphospholipid antibodies.	INC: Heparin, thrombolytic agents, naloxone, drugs interfering with vitamin K. DEC: Estrogens, oral contraceptives.	Used to detect abnormalities of most soluble coagulation factors, particularly inherited coagulation factor defects. Used to monitor heparin therapy; values should be 1.5–2.5 × baseline when therapeutic. Test markedly affected by heparin; must not be drawn from indwelling catheters if heparin is used to retard *in vivo* clotting. Also used to screen for anticardiolipin antibodies. Not useful to screen for coagulation defects in patients with no history of bleeding or thrombosis.

Pb (see Lead)

pCO₂

Arterial: 36–44 mm Hg

0.133

3.5–5.9 kPa

Interday variation 5%.
DEC: Anxiety, exercise, excess air or heparin in syringe, fever, hyperventilation.
In pregnancy, decreased 5 mm Hg from early first trimester to term. About 3–5 mm Hg lower in neonates and infants.

INC: Respiratory failure, chronic obstructive lung disease, cerebral depression, metabolic alkalosis.
DEC: Interstitial lung disease, pulmonary emboli, right to left shunt, cirrhosis, metabolic acidosis, hyperthyroidism.

INC: Drugs depressing respiratory rate (barbiturates, opiates, benzodiazepines).
DEC: Aspirin.

Used to evaluate the respiratory component of acid-base disorders. Can be measured in venous or arterial blood; venous values will be about 4–6 mm Hg higher than values given for arterial blood.

pH

Arterial blood: 7.36–7.44

1

7.36–7.44

Interday variation 3–5%.
INC: After meals, excess heparin, blood transfusions, anxiety, nasogastric suction.
DEC: Fever (unless nomogram correction used), exercise, prolonged fasting, delay in specimen analysis. Decreases slightly after age 60 years.

INC: Vomiting, volume contraction, hyperaldosteronism, Cushing's syndrome, interstitial lung disease, early congestive heart failure, right to left shunts.
DEC: Ketoacidosis, lactic acidosis, oliguric renal failure, diarrhea, renal tubular acidosis, adrenal insufficiency, respiratory failure, chronic obstructive lung disease.

INC: Drugs causing alkalosis (antacids, carbenicillin, diuretics, glucocorticoids, phenylbutazone).
DEC: Drugs causing acidosis (acetazolamide, aspirin, captopril, cholestyramine, cyclosporine, nalidixic acid, spironolactone).

Used to evaluate acid-base status. Because pH is affected by mixed disorders, must be evaluated in light of anion gap, bicarbonate, and pCO₂ changes (Figure 4.3). Can be obtained from venous blood, but values about 0.03 lower than values given for arterial blood; the difference is greater with hypoperfusion.

(continued)

Table 38.1 (continued)

Test Name	Reference Range			Nondisease Causes of Changes	Disease Related Changes	Drug Related Changes	Common Conditions for Use of Test
	Standard	Factor	SI Units				
pO₂	83–108 mm Hg	0.133	11.0–14.4 kPa	INC: Extensive air bubbles in specimen, hyperventilation, exercise. DEC: Marked delay in analysis, collection of venous blood. Markedly reduced in neonates, increases to near normal by 1 day. After age 60, upper reference limit declines by 10 mm Hg per decade.	DEC: Chronic obstructive lung disease, pneumonia, interstitial lung disease, pulmonary embolism, congestive heart failure, pulmonary malignancies, shock, CNS depression, right to left shunts.	INC: Aspirin. DEC: Drugs depressing respiratory rate (barbiturates, opiates, benzodiazepines).	Used to evaluate oxygenation of blood. Most useful when oxygen saturation <80% or >98%; in other situations, oxygen saturation determined by pulse oximeters is often adequate.

Phosphatase, acid (see Acid phosphatase)
Phosphatase, alkaline (see Alkaline phosphatase)

Test Name	Reference Range			Nondisease Causes of Changes	Disease Related Changes	Drug Related Changes	Common Conditions for Use of Test
	Standard	Factor	SI Units				
Phosphate	Serum: 2.5–4.5 mg/dL	0.32	0.81–1.45 mmol/L	Interday variation 5–10% (serum), 15–20% (urine). Usually highest at 8 AM, falls during day. Highest in summer, lowest in winter. INC: Immediately after meals, starvation, immobilization, delayed separation. DEC: After meals, refeeding after starvation, ethanol. In females, 0.3 mg/dL lower during menstruation.	INC: Severe acute illness, starvation, ketoacidosis, lactic acidosis, fracture healing, cell lysis, renal failure, vitamin D excess, sarcoidosis, hypoparathyroidism, acromegaly, hyperthyroidism. DEC: Hyperparathyroidism, malignancies producing PTHrP, refeeding after starvation, vitamin D deficiency,	INC: Androgens, clonidine, growth hormone, vitamin D, phospho-soda enemas. DEC: Anticonvulsants, acetazolamide, estrogens, insulin, oral contraceptives, lithium, aluminum containing antacids.	Must be interpreted with caution because of marked diurnal variation. Of little use as a routine test. Most useful in patients with calcium abnormalities, where it can provide a clue to etiology; PTH or PTHrP excess causes low phosphate, vitamin D excess causes
	Urine: 0.4–1.3 g/day	32.3	12.9–32.0 mmol/day				

		In children, up to 6 mg/dL normal throughout growth, reaches adult levels by late adolescence.	malabsorption, malnutrition, respiratory alkalosis, proximal renal tubular acidosis, magnesium deficiency.	high phosphate, and metastatic carcinoma produces normal phosphate. Should be monitored frequently during treatment of ketoacidosis and in refeeding after starvation. Rarely, myeloma proteins cause falsely high or low phosphate.
Phosphatidyl glycerol	Negative: <0.5 mg/L Borderline: 0.5–2.0 mg/L Positive: >2.0 mg/L	1	Negative: <0.5 mg/L Borderline: 0.5–2.0 mg/L Positive: >2.0 mg/L	INC: Heavy contamination with meconium.	INC: Fetal maturity.	INC: Glucocorticoids.	Used to detect fetal lung maturity. Presence of PG reliably indicates presence of surfactant, but up to 40% of infants with borderline or negative PG actually produce surfactant. Appears more reliable than L/S ratio in infants of diabetic mothers.

(continued)

Table 38.1 *(continued)*

Test Name	Reference Range — Standard	Reference Range — Factor	Reference Range — SI Units	Nondisease Causes of Changes	Disease Related Changes	Drug Related Changes	Common Conditions for Use of Test
Platelet count	150–400×10^3/nL	10^6	150–400×10^9/L	Interday variation 8–10%. INC: Exercise, cell fragments. DEC: Cold agglutinins, platelet aggregation, ethanol. Increased during pregnancy. In females, highest at mid-cycle.	INC: Myeloproliferative disorders, iron deficiency, malignancy, following thrombocytopenia. DEC: Aplastic anemia, bone marrow suppression or replacement, idiopathic thrombocytopenic purpura, thrombotic thrombocytopenic purpura, disseminated intravascular coagulation, sepsis, hypersplenism, myelodysplastic syndromes.	INC: Glucocorticoids, propranolol. DEC: Agents causing bone marrow suppression (particularly antineoplastic agents), drugs causing platelet antibodies (cephalosporins, heparin, quinidine, rifampin).	Used to detect low platelets as a cause of bleeding disorders. Does not evaluate platelet function directly. Typically included as part of CBC. As with red cells, the mean cell size (mean platelet volume or MPV) indicates relative age of cells; older platelets are small, while young platelets are large.
Potassium	Serum: 3.5–5.0 mEq/L Urine: 25–105 mEq/day	1	3.5–5.0 mmol/L 25–125 mmol/day	Interday variation 1–2%. Highest at 8 AM, 20% lower at night. INC: Fist clenching during tourniquet, delayed transport to lab, prolonged tourniquet use, high platelet count (serum), EDTA contamination, IV fluid contamination, blood transfusion, hemolyzed specimens. DEC: Exercise, dehydration, ethanol, supine position.	INC: Acidosis, insulin deficiency, renal failure, Addison's disease, hyporeninemic hypoaldosteronism (usually in diabetes), cell lysis syndromes, type IV renal tubular acidosis. DEC: Alkalosis, malnutrition, vomiting, diarrhea, Cushing's syndrome, hyperaldosteronism, type I and type II renal tubular acidosis, villous	INC: Drugs causing renal impairment, angiotensin converting enzyme inhibitors, heparin, lithium, spironolactone, salt substitutes, triamterene, nonsteroidal anti-inflammatory agents. DEC: Diuretics, acetazolamide, glucocorticoids, florinef, antibiotics (aminoglycosides, carbenicillin), insulin,	Usually included as part of electrolytes, used to assess plasma potassium as an indicator of total potassium. Because clinical signs and symptoms of hypokalemia and hyperkalemia are inconsistent and nonspecific, potassium should be ordered in any patient on

Prealbumin	10–40 mg/dL	10	100–400 mg/L	Slight decrease with age: About 0.1–0.2 mmol/L lower by age 60 years.	cisplatin, amphotericin.
				In pregnancy, decreases by 10%. Decreases after age 60, up to 20% lower in younger adults. Lower in females than males, until menopause.	adenoma of colon, magnesium deficiency.

INC: Cushing's syndrome, Hodgkin's disease. DEC: Malnutrition, acute inflammation, cirrhosis, nephrotic syndrome.

INC: Androgens, glucocorticoids, oral contraceptives. DEC: Amiodarone, estrogens.

Used primarily as an indicator of nutritional status. Because of short half-life of about 1 day, will rapidly change with alteration in protein nutritional state. Has been used on admission to evaluate nutritional state, but not as much data on usefulness as for albumin.

medications possibly affecting potassium and any patient with unexplained symptoms such as muscle weakness.

Progesterone	M: 0–0.4 µg/L F (follicular phase): < 1.5 µg/L F (luteal phase): 5.7–28.1 µg/L	3.18	0–1.2 nmol/L < 4.8 nmol/L 18.1–89.4 nmol/L	Interday variation 20%. Highest at bedtime, lowest at 8 AM. DEC: Exercise, after meals. In females, gradual increase after ovulation, peaks about 10 days later. Luteal phase levels increase with increasing age. In pregnancy, gradually increases to peak at term. In children, undetectable until after puberty.	INC: Congenital adrenal hyperplasia, ovarian stromal tumors, hydatidiform mole. DEC: Hypogonadism, hypopituitarism, luteal phase deficiency, toxemia, miscarriage, fetal death.

INC: Clomiphene, ketoconazole. DEC: Ampicillin, androgens, danazol, oral contraceptives, RU 486.

Used mainly to determine adequacy of function of corpus luteum, and to monitor course of assisted reproduction. Low levels of progesterone are associated with infertility and recurrent miscarriage.

(continued)

Table 38.1 *(continued)*

Test Name	Reference Range			Nondisease Causes of Changes	Disease Related Changes	Drug Related Changes	Common Conditions for Use of Test
	Standard	Factor	SI Units				
Prolactin	M: 2–16 ng/L F: 1–20 ng/L	44.4	M: 89–720 pmol/L F: 44–880 pmol/L	Interday variation 5–10% in males, 40% in females. 2–3× higher at night, lowest in early afternoon. Slightly higher in winter. INC: Stress, exercise, smoking (males), after meals, hemoconcentration, high altitude. DEC: Smoking (in females), ethanol, fasting. In females, increases during follicular phase to peak at ovulation. Increases gradually throughout pregnancy, peaks near term at up to 40× baseline, remains elevated during initial phases of lactation. Lower in females who have borne children. In children, 2–4× higher in neonates, reaches adult levels by 1 year. Up to 20% higher after age 60 years.	INC: Prolactin producing tumors, pituitary stalk compression, renal failure, hypothyroidism, anorexia nervosa, polycystic ovary syndrome, chest wall lesions, seizures. DEC: Malnutrition, acute illness, hypopituitarism.	INC: Cimetidine, estrogens, haloperidol, methadone, phenothiazines, tricyclic antidepressants, reserpine, danazol, phenytoin, opiates. DEC: L-Dopa, bromcriptine, rifampin, valproic acid, tamoxifen; erythropoietin (in renal failure).	Used primarily in females with amenorrhea or galactorrhea, or in males with impotence. Also used in evaluation of patients with pituitary tumors. Prolactin between normal and 100 ng/L is often due to medications or compression of pituitary stalk. Levels > 200 ng/L usually indicate presence of a prolactin producing tumor.
Prostate-specific antigen	M: 0–4.0 ng/mL F: 0–0.1 ng/mL	1	M: 0–4.0 µg/L F: 0–0.1 µg/L	Interday variation 15–20%. INC: After prostatic examination (<20%), prostate biopsy. DEC: Hospitalization. Increases with age after 50, usually <2.5 ng/mL <age 40 years, up to 6.8 ng/mL > age 65 years.	INC: Acute renal failure, prostatic hyperplasia, acute prostatitis, prostatic infarction, prostatic carcinoma. DEC: After prostatectomy.	DEC: GnRH analogues, estrogens, finasteride.	Used to screen for prostate cancer and to follow patients with known prostatic carcinoma. Screening is controversial because of unproven benefit of

	2.8–5.6 μg/mL	1	2.8–5.6 mg/L	early detection (see Chapter 3 for screening biases). PSA between 4 and 10 ng/mL is due to benign disease in 80% of cases; between 10 and 20 ng/mL is due to benign disease in about half of cases, and >20 ng/mL is almost always due to prostate cancer. After radical prostatectomy, PSA should fall to undetectable, while radiation will lower levels to normal. Antiandrogen therapy may cause a fall in PSA without any effect on tumor mass.
Protein C			DEC: High factor VII levels. Increases moderately in pregnancy. In children, levels 25% of adult in neonates, remains low through first month of life.	DEC: Congenital deficiency, liver disease, renal failure, sepsis.
				INC: Heparin, oral contraceptives. DEC: Coumadin. Used in evaluation of patients with thrombotic disorders. Heterozygous deficiency of protein C often does not present until adult life.

(continued)

Table 38.1 *(continued)*

Test Name	Reference Range			Nondisease Causes of Changes	Disease Related Changes	Drug Related Changes	Common Conditions for Use of Test
	Standard	Factor	SI Units				
Protein, CSF	15–45 mg/dL	10	150–450 mg/L	INC: Methotrexate (interference in some assays). Normal up to 120 mg/dL in neonates, reaches adult levels by 1 month, increases gradually with age over 30 years, about 1–2 mg/dL per decade (up to 60 mg/dL after age 60 years).	INC: CNS infection, CNS inflammation, CNS malignancies, CNS degenerative disease, lead poisoning. DEC: CSF leakage, Reye's syndrome.	INC: Ibuprofen.	Used most commonly along with other tests to detect inflammation in the CNS. Will be elevated with most CNS infections, many degenerative CNS diseases, and most examples of multiple sclerosis.
Protein electrophoresis, CSF	No oligoclonal bands.		No oligoclonal bands.		Oligoclonal bands present: Multiple sclerosis, Guillain-Barre syndrome, subacute sclerosing panencephalitis, CNS syphilis, Lyme disease, AIDS.		Used in suspected multiple sclerosis (MS). Because patients with MS often have normal total protein, should be done even if total protein normal. In addition to oligoclonal band pattern, may also see increase in serum proteins and decrease in CSF specific proteins (prealbumin, second transferrin band) in patients with increased vascular permeability, although this is of little use diagnostically.
Protein electrophoresis, serum	Albumin: 3.5–5.0 g/dL	10	Albumin: 35–50 g/L	Interday variation 10% for each fraction.	DEC (albumin): Malnutrition,	INC (α_1): Androgens. INC (α_2): Estrogens, oral	Used primarily in evaluation of

α₁-globulins: 0.1–0.3 g/dL
α₂-globulins: 0.6–1.0 g/dL
β-globulins: 0.7–1.1 g/dL
γ-globulins: 0.8–1.6 g/dL

α₁-globulins: 1–3 g/L
α₂-globulins: 6–10 g/L
β-globulins: 7–11 g/L
γ-globulins: 8–16 g/L

INC (albumin): Hemoconcentration.
DEC (albumin): Pregnancy.
INC (α₁): Pregnancy.
DEC (α₁): Prolonged storage of specimen.
INC (α₂): Pregnancy.
INC (β): Pregnancy.
DEC (β): (C3 band) prolonged storage of specimen.
INC (γ): Hemolyzed specimens, plasma samples (may produce false monoclonal bands).
DEC (γ): Plasmapheresis, pregnancy.

malabsorption, acute inflammation, malignancy, cirrhosis, nephrotic syndrome.
INC (α₁): Acute inflammation, infection, malignancy.
DEC (α₁): Congenital deficiency, nephrotic syndrome, cirrhosis.
INC (α₂): Acute inflammation, malignancy, nephrotic syndrome.
DEC (α₂): Hemolytic anemia, congenital deficiency of haptoglobin, cirrhosis, liver failure.
INC (β): Nephrotic syndrome, hypercholesterolemia, iron deficiency, obstructive jaundice, some cases of multiple myeloma (especially IgA).
DEC (β): Acute inflammation, cirrhosis, liver failure, hemochromatosis, malnutrition.
INC (γ): (polyclonal) AIDS, autoimmune disease, sarcoidosis, cirrhosis, chronic infections, parasitic disease; (monoclonal) multiple myeloma, Waldenstrom's macroglobulinemia, monoclonal gammopathy of undetermined significance, mycosis fungoides.

contraceptives, phenytoin.
INC (β): Drugs increasing low density lipoprotein.
DEC (β): Drugs lowering low density lipoprotein.
INC (γ): Propylthiouracil.
DEC (γ): Glucocorticoids.

abnormal globulins. Also used to follow patients with monoclonal gammopathies; quantitation of the monoclonal protein from the electrophoretic separation is the preferred method for detecting changes in tumor mass. Of limited usefulness in patients with normal total protein and normal globulins. Use of quantitative results for bands other than monoclonal immunoglobulins is less helpful than visual inspection of the gel and interpretation of the pattern of changes, as discussed in Chapter 9, especially Table 9.1 and Figure 9.2.

(continued)

Table 38.1 *(continued)*

Test Name	Reference Range			Nondisease Causes of Changes	Disease Related Changes	Drug Related Changes	Common Conditions for Use of Test
	Standard	Factor	SI Units				
Protein electrophoresis, serum *continued*					DEC (γ): Bruton's agammaglobulinemia, multiple myeloma (other than monoclonal band), chronic lymphocytic leukemia, nephrotic syndrome, burns.		
Protein electrophoresis, urine	Only albumin present.			INC: Glomerular type pattern: exercise, fever, acute illness.	Glomerular pattern: (selective) Increased α_1-globulins and β-globulins, with albumin also present; (nonselective) above plus γ-globulins. Tubular pattern: Albumin, three bands not seen in serum (pre-α_1, two α_2). Overflow proteinuria: One or more abnormal bands (usually monoclonal-type) especially in β-globulins and γ-globulins, multiple myeloma, hemolysis, rhabdomyolysis, monocytic leukemia.	INC (tubular pattern): Drugs injuring the proximal renal tubule (particularly cisplatin, amphotericin B, aminoglycosides, nonsteroidal anti-inflammatory agents, penicillins, sulfonamides). INC (overflow pattern): Drugs causing hemolysis or rhabdomyolysis.	Used to evaluate patients with proteinuria when the cause is not readily apparent. Not required in adults with nephrotic syndrome, but may be helpful in children (since those with nonselective proteinuria typically have other causes than minimal change disease). Useful for recognition of Bence Jones protein and used for monitoring patients with light chain disease; total Bence Jones protein excretion per day is related to tumor mass.

Protein S	21–42 μg/mL	1	21–42 mg/L	INC: Coagulation factor deficiencies. In neonates, levels about 20% of adult.	DEC: Congenital deficiency, liver disease, acute inflammation, sepsis.	DEC: Coumadin, heparin, oral contraceptives.	Used in evaluation of patients with thrombotic disorders. Deficiency of protein S often does not present until adult life.
Protein, total	6.2–8.0 g/dL	10	62–80 g/L	Interday variation 2–4%. Highest in afternoon, lowest in AM. INC: Hemoconcentration, prolonged tourniquet use, upright posture, hemolyzed specimens. Approximately 0.3 g/dL higher in plasma than serum. DEC: Low protein diet, drawing blood above IV sites, blindness. In pregnancy, gradually decreases an average of 15% by 20 weeks, decreases by 33% by third trimester. In children, about 33% lower in neonates, reaches adult levels by 1 year. Slightly higher in adolescents, young adults. Decreases an average of 0.2–0.3 g/dL after age 40 years.	INC: Multiple myeloma, Waldenstrom's macroglobulinemia, chronic inflammatory disorders (particularly autoimmune diseases), chronic infections, AIDS, some cases of cirrhosis. DEC: Malnutrition, malabsorption, nephrotic syndrome, protein losing enteropathy, burns.	INC: Androgens, glucocorticoids, epinephrine, oral contraceptives, thyroid hormone. DEC: Allopurinol, carbamazepine, estrogens.	Used most commonly (along with albumin) to screen for monoclonal gammopathies; total globulins (protein-albumin) reflects primarily changes in γ-globulin levels. Globulins are increased with monoclonal gammopathies in myeloma and Waldenstrom's, and in a polyclonal fashion with chronic inflammation or infection, cirrhosis, and AIDS. Patients with cirrhosis and nephrotic syndrome often have normal total protein but decreased albumin.

(continued)

Table 38.1 *(continued)*

Test Name	Reference Range			Nondisease Causes of Changes	Disease Related Changes	Drug Related Changes	Common Conditions for Use of Test
	Standard	Factor	SI Units				
Protein, urine	<150 mg/day	0.001	<0.15 g/day	Interday variation 30–40%. Lowest in morning, highest in afternoon. INC: Fever, upright posture, exercise, stress, ethanol, high fat diet. DEC: High fiber diet.	INC: Nephrotic syndrome, glomerulonephritis, diabetic nephropathy, multiple myeloma, renal tubular damage, urinary tract infection, hematuria, congestive heart failure, toxemia.	INC: Drugs causing renal tubular damage, corticosteroids. DEC: Angiotensin converting enzyme inhibitors.	Used to quantify urine protein excretion. Dipstick methods detect primarily albumin, and are falsely low with Bence Jones protein. While total protein is the preferred method for quantifying protein excretion, it requires 24 hour urine collection which may be problematic. There is a general equivalence between the ratio of the concentrations of urine protein and creatinine (in mg/dL) and 24 hour protein excretion; this is of more use in following protein excretion in an individual than in estimating excretion at initial evaluation. Urine protein >1 g/day is almost always due to glomerular losses or Bence Jones protein. Lower levels of

Test					Comments
					proteinuria may be due to many causes, and urine protein electrophoresis is most useful in these cases.
Prothrombin time (PT)	11–13 s	1	11–13 s	Interday variation 3–5%. In neonates, 2–3 s longer; reaches adult levels by 3–4 days.	INC: Liver disease, vitamin K deficiency, malabsorption, congenital factor deficiencies, antiphospholipid antibodies. INC: Coumadin, androgens, drugs altering Coumadin metabolism, antibiotics, propylthiouracil. DEC: Androgens, drugs increasing Coumadin metabolism.	Used to detect defects in liver coagulation protein synthesis, which is often the earliest laboratory abnormality in cirrhosis. Also often used to screen for coagulation factor deficiencies before surgery, but of limited utility for this purpose in patients with no history of liver disease or bleeding problems. Also widely used to monitor therapy with Coumadin. Results usually expressed as the International Normalized Ratio (INR), which should be between 2 and 3 for effective anticoagulation with low risk of bleeding.

(continued)

Table 38.1 *(continued)*

Test Name	Reference Range			Nondisease Causes of Changes	Disease Related Changes	Drug Related Changes	Common Conditions for Use of Test
	Standard	Factor	SI Units				
Protoporphyrin, zinc (free erythrocyte protoporphyrin)	17–77 µg/dL	0.016	0.27–1.23 µmol/L	INC: Hemolyzed specimens, increased bilirubin. In pregnancy, increases 25% in first trimester, 75% by term.	INC: Iron deficiency, chronic lead poisoning, anemia of chronic disease, renal failure.		Used to screen for iron deficiency in children; can readily be performed using blood from a fingerstick. Formerly used to screen for lead poisoning, but only reliably detects blood levels >25 µg/dL; this is not sensitive enough to detect mild lead poisoning in children.
PTT (see Partial thromboplastin time)							
Pyridimoline cross-links	Pyridinoline: 20–61 nmol/mmol creatinine Deoxypyridin- oline: 4–19 nmol/mmol creatinine	1	Pyridinoline: 20–61 nmol/mmol creatinine Deoxypyridin- oline: 4–19 nmol/mmol creatinine	Interday variation 15%. Highest in AM, 25–35% lower in PM. INC: Heavy exercise. In females, increases markedly after menopause. Lowest in children, increases markedly during puberty and then falls to adult levels. Increases after age 40 years. Slightly higher in females than males.	INC: Increased turnover metabolic bone diseases (hyperparathyroidism, osteomalacia, Paget's disease, hyperthyroidism, rarely in osteoporosis), acute illness, malignancy. DEC: Renal failure.	INC: Estrogens. DEC: Bisphosphonates.	Used to recognize increased bone turnover and to monitor treatment of metabolic bone diseases. Preferred over hydroxyproline. There is a discrepancy between this test and collagen cross-linked telopeptides in patients with osteoporosis under treatment; it is not yet clear which test will be more reliable.

Radioactive iodine uptake (RAIU)	6 h: 3–20% 24 h: 8–30%	0.011	6 h: 0.03–0.20 24 h: 0.08–0.30	INC: Iodide deficiency. DEC: High iodide diet, following use of x-ray contrast agents.	INC: Grave's disease, toxic nodules, iodide deficiency, nephrotic syndrome, acute renal failure, cirrhosis. DEC: Thyroiditis, hypopituitarism, chronic renal failure.	INC: Barbiturates, lithium. DEC: Aspirin, amiodarone, iodine, thyroid hormone, propylthiouracil, methimazole, glucocorticoids, phenylbutazone, sulfonylureas.	Used to assess functional state of the thyroid gland; high, diffuse uptake is typical of Grave's disease, while low uptake occurs with thyroid hormone ingestion, thyroiditis, and central hypothyroidism due to pituitary or hypothalamic dysfunction.
Red blood cell count	M: 4.3–5.7 $\times 10^6/\mu L$ F: 3.8–5.1 $\times 10^6/\mu L$	10^6	M: 4.3–5.7 $\times 10^{12}/L$ F: 3.8–5.1 $\times 10^{12}/L$	Interday variation 3%. Higher by 5% in AM. INC: High altitude, hemoconcentration, upright posture, tourniquet use, strenuous exercise, stress. DEC: Supine posture, after meals. In pregnancy, falls by 15% by second trimester. In children, slightly higher in neonates, 10% below adult levels by 1 year, then gradually reach adult levels by late adolescence.	INC: Polycythemia vera, erythropoietin producing tumors (kidney, liver), chronic hypoxemia, high oxygen affinity hemoglobins, thalassemia minor (mildly increased or normal). DEC: Decreased red cell production, hemolytic anemia, bleeding, chronic renal failure.	INC: Erythropoietin. DEC: Drugs causing hemolysis or bone marrow suppression.	Usually measured as part of CBC, but provides little additional information in most cases. Most helpful in microcytosis, where low RBC is typical of iron deficiency and high normal or slightly elevated RBC is seen in thalassemia minor. May be falsely decreased in presence of cold agglutinins, as occurs with mycoplasma infections.

(continued)

Table 38.1 *(continued)*

Test Name	Reference Range			Nondisease Causes of Changes	Disease Related Changes	Drug Related Changes	Common Conditions for Use of Test
	Standard	Factor	SI Units				
Red blood cell distribution width (RDW)	10.0–16.4%	0.01	0.100–0.164	INC: Cold agglutinins, hyperglycemia, reticulocytosis. DEC: After blood transfusion.	INC: Most forms of acquired anemia. Normal: Aplastic anemia, thalassemia minor, hereditary spherocytosis.	INC: Drugs causing hemolysis.	Usually included in complete blood count. Generally of little value for differential diagnosis except in patients with microcytic anemia, where a normal RDW suggests thalassemia minor as the diagnosis.
Renin	Supine: 0.5–1.6 ng/mL per h Upright: 1.9–3.6 ng/mL per h	0.278	Supine: 0.1–0.4 ng/L per s Upright: 0.5–1.0 ng/L per s	Highest 4 AM, lowest 4–6 PM. INC: Upright posture, stress, exercise, dehydration, hemoconcentration, ethanol. DEC: High altitude, volume overload, supine posture, weight loss. In females, increases during menses. Gradually increases during pregnancy to peak in third trimester. In children, markedly elevated in neonates. In adults, basal level and response to volume depletion decrease with increasing age. Higher in males than females and in whites than blacks.	INC: Dehydration, renal artery stenosis, accelerated hypertension, Bartter's syndrome, renin producing tumors, cirrhosis, nephrotic syndrome, congestive heart failure, hyperthyroidism. DEC: Cushing's syndrome, primary hyperaldosteronism, salt retaining congenital adrenal hyperplasia, low renin essential hypertension, hypothyroidism, hypopituitarism, toxemia, diabetes.	INC: Diuretics, estrogens, oral contraceptives, angiotensin converting enzyme inhibitors, albuterol, calcium channel blockers. DEC: Clonidine, cyclosporine, licorice, guanethidine, digoxin, prazosin, β-blockers, methyldopa, nonsteroidal anti-inflammatory agents.	Used primarily in evaluation of patients with hypertension, particularly when associated with hypokalemia and metabolic alkalosis; ideally, it should be measured along with plasma aldosterone. Must always be drawn when patient's volume status, salt intake, and posture are known (values given are for patients on a normal salt intake). Drugs affecting renin or aldosterone should be discontinued, preferably for 1–2 weeks, before testing is performed.

Reticulocyte count

24–84 × $10^3/\mu L$ 0.5–1.5%	10^6 0.01	24–84 × $10^9/L$ 0.005–0.015	INC: Ethanol, exercise.	INC: Hemolytic anemias, recovery from blood loss, repletion of deficient factors. DEC: Aplastic anemia, bone marrow replacement, iron deficiency, megaloblastic anemia, anemia of chronic disease, chronic renal failure, hypothyroidism, adrenal insufficiency.	INC: Drugs causing hemolysis. DEC: Drugs causing bone marrow suppression.	Used in patients with anemia to determine adequacy of marrow response, which serves as a rough guide to whether anemia is due to decreased production or red cell destruction (hemolysis, blood loss). If percent is used, must be corrected for the patient's hematocrit.

Reverse T_3 (see Triiodothyronine, reverse)

Rheumatoid factor (RF)

Negative	Negative	INC: Lipemic serum, acute illness, smoking. Frequency of positive rheumatoid factor increases with age >50 years.	INC: Rheumatoid arthritis, Sjogren's syndrome, other autoimmune diseases, Waldenstrom's macroglobulinemia, sarcoidosis.	INC: Aldomet.	Used in evaluation of patients with suspected rheumatoid arthritis. Increased in about 80–90% of patients with this disease and in Sjogren's syndrome, 50% of patients with systemic lupus erythematosus or mixed connective tissue disease, less frequently in other autoimmune disorders. Positive results with titer <1:80 are usually not clinically important.

(continued)

Table 38.1 *(continued)*

Test Name	Reference Range			Nondisease Causes of Changes	Disease Related Changes	Drug Related Changes	Common Conditions for Use of Test
	Standard	Factor	SI Units				
Schilling test	>7.5% of radioactive labeled B$_{12}$ excreted in 24 h urine.	0.01	0.075 of radioactive labeled B$_{12}$ excreted in 24 h urine.	DEC: Failure to administer B$_{12}$ before test performance.	DEC: Pernicious anemia, pancreatic insufficiency, malabsorption, bowel resection, Crohn's disease, liver disease, intestinal bacterial overgrowth, fish tapeworm infestation, renal insufficiency.	DEC: Barbiturates, aspirin, ranitidine. INC: Cimetidine.	Used to evaluate patients with low vitamin B$_{12}$ levels to determine etiology. In patients with early pernicious anemia, normal results may occur unless the radioactive labeled B$_{12}$ is administered in food. Often, a second stage (repeating the test giving intrinsic factor orally along with B$_{12}$) is used; absorption should normalize in pernicious anemia, but remain low in other causes of B$_{12}$ malabsorption. This second stage may be falsely abnormal in patients with antibodies to intrinsic factor, which occur in about 50–75% of patients with pernicious anemia.

SG (see Specific gravity)

SGOT (see Aspartate aminotransferase)

SGPT (see Alanine aminotransferase)

Smooth muscle antibodies (see Antismooth muscle antibodies)

Test	Conventional	Factor	SI	Physiologic Influences	Disease Influences	Drug Influences	Interpretation
Sodium	Serum: 135–143 mEq/L Urine: 43–260 mEq/day	1	135–143 mmol/L 43–260 mmol/day	Interday variation <1%. Highest at noon, falls 1–2% by evening. Highest in summer, lowest in winter. INC: Exercise, dehydration. DEC: Ethanol, hyperglycemia; increased lipids, protein (some assays). In females, 1.5% lower during menses. In pregnancy, decreases average 2–3 mmol/L by term. Lower in blind individuals by 5 mmol/L. Urine sodium decreases gradually after age 60 years.	INC: Dehydration, diabetes insipidus, rarely with hyperaldosteronism or Cushing's syndrome. DEC: Addison's disease, hypoaldosteronism, inappropriate antidiuresis (CNS diseases, pulmonary diseases, malignancies), polydipsia, cirrhosis, congestive heart failure, nephrotic syndrome.	INC: Agents causing salt retention: fludrocortisone, anabolic steroids, estrogens, oral contraceptives, phenylbutazone, licorice, guanethidine, clonidine, lithium. DEC: Diuretics, heparin, chlorpropamide, aminoglutethemide, amphotericin, vincristine, cyclophosphamide, carbamazepine, miconazole.	Used to evaluate disorders of volume status. Widely performed as part of routine screening tests (such as electrolytes, "chemistry panels"). Abnormal serum sodium must always be evaluated in light of the fluid status of the patient. Urine electrolytes and osmolality are usually helpful in evaluating hyponatremic patients; "normal" values are not given for urine electrolytes or osmolality; rather, values are interpreted in light of what is appropriate for the patient's volume status.

(continued)

Table 38.1 (continued)

Test Name	Reference Range			Nondisease Causes of Changes	Disease Related Changes	Drug Related Changes	Common Conditions for Use of Test
	Standard	Factor	SI Units				
Somatomedin C (see Insulin-like growth factor-1)							
Somatotropin (see Growth hormone)							
Specific gravity (SG), urine	1.002–1.030	1	1.002–1.030	Marked variation within "normal" range during the course of a day; highest in AM, lowest in PM. INC: Exercise, upright posture, proteinuria, glucosuria, x-ray contrast agents. DEC: Water intake, ethanol.	INC: Dehydration, diabetes mellitus, inappropriate antidiuresis, congestive heart failure, cirrhosis. DEC: Diabetes insipidus, ADH resistance, polydipsia, hypercalcemia, hypokalemia, renal tubular injury.	INC: Isotretinoin. DEC: Aminoglycosides, cyclosporine, lithium.	Methods for measuring specific gravity vary. Dipsticks measure ionic strength, and frequently give erroneous results in acutely ill patients. Refractometer measurements are more accurate, but overestimate urine concentration with proteinuria, glucosuria, or after x-ray contrast agents. Both are rough measures of renal concentrating ability. Urine concentration must always be interpreted in light of what the kidneys should do to maintain normal serum sodium and volume. Wide variation in values in normal individuals means there are no absolute "abnormal" results.

T_3 *(see Triiodothyronine)*
T_3RU *(see Triiodothyronine resin uptake)*
T_4 *(see Thyroxine)*

Test	Reference range	Factor	SI units	Physiologic INC/DEC	Pathologic INC/DEC	Drug effects	Comments
Testosterone, total	M: 300–1,000 ng/dL F: 15–60 ng/dL	0.035	10.4–34.7 nmol/L 0.52–2.08 nmol/L	Interday variation 10–20%. Over 100% higher in AM than at 10 PM. INC: Exercise, after meals, obesity (in females). DEC: Stress, immobilization, heavy exercise, obesity (in males), ethanol, blindness. In females, peaks at ovulation. Increases during pregnancy. In children, markedly decreased until puberty. In males, decreases with age, but in females increases after menopause. Higher in blacks than whites.	INC (in females): Sertoli-Leydig cell tumors, polycystic ovary syndrome, adrenal carcinoma, androgen insensitivity syndrome. DEC: Hypogonadism, hypopituitarism, cirrhosis, renal failure, orchitis, acute illness, immobilization.	INC: Barbiturates, bromcriptine, cimetidine, clomiphene, estrogens, oral contraceptives, phenytoin. DEC: Androgens, diethylstilbestrol, digoxin, danazol, finasteride, glucocorticoids, GnRH agonists, ketoconazole, spironolactone.	Used in evaluation of infertility or impotence in males, and in evaluation of hirsutism in females. Total testosterone is less sensitive than free testosterone because production of binding protein increases as testosterone falls. SHBG is also increased by antiepileptics, and decreased with malnutrition, in obesity, and with hypothyroidism.
Testosterone, free	M: 5.1–41.0 ng/dL F: 0.1–2.0 ng/dL	0.035 34.7	0.18–1.42 nmol/L 3.5–70 pmol/L	Same as for total testosterone, although exercise, obesity, and hemoconcentration do not affect results.	Same as for total testosterone.	Same as for total testosterone, although antiepileptics and oral contraceptives decrease free while danazol increases free.	Same as for total testosterone.

(continued)

Table 38.1 *(continued)*

Test Name	Reference Range			Nondisease Causes of Changes	Disease Related Changes	Drug Related Changes	Common Conditions for Use of Test
	Standard	Factor	SI Units				
Thrombin time	9–15s	1	9–15s	No interday variation. INC: Heparin containing tubes, multiple transfusions of RBC.	INC: Disseminated intravascular coagulation, multiple myeloma, Waldenstrom's macroglobulinemia, dysfibrinogenemia, fibrinogen deficiency (cirrhosis, malnutrition).	INC: Thrombolytic agents, heparin.	Used to detect inhibitors of fibrin formation; usually used to detect dysfinbrinogenemia or, when heparin assays are not available, presumptively identify the presence of heparin. Not needed to recognize DIC, where D-dimer or fibrin split products are preferred tests.
Thyroglobulin	2–60 ng/mL	1	2–60 μg/L	Interday variation 5%. INC: Hemoconcentration, after fine needle aspiration. In females, slight decline at time of ovulation. Increases 100% during pregnancy. Highest in neonates, higher in premature than term infants; decreases to adult levels by adolescence.	INC: Thyroid carcinoma (follicular or papillary), thyroiditis, Graves' disease. DEC: Hyperthyroidism due to thyroid hormone ingestion.	DEC: Neomycin.	Used primarily to monitor patients following resection of papillary or follicular thyroid cancers; useful only if total thyroidectomy was performed. Many patients have antithyroglobulin antibodies, which invalidate the test. If antibodies are present, they should be retested 6–12 months after surgery; disappearance of antibody usually

Thyroglobulin antibodies (see Antithyroglobulin)

Thyroid microsomal antibodies (see Antithyroid peroxidase)

				signifies complete tumor removal, but in any case indicates that thyroglobulin measurements can be used to monitor the patient.
Thyrotropin	0.3–5.0 µIU/mL	1 0.3–5.0 mIU/L	Interday variation 20%. Highest at midnight, 40% lower at 4 PM. Highest in winter, lowest in summer. INC: Smoking hemoconcentration, stress. DEC: Fasting. In pregnancy, increases 10–20%. In children, up to 3× increased in neonates; reaches adult levels by 5 years. Increases with age >40 years; average 50% higher >age 55 years, within day variation decreases after age 55 years. Higher in males than females and in whites than blacks.	INC: Primary hypothyroidism, renal failure, recovery from acute illness, recovery from painless, subacute thyroiditis. DEC: Hyperthyroidism, some cases of hypopituitarism, prolonged malnutrition, acute illness. INC: Drugs decreasing thyroxine production (see thyroxine for list), dopamine antagonists, prednisone. DEC: Aspirin, thyroid hormones, dopamine, L-dopa, most glucocorticoids, octreotide, danazol.	Used in many cases as the sole test to screen for thyroid dysfunction; low levels (below detection limits) usually indicate hyperthyroidism or excess thyroid hormone ingestion, while increased levels usually indicate primary hypothyroidism. For optimal performance, should measure to at least 0.05 mU/L. If TSH normal, no other thyroid tests indicated unless clinical features strongly suggest hyperthyroidism or hypothyroidism and a pituitary cause of thyroid dysfunction is suspected.

(continued)

Table 38.1 *(continued)*

Test Name	Reference Range			Nondisease Causes of Changes	Disease Related Changes	Drug Related Changes	Common Conditions for Use of Test
	Standard	Factor	SI Units				
Thyrotropin receptor antibodies	<10% inhibition	1	<10% inhibition		INC: Graves' disease, rarely with thyroiditis.		Used in equivocal cases to confirm a diagnosis of Graves' disease. In pregnant Graves' patients, titer correlates with degree of thyroid enlargement in neonate.
Thyroxine, total	4.5–12.5 μg/dL	12.9	58–161 nmol/L	Interday variation 15%. Up to 50% intraday variation. Highest in winter, lowest in summer. INC: Hemoconcentration. DEC: Heavy exercise, smoking. In pregnancy, increases 10–20% early, returns to baseline by third trimester. In children, reference range wider in neonates, reaches adult levels by 1 y. Decreases 10% with age >40 years. Higher in males than females.	INC: Hyperthyroidism, high TBG (active liver disease, pregnancy), dysalbuminemic hyperthyroxinemia. DEC: Hypothyroidism, hypopituitarism, malnutrition, nephrotic syndrome, severe illness, renal failure.	INC: Propranolol, drugs increasing TBG (estrogens, oral contraceptives, phenothiazines, tamoxifen), thyroxine, amiodarone (most cases). DEC: Rifampin, lithium, isotretinoin, salsalate, drugs decreasing TBG (androgens, glucocorticoids, danazol), drugs decreasing hormone binding to TBG (diazepam, heparin, antiepileptics, phenylbutazone).	Used in some laboratories instead of free thyroxine. Abnormal results must be correlated with T₃ resin uptake to detect abnormalities in TBG; T₄ and T₃RU will change in the same direction with thyroid disease, will change in opposite directions with changes in TBG.
Thyroxine, free	0.7–1.5 ng/dL	12.9	9.0–19.4 pmol/L	Interday variation 15%. Highest in winter, lowest in summer. INC: Fasting. DEC: Dialysis. In pregnancy, decreases 30%. In children, up to 2× higher in neonates,	INC: Hyperthyroidism. DEC: Hypothyroidism, hypopituitarism, severe illness.	INC: Heparin, propranolol, valproic acid. DEC: Lithium, trimethoprim-sulfamethoxazole, nitroprusside, salsalate, phenytoin, carbamazepine,	Used in some laboratories as the major test of thyroid hormone concentration. Less subject to interpretation problems than total

Test	Conventional range	Factor	SI range	Physiological factors	Drug effects	Comments
				reaches adult levels by 1 year. Decreases 10% with age >40 years. Higher in males than females.	valproic acid, cholestipol, rifampin.	T_4. Some assays (particularly analog assays) give falsely low results with acute illness. Practitioners should be aware of the type of assay used in the laboratory.
Thyroxine index, free	1.0–4.3	1	1.0–4.3	Same as for free thyroxine.	Same as for free thyroxine.	Calculated using the formula: Free thyroxine index = $T_4 \times T_3RU$. Agrees moderately well with actual free T_4 except in patients with acute illness or in patients with dysalbuminemic hyperthyroxinemia.
TIBC (see Iron binding capacity)						
Transferrin	215–375 mg/dL	0.01	2.15–3.75 g/L	Interday variation 1–3%. INC: Hemoconcentration, exercise. In pregnancy, increases 50% by third trimester. In children, 33% lower during first decade. Decreases 10% by age 65 years, another 10% by age 80 years. 10–20% higher in females than males.	INC: Iron deficiency. DEC: Chronic inflammation, hemochromatosis, malnutrition, malabsorption, cirrhosis, nephrotic syndrome.	INC: Estrogens, oral contraceptives. DEC: Androgens, glucocorticoids.	Used along with serum iron to evaluate patients with anemia and in screening for hemochromatosis. Can be estimated from TIBC using formula: Transferrin = (0.8 × TIBC) − 44.

(continued)

Table 38.1 *(continued)*

Test Name	Reference Range			Nondisease Causes of Changes	Disease Related Changes	Drug Related Changes	Common Conditions for Use of Test
	Standard	Factor	SI Units				

Transthyretin (see Prealbumin)

Triglycerides	NCEP Decision Levels: Normal: <200 mg/dL Borderline: 200–400 mg/dL High: 400–1,000 mg/dL Very High: >1,000 mg/dL	0.0113	NCEP Decision Levels: Normal: <2.26 mmol/L Borderline: 2.26–4.52 mmol/L High: 4.52–11.3 mmol/L Very High: >11.8 mmol/L	Interday variation 30–50%. Highest in winter, lowest in fall. INC: After meals (60%), stress, hemoconcentration, smoking, ethanol. DEC: Exercise, prolonged fast. In females, highest at mid-cycle. In pregnancy, increases 3–4× by third trimester. About 10% higher by age 60 years in males, 20% higher in females. Higher in males than females and in whites than blacks.	INC: Hyperlipidemia, diabetes, renal failure, gout, obstructive jaundice, nephrotic syndrome, hypothyroidism, pancreatitis, myocardial infarction. DEC: Hypolipoproteinemias, malnutrition, malabsorption, hyperthyroidism, hyperparathyroidism.	INC: β-Adrenergic antagonists, danazol, furosemide, isotretinoin, ketoconazole, glucocorticoids, oral contraceptives, spironolactone, aspirin, cholestyramine (in some patients). DEC: Androgens, amiodarone, cholestyramine, fibric acids, glyburide, heparin, probucol, sulfonylureas, vitamin C.	Used mainly in evaluating risk of atherosclerosis, and is needed to calculate LDL-cholesterol. Markedly elevated triglyceride levels can be detected by laboratory as lipemic specimens. Seldom needed as an isolated test. In pleural or peritoneal fluid, can be used on turbid specimens to differentiate chylous effusions due to lymphatic obstruction (high triglyceride) from pseudochylous effusion due to degenerating cells (low triglyceride and high cholesterol).
Triiodothyronine, total	80–220 ng/dL	0.0154	1.23–3.39 nmol/L	Interday variation 20%. Highest in winter, lowest in summer. INC: Obesity, other factors similar to thyroxine. DEC: Acute stress, fasting, smoking. In pregnancy, increases	INC: Hyperthyroidism, high TBG (active liver disease, pregnancy). DEC: Hypothyroidism, malnutrition, cirrhosis, acute illness, renal failure.	INC: Rifampin, terbutaline, valproic acid; parallels T_4 (see above). DEC: Salsalate; as for T_4; in addition, drugs which inhibit conversion of T_4 to T_3	Used primarily in patients with suppressed TSH and normal T_4. In hypothyroidism, low levels occur in more severe cases, but are normal in

Test	Reference interval (conventional)	Factor	Reference interval (SI)	Physiologic variation	Increase/Decrease (conditions)	Drugs	Comments
(continued from previous page)				10–20%. In children, lower in neonates, reaches adult levels by 1 year. Decreases 33% with age >40 years. Higher in males than females.		(propranolol, glucocorticoids, cimetidine, thiouracil).	about 30% of cases. Not useful in acutely ill patients. When abnormal, must be interpreted in light of TBG (as estimated by T_3RU).
Triiodothyronine, free	1.9–5.0 ng/L	1.54	2.9–7.7 pmol/L	Similar to total T_3.	Similar to total T_3, not affected by changes in TBG, cirrhosis, or malnutrition.	Parallels free T_4 for increases, T_3 for decreases.	Used primarily in patients with suppressed TSH and normal T_4; not as widely available as free T_4. Less is known about effects of assay type on results.
Triiodothyronine resin uptake	22–34%	0.01	0.22–0.34	In general, changes are proportional to changes in thyroid binding globulin (TBG) but in a reciprocal fashion. Increases 10% with age >40 years. DEC: Pregnancy	INC: Cirrhosis, malnutrition, malabsorption, nephrotic syndrome, hyperthyroidism. DEC: Active liver disease, hypothyroidism.	INC: Androgens, glucocorticoids, danazol. DEC: Estrogens, oral contraceptives, phenothiazines, tamoxifen.	Used to estimate unsaturated binding capacity on TBG; resin uptake is inversely related to free binding sites. Not generally needed if total T_4 is normal. Used to calculate free thyroxine index by multiplying T_4 with T_3RU.

(continued)

Table 38.1 *(continued)*

Test Name	Reference Range			Nondisease Causes of Changes	Disease Related Changes	Drug Related Changes	Common Conditions for Use of Test
	Standard	Factor	SI Units				
Troponin-I	0–2 ng/mL	1	0–2 µg/L		INC: Myocardial infarction, unstable angina, renal failure (rarely).		Used to detect myocardial injury in patients presenting late after onset of symptoms, or in patients with coexistent skeletal muscle damage. Some data suggest improved ability to detect myocardial injury in patients with unstable angina (when compared to CK MB), and worse prognosis in patients with myocardial infarction and positive troponin at time of presentation.
Troponin-T	0–3.1 ng/mL	1	0–3.1 µg/L	In neonates, cardiac troponin T may be normally present.	INC: Myocardial infarction; unstable angina, renal failure, chronic myopathy, severe skeletal muscle injury.		Used to detect myocardial injury in patients presenting late after onset of symptoms, or in patients with coexistent skeletal muscle damage. Some data suggest improved ability to detect myocardial injury in patients with unstable angina (when

TSH (see Thyrotropin)

TSI (see Thyrotropin receptor antibodies)

Urea nitrogen (see BUN)

Test					Comments
Uric acid	0.059	M: 4–8 mg/dL F: 3–7 mg/dL	0.24–0.47 mmol/L 0.18–0.41 mmol/L	Interday variation 10%. Highest in AM, 5% lower in afternoon. Higher in summer than in winter. INC: Exercise, ethanol, blindness, obesity, blood transfusions. DEC: Smoking, refeeding after starvation. In pregnancy, falls 30% by 12 weeks, rises later in pregnancy to 20% over baseline by term. In children, lower until puberty; levels similar in males and females until puberty. Increases after menopause in females to values similar to males by age 60, no differences in males.	INC: Gout, renal failure, tumors with rapid cell turnover (leukemia, lymphoma, small cell carcinoma), toxemia, chronic lead poisoning, diabetes, acromegaly, pernicious anemia. DEC: Congenital enzyme deficiencies, Wilson's disease, Hodgkin's disease, proximal renal tubular defects, inappropriate antidiuresis.	INC: Drugs impairing renal excretion (diuretics, aspirin), androgens, cisplatin, cyclosporine, ethambutol, disopyramide, piroxicam, propranolol, pyrazinamide, theophylline. DEC: Coumadin, x-ray contrast agents, guaifenesin, glucocorticoids, allopurinol, azathioprine, lithium, indomethacin.	Used primarily to monitor treatment in patients with gout and to prevent uric acid nephropathy in patients with malignancies undergoing chemotherapy. Often included in panels, but of little value as a screening test.

(Note: the first entry column shows "compared to CK MB), and worse prognosis in patients with myocardial infarction and positive troponin at time of presentation." as continuation of the previous page's comments column.)

(continued)

Table 38.1 *(continued)*

Test Name	Reference Range			Nondisease Causes of Changes	Disease Related Changes	Drug Related Changes	Common Conditions for Use of Test
	Standard	Factor	SI Units				
Urobilinogen	0–1.0 Erlich Unit	1	0–1.0 Erlich Unit	Excretion higher in afternoon. INC: Alkaline urine; foods increasing 5-HIAA (see above), ketoacidosis, salicylates, phenothiazines, phenazopyridine (interference).	INC: Cirrhosis, recovery stage of hepatitis, congestive heart failure, hemolytic anemia, megaloblastic anemia, fever. DEC: Obstructive jaundice, early hepatitis.	INC: Drugs causing hemolysis. DEC: Antibiotics, ascorbic acid, drugs causing cholestasis.	Usually included as one of dipstick urinalysis tests. May provide a clue to hemolysis as a cause of anemia. Of little use for detection or characterization of liver disease.
Vanillylmandelic acid	1–8 mg/day	5.05	5–44 µmol/day	Excretion highest at night. INC: Caffeine, exercise, starvation, stress, iron deficiency. DEC: Ethanol, x-ray contrast agents. In children, markedly elevated (up to 5×) in neonates, remains 2–4× higher throughout childhood, adult levels after puberty.	INC: Pheochromocytoma, neuroblastoma, acute illness. DEC: Renal insufficiency.	INC: Phenothiazines, lithium, drugs releasing catecholamines (see above). DEC: Drugs inhibiting catecholamine production (see above), disulfiram, phenothiazines, α-methyldopa.	Used in diagnosis or follow-up of patients with pheochromocytoma or neuroblastoma. In pheochromocytoma, VMA is less sensitive than other markers, but is preferred in patients with large adrenal tumors (which may not release intact catecholamines, only metabolites).
Vasopressin (antidiuretic hormone, ADH)	1–20 pg/mL	0.99	1–19.8 pmol/L	Increases during night to maximum on rising, falls during day. INC: Upright posture, nausea, smoking, exercise, fasting. DEC: Overhydration, ethanol, supine posture. In females, peaks at time of ovulation. In pregnancy, increases	INC: Dehydration, inappropriate antidiuresis, nephrogenic diabetes insipidus, renal failure, toxemia, polydipsia, nephrotic syndrome. DEC: Diabetes insipidus, primary polydipsia.	INC: Carbamazepine, phenothiazines, cyclophosphamide, lithium, tricyclic antidepressants, vincristine.	Used in evaluation of patients with polyuria. Measurement of ADH at start and end of water deprivation test can help to determine adequacy of ADH response. Must be interpreted in light

Test	Conventional	Factor	SI				Comments
						during first and second trimester, returns to baseline in third trimester.	of plasma osmolality; high osmolality stimulates ADH production while low osmolality inhibits it.
Vitamin B$_{12}$	280–1,500 pg/mL	0.74	163–1,107 pmol/L	INC: Hemoconcentration, leukocytosis. DEC: Ethanol. In pregnancy, decreases 33% by third trimester. Decreases with increasing age in males. Highest in blacks, intermediate in Hispanics, lowest in whites.	INC: Myeloproliferative disorders, leukocytosis, liver disease, malignancies, renal failure, malnutrition. DEC: Pernicious anemia, intestinal malabsorption, fish tapeworm infestation, folate deficiency, hyperthyroidism.	INC: Valproic acid. DEC: Most anticonvulsants, aminoglycosides, aspirin, cholestyramine, colchicine, neomycin, H$_2$-antagonists, oral contraceptives, ranitidine, vitamin C.	Used to recognize B$_{12}$ deficiency. There is significant overlap between normal and deficient levels. Persons with values from 100–200 are usually deficient, while those with values from 200–300 are usually not deficient; however, exceptions are common. If macrocytosis or hypersegmentation of neutrophils are not present, further tests may help to clarify whether deficiency actually exists. Methylmalonic acid is most sensitive for this purpose.

(continued)

Table 38.1 *(continued)*

Test Name	Reference Range			Nondisease Causes of Changes	Disease Related Changes	Drug Related Changes	Common Conditions for Use of Test
	Standard	Factor	SI Units				
Vitamin C	0–2.0 mg/dL	56.78	0–114 μmol/L	Interday variation 25%. Highest in early AM, falls during day. Highest in summer, lowest in winter. INC: Hemolyzed specimens. DEC: Ethanol, smoking, obesity. In females, peaks at time of ovulation. Decreases during pregnancy. In adults, decreases with increasing age. Higher in females than males.	DEC: Dietary deficiency, malabsorption, renal failure, hyperthyroidism, autoimmune disease, malignancies.	DEC: Aspirin, estrogens, oral contraceptives.	Used to diagnose vitamin C deficiency.
Vitamin D, 1,25-dihydroxy	18–62 ng/L	2.40	43–149 pmol/L	Interday variation 20%. Higher in winter than summer. INC: Obesity, hemoconcentration. DEC: Immobilization. In females, sharp increase (4–5×) at ovulation. Increases during pregnancy and remains high during lactation. In children, highest in infants; falls during childhood, but rises to second peak in teens. Higher in blacks and Hispanics than whites.	INC: Primary hyperparathyroidism, sarcoidosis, other granulomatous diseases, lymphoma. DEC: Late vitamin D deficiency, hypoparathyroidism, renal insufficiency, vitamin D dependent rickets, tumoral osteomalacia.	INC: Estrogens, octreotide, prednisone. DEC: Aluminum hydroxide, isotretinoin, ketoconazole.	Used in evaluation of patients with abnormal calcium, particularly in patients whose phosphate is abnormal in the same direction as calcium. Often normal in early stages of dietary vitamin D deficiency because of increased rate of synthesis of 1,25-dihydroxyvitamin D due to high PTH levels because of hypocalcemia. Not routinely needed in confirmation of

primary hyper-parathyroidism or in documenting decreased production prior to starting treatment in patients with renal failure.

Test	Reference range	Factor	SI range	Physiologic/Analytic factors	Disease factors	Drug factors	Comments
Vitamin D, 25-hydroxy	10–55 µg/L	2.40	24–132 nmol/L	Higher in summer than winter. INC: Exercise, hemoconcentration. DEC: Ethanol. In children, values decrease slightly with increasing age. In adults, decreases with age >65 years. Lower in Hispanics than whites.	INC: Vitamin D intoxication. DEC: Dietary vitamin D deficiency, liver disease, malabsorption, malnutrition, pancreatic insufficiency, hyperthyroidism, nephrotic syndrome.	DEC: Phenytoin, carbamazepine, glucocorticoids, rifampin.	Used to determine adequacy of dietary vitamin D and its absorption. Will be abnormal before 1,25-dihydroxyvitamin D in patients with developing vitamin D deficiency states. Most useful in patients with low calcium and low phosphate.
VMA (see Vanillylmandelic acid)							
Von Willebrand factor	0.6–1.5 U/mL	1	0.6–1.5 kU/L	INC: Ethanol.	INC: Acute inflammation, renal failure. DEC: Von Willebrand's disease.	INC: Triiodothyronine.	Used to diagnose Von Willebrand's disease. Usually measured by ristocetin cofactor assay, but may also be measured by immunoassays; in these, some variants of Von Willebrand factor will have normal levels.

(continued)

Table 38.1 (continued)

Test Name	Reference Range			Nondisease Causes of Changes	Disease Related Changes	Drug Related Changes	Common Conditions for Use of Test
	Standard	Factor	SI Units				
White blood cell count, blood	Total: 4.5–11.0 × 10³/μL Neutrophils: 1.5–6.7 × 10³/μL Lymphocytes: 1.5–4.0 × 10³/μL Monocytes: 0.2–1.0 × 10³/μL Eosinophils: 0–0.7 × 10³/μL Basophils: 0–0.2 × 10³/μL	10⁶	Total: 4.5–11.0 × 10⁹/L Neutrophils: 1.5–6.7 × 10⁹/L Lymphocytes: 1.5–4.0 × 10⁹/L Monocytes: 0.2–1.0 × 10⁹/L Eosinophils: 0–0.7 × 10⁹/L Basophils: 0–0.2 × 10⁹/L	Interday variation 10–15%. Total, monocytes, and eosinophils 25% lower in early AM, maximum in evening. Lymphocytes are highest in AM, lowest in PM. INC (neutrophils): Cold, heat, exercise, stress. INC (lymphocytes): Smoking. DEC (lymphocytes): Ethanol. INC (monocytes): Smoking. INC (eosinophils): X-ray contrast agents. DEC (eosinophils): Smoking. In pregnancy, total increases 50% by 12 weeks, remains stable until near term, with increases in neutrophils and basophils; during labor, eosinophils decrease. In childhood, highest in neonates, falls to lowest by teens. In adults, gradually decreases with age. Higher in females in males and in whites than blacks.	INC (neutrophils): Bacterial infections, tissue injury, diabetic ketoacidosis, Cushing's syndrome, chronic myeloproliferative disorders, malignancies, toxemia. DEC (neutrophils): Severe infections, aplastic anemia, bone marrow replacement, hypothyroidism, hypopituitarism, cirrhosis. INC (lymphocytes): Mononucleosis, viral infections, lymphocytic leukemias. DEC (lymphocytes): Acute infections, tuberculosis, aplastic anemia, Cushing's syndrome, autoimmune disease, AIDS, malnutrition. INC (monocytes): Chronic infections, viral infections, granulomatous diseases, monocytic leukemias, autoimmune disease. DEC (monocytes): Bone marrow suppression. INC (eosinophils): Allergies, parasitic infections, bronchopulmonary aspergillosis,	INC (neutrophils): Heparin, glucocorticoids. DEC (neutrophils): Drugs causing bone marrow suppression. INC (lymphocytes): Albuterol, L-dopa, phenytoin, salicylates, valproic acid. DEC (lymphocytes): Antineoplastics, glucocorticoids, lithium. INC (monocytes): Haloperidol, glucocorticoids. INC (eosinophils): Reaction to many drugs; allopurinol, dapsone, methotrexate, α-methyldopa, penicillamine, triamterene. DEC (eosinophils): Glucocorticoids, procainamide. INC (basophils): Desipramine, estrogens, antithyroid drugs. DEC (basophils): Glucocorticoids, procainamide, chemotherapeutic agents.	Used primarily to screen for infections and in evaluation of patients with signs and symptoms such as fever. Until recently, manual differential count was performed routinely along with total WBC. In most laboratories, automated cell counters quantify each of the cell populations listed much more precisely than manual differential, which is no longer performed routinely. Manual differential is still preferred for identification of immature or blast cells, and in monitoring patients with known myeloproliferative disorders. Manual differentials also allow determination of "band" neutrophils, which are young neutrophils; however, this distinction adds

	Conventional	Factor	SI Units		
				little to the total neutrophil count.	
				myeloproliferative disease, hypereosinophilic syndrome, Hodgkin's disease, adrenal insufficiency. DEC (eosinophils): Infections, toxemia, surgery, shock, Cushing's syndrome. INC (basophils): Hypothyroidism, myeloproliferative syndromes, Hodgkin's disease, hypersensitivity reactions. DEC (basophils): Hyperthyroidism, acute infections, Cushing's syndrome. INC (neutrophils): Bacterial meningitis, brain abscess, early viral meningitis or encephalitis, CNS hemorrhage, metastatic carcinoma to CNS, cerebral infarction, brain abscess.	
White blood cell count, CSF	0–5/µL	10^6	0–5 × 10^6/L	Higher in neonates (up to 30/µL) with neutrophils a normal finding; normal count may be up 20/µL in children <4 years, up to 10/µL in children throughout adolescence.	Used in evaluation of patients with CNS symptoms in whom LP is performed. Increased WBC also varies in significance depending on cell count; counts are

(continued)

Table 38.1 (continued)

Test Name	Reference Range			Nondisease Causes of Changes	Disease Related Changes	Drug Related Changes	Common Conditions for Use of Test
	Standard	Factor	SI Units				
					INC (lymphocytes): Viral, fungal meningitis, multiple sclerosis, Guillain-Barre syndrome, brain abscess, partially treated bacterial meningitis. INC (monocytes): *Listeria monocytogenes*, tuberculous, fungal meningitis.		rarely >1,000/μL in any disorder except bacterial meningitis. In noninfectious disorders, cell counts are rarely >100/μL. In patients with suspected CNS lymphoma or leukemia, cell count and differential is inadequate to identify the presence of tumor cells; cytology is the preferred test.
D-Xylose	Blood: >25 mg/dL at 2 h Urine: >4.0 g/5h	0.067 6.66	Blood: >1.7 mmol/L at 2 h Urine: >26.64 mmol/5 h	INC: Ethanol (urine). DEC: After meals, delayed gastric emptying, vomiting. Increased in pregnancy. In children, levels are slightly higher than in adults. Urine excretion decreases with increasing age.	INC: Cystic fibrosis, renal failure (blood). DEC: Intestinal malabsorption, bacterial overgrowth, ascites, diabetes (blood and urine); hypothyroidism, renal failure (urine).	DEC: Colchicine, digitalis, gold salts, monoamine oxidase inhibitors, salicylates (blood and urine).	Xylose is a simple sugar which can be absorbed without need for digestion by pancreatic and salivary amylases. Values are based on a 25 g dose of xylose. Used to distinguish intestinal malabsorption, where results will be low, from other causes of malabsorption, or maldigestion.

Zinc

| | 0.15 | Serum: 50–160 μg/dL | 7.7–24.5 μmol/L | Interday variation 15%. Highest at 9 AM, lowest at 9 PM. INC: Exercise, hemoconcentration. DEC: Ethanol, decreased albumin, following meals. In pregnancy, 20% lower by 20 weeks, 30% lower by term. In children, slightly higher in neonates. Decreases about 30% after age 60 years. Slightly higher in males than in females. | INC: Atherosclerosis, anemia, renal failure, bone metastases. DEC: Zinc deficiency, malnutrition, infections, renal failure, liver disease, leukemia, lymphoma, acute myocardial infarction, nephrotic syndrome, cirrhosis. | INC: Chlorthalidone. DEC: Captopril, cisplatin, estrogens, interferon, oral contraceptives, penicillamine, phenytoin. | Used to screen for zinc deficiency, particularly in patients with malabsorption or malnutrition. |

Zinc protoporphyrin (see Protoporphyrin, zinc)

Index

Page numbers in *italics* refer to illustrations; numbers followed by t indicate tables.

The Best 5 Minutes in Medicine

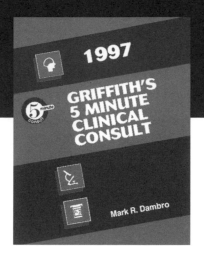

Griffith's 5 Minute Clinical Consult 1997

Mark R. Dambro, MD, FAAFP

Jo A. Griffith, Technical Editor

Five minutes isn't very long, but sometimes it's all the time you have to make the right diagnosis and get on-target treatment recommendations. That's why the *5 Minute Clinical Consult* has become so popular with your colleagues, and why it's now in a new fifth edition that incorporates all the latest advances for your practice.

Topics are arranged alphabetically, with clear sections that cover basics, diagnosis, treatment, medications, follow-up, and miscellaneous considerations. It's just the information you need, in a unique format that makes the most of your clinical time.

If you see it in your practice, chances are excellent you'll also see it in the *5 Minute Clinical Consult*. More than 1,000 medical/ surgical conditions are covered, representing 98% of the problems encountered in primary care. And to ensure the most accurate information possible, consultants from all specialty areas have carefully reviewed the material.

To keep up with recent developments, the 1997 edition includes new sections on:

- personality disorders
- somatoform disorders
- substance abuse
- parasitic problems, including leishmaniasis
- new drugs
- jet lag

There's also a comprehensive drug index that lists drugs by both their brand and generic names. At a glance you'll see how many times the drug is listed, where it appears, and what diseases it is used for.

Order the new *Griffith's 5 Minute Clinical Consult 1997* and be sure some of today's top consultants are always there when you need them.

1997/1320 pages/30182-9

We invite you to preview this book for a full month. If you're not completely satisfied, return it at no further obligation (US and Canada only).

Prices subject to change without notice. Also available at your local health science bookstore.

Phone orders accepted 24 hours a day, 7 days a week (U.S. only).

From the US call: 1-800-638-0672
From Canada call: 1-800-665-1148
From outside the US and Canada call: 410-528-4223
From the UK and Europe call 44 (171) 385-2357
From Southeast Asia call (852) 2610-2339

INTERNET:
  E-mail: custserv@wwilkins.com
  Home page: http://www.wwilkins.com